Operative Techniques in Foregut Surgery

Second Edition

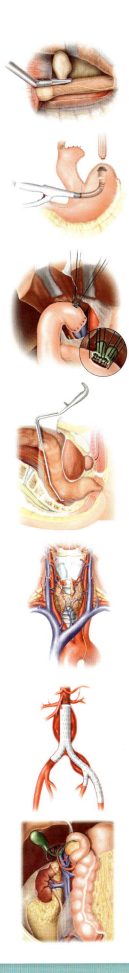

Operative Techniques in Foregut Surgery

Second Edition

Mary T. Hawn, MD, MPH
EDITOR-IN-CHIEF

Emile Holman Professor and Chair
Department of Surgery
Stanford University School of Medicine
Stanford, California

EDITOR
Aurora D. Pryor, MD, MBA, FACS, FASMBS

Professor of Surgery
Donald and Barbara Zucker School of Medicine at
   Hofstra/Northwell
Hempstead, New York
Surgeon-in-Chief
Long Island Jewish Medical Center
System Chief, Bariatric Surgery
Northwell Health
North New Hyde Park, New York

Illustrations by: Body Scientific International, LLC

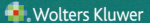
Wolters Kluwer

Philadelphia · Baltimore · New York · London
Buenos Aires · Hong Kong · Sydney · Tokyo

Senior Acquisitions Editor: Keith Donnellan
Senior Development Editor: Ashley Fischer
Development Editor: Barton Dudlick
Editorial Coordinator: Erin E. Hernandez
Marketing Manager: Kirsten Watrud
Production Project Manager: Bridgett Dougherty
Manager, Graphic Arts & Design: Stephen Druding
Manufacturing Coordinator: Beth Welsh
Prepress Vendor: TNQ Technologies

Copyright © 2024 Wolters Kluwer.

Copyright © 2015 Wolters Kluwer Health/Lippincott Williams & Wilkins. All rights reserved. This book is protected by copyright. No part of this book may be reproduced or transmitted in any form or by any means, including as photocopies or scanned-in or other electronic copies, or utilized by any information storage and retrieval system without written permission from the copyright owner, except for brief quotations embodied in critical articles and reviews. Materials appearing in this book prepared by individuals as part of their official duties as U.S. government employees are not covered by the above-mentioned copyright. To request permission, please contact Wolters Kluwer at Two Commerce Square, 2001 Market Street, Philadelphia, PA 19103, via email at permissions@lww.com, or via our website at shop.lww.com (products and services).

9 8 7 6 5 4 3 2 1

Printed in United States of America.

Library of Congress Cataloging-in-Publication Data

ISBN-13: 978-1-9751-7661-7

Cataloging in Publication data available on request from publisher.

This work is provided "as is," and the publisher disclaims any and all warranties, express or implied, including any warranties as to accuracy, comprehensiveness, or currency of the content of this work.

This work is no substitute for individual patient assessment based upon healthcare professionals' examination of each patient and consideration of, among other things, age, weight, gender, current or prior medical conditions, medication history, laboratory data and other factors unique to the patient. The publisher does not provide medical advice or guidance and this work is merely a reference tool. Healthcare professionals, and not the publisher, are solely responsible for the use of this work including all medical judgments and for any resulting diagnosis and treatments.

Given continuous, rapid advances in medical science and health information, independent professional verification of medical diagnoses, indications, appropriate pharmaceutical selections and dosages, and treatment options should be made and healthcare professionals should consult a variety of sources. When prescribing medication, healthcare professionals are advised to consult the product information sheet (the manufacturer's package insert) accompanying each drug to verify, among other things, conditions of use, warnings and side effects and identify any changes in dosage schedule or contraindications, particularly if the medication to be administered is new, infrequently used or has a narrow therapeutic range. To the maximum extent permitted under applicable law, no responsibility is assumed by the publisher for any injury and/or damage to persons or property, as a matter of products liability, negligence law or otherwise, or from any reference to or use by any person of this work.

shop.lww.com

Contributing Authors

Sherif R. Z. Abdel-Misih, MD
Associate Professor of Surgery
Program Director, General Surgery Residency
Department of Surgery
Renaissance School of Medicine at Stony Brook University
Program Director, General Surgery Residency
Department of Surgery
Stony Brook University Hospital
Stony Brook, New York

Waddah B. Al-Refaie, MD, FACS
John S. Dillon Professor of Surgical Oncology
Department of Surgery
Georgetown University School of Medicine
Regional Chief of Surgical Oncology
Surgical in-Chief
Georgetown Lombardi Comprehensive Cancer Center
MedStar Health
Washington, D.C.

Roslyn Alexander, DO
Department of Surgery
St. Luke's University Health Network
Bethlehem, Pennsylvania

Evan T. Alicuben, MD
Fellow
Department of Cardiothoracic Surgery
University of Pittsburgh Medical Center
Pittsburgh, Pennsylvania

Yewande R. Alimi, MD, MHS
Assistant Professor
Department of Surgery
Georgetown University School of Medicine
Attending Physician
Department of Surgery
Medstar Georgetown University Hospital
Washington, D.C.

Marco Ettore Allaix, MD, PhD
Associate Professor
Department of Surgical Sciences
University of Torino
Attending Surgeon
Department of Surgery
Citta della Salute e della Scienza di Torino
Torino, Italy

Melissa M. Alvarez-Downing, MD
Assistant Professor
Department of Surgery
Rutgers New Jersey Medical School
Newark, New Jersey

Scott A. Anderson, MD
Associate Professor of Surgery
Division of Pediatric Surgery
Department of Surgery
University of Alabama at Birmingham School of Medicine
Director, ECMO Program
Children's of Alabama
Birmingham, Alabama

Sullivan A. Ayuso, MD
Department of GI & Minimally Invasive Surgery
Carolinas Medical Center
Charlotte, North Carolina

Xavier Lyndell Baldwin, MD
Post-Doctoral Research Fellow
Department of Surgery
University of North Carolina at Chapel Hill
Department of Surgery
University of North Carolina Hospitals
Chapel Hill, North Carolina

Juan S. Barajas-Gamboa, MD
Postdoctoral Research Fellow
Department of General Surgery
Cleveland Clinic Abu Dhabi
Abu Dhabi, United Arab Emirates

Givi Basishvili, MD
Clinical Assistant Instructor
Renaissance School of Medicine at Stony Brook University
Department of Surgery
Stony Brook University Hospital
Stony Brook, New York

Andrew T. Bates, MD
Assistant Professor
Department of Surgery
Zucker School of Medicine at Hofstra/Northwell
Hempstead, New York
Director, Minimally-Invasive Surgery
Department of Surgery
South Shore University Hospital
Bay Shore, New York

Lucas R. Beffa, MD, FACS
Assistant Professor of Surgery
Digestive Diseases and Surgery Institute
Cleveland Clinic, Cleveland, Ohio

Thomas J. Birdas, MD, MBA
Associate Professor
Department of Surgery
Indiana University School of Medicine
Indianapolis, Indiana

Andrew M. Brown, MD
Clinical Assistant Professor of Surgery
Department of Surgery
Lewis Katz School of Medicine at Temple University
Philadelphia, Pennsylvania
Bethlehem, General Surgeon
Department of Surgery
St. Luke's University Health Network
Bethlehem, Pennsylvania

James P. Byrne, MD, PhD
Assistant Professor of Surgery
Division of Trauma and Acute Care Surgery
Department of Surgery
Johns Hopkins Hospital
Baltimore, Maryland

John M. Campbell, MD
Department of Surgery
Renaissance School of Medicine at Stony Brook University
Stony Brook University Hospital
Stony Brook, New York

DuyKhanh P. Ceppa, MD
Associate Professor of Surgery
Division of Cardiothoracic Surgery
Department of Surgery
Indiana University School of Medicine
Indianapolis, Indiana

Susan M. Cera, MD, FACS, FASCRS
Colorectal Surgeon
Clinical Associate
Cleveland Clinic Florida
Department of Surgery
Physicians Regional Medical Center
Naples, Florida

Ernest G. Chan, MD, MPH
Department of Cardiothoracic Surgery
University of Pittsburgh Medical Center
Pittsburgh, Pennsylvania

Mike K. Chen, MD, MBA
Professor and Chief of Pediatric Surgery
Division of Pediatric Surgery
Department of Surgery
University of Alabama at Birmingham School of Medicine
Surgeon-in-Chief
Children's of Alabama
Birmingham, Alabama

S. Ariane Christie, MD
Trauma, Acute and Critical Care Surgery Fellow
Department of Trauma and Acute Care Surgery
University of Pittsburgh Medical Center
Pittsburgh, Pennsylvania

Paul D. Colavita, MD, FACS
Associate Professor of Surgery
Department of Surgery
Carolinas Medical Center
Charlotte, North Carolina

Jazmín M. Cole, MD
Assistant Professor
Department of Surgery
Emory University School of Medicine
Emory University Hospital Midtown
Atlanta, Georgia

Courtney E. Collins, MD, MS
Assistant Professor
Department of Surgery
The Ohio State University School of Medicine
Columbus, Ohio

Tuesday F. A. Cook, MD
Director
Department of Minimally Invasive, Foregut and Bariatric Surgery
Adventist HealthCare Fort Washington Medical Center
Fort Washington, Maryland

Jennifer Colvin, MD
Assistant Professor
Department of Surgery
University of Cincinnati
Cincinnati, Ohio

Salvatore Docimo, Jr., DO, FACS, FASMBS
Associate Professor
Department of Surgery
Morsani College of Medicine
University of South Florida
Tampa, Florida

Erin E. Devine, MD, PhD
Department of Surgery
Stanford University School of Medicine
Stanford Hospital and Clinics
Stanford, California

Elizabeth A. Dovec, MD, FACS, FASMBS, DBOM
Medical Director and Bariatric Surgeon
Department of Weight Loss and Bariatric Surgery
Digestive Health and Surgery Institute
AdventHealth at Orlando
AdventHealth Medical Group
Orlando, Florida

Christopher DuCoin, MD, MPH
Associate Professor of Surgery
Division of GI Surgery
University of South Florida
Chief, Division of Gastrointestinal Surgery
Department of Surgery
Tampa General Hospital
Tampa, Florida

Sharbel A. Elhage, MD
Department of Surgery
Carolinas Medical Center
Charlotte, North Carolina

Luke M. Funk, MD, MPH
Associate Professor of Surgery
Department of Surgery
University of Wisconsin-Madison School of Medicine and Public Health
Chief, Division of General Surgery
Department of Surgery
William S. Middleton VA
Madison, Wisconsin

Robert E. Glasgow, MD, MBA, FACS
Professor and Interim Chair
Department of Surgery
University of Utah
Salt Lake City, Utah

Abigail Gotsch, MD
Department of General Surgery
St. Luke's University Health Network
Bethlehem, Pennsylvania

Meredith A. Harrison, MD, FACS
Assistant Professor Thoracic Surgery
Department of General Surgery
St. Luke's University Health Network
Bethlehem, Pennsylvania

Mary T. Hawn, MD, MPH
Emile Holman Professor and Chair
Department of Surgery
Stanford University School of Medicine
Stanford, California

Alex Helkin, MD
Assistant Professor
Department of Surgery
The Ohio State University Wexner Medical Center
Columbus, Ohio

B. Todd Heniford, MD, FACS
Professor of Surgery
Chief, Gastrointestinal and Minimally Invasive Surgery
Chief, Carolinas Hernia Center
Department of Surgery
Carolinas Medical Center, Charlotte, North Carolina

Martin J. Heslin, MD, MSHA
Professor of Surgery
Executive Director Mitchell Cancer Institute
Department of Surgery
University of South Alabama School of Medicine
Mobile, Alabama

David I. Hindin, MD, MS
Surgical Critical Care Fellow
Department of Surgery
Stanford University Hospital
Stanford, California

Charlotte M. Horne, MD
Assistant Professor of Surgery
Department of General Surgery
Pennsylvania State University
Milton S. Hershey Medical Center
Hershey, Pennsylvania

John G. Hunter, MD, FACS
Professor of Surgery
Oregon Health & Sciences University School of Medicine
Executive Vice President, OHSU
Chief Executive Officer
OHSU Health System
Portland, Oregon

CONTRIBUTING AUTHORS

Matthew M. Hutter, MD, MBA, MPH
Professor of Surgery
Harvard Medical School
Director, Codman Center for Clinical Effectiveness in Surgery
Department of Surgery
Massachusetts General Hospital
Boston, Massachusetts

Kamal M.F. Itani, MD
Professor of Surgery
Boston University
Chief of Surgery
Department of Surgery
VA Boston Health Care System
Boston, Massachusetts

Hope T. Jackson, MD, FACS
Associate Professor of Surgery
Department of Surgery
George Washington University School of Medicine and Health Sciences
Washington, D.C.

Patrick G. Jackson, MD
Professor of Surgery
Department of Surgery
Georgetown University School of Medicine
Chief of General Surgery
MedStar Georgetown University Hospital
Washington, D.C.

Harel Jacoby, MD
Fellow
Department of Advanced Gastrointestinal Surgery
AdventHealth
Tampa, Florida

Kunoor Jain-Spangler, MD
Assistant Professor
Director, Advanced GI/MIS and Bariatric Surgery Fellowships
Department of Surgery
Duke University School of Medicine
Durham, North Carolina

Susan Laura Jao, BA
Renaissance School of Medicine at Stony Brook University
Stony Brook University Hospital
Stony Brook, New York

Shaneeta M. Johnson, MD, MBA, FACS, FASMBS
Professor of Surgery
Chief, Minimally Invasive and Bariatric Surgery
Department of Surgery
Morehouse School of Medicine
Atlanta, Georgia

Saher-Zahra Khan, MD
Department of Surgery
The Cleveland Clinic Lerner College of Medicine of Case Western University
University Hospitals Cleveland Medical Center
Cleveland, Ohio

Matthew Kroh, MD
Professor of Surgery
Vice Chair, Innovation and Technology
Digestive Disease and Surgery Institute
Cleveland Clinic
Cleveland, Ohio

Ryan M. Levy, MD, FACS
Assistant Professor of Thoracic Surgery
University of Pittsburgh School of Medicine
Chief of Thoracic Surgery
Department of Cardiothoracic Surgery
University of Pittsburgh Medical Center
Pittsburgh, Pennsylvania

James D. Luketich, MD
Professor of Surgery
Department of Cardiothoracic Surgery
University of Pittsburgh School of Medicine
Chair, Department of Cardiothoracic Surgery
University of Pittsburgh Medical Center
Pittsburgh, Pennsylvania

Megan P. Lundgren, MD
Surgical Fellow
Digestive Disease Institute
Cleveland Clinic
Cleveland Ohio

Ugwuji N. Maduekwe, MD, MMSc, MPH
Associate Professor
Division of Surgical Oncology
Department of Surgery
The Medical College of Wisconsin
Milwaukee, Wisconsin

Jeffrey M. Marks, MD
Professor of Surgery
The Cleveland Clinic Lerner College of Medicine of Case Western University
Director of Surgical Endoscopy
Department of Surgery
University Hospitals Cleveland Medical Center
Cleveland, Ohio

Elizabeth G. McCarthy, MD
MIS/Bariatric Fellow
Department of Surgery
Stony Brook University Hospital
Stony Brook, New York

Ozanan R. Meireles, MD
Assistant Professor of Surgery
Harvard Medical School
Bariatric, Foregut, and Advanced Endoluminal Surgeon
Department of Surgery
Massachusetts General Hospital
Boston, Massachusetts

Marcovalerio Melis, MD, FACS
Associate Professor of Surgery
Division of Surgical Oncology
Zucker School of Medicine at Hofstra/Northwell
Lenox Hill Hospital
Chief, Division of Surgical Oncology
Phelps Hospital
New York, New York

W. Scott Melvin, MD
Vice Chair, Professor of Surgery
Albert Einstein School of Medicine
Montefiore Medical Center
New York, New York

Robert E. Merritt, MD
Division Director of Thoracic Surgery
Department of Surgery
The Ohio State School of Medicine
Thoracic Surgeon
Department of Surgery
The Ohio State University Wexner Medical Center
Columbus, Ohio

Kelsey B. Montgomery, MD
Department of Surgery
University of Alabama at Birmingham
Birmingham, Alabama

Elliot Newman, MD
Professor of Surgery
Department of Surgery
Zucker School of Medicine at Hofstra/Northwell
Hempstead, New York
Chief of Surgical Oncology
Northwell Cancer Institute at Lenox Hill Hospital
New York, New York

Aanuoluwapo Obisesan, MD
Department of Surgery
St. Luke's University Health Network
Bethlehem, Pennsylvania

David D. Odell, MD
Associate Professor of Surgery
Department of Surgery
Feinberg School of Medicine
Northwestern University
Thoracic Surgeon
Northwestern Memorial Hospital
Chicago, Illinois

CONTRIBUTING AUTHORS

Brant K. Oelschlager, MD
Chief, General Surgery
Department of General Surgery
University of Washington Medical Center
Seattle, Washington

Sean Michael O'Neill, MD, PhD
Clinical Assistant Professor
Department of Surgery
University of Michigan Medical School
Ann Arbor, Michigan
General Surgeon
Department of Surgery
St. Joseph Mercy Chelsea Medical Center
Chelsea, Michigan

Gilbert Pan, MS
Boston University School of Medicine
Boston, Massachusetts

Marco G. Patti, MD
Department of Surgery
University of Virginia
Charlottesville, Virginia

David M. Pechman, MD, MBA
Assistant Professor of Surgery
Department of Surgery
Zucker School of Medicine at Hofstra/Northwell
Hempstead, New York
Minimally Invasive and Bariatric Surgeon
Department of Surgery
South Shore University Hospital
Bay Shore, New York

Andrew B. Peitzman, MD
Mark M. Ravitch Professor of Surgery
Department of Surgery
University of Pittsburgh School of Medicine
Chief, University of Pittsburgh Medical Center Trauma System
University of Pittsburgh Medical Center, Presbyterian
Pittsburgh, Pennsylvania

Kyle A. Perry, MD, MBA
Professor of Surgery
Department of Surgery
The Ohio State University School of Medicine
Columbus, Ohio

Dana Portenier, MD, FASC, FASMBS
Division Chief, Duke Center for Metabolic and Weight Loss Surgery
Duke University School of Medicine
Durham, North Carolina

John R. Porterfield, Jr., MD, MSPH, FACS
Professor of Surgery
Division of Gastrointestinal Surgery
Department of Surgery
University of Alabama at Birmingham School of Medicine
UAB University Hospital
Birmingham, Alabama

Benjamin Kuttikatt Poulose, MD, MPH
Robert M. Zollinger Lecrone-Baxter Chair
Chief, Division of General and Gastrointestinal Surgery
Department of Surgery
The Ohio State University Wexner Medical Center
Columbus, Ohio

Ajita S. Prabhu, MD, FACS
Associate Professor of Surgery
Department of General Surgery
Cleveland Clinic Foundation
Cleveland, Ohio

Aurora D. Pryor, MD, MBA, FACS, FASMBS
Professor of Surgery
Donald and Barbara Zucker School of Medicine at Hofstra/Northwell
Hempstead, New York
Surgeon-in-Chief
Long Island Jewish Medical Center
System Chief, Bariatric Surgery
Northwell Health
North New Hyde Park, New York

Carla M. Pugh, MD, PhD, FACS
Thomas Krummel Professor of Surgery
Director of the Technology Enabled Clinical Improvement (T.E.C.I.) Center
Department of Surgery
Stanford University School of Medicine
Stanford, California

Sushanth Reddy, MD
Associate Professor of Surgery
Department of Surgery
University of Alabama at Birmingham School of Medicine
Birmingham, Alabama

Patrick M. Reilly, MD, FACS
C. William Schwab Professor of Surgery
Perelman School of Medicine at the University of Pennsylvania
Philadelphia, Pennsylvania

William Richards, MD
Professor and Chair
Department of Surgery
University of South Alabama College of Medicine
Mobile, Alabama

Richard Rieske, MD
Department of Surgery
University of South Alabama College of Medicine
Mobile, Alabama

John H. Rodriguez, MD, FACS
Assistant Professor of Surgery
Department of Surgery
Cleveland Clinic Lerner College of Medicine
Cleveland, Ohio
Chair, Department of General Surgery
Cleveland Clinic Abu Dhabi
Abu Dhabi, United Arab Emirates

Alexander S. Rosemurgy, MDII
Professor
Department of Surgery
University of Central Florida
Orlando, Florida
Professor
Department of Surgery
Nova Southeastern University
Fort Lauderdale, Florida

Michael J. Rosen, MD
Professor of Surgery
Cleveland Clinic
Cleveland, Ohio

Amy Rosenbluth, MD
Clinical Assistant Professor of Surgery
Associate Program Director of Surgical Residency
Department of Surgery
Stony Brook University Hospital
Stony Brook, New York

Sharona B. Ross, MD, FACS
Professor
Department of Surgery
University of Central Florida
Orlando, Florida
Director, Minimally Invasive Robotic Surgery and Surgical Endoscopy
Digestive Health Institute Tampa
AdventHealth Tampa
Tampa, Florida

George A. Sarosi, Jr., MD
Robert H. Hux MD Professor
Vice Chair for Education
Department of Surgery
University of Florida College of Medicine
Gainesville, Florida

Samer Sbayi, MD, MBA, FACS
Assistant Professor
Department of General Surgery
Renaissance School of Medicine at Stony Brook University
Director, Emergency General Surgery
Chief, Mastery in General Surgery Fellowship
Deputy Chief Medical Information Officer
Department of General Surgery
Stony Brook University Hospital
Stony Brook, New York

Scott W. Schimpke, MD, FACS
Assistant Professor
Program Director, General Surgery Residency
Associate Program Director, MIS/Bariatric Fellowship
Department of Surgery
Rush University Medical Center
Chicago, Illinois

Eric G. Sheu, MD, PhD
Assistant Professor of Surgery
Harvard Medical School
Associate Program Director
Minimally Invasive and Bariatric Surgery Fellowship
Department of Surgery
Brigham and Women's Hospital
Boston, Massachusetts

Carrie Sims, MD, PhD
Professor
Division Chair, Trauma, Critical Care and Burns
Department of Surgery
The Ohio State University Wexner Medical Center
Columbus, Ohio

C. Daniel Smith, MD
Director
Esophageal Institute of Atlanta
Atlanta, Georgia

David A. Spain, MD
Professor and Chief, Acute Care Surgery
Department of Surgery
Stanford University School of Medicine
Stanford, California

John H. Stewart IV, MD, MBA
Director, LSU NO/LCMC Cancer Center
Professor of Surgery
Department of Surgery
Louisiana State University School of Medicine
New Orleans, Louisiana

Andrew T. Strong, MD
Clinical Associate
Center for Metabolic and Weight Loss Surgery
Duke University Hospital
Durham, North Carolina

Ryland S. Stucke, MD
Clinical Instructor
Department of Surgery
Oregon Health & Sciences University School of Medicine
OHSU Adventist Health
Portland, Oregon

Iswanto Sucandy, MD, FACS
Associate Professor of Surgery
Department of Surgery
University of Central Florida
Director, Liver Surgery and Disorders Program
Digestive Health Institute
AdventHealth Tampa
Tampa, Florida

Joseph Adam Sujka, MD
Assistant Professor of Surgery
Division of GI Surgery
University of South Florida
Attending Surgeon
Division of GI Surgery
Department of Surgery
Tampa General Hospital
Tampa, Florida

Cameron Syblis, BS
Digestive Health Institute
AdventHealth Tampa
Tampa, Florida

Dana A. Telem, MD, MPH
Lazar J Greenfield Professor of Surgery
Section Chief, General Surgery
Department of Surgery
University of Michigan Medical School
Ann Arbor, Michigan

Jennifer F. Tseng, MD, MPH, FACS
James Utley Professor and Chair of Surgery
Department of Surgery
Boston University School of Medicine
Surgeon-in-Chief
Department of Surgery
Boston Medical Center
Boston, Massachusetts

Anthony M. Villano, MD
Fellow
Department of Surgical Oncology
Fox Chase Cancer Center
Philadelphia, Pennsylvania

Jordan A. Wilkerson, MD
Thoracic Surgery Fellow
Division of Cardiothoracic Surgery
Department of Surgery
Indiana University School of Medicine
Indianapolis, Indiana

Jin Soo Yoo, MD
Associate Professor
Department of Surgery
Duke University School of Medicine
Duke University Health System
Durham, North Carolina

Series Preface

Operative interventions are complex, technically demanding, and rapidly evolving. *Operative Techniques in Surgery* seeks to provide highly visual step-by-step instructions to perform these complex tasks. The series is organized anatomically with volumes covering foregut surgery, hepato-pancreato-biliary surgery, and colorectal surgery. Breast and endocrine surgery as well as other topics related to surgical oncology are included in a separate volume. Modern approaches to vascular surgery are covered in a standalone volume. We also have a first edition standalone volume dedicated to trauma surgery. Additionally, many chapters are augmented by video clips dynamically demonstrating the critical steps of the procedure throughout the series.

The series editors are renowned surgeons with expertise in their respective fields. Each is a leader in the discipline of surgery, each recognized for superb surgical judgment and outstanding operative skill. Breast surgery, endocrine procedures, and surgical oncology topics were edited by Dr. Michael S. Sabel of the University of Michigan. Thoracic and upper gastrointestinal surgery topics were edited by Dr. Aurora D. Pryor of Donald and Barbara Zucker School of Medicine at Hofstra/Northwell, with Dr. Steven J. Hughes of the University of Florida directing the section on hepato-pancreatico-biliary surgery. Dr. Daniel Albo of University of Texas Rio Grande directed the section dedicated to colorectal surgery. Dr. Kellie R. Brown of Medical College of Wisconsin edited topics related to vascular surgery, including both open and endovascular approaches. New this year, we have added a section on Trauma and Critical Surgery, led by Dr. Amy J. Goldberg of Temple University.

In turn, the series editors recruited contributors that are world-renowned; the resulting volumes have a distinctly international flavor. Surgery is a visual discipline. *Operative Techniques in Surgery* is lavishly illustrated with a compelling combination of line art and intraoperative photography. The illustrated material provides a uniform style emphasizing clarity and strong, clean lines. Intraoperative photographs are taken from the perspective of the operating surgeon so that operations might be visualized as they would be performed.

The accompanying text is intentionally sparse, with a focus on crucial operative details and important aspects of postoperative management and potential complications. The series is designed for surgeons at all levels of practice, from surgical residents to advanced practice fellows to surgeons of wide experience.

Operative Techniques in Surgery would be possible only at Wolters Kluwer, an organization of unique vision, organization, and talent of Brian Brown, executive editor, Keith Donnellan, senior acquisition editor, and Ashley Fischer, senior development editor.

I am deeply indebted to Dr. Michael W. Mulholland, a master surgeon and leader and the editor in chief of the first series for *Operative Techniques in Surgery*. Without his leadership, this project would not have been successful. I am grateful to our new and returning series editors for their vision on how to make the second edition even more impactful. Curating and editing a major surgical techniques textbook during a worldwide pandemic has not been seamless, yet the outcome is masterful.

Mary T. Hawn, MD, MPH

Preface

This volume on foregut surgery is from the second edition of *Operative Techniques in Surgery*. This book has quickly become an essential reference for surgeons and surgical trainees. We trust this addition will be equally well received. In this book, we have expanded on minimally invasive and open techniques for the management of foregut disease, including detailed sections on hernia and the surgical management of obesity and metabolic diseases. We have new chapters on endoscopic management of complications, robotic approaches to surgery, and duodenal switch procedures. Many of the chapters have supporting video clips to provide additional technical insights.

The authors in this volume represent some of the top innovative and respected foregut surgeons in the world. They share with readers an easily palatable approach to the management of surgical disease focusing on the technical steps of each procedure with step-by-step graphical illustrations. I would like to thank each of our authors for sharing their tricks for surgical excellence. This book is designed to be an easy reference for surgeons at all levels to prepare for surgery and optimize patient care.

This book would not be possible without the support of our fabulous editor-in-chief Dr. Mary T. Hawn and the amazingly supportive publishing team at Wolters Kluwer. Executive editor Brian Brown, senior acquisition editor Keith Donnellan, and senior development editor Ashley Fischer were invaluable in their organization and follow through. They have helped us achieve a truly remarkable book that I hope you'll enjoy for years to come.

Aurora D. Pryor, MD, MBA, FACS, FASMBS

Contents

Contributing Authors   v
Series Preface   xi
Preface   xiii
Video Contents List   xvii

Section I Esophagus

1 **Epiphrenic Diverticulum**   1
   Evan T. Alicuben, James D. Luketich, and Ryan M. Levy

2 **Long Myotomy for Distal Esophageal Spasm**   8
   Gilbert Pan, Ernest G. Chan, David D. Odell, and James D. Luketich

3 **Laparoscopic Heller Myotomy and Anterior Fundoplication for Esophageal Achalasia**   15
   Marco Ettore Allaix and Marco G. Patti

4 **Per-Oral Endoscopic Myotomy for Achalasia and Hypercontractile Esophagus**   21
   Jazmín M. Cole, Saher-Zahra Khan, and Jeffrey M. Marks

Section II Diaphragm

5 **Repair of Congenital Defects: Morgagni Diaphragmatic Hernia**   26
   Scott A. Anderson and Mike K. Chen

6 **Repair of Congenital Defects: Bochdalek Congenital Diaphragmatic Hernia**   33
   Scott A. Anderson and Mike K. Chen

Section III Treatment of Paraesophageal Hernias

7 **Paraesophageal Hernia Repair: Laparoscopic Technique**   41
   Yewande R. Alimi and Mary T. Hawn

8 **Collis Gastroplasty**   53
   Ryland S. Stucke and John G. Hunter

Section IV Treatment of Gastroesophageal Reflux

9 **Laparoscopic Nissen Fundoplication**   59
   Hope T. Jackson and Brant K. Oelschlager

10 **Laparoscopic Partial Fundoplication for Gastroesophageal Reflux Disease**   70
   Jennifer Colvin and Kyle A. Perry

11 **The Endoscopic Approach to Gastroesophageal Reflux Disease**   75
   W. Scott Melvin and Luke M. Funk

12 **Magnetic Sphincter Augmentation for GERD**   84
   William Richards and Richard Rieske

13 **Redo Fundoplication**   93
   C. Daniel Smith

14 **Roux-en-Y (Roux Limb Reconstruction) for Recurrent Hiatal Hernia**   103
   Joseph Adam Sujka and Christopher DuCoin

Section V Treatment of Esophageal Cancer

15 **Esophagectomy: Transhiatal and Reconstruction**   110
   Robert E. Glasgow

16 **Ivor Lewis Esophagectomy**   124
   Robert E. Merritt

17 **Minimally Invasive Esophagectomy**   133
   Jordan A. Wilkerson, Thomas J. Birdas, and DuyKhanh P. Ceppa

Section VI Treatment of Esophageal Perforation

18 **Treatment of Esophageal Perforation: Cervical, Thoracic, and Abdominal**   138
   Roslyn Alexander, Abigail Gotsch, Aanuoluwapo Obisesan, Andrew M. Brown, and Meredith A. Harrison

19 **Endoscopic Management of Esophageal Perforation**   146
   John M. Campbell and Salvatore Docimo Jr.

Section VII Surgery of the Abdominal Wall

20 **Inguinal Hernia: Open Approaches** 156
Kamal M.F. Itani and Samer Sbayi

21 **Inguinal Hernia: Laparoscopic Approaches** 169
Courtney E. Collins and Benjamin Kuttikatt Poulose

22 **Robotic Inguinal Hernia Repair** 179
Andrew T. Bates and David M. Pechman

23 **Incisional Hernia: Open Approaches** 183
Sean Michael O'Neill and Dana A. Telem

24 **Incisional Hernia: Laparoscopic Approaches** 201
Sullivan A. Ayuso, Sharbel A. Elhage, Paul D. Colavita, and B. Todd Heniford

25 **Incisional Hernia Repair: Abdominal Wall Reconstruction Options** 210
Lucas R. Beffa and Michael J. Rosen

26 **Robotic Ventral Hernia Repair: Transversus Abdominis Release** 219
Charlotte M. Horne and Ajita S. Prabhu

27 **Parastomal Hernia** 228
Melissa M. Alvarez-Downing and Susan M. Cera

28 **Umbilical, Epigastric, Spigelian, and Lumbar Hernias** 234
Andrew T. Strong and Jin Soo Yoo

Section VIII Surgery of the Stomach and Duodenum

29 **Vagotomy: Truncal and Highly Selective** 246
George A. Sarosi Jr. and Mary T. Hawn

30 **Drainage Procedures: Pyloromyotomy, Pyloroplasty, Gastrojejunostomy** 256
George A. Sarosi Jr

31 **Endoscopic Management of Gastroparesis and Gastric Outlet Obstruction** 268
Juan S. Barajas-Gamboa and John H. Rodriguez

32 **Surgical Management of Gastroduodenal Perforation** 275
Amy Rosenbluth and Givi Basishvili

33 **Trauma Laparotomy** 280
S. Ariane Christie and Andrew B. Peitzman

34 **Gastric and Small Bowel Injury: Primary Repair, Resection, Anastomosis, Wedge Resection** 290
Alex Helkin and Carrie Sims

35 **Operative Management of Duodenal Injury** 299
David I. Hindin and David A. Spain

36 **Antrectomy** 305
Sherif R. Z. Abdel-Misih

37 **Subtotal Gastrectomy for Cancer** 315
Anthony M. Villano, Patrick G. Jackson, and Waddah B. Al-Refaie

38 **Minimally Invasive Total Gastrectomy** 326
Elliot Newman and Marcovalerio Melis

39 **Robotic/Minimally Invasive Distal Gastrectomy** 333
Sharona B. Ross, Harel Jacoby, Cameron Syblis, Iswanto Sucandy, and Alexander S. Rosemurgy

40 **Proximal Gastrectomy** 339
Sushanth Reddy and Martin J. Heslin

41 **Total Gastrectomy for Cancer** 347
Anthony M. Villano, Jennifer F. Tseng, and Waddah B. Al-Refaie

42 **Surgical Management of Injuries to the Cervical Esophagus** 358
James P. Byrne and Patrick M. Reilly

43 **Gastrostomy** 365
Erin E. Devine, David I. Hindin, and Carla M. Pugh

44 **Feeding Jejunostomy** 376
Kelsey B. Montgomery and John R. Porterfield Jr.

45 **Surgical Management of Postgastrectomy Syndrome** 387
Xavier Lyndell Baldwin, Ugwuji N. Maduekwe, and John H. Stewart IV

46 **Laparoscopic Gastric Bypass** 390
Tuesday F. A. Cook, Elizabeth A. Dovec, and Shaneeta M. Johnson

47 **Laparoscopic Sleeve Gastrectomy** 397
Ozanan R. Meireles, Eric G. Sheu, and Matthew M. Hutter

48 **Removal and Revision of Laparoscopic Adjustable Gastric Banding** 405
Scott W. Schimpke and Kunoor Jain-Spangler

49 **Laparoscopic Biliopancreatic Diversion With Duodenal Switch and Single Anastomosis Duodenal-Ileal Bypass** 411
Dana Portenier

50 **Surgical Management of Bariatric Complications: Internal Hernia and Leak** 418
Elizabeth G. McCarthy, Susan Laura Jao, and Aurora D. Pryor

51 **Endoscopic Management of Bariatric Complications: Leak and Stricture** 423
Megan P. Lundgren and Matthew Kroh

Index I-1

Video Contents List

Section **I**	Esophagus

Chapter 1 — Epiphrenic Diverticulum
- Video 1 VATS for esophageal diverticulectomy and esophagomyotomy

Chapter 4 — Per-Oral Endoscopic Myotomy for Achalasia and Hypercontractile Esophagus
- Video 1 Per-oral endoscopic myotomy

Section **IV**	Treatment of Gastroesophageal Reflux

Chapter 10 — Laparoscopic Partial Fundoplication for Gastroesophageal Reflux Disease
- Video 1 Hiatal dissection
- Video 2 Division of short gastric vessels
- Video 3 Creation of retroesophageal window
- Video 4 Mediastinal dissection
- Video 5 Crural closure
- Video 6 Fundoplication set-up and shoeshine maneuver
- Video 7 Initial fundoplication suture placement
- Video 8 Initial sutures left side of fundoplication
- Video 9 Final sutures fundoplication in creation

Chapter 12 — Magnetic Sphincter Augmentation for GERD
- Video 1 MSA minimal hiatal dissection

Section **V**	Treatment of Esophageal Cancer

Chapter 17 — Minimally Invasive Esophagectomy
- Video 1 MIE hiatal dissection
- Video 2 MIE gastric mobilization
- Video 3 MIE lymph node dissection
- Video 4 MIE conduit cormation
- Video 5 MIE esophageal mobilization
- Video 6 MIE anastomosis

Section **VII**	Surgery of the Abdominal Wall

Chapter 20 — Inguinal Hernia: Open Approaches
- Video 1 Shouldice repair of groin hernias
- Video 2 Shouldice repair (with McVey repair techniques) of a femoral hernia
- Video 3 Lichtenstein repair of groin hernias

Chapter 26 — Robotic Ventral Hernia Repair: Transversus Abdominis Release
- Video 1 Retrorectus dissection
- Video 2 Neurovascular bundles.
- Video 3 TAR-Up
- Video 4 TAR-Down
- Video 5 Posterior sheath closure
- Video 6 Anterior sheath closure

Chapter 28 — Umbilical, Epigastric, Spigelian, and Lumbar Hernias
- Video 1 Hybrid umbilical hernia repair

Section **VIII**	Surgery of the Stomach and Duodenum

Chapter 31 — Endoscopic Management of Gastroparesis and Gastric Outlet Obstruction
- Video 1 Per-oral pyloromyotomy

Chapter 39 — Robotic/Minimally Invasive Distal Gastrectomy
- Video 1 Gastrocolic dissection with elevation
- Video 2 Duodenal dissection and transection
- Video 3 Ligation of LGA and coronary vein
- Video 4 Proximal gastric transection
- Video 5 Gastrojejunostomy anastomosis

Chapter 44 — Feeding Jejunostomy
- Video 1 Laparoscopic J-tube placement

xvii

Chapter 48 Removal and Revision of Laparoscopic Adjustable Gastric Banding

Video 1   Adjustable gastric band to a Roux-En-Y gastric bypass
Video 2   Adjustable gastric band to a sleeve gastrectomy

Chapter 50 Surgical Management of Bariatric Complications: Internal Hernia and Leak

Video 1   Techniques for diagnostic laparoscopy

SECTION I: Esophagus

Chapter 1: Epiphrenic Diverticulum

Evan T. Alicuben, James D. Luketich, and Ryan M. Levy

DEFINITION
- Epiphrenic diverticula are those that occur in the distal 10 cm (lower third) of the esophagus. They constitute approximately 20% of all esophageal diverticula. The underlying pathophysiologic mechanism is a result of increased intraluminal pressure, presumably secondary to an esophageal motility disorder. Most commonly, epiphrenic diverticula occur in the setting of achalasia or diffuse esophageal spasm. A high-pressure environment in the esophageal lumen is created by some form of distal functional or mechanical obstruction, such as a nonrelaxing, hypertensive lower esophageal sphincter (LES); repetitive normal to high-amplitude simultaneous contractions; or a distal peptic stricture. A prior fundoplication for the treatment of reflux may also lead to epiphrenic diverticula in the setting of an esophageal motility disorder. Any of these processes may lead to herniation of the mucosa and submucosa through an area of weakness in the muscle layers of the esophagus. Epiphrenic diverticula are thus false, or pulsion, diverticula.

DIFFERENTIAL DIAGNOSIS
- The differential diagnosis of epiphrenic diverticula includes hiatal hernia, esophageal webs and strictures, esophageal duplication cyst, and esophageal carcinoma. Equally relevant is the differential diagnosis of the underlying cause of the epiphrenic diverticulum, which includes achalasia, distal esophageal spasm, ineffective esophageal motility, esophagogastric junction outflow obstruction, end-stage gastroesophageal (GE) reflux disease with a "burnt out" esophagus, peptic stricture, or failed previous fundoplication.

PATIENT HISTORY AND PHYSICAL FINDINGS
- Epiphrenic diverticula are estimated to be symptomatic in only 15% to 20% of cases. Typical symptoms include dysphagia and regurgitation. Reflux and chest pain may also commonly occur. Pulmonary symptoms may include chronic cough, productive or purulent sputum, or chronic dyspnea. Malodorous breath may also be present.
- On history, it is important to elicit whether the patient experiences symptoms of GE reflux disease, regurgitation, chest pain, or dysphagia. Additional medical history such as recurrent pneumonia, lung abscesses, or repeated aspiration episodes is pertinent. A history of weight loss is not uncommon.
- Prior procedures such as esophageal dilations or botulinum toxin injection are also pertinent.

IMAGING AND OTHER DIAGNOSTIC STUDIES
- Epiphrenic diverticula are associated with an underlying esophageal motility disorder in most cases. It is imperative to not only assess the size and location of the diverticulum but also characterize the motor function of the esophagus.
- A barium esophagram is the initial test performed to define the anatomy of the diverticulum and esophagus. Size, location, and right or left sidedness can be determined from the esophagram. This provides a "road map" for operative planning, as diverticula more than 7 to 10 cm above the diaphragm are not easily accessible through the transhiatal route and may be better approached from the chest. Barium esophagram may also offer information about motility.
- High-resolution manometry, the current gold standard, is necessary to evaluate for an underlying esophageal motility disorder. In the setting of achalasia, manometry demonstrates aperistalsis with a nonrelaxing LES. Other manometric patterns seen in the setting of epiphrenic diverticula include distal esophageal spasm, hypercontractile esophagus, esophagogastric outflow obstruction, and ineffective esophageal motility. Failure to identify and treat the underlying motility disorder during diverticulum resection has been associated with high rates of recurrence and leak along the staple line in the range of 10% to 20%.[1] Specifically, failure to perform an adequate myotomy in such patients has yielded leak rates exceeding 25% when diverticulectomy alone is performed.
- Preoperative upper endoscopy is necessary to examine the esophagus and stomach for the presence of Barrett esophagus and esophagitis and to exclude malignancy.[2] In addition, the presence of a pop upon passage of the scope across the LES may further suggest the diagnosis of achalasia. Lastly, it is important to remove debris from the diverticulum on the day of surgery.

SURGICAL MANAGEMENT
- The need for surgical resection of epiphrenic diverticula largely depends on the patient's symptoms. Small, asymptomatic diverticula (less than 3 cm) often do not require intervention. Symptomatic patients with small diverticula may benefit from myotomy (with concomitant partial fundoplication) to correct the underlying motility disorder. Larger diverticula require diverticulectomy in addition to myotomy (with concomitant partial fundoplication).

Preoperative Planning

- A review of the barium esophagram is helpful to confirm the size and location of the diverticulum relative to the diaphragm and GE junction. It also defines the esophageal anatomy in terms of degree of esophageal dilation and presence of megaesophagus or sigmoid appearance in the setting of achalasia.
- The patient's diet should be restricted to clear liquids for 2 days prior to surgery to minimize the accumulation of food debris in the diverticulum prior to operation.
- The anesthesiologist must be informed that rapid sequence induction is needed to minimize risk of aspiration.
- After induction of anesthesia, upper endoscopy should be performed to delineate esophageal anatomy, rule out malignancy, and remove debris from the pouch. Esophagogastroduodenoscopy should also evaluate for the presence of a "pop," which is consistent with achalasia.
- Prophylactic antibiotics should be administered prior to skin incision, with consideration given to covering for oral flora, anaerobes, and yeast.
- Standard procedures such as sequential compression devices and Foley catheter are employed.

Positioning

- Positioning of the patient varies with surgical approach. When approaching epiphrenic diverticula from the abdomen, the patient is positioned supine. If a thoracic approach is chosen, the patient is placed in either a right or left lateral decubitus position. The authors prefer a right-sided video-assisted thoracic surgery (VATS) approach and therefore use the left lateral decubitus position. If a thoracic approach is used, single-lung ventilation is needed with use of a double lumen endotracheal tube or bronchial blocker.

TECHNIQUES

VIDEO-ASSISTED THORACIC SURGERY
(▶ VIDEO 1)

- Either right or left VATS may be used for a minimally invasive thoracic approach to the diverticulum. The location of the diverticulum typically dictates the side of the approach. Classically, distal diverticula have been approached from the left side, whereas more proximal diverticula are more readily approached from the right. However, in the authors' experience, a right-sided VATS approach works equally well for the classic, distally located right- or left-sided epiphrenic diverticula.

Video-Assisted Thoracic Surgery Port Placement

- We commonly employ a five-port approach to VATS resection of epiphrenic diverticula. The port placement is identical to the ports we employ for minimally invasive esophagectomy. Specifically, the surgeon works from the posterior ports, which include an infrascapular tip 5-mm port and a 10-mm port in the 9th interspace along a line parallel to the infrascapular tip port. The remaining three ports are assistant ports and include a 10-mm camera port in the 9th interspace along the posterior axillary line, a 5-mm port for endoscopic suction in the 7th interspace in the midaxillary to posterior axillary line, and a lung retraction 10-mm port in the 5th interspace in the posterior axillary line. See **FIGURE 1** for ideal placement of ports.[3]

Entering the Chest and Mobilizing the Esophagus

- Upon entering the chest, the inferior pulmonary ligament is divided and the lung is retracted superiorly and anteriorly.
- A diaphragm stitch is placed through the central tendon of the diaphragm with a 48-in 0-Surgidac Endo Stitch. It is brought out the right flank at the level of the inferior diaphragm insertion using an endoscopic Endo Close device. Tension is applied to the retraction stitch to retract the diaphragm caudally, exposing the distal esophagus and esophageal hiatus.
- Alternatively, use of carbon dioxide insufflation can result in downward displacement of the diaphragm and in our experience has obviated the need for the diaphragm stitch in most cases.
- Using sharp dissection with a heat source such as an ultrasonic scalpel, the mediastinal pleura overlying the esophagus is opened. As much of the pleura as possible is kept intact so that it may be reapproximated over the repair at the end of the procedure. As such, the pleura is gently dissected away from the esophagus. Opening of the mediastinal pleura from the diaphragm up to the azygous vein is beneficial, as it will be necessary for the performance of a long myotomy. The azygous vein can be divided as needed with an endoscopic stapler.
- Once the pleura has been opened adequately, esophageal mobilization is carried out. If an ipsilateral approach is taken

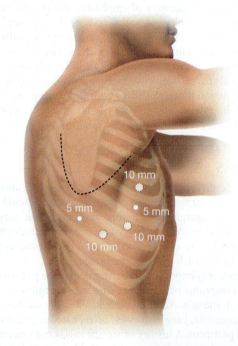

FIGURE 1 • Right VATS thoracoscopic port placement.

to the diverticulum (eg, right VATS for a right-sided diverticulum), minimal mobilization is needed. However, if the diverticulum protrudes on the contralateral aspect of the esophagus, the esophagus must be mobilized so that it may be rotated to provide adequate exposure for dissection of the diverticulum and its neck.
- A Penrose drain may be used to encircle the esophagus and aid in esophageal mobilization.
- Both vagus nerves should be identified and preserved whenever possible.
- It is necessary to expose the entire diverticulum and its neck. The diverticulum may be grasped with an endoscopic Babcock grasper (Snowden-type endoscopic forceps). Alternatively, a long stitch may be placed in the apex of the diverticulum to aid with retraction during dissection. Subsequently, the diverticulum is circumferentially dissected free from its surrounding attachments. It is not uncommon for there to be significant inflammatory-type adhesions from the diverticulum to surrounding structures. It is essential to dissect the surrounding esophageal muscle fibers down to the neck of the diverticulum. This maneuver is critical to ensure complete resection of the diverticulum at the time of stapling. A common technical error is failure to expose the true neck of the diverticulum, which subsequently results in improper positioning of the stapling device and therefore leaves a residual diverticulum.

Diverticulectomy

- Once the neck of the diverticulum is clearly visualized, either the endoscope or a 48- to 54-Fr bougie should be inserted into the esophagus beyond the GE junction. This prevents narrowing of the esophageal lumen during stapling of the diverticulum. If difficulty is encountered passing the bougie, intraoperative upper endoscopy should be performed and a wire passed distally through the true lumen of the esophagus into the stomach. The bougie may then be passed over the wire to minimize risk of perforation.
- With minimal tension on the diverticulum, the stapling device is positioned along the base (neck), parallel to the longitudinal axis of the esophagus (**FIGURE 2**).
- The diverticulum is then transected with a reticulating endoscopic stapler. The authors prefer to use a vascular load for transection of the mucosa and submucosa that comprises the diverticulum.

Esophagomyotomy

- It is preferable to perform the myotomy at least 90° away from the diverticular staple line if possible. The longitudinal esophageal muscle fibers are incised initially with either an ultrasonic scalpel or hook cautery along the direction of the fibers. Alternatively, the myotomy may also be started with a blunt technique by pulling apart the longitudinal muscle fibers. Once the underlying circular muscle fibers are exposed, they are sharply divided. It is critical to lift the circular muscle fibers away from the underlying mucosa to avoid perforation of the mucosa layer (**FIGURE 3**).
- The main vagal trunks should be preserved while performing the myotomy.
- The total length of the myotomy should extend several centimeters (3-5 cm) above the proximal extent of the diverticulum. Distally, the myotomy should extend to or across the GE

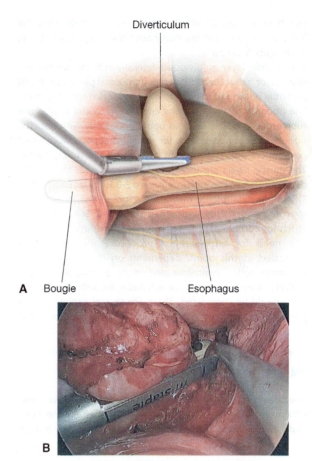

FIGURE 2 • **A**, Circumferential dissection of the diverticulum, bougie in the esophagus, and endoscopic stapler excising the diverticulum. **B**, Excision of the diverticulum with the stapler placed at the neck of diverticulum.

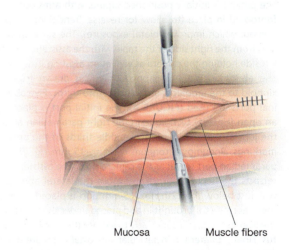

FIGURE 3 • Esophageal myotomy with gastric cardia extension.

junction, depending on the preoperative manometry results and the underlying pathologic diagnosis. For example, a LES that has a normal resting pressure and normal relaxation may not require myotomy across the GE junction, preserving its natural antireflux function. If the patient has achalasia,

- the myotomy should ideally extend to 3 cm below the GE junction, carrying the myotomy onto the sling muscle fibers of the gastric cardia.
- The muscle layer is dissected laterally off the underlying mucosa for a short distance in the submucosal plane to prevent potential healing of the myotomy site (muscle reconstitution).
- The integrity of the myotomy and diverticulectomy sites are submerged under saline, and upper endoscopy with insufflation of air is done to check for leaks. Intraoperative mucosal perforations are repaired with interrupted absorbable suture. The muscle layers are then reapproximated over the diverticulectomy staple line with interrupted 2-0 Surgidac Endo Stitch.
- The mediastinal pleura may also be loosely reapproximated over the esophagus with interrupted 2-0 Surgidac Endo Stitch for additional protection of the staple line.
- The need for an antireflux procedure should also be addressed at this point, depending on the patient's preoperative reflux symptoms and motility studies.[1,4] If the patient carries a diagnosis of achalasia, an antireflux operation should be considered. There are several options at this point. If performing the case from a left VATS approach, one may attempt a Belsey Mark IV fundoplication. This can be quite challenging and technically demanding from a VATS approach as this operation is traditionally performed via left thoracotomy. A second option is to combine VATS with laparoscopy and perform a standard laparoscopic Dor or Toupet (partial) fundoplication. Partial fundoplications are favored in the setting of esophageal motility disorders, as a complete (Nissen) fundoplication may lead to obstruction of the dysmotile esophagus and recurrent diverticula. Lastly, one could forego the antireflux procedure and treat any reflux symptoms with proton pump inhibitors, opting to perform a fundoplication selectively at a later time depending on patient symptoms and response to medical therapy.

Closure

- Once hemostasis is achieved, a pleural drain (chest tube, Blake drain, or pigtail catheter) is placed.
- A Jackson-Pratt (JP) drain is also placed along the posterior mediastinum near the diverticula staple line to control any leak that can potentially occur postoperatively.
- Intercostal bupivacaine is injected for analgesia.

OPEN THORACIC APPROACH

- The operative steps for an open transthoracic epiphrenic diverticulum resection are similar to those described for the minimally invasive approach. A 7th interspace thoracotomy is used.

An open left thoracic approach is ideal when a fundoplication is to be performed from the chest (Belsey Mark IV). Use of a thoracoabdominal stapler or resection and hand-sewn closure of the mucosa are commonly used techniques for resection of the diverticulum when an open approach is used.

LAPAROSCOPIC TRANSHIATAL APPROACH

Port Placement

- The patient is initially positioned supine, with arms out and a footboard in place (to allow for reverse Trendelenburg positioning, which improves hiatal exposure). The surgeon operates from the right side of the table with the assistant from the left side holding the camera as well as an assisting instrument.
- The abdomen is then mapped. A line is drawn from the xiphoid to the umbilicus and divided into thirds. Five abdominal ports are used (FIGURE 4). The initial port is placed via an open (Hasson) technique in the right paramedian area at the junction of the upper and middle thirds of the previous markings. Pneumoperitoneum is set to 15 mm Hg. The left paramedian port serves as the camera port. The assistant then retracts the hepatic flexure to expose the lateral abdominal wall just below the 12th rib. A 5-mm port is placed here and the liver retractor brought in and placed under the left lobe of the liver, retracting it superiorly to expose the esophageal hiatus. Finally, bilateral midclavicular subcostal ports are placed. All ports should be a handbreadth apart to avoid unwanted contact between the surgeon's and assistant's instruments. Skin incisions must be made as small as possible to help ports remain in place and minimize accumulation of subcutaneous emphysema. See FIGURE 4 for ideal placement of ports.[2,5]

Mobilizing the Esophagus

- The gastrohepatic ligament is opened with an ultrasonic scalpel or other energy device to expose the right crus.
- The phrenoesophageal membrane is divided circumferentially around the esophageal hiatus to gain access to the mediastinum and intrathoracic esophagus. The peritoneal lining along the left and right crura should be preserved.

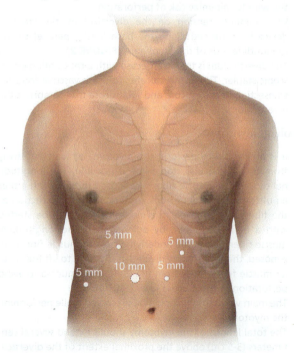

FIGURE 4 • Laparoscopic port placement for abdominal approach.

- Mediastinal mobilization of the esophagus, GE junction, and any associated hiatal hernia is then performed. The anterior and posterior vagal nerves should be identified and preserved during this dissection.
- The short gastric vessels and gastrosplenic attachments are divided so that the upper third of the fundus along the greater curvature is completely mobile for creation of the fundoplication.

Diverticulectomy

- As described earlier, it is necessary to expose the entire diverticulum and its neck. The diverticulum is circumferentially dissected free from its surrounding attachments. Again, it is essential to dissect off the surrounding esophageal muscle fibers down to the neck of the diverticulum. This maneuver is critical to ensure complete resection of the diverticulum at the time of stapling.
- Once the neck of the diverticulum is clearly visualized, either the endoscope or a 48- to 54-Fr bougie should be inserted into the esophagus beyond the GE junction. This prevents narrowing of the esophageal lumen during stapling of the diverticulum.
- With minimal tension on the diverticulum, the stapling device is positioned along the base (neck) parallel to the longitudinal axis of the esophagus.
- The diverticulum is transected with a reticulating endoscopic stapler at its neck.

Esophagomyotomy

- It is preferable to perform the esophagomyotomy 180° from the staple line. However, if this is not possible, then it is preferable to perform the myotomy at least 90° away from the diverticulectomy site.
- The authors prefer to start the myotomy by separating the longitudinal muscle fibers with a blunt technique using Snowden forceps. It is important to pull with equal tension along each side during this maneuver. Once the myotomy is started, we often switch to sharp division of the remaining longitudinal and circular fibers using the ultrasonic scalpel or hook electrocautery. The proximal extent of the myotomy should extend several centimeters above the proximal extent of the diverticulum. If the patient has achalasia, the distal extent of the myotomy should be 3 cm distal to the GE junction so as to include the sling fibers of the proximal most aspect of the gastric cardia.

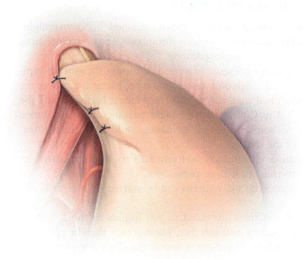

FIGURE 5 • Laparoscopic Dor anterior fundoplication.

- Once again, the muscle layer is dissected off the underlying mucosa laterally on each side for a short distance in the submucosal plane to prevent potential healing of the myotomy site (muscle reconstitution).
- Mucosal integrity can be examined by submerging the esophagus in saline and insufflating with the endoscope to look for an air leak. Small leaks can be closed with a simple stitch.
- Along the diverticulectomy site, the muscle layers of the esophagus are reapproximated over the staple line with 2-0 Surgidac Endo Stitch.
- At the end of the esophagomyotomy, an antireflux procedure is often performed, which is most commonly a partial fundoplication (Dor or Toupet). The authors prefer an anterior 180° fundoplication (Dor) for most cases of achalasia and epiphrenic diverticula (**FIGURE 5**).

Closure

- A JP drain is placed through the hiatus along the diverticulum staple line to control any potential leak that may occur postoperatively.

PEARLS AND PITFALLS

Diverticulectomy	▪ Staple over a bougie or endoscope to prevent esophageal luminal narrowing. ▪ Incomplete dissection of the diverticular neck can lead to stapling too high, leaving a residual diverticulum.
Esophagomyotomy	▪ Failure to perform an adequate esophagomyotomy is associated with up to a 20% rate of recurrence and/or leak. Be sure to extend the myotomy beyond the borders of the staple line longitudinally and to address the original motility disorder. ▪ Reapproximate the esophageal wall muscle loosely over the diverticulum resection site. This can help minimize the development of pseudodiverticulum at the site. ▪ Attempt to preserve the mediastinal pleura that overlies the esophagus. It is helpful to have this layer to close at the end of the case.
Fundoplication	▪ Choice of antireflux procedure should be based on patient's reflux symptoms, anatomy, and esophageal motility.

POSTOPERATIVE CARE

- Postoperatively, patients are maintained NPO overnight. Standard use of deep venous thrombosis and gastrointestinal prophylaxis is employed.
- Owing to the presence of a fresh myotomy, the authors typically avoid usage of a nasogastric tube. Hang a sign over the patient's bed that states, "Do Not Place a Nasogastric Tube Under Any Circumstance." Blind passage of a nasogastric tube without endoscopic guidance could result in perforation of the mucosa.
- Barium esophagram is performed 24 to 48 hours after surgery to rule out leak or perforation.
- After esophagram, patients can be started on a clear liquid diet.
- The diet is then advanced to full liquids in the following days, followed by a soft diet. The diet may then be advanced further when the patient is seen in the clinic 2 weeks later.

OUTCOMES

- Interpretation of the literature regarding surgical management of epiphrenic diverticula is difficult owing to the variability in the following:
  - Approach (thoracotomy, VATS, laparoscopic, or combination of approaches)
  - Direction from which the esophagus is approached (right transthoracic, left transthoracic, or transabdominal)
  - Procedures performed (diverticulectomy alone, myotomy alone, diverticulectomy + myotomy, diverticulectomy + myotomy + fundoplication)
  - Choice of fundoplication (Dor, Toupet, Nissen, Belsey Mark IV)
  - Only small case series being reported
- Controversy exists regarding whether or not all epiphrenic diverticula should be treated surgically. Some surgeons have advocated for a more selective approach,[6] whereas others have supported surgical treatment of all patients with epiphrenic diverticula.[1] The common current practice is to only operate on patients with severe symptoms (eg, dysphagia, regurgitation, aspiration) owing to the low rate in progression of symptoms noted in asymptomatic/mildly symptomatic diverticula, 2.8% in a review by Zaninotto and colleagues.[7]
- There are currently no reports in the literature directly comparing open with minimally invasive approaches; however, reviews have concluded that better outcomes are obtained with a minimally invasive approach in regard to morbidity, mortality, and length of stay (greater than 1 week in open series and less than 1 week in most minimally invasive series).[8,9]
- Reported morbidity rates in open series range from 5% to 38%[1-3,10-14] with leaks rates ranging from 0%[1,10] to as high as 21%.[2] Thirty-day mortality rates ranging from 0% to 15% demonstrate that surgical treatment of epiphrenic diverticula is not without risk.
- Although minimally invasive approaches (VATS, laparoscopic, or a combination of the two) appear to have similar morbidity rates, ranging from 7% to 45% in series with more than 10 patients,[4,5,15-21] mortality appears to be significantly lower with only one reported 30-day death[5] and one additional in-hospital death.[4] Leaks rates again are similar in these series, ranging from 0% to 23%.
- There are currently two published small series[22,23] reporting the results of VATS treatment of epiphrenic diverticula. Six of eight patients operated on were completed thoracoscopically in the series reported by Perrachia,[22] whereas one of five patients required laparoscopy to complete the procedure in van der Peet's series.[23] The few other series reporting use of a VATS approach include a mix of other approaches as well,[4,13,16,24,25] making it impossible to make comparisons between minimally invasive approaches. The authors favor a right VATS approach for diverticula 7 cm or more above the hiatus, diverticula with anticipated dense adhesions, and redo operations for treatment of recurrent diverticula previously treated with a transabdominal approach.
- The literature reporting use of a laparoscopic approach is more robust,[4,5,16,17,19,25,26] with some authors proposing that the laparoscopic approach be considered the standard initial approach for surgical treatment of epiphrenic diverticula.[25]
- The growing use of robotic technology in minimally invasive surgery has also been applied to management of epiphrenic diverticula.[27] While reports of its use are currently limited to small case series, early outcomes appear to be similar to that of the laparoscopic approach. The added dexterity of the robotic arms may prove to be useful in an especially crowded hiatus due to a large diverticulum.
- There also remains controversy about what procedures need be performed for adequate surgical treatment of epiphrenic diverticula. Those in favor of both diverticulectomy and myotomy note that recurrence and suture line leaks appear to be more common in patients who have not had a myotomy.[2,3] There are also proponents who favor a more selective approach for myotomy, particularly in patients with hypotonic esophageal body motor function and/or LES as well as normal esophageal motility.[11,28]
- The length/extent of myotomy required also remains to be clarified. Some authors prefer not to carry the myotomy across the GE junction in case where there is normal LES function, although others favor a long myotomy that is carried across the GE junction and onto the gastric cardia in all cases.[29,30] The reason for this is that some esophageal motility disorders may occur intermittently and therefore may not be revealed on preoperative manometry testing.[12] The authors favor a long myotomy in all cases, except for those in which there is a distal mechanical obstruction (peptic stricture, stenotic previous fundoplication) with normal esophageal motility. In cases such as this, removal of the distal obstruction (dilation, revision to a partial fundoplication) and diverticulectomy may be all that is needed.
- Inclusion of an antireflux procedure and which type of fundoplication should be employed are additional areas of debate. Some believe that an antireflux procedure should be included in all cases in which the myotomy is carried across the LES and onto the stomach, as these patients are more prone to reflux. Most surgeons favor a partial fundoplication (Dor, Toupet, or Belsey Mark IV) owing to the high prevalence of ineffective esophageal motility. It should be noted that performing a fundoplication via a VATS approach is technically challenging. The authors favor a laparoscopic Dor fundoplication, either from an initial laparoscopic

approach or in combination with a right VATS approach, for patients with significant GE reflux preoperatively, achalasia, hiatal hernia or when significant dissection in the area of the GE junction performed.
- With increasing performance of the peroral endoscopic myotomy (POEM) procedure worldwide, some have described its use as the primary treatment for epiphrenic diverticulum.[31] While this approach does not resect the diverticulum, small outpouchings may resolve on their own following relief of distal obstruction. In addition, a diverticular-POEM technique has been used to perform a septotomy endoscopically for management of larger diverticuli.[32] This has been limited to small case series, and long-term follow-up is pending.

COMPLICATIONS
- Leak
- Perforation
- Pleural effusion
- Pneumothorax
- Empyema
- Bleeding
- Recurrence
- Death

REFERENCES

1. Altorki NK, Sunagawa M, Skinner DB. Thoracic esophageal diverticula. Why is operation necessary? *J Thorac Cardiovasc Surg.* 1993;105(2):260-264.
2. Benacci JC, Deschamps C, Trastek VF, Allen MS, Daly RC, Pairolero PC. Epiphrenic diverticulum: results of surgical treatment. *Ann Thorac Surg.* 1993;55(5):1109-1113; discussion 1114. doi:10.1016/0003-4975(93)90016-b
3. Fekete F, Vonns C. Surgical management of esophageal thoracic diverticula. *Hepatogastroenterology.* 1992;39(2):97-99.
4. Fernando HC, Luketich JD, Samphire J, et al. Minimally invasive operation for esophageal diverticula. *Ann Thorac Surg.* 2005;80(6):2076-2080. doi:10.1016/j.athoracsur.2005.06.007
5. Del Genio A, Rossetti G, Maffetton V, et al. Laparoscopic approach in the treatment of epiphrenic diverticula: long-term results. *Surg Endosc.* 2004;18(5):741-745. doi:10.1007/s00464-003-9044-6
6. Orringer MB. Epiphrenic diverticula: fact and fable. *Ann Thorac Surg.* 1993;55(5):1067-1068. doi:10.1016/0003-4975(93)90007-5
7. Zaninotto G, Portale G, Costantini M, Zanatta L, Salvador R, Ruol A. Therapeutic strategies for epiphrenic diverticula: systematic review. *World J Surg.* 2011;35(7):1447-1453. doi:10.1007/s00268-011-1065-z
8. Kilic A, Schuchert MJ, Awais O, Luketich JD, Landreneau RJ. Surgical management of epiphrenic diverticula in the minimally invasive era. *J Soc Laparoendosc Surg.* 2009;13(2):160-164
9. Soares R, Herbella FA, Prachand VN, Ferguson MK, Patti MG. Epiphrenic diverticulum of the esophagus. From pathophysiology to treatment. *J Gastrointest Surg.* 2010;14(12):2009-2015. doi:10.1007/s11605-010-1216-9
10. D'Journo XB, Ferraro P, Martin J, Chen LQ, Duranceau A. Lower oesophageal sphincter dysfunction is part of the functional abnormality in epiphrenic diverticulum. *Br J Surg Aug.* 2009;96(8):892-900. doi:10.1002/bjs.6652
11. Jordan Jr PH, Kinner BM. New look at epiphrenic diverticula. *World J Surg.* 1999;23(2):147-152. doi:10.1007/pl00013158
12. Reznik SI, Rice TW, Murthy SC, Mason DP, Apperson-Hansen C, Blackstone EH. Assessment of a pathophysiology-directed treatment for symptomatic epiphrenic diverticulum. *Dis Esophagus.* 2007;20(4):320-327. doi:10.1111/j.1442-2050.2007.00716.x
13. Varghese Jr TK, Marshall B, Chang AC, Pickens A, Lau CL, Orringer MB. Surgical treatment of epiphrenic diverticula: a 30-year experience. *Ann Thorac Surg.* 2007;84(6):1801-1809; discussion 1801-9. doi:10.1016/j.athoracsur.2007.06.057
14. Tapias LF, Morse CR, Mathisen DJ, et al. Surgical management of esophageal epiphrenic diverticula: a transthoracic approach over four decades. *Ann Thorac Surg.* 2017;104(4):1123-1130. doi:10.1016/j.athoracsur.2017.06.017
15. Fumagalli Romario U, Ceolin M, Porta M, Rosati R. Laparoscopic repair of epiphrenic diverticulum. *Semin Thorac Cardiovasc Surg.* 2012;24(3):213-217. doi:10.1053/j.semtcvs.2012.10.003
16. Klaus A, Hinder RA, Swain J, Achem SR. Management of epiphrenic diverticula. *J Gastrointest Surg.* 2003;7(7):906-911. doi:10.1007/s11605-003-0038-4
17. Melman L, Quinlan J, Robertson B, et al. Esophageal manometric characteristics and outcomes for laparoscopic esophageal diverticulectomy, myotomy, and partial fundoplication for epiphrenic diverticula. *Surg Endosc.* 2009;23(6):1337-1341. doi:10.1007/s00464-008-0165-9
18. Palanivelu C, Rangarajan M, Maheshkumaar GS, Senthilkumar R. Minimally invasive surgery combined with peroperative endoscopy for symptomatic middle and lower esophageal diverticula: a single institute's experience. *Surg Laparosc Endosc Percutan Tech.* 2008;18(2):133-138. doi:10.1097/SLE.0b013e31815acb97
19. Rosati R, Fumagalli U, Bona S, et al. Laparoscopic treatment of epiphrenic diverticula. *J Laparoendosc Adv Surg Tech A.* 2001;11(6):371-375. doi:10.1089/10926420152761897
20. Rosati R, Fumagalli U, Elmore U, de Pascale S, Massaron S, Peracchia A. Long-term results of minimally invasive surgery for symptomatic epiphrenic diverticulum. *Am J Surg.* 2011;201(1):132-135. doi:10.1016/j.amjsurg.2010.03.016
21. Hirano Y, Takeuchi H, Oyama T, et al. Minimally invasive surgery for esophageal epiphrenic diverticulum: the results of 133 patients in 25 published series and our experience. *Surg Today.* 2013;43(1):1-7. doi:10.1007/s00595-012-0386-3
22. Peracchia A, Bonavina L, Rosati R, Bona S. Thoracoscopic resection of epiphrenic esophageal diverticula. In: Peters JH, DeMeester TR, eds. *Minimally Invasive Surgery of the Foregut.* Quality Medical Publishing; 1994:100-116.
23. van der Peet DL, Klinkenberg-Knol EC, Berends FJ, Cuesta MA. Epiphrenic diverticula: minimal invasive approach and repair in five patients. *Dis Esophagus.* 2001;14(1):60-62. doi:10.1111/j.1442-2050.2001.00151.x
24. Matthews BD, Nelms CD, Lohr CE, Harold KL, Kercher KW, Heniford BT. Minimally invasive management of epiphrenic esophageal diverticula. *Am Surg.* 2003;69(6):465-470; discussion 470.
25. Soares RV, Montenovo M, Pellegrini CA, Oelschlager BK. Laparoscopy as the initial approach for epiphrenic diverticula. *Surg Endosc.* 2011;25(12):3740-3746. doi:10.1007/s00464-011-1779-x
26. Zaninotto G, Parise P, Salvador R, et al. Laparoscopic repair of epiphrenic diverticulum. *Semin Thorac Cardiovasc Surg.* 2012;24(3):218-222. doi:10.1053/j.semtcvs.2012.10.009
27. Hukkeri VS, Jindal S, Qaleem M, Tandon V, Govil D. Robotic transhiatal excision of epiphrenic diverticula. *J Robot Surg.* 2016;10(4):365-368. doi:10.1007/s11701-016-0595-7
28. Streitz Jr JM, Glick ME, Ellis Jr FH Selective use of myotomy for treatment of epiphrenic diverticula. Manometric and clinical analysis. *Arch Surg.* 1992;127(5):585-587; discussion 587-588. doi:10.1001/archsurg.1992.01420050109014
29. Allen TH, Clagett OT. Changing concepts in the surgical treatment of pulsion diverticula of the lower esophagus. *J Thorac Cardiovasc Surg.* 1965;50(4):455-462.
30. Nehra D, Lord RV, DeMeester TR, et al. Physiologic basis for the treatment of epiphrenic diverticulum. *Ann Surg.* 2002;235(3):346-354. doi:10.1097/00000658-200203000-00006
31. Sato H, Takeuchi M, Hashimoto S, et al. Esophageal diverticulum: new perspectives in the era of minimally invasive endoscopic treatment. *World J Gastroenterol.* 2019;25(12):1457-1464. doi:10.3748/wjg.v25.i12.1457
32. Yang J, Zeng X, Yuan X, et al. An international study on the use of peroral endoscopic myotomy (POEM) in the management of esophageal diverticula: the first multicenter D-POEM experience. *Endoscopy.* 2019;51(4):346-349. doi:10.1055/a-0759-1428

Chapter 2 Long Myotomy for Distal Esophageal Spasm*

Gilbert Pan, Ernest G. Chan, David D. Odell, and James D. Luketich

DEFINITION

- Distal esophageal spasm (DES) is a rare esophageal motility disorder characterized by premature, simultaneous, and/or irregular smooth muscle contractions in the distal esophagus.
- Patients may demonstrate both nonocclusive and occlusive high-amplitude tertiary contractions and are often nonpropulsive, resulting in substernal chest pain and debilitating dysphagia.
- This disease is still commonly referred to as "diffuse esophageal spasm." However, due to the advances in diagnostic modalities such as high-resolution manometry (HRM), the proper term has been changed to distal esophageal spasm as seen in the Chicago Classification of esophageal motility disorders in 2015.[1,2]

DIFFERENTIAL DIAGNOSIS

- DES is part of a spectrum of spastic esophagus disorders causing esophageal hyperactivity and dysmotility.
- Evaluation of clinical presentation and diagnostic studies provide critical information to facilitate an accurate diagnosis and appropriate treatment.
- Examination of the motility phase of the esophagus may result in no demonstrable abnormality.
- Despite differences in pathophysiology, several esophageal disorders share similar presentations and can lead to misdiagnosis.
  - Achalasia[3,4]: Pathologically arises from degeneration of neurons in the lower esophageal wall, which leads to the inability of the lower esophageal sphincter (LES) to relax. Nonsurgical treatment modalities include pharmacotherapy or endoscopic therapy to aid in relaxation of the LES while surgical modalities include a Heller myotomy extending onto the gastric cardia.
  - Chagas disease[5]: Caused by an infection from *Trypanosoma cruzi*, which has become increasingly common in nonendemic countries due to increased accessibility of migratory travel. Chronic manifestations of disease in about 10% to 15% of patients involve peristaltic and esophageal dysfunction, leading to nonpathognomonic manifestation of dysphagia. Antitrypanosomal pharmacotherapy is first-line treatment.
  - Connective tissue disorder: Diseases such as systemic lupus erythematosus, systemic sclerosis, and rheumatoid arthritis frequently impact esophageal motility. Dysphagia, regurgitation, and chest pain are common presenting symptoms and should be evaluated for an autoimmune etiology.
  - Gastroesophageal reflux disease (GERD)[6]: Chronic severe regurgitation and refluxate irritates the esophagus, leading to esophagitis and subsequent dysmotility. HRM and 24-hour pH studies are useful in assessing the severity of disease. Patients with GERD will also develop simultaneous contractions similar to patients with symptomatic DES. Esophageal dysmotility symptoms typically resolve upon successful control of reflux.
  - Jackhammer/Nutcracker esophagus[7,8]: Characterized by hypertensive, but normal esophageal peristaltic contractions that often presents as noncardiac chest pain. Calcium channel blockers, botulinum toxin injections, and pneumatic dilation are appropriate therapies to consider for symptom management.
  - Pseudoachalasia: Mechanical obstruction of the esophagus (neoplasms, stenosis, foreign bodies, esophagitis, prior operative adhesions, etc) can manifest symptoms of dysphagia, chest pain, esophageal dysmotility characterized by simultaneous contractions, and esophageal dilation. Correction of underlying pathology typically resolves symptoms.

PATIENT HISTORY AND PHYSICAL FINDINGS

- Patients presenting with a history of noncardiac chest pain and dysphagia should be carefully evaluated for DES. Assessment of frequency (every meal vs daily vs weekly) and severity (salivary secretions vs liquids vs solids) can help characterize the etiology of dysphagia. Occasional regurgitation of solid food is common. Characterization of the quality and duration of substernal chest pain provide important context for diagnosis, especially in relation to swallowing.
- Typical and atypical reflux symptoms should be directly question and evaluated:
  - Typical: globus sensation, heartburn, history of dysphagia/stricture, water brash
  - Atypical: aspiration, cough, dysphonia, recurrent pulmonary infections
- Psychiatric history (anxiety and depression commonly co-manifest with DES)
- Cardiac history (prior myocardial infarction, exertional chest pain, cardiac procedures)
- Connective tissue disease history (evaluation of healing difficulties, cutaneous lesions, and/or concomitant visual problems)

---

*Former nomenclature Diffuse Esophageal Spasm.

IMAGING AND OTHER DIAGNOSTIC STUDIES

- Barium esophagram[9,10]—findings will illustrate a classic "corkscrew" or "rosary bead" appearance suggestive of abnormal contractions in the esophagus. Presence of findings is highly indicative of spastic esophageal disorders while absence is nonspecific. Results are supplemental, and additional studies are necessary for diagnosing DES.
- Esophageal manometry[1,2]—considered the gold standard, the diagnostic criterion for DES is characterized by the occurrence of simultaneous/premature contractions with amplitudes of more than 30 mm Hg in the presence of normal peristalsis. These simultaneous/premature contractions are accompanied with the presence of symptoms after greater than 10% to 30% of wet swallows. LES pressures can either be normal or abnormal when interrogated during manometry. If 100% of the esophageal contractions are simultaneous, then the diagnosis is more indicative of achalasia.
- Esophagogastroduodenoscopy[11]—affords limited diagnostic value, but required to visualize the anatomy prior to treatment interventions and exclude the alternative diagnosis of pseudoachalasia. The uncoordinated esophageal spasms and corkscrew appearance can be seen on endoscopy. Biopsies can be obtained to rule out inflammatory causes of dysphagia including esophagitis. Visualization also permits assessment of reflux-related metaplastic changes such as Barrett esophagus that may warrant subsequent observation and/or treatment.
- Endoscopic ultrasound[7]—can be used to quantify thickening of the esophageal muscular layers, visualize intramural or mediastinal abnormalities, and function as an adjunct in surgical planning.
- 24-hour pH studies[7,12]—useful in patients experiencing noncardiac chest pain to confirm the presence of pathologic reflux which helps elucidate the overlap between DES and GERD. Evidence of reflux can guide surgical decisions to include a fundoplication at the time of correction.

SURGICAL MANAGEMENT

- Surgical management is purely palliative and should be considered after unsuccessful medical therapy.[13]
- It is primarily aimed at addressing symptoms of dysphagia and chest pain.[14]
- While both medical and surgical treatments are associated with disappointing outcomes in some patients, surgical interventions have demonstrated improved outcomes which have been hypothesized to be due to surgical selection criteria.[15,16]
- Utilization of a surgical myotomy as treatment for various esophageal dysmotility disorders has been documented to be highly successful in minimizing symptomatology and progression of disease.[17-19]
- An extended esophagomyotomy is traditionally considered the gold standard procedure to address the spastic portion of the esophagus refractory to alternative therapies. Recent studies have also demonstrated similar outcomes utilizing peroral endoscopic myotomy (POEM) for DES.[20-23]

Preoperative Planning

- Medical[24] and endoscopic interventions should have been unsuccessful in relieving symptoms. Attempted alternative therapies should include calcium channel blockers, tricyclic antidepressants, serotonin reuptake inhibitors, and phosphodiesterase inhibitors for smooth muscle relaxation and/or endoscopic procedures such as pneumatic dilation or endoscopic administration of botulinum toxin.
- Patients should be counseled of operative risks such as esophageal perforations, pneumothorax, persistence of symptoms, and exacerbation of reflux.
- A liquid diet should be maintained for 2 days prior to the procedure with no dietary intake (solid or liquid) in the 12 hours immediately prior to the procedure.

Position

- The patient is turned to the left lateral decubitus position. A beanbag is placed underneath the patient to afford additional support and to fi the patient in position. An axillary roll is positioned at the base of the axilla to minimize nerve compression. Positions of the double lumen endotracheal tube, placed prior to turning the patient lateral, is reconfirmed using a pediatric endoscope. The operating surgeon stands on the right side of the table (facing the patient's back) while the assistant stands on the left side of the table.

Airway Management

- The patient is intubated with a double lumen endotracheal tube. This allows for lung isolation on the operative side to provide adequate exposure.

THORACOSCOPIC APPROACH

Port Placement

Once the patient is placed in left lateral decubitus position, a total of five thoracoscopic ports are placed including three 10-mm ports (camera, working port, retraction port for a fan-shaped retractor) and two 5-mm ports (**FIGURE 1**). The camera port is placed in the eighth or ninth intercostal space in the midaxillary line. The working port is placed in the eighth or ninth intercostal space in the posterior axillary line. The last 10-mm port is placed in the fourth intercostal space in the anterior axillary line. The two 5-mm ports are placed inferior to the tip of the scapula and in the fifth interspace at the anterior axillary line for the surgeon's left hand and assistant's suction port, respectively.

Exposure

Adhesions between the lung and its surrounding structures are taken down to expose the pleura overlaying the esophagus. In some patients, a high riding diaphragm may impede adequate visualization of the lower portion of the esophagus. This may be remedied either with the use of CO_2 insufflation or placement of a diaphragmatic retraction suture. We place a 48 in 0-Surgidac suture through the central tendon (**FIGURE 2**). This suture is brought out through the lateral chest wall where the diaphragm inserts into the chest wall and held in place with a surgical clamp.

Esophageal Mobilization

Once the inferior pulmonary ligament is incised, the pleura overlying the esophagus is then sharply incised with energy (**FIGURE 3A**). The dissection is continued in the avascular pleural plan along the pericardium to expose the esophagus (**FIGURE 3B**). This is further continued to the level of the subcarinal space. Once the level 7 lymph nodes are identified, care is taken to identify the membranous wall of the right mainstem bronchus (**FIGURE 3C**). During this dissection, attention is needed to ensure the heated portion of the energy device does not touch the membranous portion of the airway to avoid any thermal injury.

As the dissection is carried cranially, retraction of the lung anteriorly will help further expose the proper plane to mobilize the esophagus. Once the airway is safely identified, the azygous vein is approached and can be divided with a vascular surgical stapler if the spasmodic segment of the esophagus extends above this level (**FIGURE 3D** and **E**). The vagus nerve is identified and preserved at this level to maintain normal gastric function.

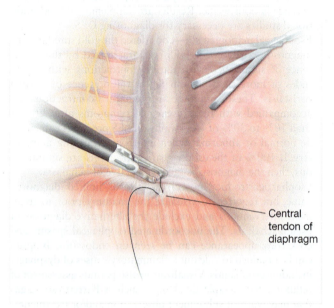

FIGURE 2 • Diaphragm retraction suture. Placement of a suture in the central tendon of the diaphragm facilitates retraction and improves visualization of the esophagus.

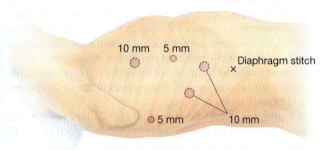

FIGURE 1 • Port placement: positioning of the thoracoscopic ports used for esophageal myotomy.

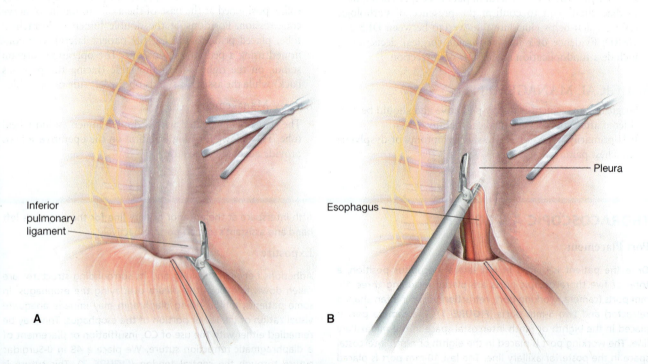

FIGURE 3 • Pleural dissection. **A,** Mobilization of the inferior pulmonary ligament. **B,** Beginning of the dissection along the pericardium. **C,** Pleura is incised overlying the esophagus and a Penrose drain used to encircle the esophagus for retraction. The anterior boundary of dissection along the bronchus intermedius. **D,** Division of the azygous vein using an endoscopic stapler. **E,** Dissection above the azygous directly on the esophagus to avoid recurrent nerve injury.

Chapter 2 LONG MYOTOMY FOR DISTAL ESOPHAGEAL SPASM 11

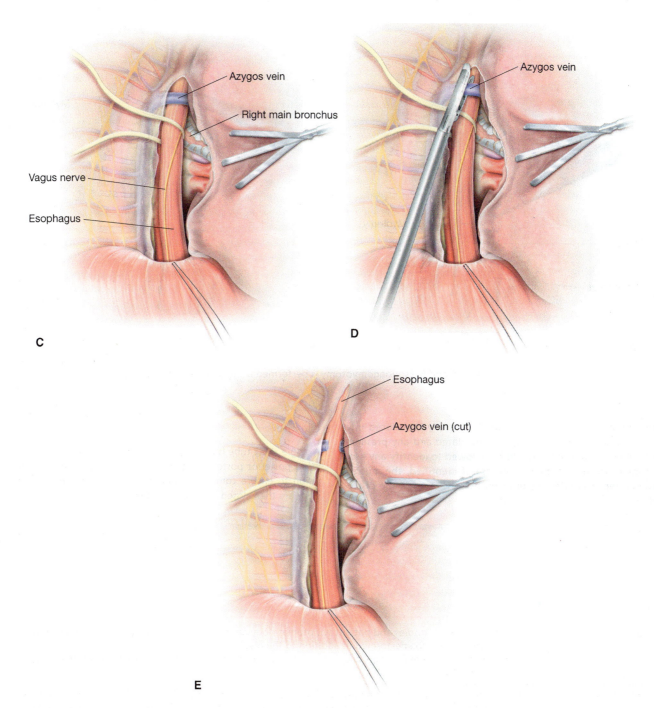

FIGURE 3 • Continued

Esophagomyotomy

Once the diseased portion of the esophagus is completely exposed, the myotomy can be performed. The myotomy is started 6 to 7 cm above the diaphragm. This begins with the identification of the longitudinal muscle layer of the esophagus. The longitudinal muscle layer can be incised with either hook electrocautery or an energy dissection device (FIGURE 4A and B). This maneuver will help expose the circular muscle layer which is also incised. The cut ends of the muscle layer should be gently separated from one another to prevent early reapproximation as the myotomy heals. Care is taken to minimize thermal injury to the esophageal mucosa by situating the Teflon of the energy device down toward the mucosa. In the presence of dysfunctional LES relaxation, the myotomy can also be carried onto the stomach.

Leak Test

Once the myotomy is complete, a leak test is performed to identify any area of injury to the esophageal mucosa. The right hemithorax is filled with enough water or saline to submerge

SECTION I ESOPHAGUS

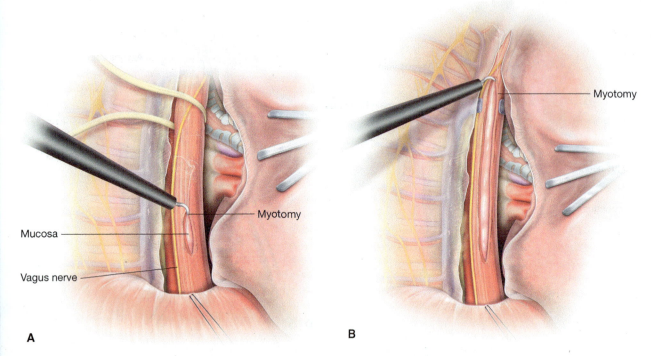

FIGURE 4 • A and B, Esophagomyotomy is performed using an energy device.

the esophagus and an endoscope is carefully introduced into the esophagus. The esophagus is insufflated and any presence of bubbles in the chest should be followed to identify any area of injury to the esophageal mucosa. If identified, the mucosa can be repaired primarily prior to the conclusion of the procedure.

Closure

A single chest tube is left in place at the completion of the operation posterior posteriorly and the lung is aerated under direct vision to ensure complete parenchymal re-expansion. Skin incisions are then closed in standard fashion.

PEARLS AND PITFALLS

Reflux	▪ Preoperative pH studies and patient symptomatology are necessary to identify whether an antireflux procedure should be performed in addition to the myotomy. ▪ Controversy still remains regarding the need for an antireflux procedure when the myotomy is carried across the EGJ.
Chylothorax	▪ Due to the variability in the anatomy of the thoracic duct and difficulty in its visualization, care is taken to avoid the need to enter the plain between the vertebral bodies and aorta posterior to the esophagus.
Extent of myotomy	▪ Myotomy should be taken above the level of the aortic arch and ideally, to the thoracic inlet, as smooth muscle fibers may comprise as much as one-third of the upper thoracic esophageal muscle.
Esophageal leak	▪ Once the myotomy is complete, an intraoperative leak test should be performed. We will typically perform a water-soluble contrast esophagram on postoperative day 1 prior to starting any postoperative diet. Unexplained postoperative tachycardia, fever, or chest pain should prompt further workup.

POSTOPERATIVE CARE

- Postoperative hospital stay is usually limited to about 1 or 2 days.[17-19,25]
- No nasogastric tube is typically required.
- Barium esophagrams are typically performed on postoperative day 1 prior to initiation of oral intake to ensure patency as well as confirm free passage of contrast from distal esophagus into stomach. This helps in establishing a postoperative baseline for future follow-up reference.
- Pain control can be adequately achieved using oral nonopioid analgesics; additional opioid pain medications paired with stool softeners can be prescribed for any remaining discomfort.
- A liquid diet may be initiated following confirmation of esophageal integrity with an esophagram. Diet can be gradually progressed to a soft diet over the course of the first week.

OUTCOMES

Extended myotomy procedures for DES have excellent reported outcomes for symptom alleviation. Improvement and/or resolution of dysphagia and noncardiac chest pain range from 70% to 94% postoperatively.[12,14,26,27] Alternative surgical modalities and approaches have yielded similar results.

POEM has become a popular therapeutic option for DES due to its minimally invasive nature. Clinical success rate has been reported to be as high as 98%.[21,28,29] However, technical difficulties can arise due to hyperactive spastic contractions during the procedure, prolonging the operative time and increasing the risk of complications.[30] Reports also suggest an increased incidence of postoperative GERD following POEM since there an antireflux procedure is not performed.[28,31]

A transabdominal approach via a laparoscopic myotomy is an emerging surgical alternative as the thoracoscopic approach is considered more technically demanding. Access to the LES and distal esophagus is easily obtained. Outcomes were similar, if not slightly better for the laparoscopic approach when compared to the thoracoscopic approach.[32,33] However, the proximal esophagus is not readily accessible via laparoscopy, which limits the length of the myotomy.

COMPLICATIONS

Dysphagia

Dysphagia following surgical myotomy and fundoplication is frequently related to an incomplete myotomy and/or fibrosis at the distal esophagus. Endoscopy and barium esophagrams are useful diagnostic tools to visualize potential sites of obstruction and rule out alternative pathologies such as malignancy, strictures, or herniations. Edema at myotomy site should also be considered. Treatment with endoscopic pneumatic dilation is the first-line choice.[34,35]

Perforation/Leak

Esophageal perforations can result from mobilization of the mediastinal esophagus during surgical dissection. Injuries recognized at the time of operation can be repaired with sutures or a Dor fundoplication (if the injury was anterior at the GE junction). If a postmyotomy leak is suspected, an endoscopic examination is a valuable diagnostic tool. Unrecognized mucosal injury will often present within 24 to 72 hours with peritonitis, mediastinitis, dyspnea and pleuritic pain from pleural effusion, fever, leukocytosis, and/or overt sepsis. A high index of suspicion is necessary for early diagnosis, and aggressive surgical intervention is warranted to facilitate adequate drainage and repair the injury. A feeding jejunostomy should be considered if a prolonged healing time is anticipated. The specific approach is dictated by the location of injury and presentation of the patient.[25]

Reflux

Reflux symptoms following myotomy with fundoplication are common and even more common in patients receiving myotomy alone procedures. The decision to perform an antireflux operation at the time of the index operative must be individualized to the patient. pH monitoring should be performed after myotomy in patients experiencing symptoms to assess the extent of reflux. Medical treatment with proton pump inhibitors has demonstrable efficacy for symptom management. Effective lifestyle modifications may include the avoidance of late evening meals and head of bed elevation while sleeping. Antireflux operative repair can be considered in rare circumstances when symptoms are refractory to alternative therapies.[35-37]

Vagus Nerve Division

While rare, the anterior and posterior vagus nerves are at risk of injury during several steps of the operation. If only one is injured, repair is generally not indicated as symptoms are rare with unilateral vagotomy.[38]

Other Complications

Atelectasis, bleeding, infection, and pneumothorax are uncommon complications that occur in approximately 3% to 4% of all patients.[39,40] Pneumothorax resulting from injury to the pleura often occurs during mobilization of the esophagus. Repairs can be made intraoperatively if warranted; otherwise, careful observation of hemodynamic stability and oxygen saturation will suffice.

REFERENCES

1. Kahrilas PJ, Bredenoord AJ, Fox M, et al. The Chicago Classification of esophageal motility disorders, v3.0. *Neuro Gastroenterol Motil.* 2015;27(2):160-174. doi:10.1111/NMO.12477
2. Yadlapati R, Kahrilas PJ, Fox MR, et al. Esophageal motility disorders on high-resolution manometry: Chicago classification version 4.0©. *Neuro Gastroenterol Motil.* 2021;33(1):e14058. doi:10.1111/NMO.14058
3. Andrási L, Paszt A, Simonka Z, et al. Surgical treatment of esophageal achalasia in the era of minimally invasive Surgery. *JSLS J Soc Laparosc Robot Surg.* 2021;25(1). doi:10.4293/JSLS.2020.00099
4. Fontes LHS, Herbella FAM, Rodriguez TN, Trivino T, Farah JFM. Progression of diffuse esophageal spasm to achalasia: incidence and predictive factors. *Dis Esophagus.* 2013;26(5):470-474. doi:10.1111/J.1442-2050.2012.01377.X
5. Pinazo M-J, Lacima G, Elizalde JI, et al. Characterization of digestive involvement in patients with chronic T. Cruzi infection in Barcelona, Spain. *PLoS Negl Trop Dis.* 2014;8(8):e3105. doi:10.1371/JOURNAL.PNTD.0003105
6. Liu L, Li S, Zhu K, et al. Relationship between esophageal motility and severity of gastroesophageal reflux disease according to the Los Angeles classification. *Medicine (Baltim).* 2019;98(19):e15543. doi:10.1097/MD.0000000000015543
7. Roman S, Kahrilas PJ. Management of spastic disorders of the esophagus. *Gastroenterol Clin North Am.* 2013;42(1):27. doi:10.1016/J.GTC.2012.11.002

8. Voulgaris TA, Karamanolis GP. Esophageal manifestation in patients with scleroderma. *World J Clin cases.* 2021;9(20):5408-5419. doi:10.12998/wjcc.v9.i20.5408
9. Fonseca EKUN, Yamauchi FI, Tridente CF, Baroni RH. Corkscrew esophagus. *Abdom Radiol.* 2017;42(3):985-986. doi:10.1007/s00261-016-0965-7
10. Sugihara Y, Sakae H, Hamada K, Okada H. Peroral endoscopic myotomy is an effective treatment for diffuse esophageal spasm. *Clin Case Reports.* 2020;8(5):927. doi:10.1002/CCR3.2755
11. Valdovinos MA, Zavala-Solares MR, Coss-Adame E. Esophageal hypomotility and spastic motor disorders: current diagnosis and treatment. *Curr Gastroenterol Rep.* 2014;16(11):1-10. doi:10.1007/S11894-014-0421-1
12. Henderson RD, Ryder DE. Reflux control following myotomy in diffuse esophageal spasm. *Ann Thorac Surg.* 1982;34(3):230-236. doi:10.1016/S0003-4975(10)62491-5
13. Salvador R, Costantini M, Rizzetto C, Zaninotto G. Diffuse esophageal spasm: the surgical approach. *Dis Esophagus.* 2012;25(4):311-318. doi:10.1111/J.1442-2050.2010.01172.X
14. Leconte M, Douard R, Gaudric M, Dumontier I, Chaussade S, Dousset B. Functional results after extended myotomy for diffuse oesophageal spasm. *Br J Surg.* 2007;94(9):1113-1118. doi:10.1002/bjs.5761
15. Herbella FA, Tineli AC, Wilson JL, Del Grande JC. Surgical treatment of primary esophageal motility disorders. *J Gastrointest Surg.* 2007;12(3):604-608. doi:10.1007/S11605-007-0379-5
16. Patti MG, Pellegrini CA, Arcerito M, Tong J, Mulvihill SJ, Way LW. Comparison of medical and minimally invasive surgical therapy for primary esophageal motility disorders. *Arch Surg.* 1995;130(6):609-616. doi:10.1001/ARCHSURG.1995.01430060047009
17. Kilic A, Schuchert MJ, Pennathur A, et al. Minimally invasive myotomy for achalasia in the elderly. *Surg Endosc.* 2008;22(4):862-865. doi:10.1007/S00464-007-9657-2
18. Kilic A, Schuchert MJ, Pennathur A, Gilbert S, Landreneau RJ, Luketich JD. Long-term outcomes of laparoscopic Heller myotomy for achalasia. *Surgery.* 2009;146(4):826-833. doi:10.1016/J.SURG.2009.06.049
19. Schuchert MJ, Luketich JD, Landreneau RJ, et al. Minimally-invasive esophagomyotomy in 200 consecutive patients: factors influencing postoperative outcomes. *Ann Thorac Surg.* 2008;85(5):1729-1734. doi:10.1016/J.ATHORACSUR.2007.11.017
20. Khashab MA, Benias PC, Swanstrom LL. Endoscopic myotomy for Foregut motility disorders. *Gastroenterology.* 2018;154(7):1901-1910. doi:10.1053/j.gastro.2017.11.294
21. Khan MA, Kumbhari V, Ngamruengphong S, et al. Is POEM the answer for management of spastic esophageal disorders? A systematic review and meta-analysis. *Dig Dis Sci.* 2017;62(1):35-44. doi:10.1007/s10620-016-4373-1
22. Minami H, Inoue H, Haji A, et al. Per-oral endoscopic myotomy: emerging indications and evolving techniques. *Dig Endosc.* 2015;27(2):175-181. doi:10.1111/den.12328
23. Schaheen LW, Sanchez MV, Luketich JD. Peroral endoscopic myotomy for achalasia. *Thorac Surg Clin.* 2018;28(4):499-506. doi:10.1016/J.THORSURG.2018.07.005
24. Miller DR, Averbukh LD, Kwon SY, et al. Phosphodiesterase inhibitors are viable options for treating esophageal motility disorders: a case report and literature review. *J Dig Dis.* 2019;20(9):495-499. doi:10.1111/1751-2980.12802
25. Vaziri K, Soper NJ. Laparoscopic heller myotomy: technical aspects and operative Pitfalls. *J Gastrointest Surg.* 2008;12(9):1586-1591. doi:10.1007/S11605-008-0475-1
26. Henderson RD, Ryder D, Marryatt G. Extended esophageal myotomy and short total fundoplication hernia repair in diffuse esophageal spasm: five-year review in 34 patients. *Ann Thorac Surg.* 1987;43(1):25-31. doi:10.1016/S0003-4975(10)60161-0
27. Nastos D, Chen LQ, Ferraro P, Taillefer R, Duranceau AC. Long myotomy with antireflux repair for esophageal spastic disorders. *J Gastrointest Surg.* 2002;6(5):713-722. doi:10.1016/S1091-255X(02)00016-1
28. Wong I, Law S. Peroral endoscopic myotomy (POEM) for treating esophageal motility disorders. *Ann Transl Med.* 2017;5(8):192. doi:10.21037/ATM.2017.04.36
29. Shiwaku H, Inoue H, Beppu R, et al. Successful treatment of diffuse esophageal spasm by peroral endoscopic myotomy. *Gastrointest Endosc.* 2013;77(1):149-150. doi:10.1016/J.GIE.2012.02.008
30. Ponds FA-M, Smout AJPM, Fockens P, Bredenoord AJ. Challenges of peroral endoscopic myotomy in the treatment of distal esophageal spasm. *Scand J Gastroenterol.* 2018;53(3):252-255. doi:10.1080/00365521.2018.1424933
31. Familiari P, Gigante G, Marchese M, et al. EndoFLIP system for the intraoperative evaluation of peroral endoscopic myotomy. *UEG J.* 2014;2(2):77-83. doi:10.1177/2050640614521193
32. Patti MG, Gorodner MV, Galvani C, et al. Spectrum of esophageal motility disorders: implications for diagnosis and treatment. *Arch Surg.* 2005;140(5):442-449. doi:10.1001/ARCHSURG.140.5.442
33. Champion J, Delisle N, Hunt T. Comparison of thoracoscopic and laproscopic esophagomyotomy with fundoplication for primary motility disorders. *Eur J Cardio Thorac Surg.* 1999;16(suppl 1):S34-S36. doi:10.1016/S1010-7940(99)00181-5
34. Zaninotto G, Costantini M, Rizzetto C, et al. Four hundred laparoscopic myotomies for esophageal achalasia. *Ann Surg.* 2008;248(6):986-993. doi:10.1097/SLA.0b013e3181907bdd
35. Wright AS, Williams CW, Pellegrini CA, Oelschlager BK. Long-term outcomes confirm the superior efficacy of extended Heller myotomy with Toupet fundoplication for achalasia. *Surg Endosc.* 2007;21(5):713-718. doi:10.1007/S00464-006-9165-9
36. Luketich JD, Fernando HC, Christie NA, et al. Outcomes after minimally invasive esophagomyotomy. *Ann Thorac Surg.* 2001;72(6):1909-1913. doi:10.1016/S0003-4975(01)03127-7
37. Ness-Jensen E, Hveem K, El-Serag H, Lagergren J. Lifestyle intervention in gastroesophageal reflux disease. *Clin Gastroenterol Hepatol.* 2016;14(2):175. doi:10.1016/J.CGH.2015.04.176
38. Oelschlager BK, Chang L, Pellegrini CA. Improved outcome after extended gastric myotomy for achalasia. *Arch Surg.* 2003;138(5):490-497. doi:10.1001/ARCHSURG.138.5.490
39. Finley RJ, Clifton JC, Stewart KC, et al. Laparoscopic Heller myotomy improves esophageal emptying and the symptoms of achalasia. *Arch Surg.* 2001;136(8):892-896. doi:10.1001/archsurg.136.8.892
40. Ludemann R, Krysztopik R, Jamieson GG, Watson DI. Pneumothorax during laparoscopy. *Surg Endosc Other Interv Tech.* 2003;17(12):1985-1989. doi:10.1007/S00464-003-8126-9

Chapter 3 — Laparoscopic Heller Myotomy and Anterior Fundoplication for Esophageal Achalasia

Marco Ettore Allaix and Marco G. Patti

DEFINITION
Esophageal achalasia is a primary disorder of esophageal motility characterized by lack of esophageal peristalsis and failure of the lower esophageal sphincter (LES) to relax properly in response to swallowing.

DIFFERENTIAL DIAGNOSIS
- Benign peptic strictures secondary to gastroesophageal reflux disease (GERD) or strictures due to esophageal neoplasms may present with the same symptoms of esophageal achalasia.
- A cancer infiltrating the gastroesophageal junction can mimic not only the clinical and radiological findings of achalasia but also the manometric profile. This condition, called "secondary achalasia" or "pseudoachalasia," should be considered and ruled out in patients older than 60 years, with recent onset of dysphagia (less than 6 months), and with excessive weight loss.[1]

PATIENT HISTORY AND PHYSICAL FINDINGS
- Dysphagia is the main complaint. It is present in about 95% of patients and is often for both solids and liquids. Most patients are able to maintain a stable weight due to changes made in their diet.
- Regurgitation of undigested food is experienced by about 60% of patients. It occurs more frequently while in the supine position and may lead to aspiration that can cause respiratory symptoms, such as cough, hoarseness, wheezing, and episodes of pneumonia.[2]
- About 40% of patients complain of heartburn: it is secondary to stasis and fermentation of undigested food in the distal esophagus, rather than to gastroesophageal reflux (GER).
- Esophageal distention can cause chest pain in up to 40% of patients, and it is usually experienced at the time of a meal.

IMAGING AND OTHER DIAGNOSTIC STUDIES
A thorough evaluation to establish the diagnosis should be obtained in all cases when esophageal achalasia is suspected.[3] It includes the following studies:
- *Upper endoscopy* is usually the first test that is performed to rule out the presence of a mechanical obstruction secondary to a peptic stricture or cancer.
- *Barium swallow* shows a narrowing at the level of the gastroesophageal junction (the so-called *bird's beak*), slow esophageal emptying with an air-fluid level, and either absence of or tertiary contractions of the esophageal wall (**FIGURE 1**). It also helps defining the diameter and the axis of the esophagus (dilated and sigmoid in long-standing achalasia), and associated pathological findings, including an epiphrenic diverticulum.
- *Esophageal manometry* is the gold standard for the diagnosis of esophageal achalasia. Lack of peristalsis and absent or incomplete LES relaxation in response to swallowing are the key criteria for the diagnosis. The LES is hypertensive in about 50% of patients.[3] The current classification of esophageal achalasia is based on high-resolution manometry type I, classic, with minimal esophageal pressurization; type II, achalasia with panesophageal pressurization; and type III, achalasia with spasm (**FIGURE 2**).[4]

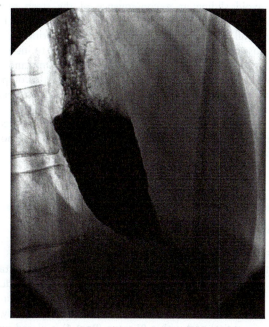

FIGURE 1 • Barium swallow: dilation of the esophageal body, retained barium, and distal esophageal narrowing (bird's beak).

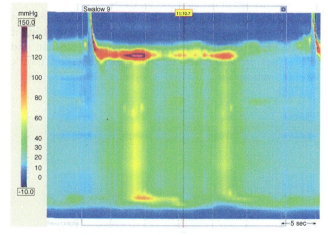

FIGURE 2 • High-resolution esophageal manometry: type II achalasia according to the Chicago classification.

- *24-hour ambulatory pH monitoring* is recommended in untreated patients when the diagnosis is uncertain in order to distinguish between GERD and achalasia.[5] Postoperatively, ambulatory pH monitoring can be performed to rule out pathologic reflux that can occur in up to 30% of cases after Heller myotomy and is often asymptomatic.[6]

SURGICAL MANAGEMENT

Preoperative Planning

A careful symptomatic evaluation and the tests described before should be performed in every patient before treatment.

Positioning

- After induction of general endotracheal anesthesia, the patient is positioned supine in low lithotomy position with the lower extremities extended on stirrups, with knees flexed 20° to 30° or straight if using a split leg table.
- To avoid sliding as a consequence of the steep reverse Trendelenburg position used during the procedure, a bean bag is inflated to create a "saddle" under the perineum.
- Because of decreased venous return secondary to increased abdominal pressure from pneumoperitoneum and the steep reverse Trendelenburg position, pneumatic compression stockings are always used to prevent deep venous thrombosis.
- An orogastric tube is placed to keep the stomach decompressed during the procedure; the orogastric tube is removed before starting the myotomy.
- The surgeon stands between the patient's legs. The first and second assistants stand on the right and left side of the operating table (**FIGURE 3**).

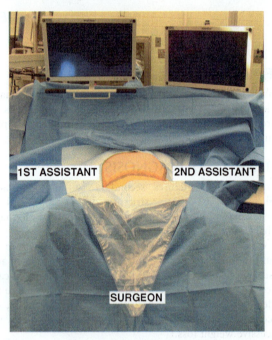

FIGURE 3 • Position of the patient and surgical team in the operating room.

TECHNIQUES

PLACEMENT OF PORTS

- Five trocars are used for the procedure (**FIGURE 4**).
    1. The first incision is made in the midline 14 cm distal to the xiphoid process and a Veress needle is introduced into the peritoneal cavity. The peritoneal cavity is insufflated to a pressure of 15 mm Hg. Subsequently, an optical port with a 0° scope (**Port 1**) is placed under direct vision. Once this port is positioned, the 0° scope is replaced with a 30° scope and the other trocars are inserted under laparoscopic vision.
    2. **Port 2** is placed in the left midclavicular line at the same level of port 1. It is used by the assistant for traction on the gastroesophageal junction and of an instrument to take down the short gastric vessels.

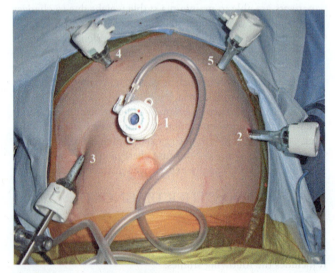

FIGURE 4 • Placement of the ports.

3. **Port 3** is placed in the right midclavicular line at the same level of the other two ports. A retractor is used through this port to lift the left lateral segment of the liver to expose the gastroesophageal junction. The retractor is held in place by a self-retaining system fixed to the operating table.
4. **Ports 4** and **5** are placed under the right and left costal margins so that their axes and the camera form an angle of about 120°. These ports are used by the operating surgeon.

TABLE 1 summarizes the instrumentation that is necessary for the laparoscopic myotomy.

Table 1: Instrumentation for Laparoscopic Heller Myotomy and Partial Fundoplication

Five 10-mm ports
0° and 30° scope
Graspers and needle holder
Babcock clamp
L-shaped hook cautery with suction-irrigation capacity
Scissors
Laparoscopic clip applier
Electrothermal bipolar vessel sealing system
Liver retractor
Suturing device
2-0 silk sutures

DISSECTION

- The gastrohepatic ligament is divided, beginning the dissection above the caudate lobe of the liver, where the ligament is thinner; it is continued toward the diaphragm until the right pillar of the crus is identified and separated from the esophagus by blunt dissection.
- Subsequently, the peritoneum and the phrenoesophageal membrane overlying the esophagus are divided, and the anterior vagus nerve is identified (**FIGURE 5A**).
- The left pillar of the crus is then separated from the esophagus (**FIGURE 5B**).
- Blunt dissection is finally performed in the posterior mediastinum, laterally and anteriorly to the esophagus in order to have about 4 to 5 cm of esophagus without any tension below the diaphragm. Posterior dissection is necessary only if a partial posterior fundoplication is planned.

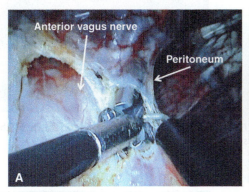
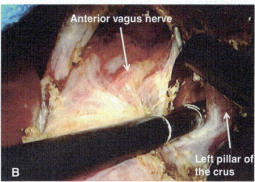

FIGURE 5 • Division of the peritoneum and the phrenoesophageal membrane overlying the esophagus with anterior vagus nerve identification **(A)**; separation of the left pillar of the crus from the esophagus **(B)**.

DIVISION OF THE SHORT GASTRIC VESSELS

- The short gastric vessels are taken down all the way to the left pillar of the crus, starting from a point midway along the greater curvature of the stomach (**FIGURE 6**).[7]

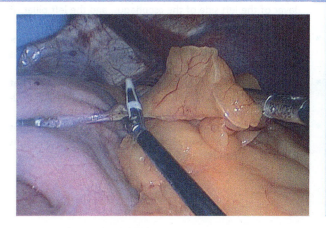

FIGURE 6 • Division of the short gastric vessels.

MYOTOMY

- The fat pad should be removed to expose the gastroesophageal junction, after identification of the anterior vagus nerve.
- Traction is then applied with a Babcock clamp, grasping below the gastroesophageal junction and pulling downward and to the left in order to expose the right side of the esophagus.
- A myotomy is performed on the right side of the esophagus in the 11-o'clock position using a hook cautery. The proper submucosal plane is found using the cautery, about 3 cm above the gastroesophageal junction.
- Once the mucosa is exposed, the myotomy is extended proximally for about 6 cm above the gastroesophageal junction and distally for 2.5 to 3 cm onto the gastric wall (**FIGURE 7**).[8]
- The edges of the muscles are then separated with a dissector in order to have 30% to 40% of the mucosa not covered by muscles.
- Intraoperative upper endoscopy is rarely necessary, particularly when the operation is performed by expert surgeons and a long myotomy onto the gastric wall is performed.

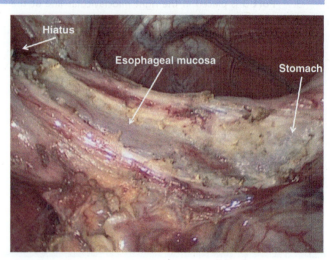

FIGURE 7 • Esophageal myotomy.

PARTIAL FUNDOPLICATION

- The main goal of the surgical treatment is relief of dysphagia while preventing GER.[9]
- A laparoscopic Heller myotomy (LHM) alone is associated with postoperative GER in about 50% to 60% of patients.[10]
- Better functional results are achieved with a partial fundoplication added to the myotomy compared to a total fundoplication that is associated with higher rates of postoperative dysphagia.[11]
- Regarding the type of partial fundoplication, no significant differences are evident in terms of control of GER after the partial anterior and partial posterior fundoplication.[5]
- We prefer the partial anterior fundoplication because it is simpler to perform as posterior dissection is not necessary, and because it covers the exposed esophageal mucosa.

Partial Anterior Fundoplication (Dor)

- The Dor fundoplication is a 180° anterior fundoplication.
- Two rows of sutures (2-0 silk) are used. The first row is on the left side of the esophagus and has three stitches. The top stitch incorporates the fundus of the stomach, the muscular layer of the left side of the esophagus, and the left pillar of the crus (**FIGURE 8**).
- The second and third stitches incorporate the gastric fundus and the muscular layer of the left side of the esophagus (**FIGURE 9**).
- The fundus is then folded over the exposed mucosa so that the greater curvature of the stomach is next to the right pillar of the crus.
- The second row of sutures on the right side of the esophagus consists of three stitches between the fundus and the right pillar of the crus (**FIGURE 10**).

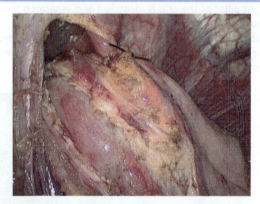

FIGURE 8 • Dor fundoplication: top stitch of the left row of sutures.

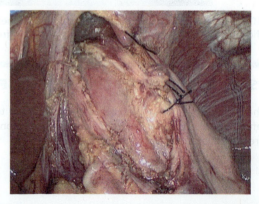

FIGURE 9 • Dor fundoplication: second and third stitches of the left row of sutures.

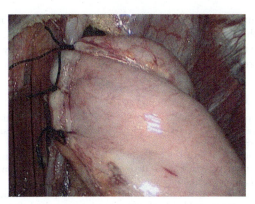

FIGURE 10 • Dor fundoplication: right row of sutures.

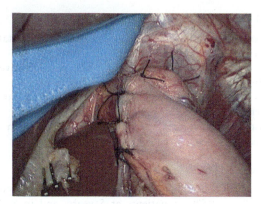

FIGURE 11 • Completed Dor fundoplication.

- Finally, two additional stitches are placed between the fundus and the rim of the esophageal hiatus to eliminate any tension from the fundoplication (**FIGURE 11**).

Partial Posterior Fundoplication

- Some authors argue that the posterior partial fundoplication should be used as it might be more effective in preventing postoperative pathologic GER and in keeping the distal edges of the myotomy separated.[12]

- The posterior fundoplication requires the creation of a posterior window between the left pillar of the crus, the stomach, and the esophagus followed by the passage of the gastric fundus under the esophagus.
- The hiatus is loosely closed posterior to the esophagus.
- Subsequently, each side of the wrap is attached to the esophageal wall lateral to the myotomy with three stitches. The resulting wrap measures about 220° to 240°.

PEARLS AND PITFALLS

Indications	■ A careful evaluation, including manometry, 24-hour pH monitoring, upper endoscopy, and barium swallow, must be done.
Placement of ports	■ Extreme care must be taken when positioning port 1, since the site of insertion is just above the aorta. ■ We recommend using an optical trocar with a 0° scope to obtain access. ■ If port 3 is too low, the left lateral segment of the liver will not be properly retracted and exposure of the esophagogastric junction may be inadequate. ■ If port 2 is too low, the esophagogastric junction or the upper short gastric vessels may be difficult to access. ■ If ports 4 and 5 are too low, the dissection at the beginning of the procedure and the suturing at the end will be challenging. ■ If port 3 is too medial, the liver retractor may interfere with the instrument used through port 4.
Dissection	■ An accessory left hepatic artery originating from the left gastric artery is frequently present in the gastrohepatic ligament. If this vessel limits the exposure, it may be safely divided. ■ The electrocautery should be used with extreme caution. Because of the lateral spread of the monopolar current, vagus nerves may be damaged, even without direct contact. A bipolar instrument represents a safer alternative.
Short gastric vessels division	■ Bleeding, either from the short gastric vessels or from the spleen, and damage to the gastric wall are possible complications. ■ Excessive traction or division of a vessel not completely coagulated are the main causes of bleeding. ■ A burn caused during dissection of the short gastric vessels or traction applied with the graspers or the Babcock clamp are the most common mechanisms of damage to the gastric wall.
Myotomy	■ In patients who have had previous treatment with botulinum toxin injection, the myotomy is technically more challenging due to the fibrosis that alters the normal anatomical planes and may increase the risk of perforation.[13] ■ If a mucosal perforation occurs, it can be repaired with 5-0 absorbable material. ■ In case of bleeding from the cut muscular fibers, gentle compression with a sponge is recommended rather than the electrocautery, which can cause thermal damage to the esophageal wall.

Partial anterior fundoplication	■ To reduce the risk of postoperative dysphagia due to the fundoplication:
	  1. The short gastric vessels should be divided.
	  2. The wrap should be performed using the fundus rather than the body of the stomach.

POSTOPERATIVE CARE

- Patients spend an average of 1 to 2 days in the hospital and return to work in 2 to 3 weeks.
- Patients are fed the morning of the first postoperative day with clear liquids and then a soft diet.
- They are instructed to avoid meat, bread, and carbonated beverages for the following 2 weeks.
- Most patients resume their regular activity within 2 to 3 weeks.

OUTCOMES

- Long-term follow-up show that symptoms are improved in 90% to 95% of patients at 5 years, and in 80% at 10 years.
- Most LHM failures present within the first 2 to 3 years of follow-up and may reflect scarring of the distal edge of the myotomy that can be successfully treated in most cases with pneumatic dilation.
- Postoperative GER occurs in about 30% to 40% of patients, and it is usually controlled by acid-reducing medications.

COMPLICATIONS

- An esophageal leak may occur during the first 24 to 36 hours postoperatively, and it is usually the result of a thermal injury of the esophageal mucosa.
  1. Typical signs and symptoms include pain, fever, and dyspnea. A chest x-ray may show a pleural effusion.
  2. An esophagogram confirms the location and the extension of the leak.
  3. Treatment options vary based on the time of diagnosis and on the location and extension of the leak. In case of early diagnosis, small leaks can be repaired directly. If the damage is too extensive or the inflammatory reaction in case of late diagnosis does not allow a direct repair, an esophagectomy may be indicated. In selected cases, wide drainage and placement of a feeding jejunostomy tube with or without the use of an esophageal stent may allow the leak to heal without esophagectomy.
- Pneumothorax occurs in case of intraoperative violation of the parietal pleura. Usually, it resolves spontaneously and does not require tube thoracostomy as the CO_2 is rapidly absorbed.
- Persistent dysphagia is usually due to technical errors, such as a too short of a myotomy or a constricting fundoplication.
- Recurrent dysphagia after a symptom-free period may be caused by scar tissue at the distal edge of the myotomy, postoperative GER, technical errors (as cited above), or by esophageal cancer. A thorough evaluation is mandatory to rule out malignancies and make a correct diagnosis. Subsequent treatment is tailored to the results of this workup and includes pneumatic dilatation, peroral endoscopic myotomy,[14,15] or an esophagectomy if no improvement is obtained.[16]

REFERENCES

1. Moonka R, Patti MG, Feo CV, et al. Clinical presentation and evaluation of malignant pseudoachalasia. *J Gastrointest Surg*. 1999;3:456-461.
2. Andolfi C, Kavitt RT, Herbella FA, Patti MG. Achalasia and respiratory symptoms. Effect of laparoscopic Heller myotomy. *J Laparoendoscop Adv Surg Tech A*. 2016;9:675-679.
3. Fisichella PM, Raz D, Palazzo F, et al. Clinical, radiological and manometric profile in 145 patients with untreated achalasia. *World J Surg*. 2008;32:1974-1979.
4. Yadlapati R, Kahrilas PJ, Fox MR, et al. Esophageal motilkity disorders on high resolution manometry: Chicago classification update (V4.0). *Neurogastroenterol Motil*. 2021;33(1):e14058.
5. Andolfi C, Bonavina L, Kavitt RT, et al. Importance of esophageal manometry and pH monitoring in the evaluation of patients with refractory gastroesophageal reflux disease. A multicenter study. *J Laparoendosc Adv Surg Tech A*. 2016;26:48-50.
6. Rawlings A, Soper NJ, Oelschlager B, et al. Laparoscopic Dor versus Toupet fundoplication following Heller myotomy for achalasia: results of a multicenter, prospective, randomized-controlled trial. *Surg Endosc*. 2012;26:18-26.
7. Patti MG, Molena D, Fisichella PM, et al. Laparoscopic Heller myotomy and Dor fundoplication for achalasia. Analysis of successes and failures. *Arch Surg*. 2001;136:870-877.
8. Oelschlager BK, Chang L, Pellegrini CA. Improved outcome after extended gastric myotomy for achalasia. *Arch Surg*. 2003;138:490-497.
9. Patti MG, Herbella FA. Fundoplication after laparoscopic Heller myotomy for esophageal achalasia: what type? *J Gastrointest Surg*. 2010;14:1453-1458.
10. Richards WO, Torquati A, Holzman MD, et al. Heller myotomy versus Heller myotomy with Dor fundoplication. A prospective randomized double-blind clinical trial. *Ann Surg*. 2004;240:405-415.
11. Rebecchi F, Giaccone C, Farinella E, et al. Randomized controlled trial of laparoscopic Heller myotomy plus Dor fundoplication versus Nissen fundoplication for achalasia. *Ann Surg*. 2008;248:1023-1030.
12. Tatum RP, Pellegrini CA. How I do it: laparoscopic Heller myotomy with Toupet fundoplication for achalasia. *J Gastrointest Surg*. 2009;13:1120-1124.
13. Smith CD, Stival A, Howell L, et al. Endoscopic therapy for achalasia before Heller myotomy results in worse outcome than Heller myotomy alone. *Ann Surg*. 2006;243:579-586.
14. Ngamruengphong S, Inoue H, Ujiki MB, et al. Efficacy and safety of peroral endoscopic myotomy for treatment of achalasia after failed Heller myotomy. *Clin Gastroenterol Hepatol*. 2017;15:1531-1537.
15. Kamal F, Ismail MK, Khan MA, et al. Efficacy and safety of peroral endoscopic myotomy in the management of recurrent achalasia after failed Heller myotomy: a systematic review and meta-analysis. *Ann Gastroenterol*. 2021;34:155-163.
16. Felix VN, Murayama KM, Bonavina L, Park MI. Achalasia: what to do in the face of failures of Heller myotomy. *Ann N Y Acad Sci*. 2020;1481:236-246.

Chapter 4

Per-Oral Endoscopic Myotomy for Achalasia and Hypercontractile Esophagus

Jazmín M. Cole, Saher-Zahra Khan, and Jeffrey M. Marks

DEFINITION
- Achalasia is an esophageal motility disorder characterized by aperistalsis in the distal esophagus, elevated resting lower esophageal sphincter (LES) tone, and lack of physiologic LES relaxation during swallowing.[1]
- Hypercontractile esophagus (HE), also known as jackhammer esophagus, is characterized by abnormally high pressures in the distal esophagus with normal LES relaxation.[1]
- Per-oral endoscopic myotomy (POEM) is a procedure defined as the endoscopic creation of an esophageal submucosal tunnel to allow disruption and division of the muscle fibers of the esophagus and the LES. Circular muscle division vs circular plus longitudinal muscle fiber division have both been described and have equal symptom response.

DIFFERENTIAL DIAGNOSIS
- The differential diagnosis of achalasia and HE includes the spectrum of esophageal motility disorders, gastroesophageal reflux disease (GERD), and mechanical obstructions such as benign or malignant masses and peptic strictures.
- The Chicago classification of esophageal motility disorders defines three primary disease categories:
  - Disorders with obstruction of the esophagogastric junction (EGJ), including achalasia and mechanical obstruction.[2] Mechanical obstruction can potentially be caused by esophageal cancer, distal peptic stricture, and pseudoachalasia (malignancy at the EGJ or a large hiatal hernia that mimics achalasia on diagnostic studies)[1]
  - Major motility disorders of the esophagus, including HE and distal esophageal spasm[2]
  - Minor motility disorders due to ineffective motility and fragmented peristalsis causing impaired clearance without meeting criteria for a major disorder[3]

PATIENT HISTORY AND PHYSICAL FINDINGS
- Dysphagia, often to both liquids and solids, is the most common symptom of achalasia, occurring in 39% to 75% of patients.[1]
- Other symptoms include regurgitation of undigested food, chest pain, heartburn, and weight loss, occurring in over 30% of patients.[1]
- Patients can also present with pulmonary symptoms including nocturnal cough, vocal hoarseness, recurrent aspiration, and pneumonia.
- The most common symptoms reported in HE are dysphagia (32%-100%), chest pain (10%-52%), and heartburn (17%-58%).[4,5] Regurgitation can occur in HE as well, although it is unclear if it is related more to heartburn vs impaired clearance of food from the esophagus.

IMAGING AND OTHER DIAGNOSTIC STUDIES
- High-resolution esophageal manometry (HREM) is the gold standard study for characterizing and diagnosing esophageal motility disorders. The manometric findings consistent with achalasia include an elevated resting LES pressure, lack of physiologic LES relaxation with swallowing, and aperistalsis with or without pressurization of the esophageal body. These findings can further be classified into achalasia types I (classic achalasia, aperistalsis without pressurization), II (panesophageal pressurization), and III (spastic achalasia with >20% swallows showing spastic contractions of the distal esophagus).
- All three types of achalasia can be treated with POEM; however, studies suggest varying degrees of symptomatic relief following POEM versus Heller myotomy depending on the disease type.[6]
- HREM findings in HE are characterized by preserved peristalsis with highly elevated distal contractile integral (DCI) over 8000 mm Hg/s/cm^3.
- Upper endoscopy is an essential component of the workup for dysphagia and esophageal dysmotility to rule out underlying malignancy. It is imperative that a complete endoscopy be performed traversing the LES, as well as retroflexion to rule out hiatal hernia or other possible sources of pseudoachalasia.
- Esophagram is often performed as part of the patient's dysphagia workup and can rule out pseudoachalasia, as well as show the contour and degree of dilation of the esophageal body. Patients with achalasia may have the classic "bird's beak" appearance of the dilated esophageal body with a tapered LES.

SURGICAL MANAGEMENT

Preoperative Planning
- Careful review of all diagnostic and imaging tests should be performed for each patient, paying particular attention to HREM results and the type of achalasia diagnosed as this will dictate the length of the submucosal tunnel and myotomy, as well as history of prior myotomy or achalasia interventions.
- Patients maintain a clear liquid diet for 2 days and are prescribed oral antifungal antibiotics for 1 day prior to surgery.
- No chemical deep vein thrombosis prophylaxis is given preoperatively.

Positioning
- Supine position with right arm out, left arm tucked, and endotracheal tube angled to the patient's right

Equipment

- Diagnostic gastroscope
- Endoscopic cautery endoscopic submucosal dissection (ESD) knife
- Injection sclerotherapy needle
- Methylene blue diluted in dextrose ± epinephrine
- Endoscopic overtube (optional)
- Endoscopic clips or sutures

STEPS (▶ VIDEO 1)

- Once the patient is intubated, a complete upper endoscopy is performed to examine the esophageal mucosa, stomach, and duodenal bulb for erosions/ulcers/masses, clear any retained food debris, and assess the LES resting tone and any sources for pseudoachalasia.
- Identify the Z-line (**FIGURE 1**), then choose a site 14 to 18 cm proximal (depending on the disease type) to begin the submucosal dissection.
- Inject methylene blue to create a submucosal wheal in the anterior or posterior surface depending on prior interventions and physician choice, then make a 2 cm longitudinal mucosotomy using an endoscopic ESD cautery knife (**FIGURE 2**).
- The submucosal tunnel is developed using a combination of blunt and electrocautery dissection (**FIGURE 3**) and continued onto the stomach.
- Once the submucosal tunnel dissection has extended at least 2 cm onto the stomach, it is completed (**FIGURE 4**) and the myotomy can then be performed.
- Myotomy is started approximately 3 cm distal to the start of the mucosotomy and extended across the LES onto the stomach along the entire length of the submucosal tunnel. It is our practice to only divide the circular muscle fibers and leave the longitudinal muscle fibers intact (**FIGURE 5**), although both techniques are commonly performed with equal symptom relief.
- Gastroscope is again returned to the true esophageal lumen and the mucosa inspected for inadvertent injury. The LES is again evaluated to ensure it is widely patent and easily traversed compared to the premyotomy endoscopy.

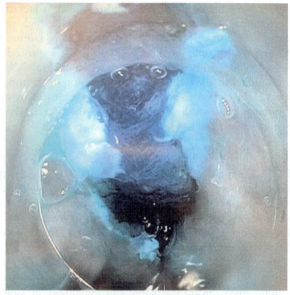

Procedure image capture

FIGURE 2 • Longitudinal mucosotomy.

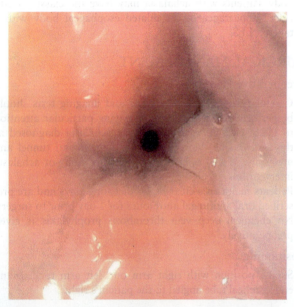

FIGURE 1 • View of the stenotic lower esophageal sphincter and Z-line on premyotomy endoscopy.

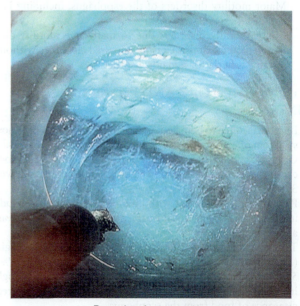

Procedure image capture

FIGURE 3 • Submucosal tunnel creation using blunt and electrocautery dissection.

Chapter 4 PER-ORAL ENDOSCOPIC MYOTOMY FOR ACHALASIA AND HYPERCONTRACTILE ESOPHAGUS

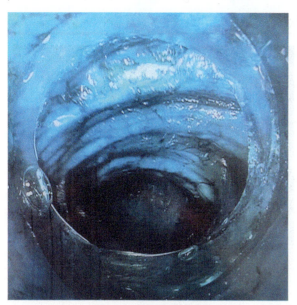

FIGURE 4 • Completed submucosal tunnel. In this case, brighter white circular muscle fibers are maintained at the 12-o'clock position during dissection for an anterior myotomy.

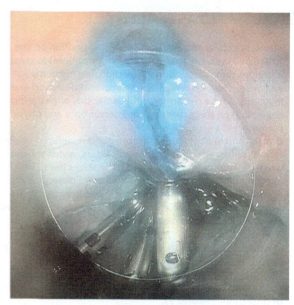

FIGURE 6 • Closure of mucosotomy with through-the-scope endoscopic metallic clips.

- The mucosotomy is then closed using through-the-scope endoscopic metallic clips (FIGURE 6), which will fall off and pass through the patient's gastrointestinal tract as mucosal healing occurs.

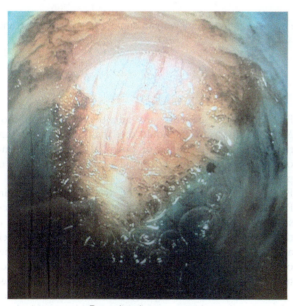

FIGURE 5 • Myotomy. This is continued along the entire length of the submucosal tunnel. It is our practice to only divide the circular muscle fibers and leave the longitudinal muscle fibers intact as shown.

PEARLS AND PITFALLS

- Maintain circular muscle fibers in a single position on the screen (ie, always at the 12- or 6-o'clock positions) to create a straight submucosal tunnel dissection and myotomy and avoid "corkscrewing." The submucosal dissection and myotomy can be performed either anteriorly or posteriorly, depending on the patient's prior interventions and physician preference.
- Gastric muscle fibers run in a more oblique, splayed orientation compared to the esophageal fibers, watch for this when extending the myotomy distally across the LES.
- Inject methylene blue into the submucosal dissection plane as the dissection is continued distally and keep this space as hemostatic as possible, as this will more clearly delineate the correct dissection plane.
- Periodically during the procedure, return to the true esophageal lumen to traverse the LES into the stomach and retroflex to check the progress of the submucosal dissection, look for pale blue mucosal changes extending from the gastroscope onto the fundus to ensure sufficient extent of dissection (FIGURE 7).
- During dissection, close attention must be paid to the patient's starting peak airway pressures and end title CO_2 levels. The physician must maintain open communication with the anesthesia team and be alerted when pressures increase while working. At this point, the physician should return the endoscope to the true lumen, traverse into the stomach, and desufflate the stomach. Decompression of capnoperitoneum and resultant abdominal compartment syndrome may also be necessary with an angiocatheter inserted at the patient's right upper quadrant and removed at the end of the case.

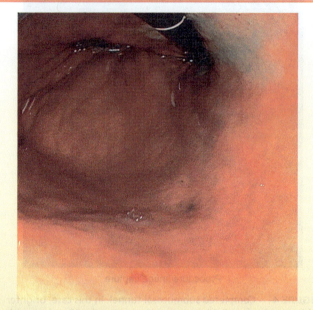

FIGURE 7 • Retroflexed view showing extent of submucosal dissection. Pale blue mucosal changes extend from the gastroscope onto the fundus to ensure sufficient extent of dissection.

OUTCOMES

- Since the introduction of POEM in 2008, the technique has become more popular as an effective treatment option for achalasia and long-term outcomes are being evaluated. Meta-analyses have been performed comparing patient outcomes following POEM with laparoscopic Heller myotomy (LHM) to better understand the optimal course of management.
- POEM is associated with higher rates of improvement in dysphagia at 1- and 2-year follow-up compared to LHM (93.5% vs 91%, and 92.7% vs 90.0%),[7] and lower Eckardt scores after surgery compared to LHM.[8]
- Patients undergoing POEM have also been shown to be more likely to develop GERD, whether evaluated by patient symptoms, the presence of erosive esophagitis, or pH monitoring results (all $P < .0001$).[7]
- Studies have shown that POEM patients use lower doses of narcotic medications while hospitalized, fewer require prescribed narcotic medications at the time of discharge, and they benefit from a shorter hospital length of stay.[9]
- Patients with type III (spastic) achalasia have improved symptomatic response to therapy following POEM compared to LHM, likely due to the ability to perform a longer endoscopic myotomy.[6]
- Overall, POEM has been shown to provide excellent symptomatic relief with low complication rates and durable efficacy at least equivalent to LHM.

POSTOPERATIVE CARE

- Postoperatively, patients are admitted for observation. Most are given a clear liquid diet the day of surgery and then monitored for signs of potential adverse outcomes overnight before being advanced to a full liquid diet on postoperative day 1.
- For patients who had a more technically challenging POEM, such as those with prior myotomy and subsequent submucosal fibrosis making dissection more difficult, or those with cognitive difficulties preventing them from reliably reporting symptoms concerning for adverse outcomes, our practice is to keep patients nil per os except medications overnight and then perform an esophagram on postoperative day 1. If the esophagram demonstrates free flow of contrast into the stomach without evidence of leak, we then begin clear liquids and advance to full liquids.
- All patients are discharged home with pain medications and on a full liquid diet for 1 week, and then advanced to a soft diet for 1 week. They are maintained on proton pump inhibitor therapy for 6 months, at which time they return to clinic for an off-medication Bravo study to quantify postmyotomy reflux.

COMPLICATIONS

- Complications are overall very rare (approximately 3%-10%), with the most common being mucosal injury. In general, complications associated with POEM can be divided into intraoperative, postoperative, and perioperative categories:

- Intraoperative—bleeding (approximately 1.1%, can occur from the mucosotomy site or perforating vessels within the submucosal tunnel), capnothorax (usually self-limited), and capnoperitoneum (may require decompression with angiocatheter)
- Perioperative—arrhythmia (due to mediastinal irritation caused by electrocautery dissection), aspiration on anesthesia induction (ideally limited by maintaining clear liquid diet preoperatively; however, open communication with the anesthesia team can help with appropriate planning and patient positioning to mitigate this risk)
- Postoperative—GERD (routinely evaluated with pH monitoring study at 6 months postoperatively), mediastinal leak (approximately 0.3%),[1] recurrence of dysphagia (can occur due to scarring, incomplete myotomy, or disease progression, and should be evaluated thoroughly with repeat upper endoscopy to rule out esophageal malignancies as well as possibly repeat HREM to correctly diagnose the source of symptoms)

REFERENCES

1. Cappell MS, Stavropoulos SN, Friedel D. Updated systematic review of achalasia, with a focus on POEM therapy. *Dig Dis Sci.* 2020;65(1):38-65. doi:10.1007/s10620-019-05784-3
2. Schlottmann F, Patti MG. Primary esophageal motility disorders: beyond achalasia. *Int J Mol Sci.* 2017;18(7):1399. doi:10.3390/ijms18071399
3. Kahrilas PJ, Bredenoord AJ, Fox M, et al. The Chicago classification of esophageal motility disorders, v3.0. *Neuro Gastroenterol Motil.* 2015;27(2):160-174. doi:10.1111/nmo.12477
4. de Bortoli N, Gyawali PC, Roman S, et al. Hypercontractile esophagus from pathophysiology to management: proceedings of the pisa symposium. *Am J Gastroenterol.* 2021;116(2):263-273. doi:10.14309/ajg.0000000000001061
5. Savarino E, Smout AJPM. The hypercontractile esophagus: still a tough nut to crack. *Neuro Gastroenterol Motil.* 2020;32(11):e14010. doi:10.1111/nmo.14010
6. Chuah SK, Lim CS, Liang CM, et al. Bridging the gap between advancements in the evolution of diagnosis and treatment towards better outcomes in achalasia. *BioMed Res Int.* 2019;2019:8549187. doi:10.1155/2019/8549187
7. Schlottmann F, Luckett DJ, Fine J, Shaheen NJ, Patti MG. Laparoscopic Heller myotomy versus peroral endoscopic myotomy (POEM) for achalasia: a systematic review and meta-analysis. *Ann Surg.* 2018;267(3):451-460. doi:10.1097/SLA.0000000000002311
8. Zhang Y, Wang H, Chen X, et al. Per-oral endoscopic myotomy versus laparoscopic Heller myotomy for achalasia: a meta-analysis of nonrandomized comparative studies. *Medicine (Baltim).* 2016;95(6):e2736. doi:10.1097/MD.0000000000002736
9. Docimo S Jr, Mathew A, Shope AJ, Winder JS, Haluck RS, Pauli EM. Reduced postoperative pain scores and narcotic use favor peroral endoscopic myotomy over laparoscopic Heller myotomy. *Surg Endosc.* 2017;31(2):795-800. doi:10.1007/s00464-016-5034-3

SECTION II: Diaphragm

Chapter 5
Repair of Congenital Defects: Morgagni Diaphragmatic Hernia

Scott A. Anderson and Mike K. Chen

DEFINITION

- A Morgagni congenital diaphragmatic hernia (CDH) refers to a defect in the anteromedial diaphragm through the foramen of Morgagni. The most common contents of the hernia include the omentum and transverse colon but can also include the stomach, liver, spleen, and other segments of bowel. Morgagni hernias often include a hernia sac.
- They account for approximately 3% of surgically repaired diaphragmatic hernias. They are more frequently seen in females, and the majority of them are right sided. Bilateral Morgagni hernias can be seen but are not common.
- Unlike Bochdalek CDHs, Morgagni hernias are more often asymptomatic, diagnosed incidentally, and are usually not associated with pulmonary hypoplasia. They are typically smaller and more frequently an isolated congenital anomaly.

DIFFERENTIAL DIAGNOSIS

- Morgagni CDH can be mistaken for a number of other thoracic anomalies, both congenital and acquired. In infancy, these can include congenital cystic lung disease, esophageal hiatal hernia, and mediastinal mass.
- Later in life, Morgagni hernia can be confused with a mediastinal mass, pericardial fat pad, atelectasis, pneumonia, or a pleural abscess.
- The various imaging and diagnostic studies used to distinguish among these are mentioned in a subsequent section.

PATIENT HISTORY AND PHYSICAL FINDINGS

- The diagnosis of a Morgagni diaphragmatic hernia can sometimes be a long and winding road. Neonates do not frequently arrive with the diagnosis already made by prenatal imaging, as is often the case with Bochdalek CDH. The signs and symptoms of Morgagni hernias are also often nonspecific. Likewise, routine radiologic imaging can also overlook the more subtle defects. Because of this, Morgagni hernias are sometimes not diagnosed until later in life.
- The most common presentation in neonates and infants is an increased work of breathing or respiratory distress. Many, however, are relatively asymptomatic. Children may present with a history of recurrent chest infections. Teenagers and adults can present with any variety of symptoms including dyspnea, chest pain, abdominal pain, nausea and vomiting, and constipation or they may be completely asymptomatic. Predisposing conditions, such as chronic cough, trauma, pregnancy, and obesity, can contribute to the likelihood of symptomatic presentation.
- The physical examination is most commonly normal. However, distant heart tones and unequal breath sounds may be present. In cases of strangulation or volvulus, the patient may demonstrate significant abdominal tenderness and signs of shock. A detailed physical examination is always indicated in newborns to assess for congenital abnormalities.
- Although most commonly isolated, Morgagni hernias can be associated with congenital heart disease, malrotation, and Down syndrome.[1] The workup should include an echocardiogram when the diagnosis is made in infancy.

IMAGING AND OTHER DIAGNOSTIC STUDIES

- Morgagni hernias are not frequently detected on prenatal imaging.
- A posteroanterior (PA) and lateral chest radiograph is the initial diagnostic study of choice. This can have different appearances depending on the contents within the hernia. It may show air-filled loops of bowel projecting over the anterior mediastinum (**FIGURE 1A** and **B**) or a well-defined opacity in the right cardiophrenic angle (**FIGURE 2**). The latter, however, is not very specific.
- The diagnosis can be more readily made on computed tomography or magnetic resonance imaging (**FIGURE 3**).
- Ultrasound, barium enema, and upper gastrointestinal series also can be a useful part of the diagnostic workup.
- Diagnostic laparoscopy is recommended if the diagnosis remains unclear after appropriate imaging studies.

SURGICAL MANAGEMENT

Preoperative Planning

- In general, elective repair of Morgagni hernias is recommended to prevent future complications such as incarceration, strangulation, or volvulus.
- Morgagni diaphragmatic hernias can be successfully repaired through either transabdominal or transthoracic approaches using open or minimally invasive techniques. We tend to favor the transabdominal approach when feasible because it allows for better visualization of the central diaphragm and for detection of bilateral hernias that may not be clearly seen on preoperative imaging. Laparoscopy is generally well tolerated in infants, even those with congenital heart disease.[2]

Chapter 5 REPAIR OF CONGENITAL DEFECTS: MORGAGNI DIAPHRAGMATIC HERNIA

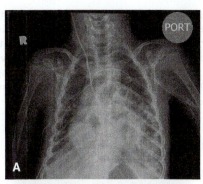

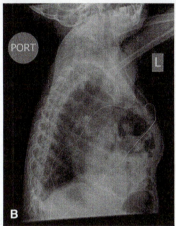

FIGURE 1 • PA **(A)** and lateral **(B)** chest x-ray demonstrating air-filled loops of bowel in the anterior mediastinum consistent with a Morgagni diaphragmatic hernia.

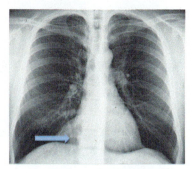

FIGURE 2 • PA chest x-ray demonstrates a Morgagni hernia indicated by the opacity *(arrow)* at the right cardiophrenic angle. This hernia most commonly contains omentum.

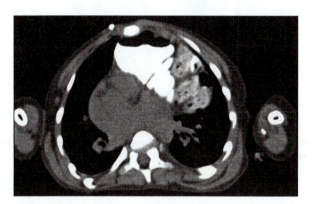

FIGURE 3 • Computed tomography of the chest in a patient with a Morgagni hernia. Note the contrast-opacified intestinal contents within the anterior mediastinum, shifting the heart posteriorly and to the right.

- In infants, who can present with respiratory distress, lung protective strategies are initiated. When a ventilator is required, spontaneous respiration and permissive hypercapnia are used. Surgery is then performed on an elective basis, once medically stable, prior to discharge.
- For the patients with Morgagni hernias that present with acute incarceration, strangulation, or volvulus, immediate surgical management is indicated. Appropriate resuscitative measures should be initiated prior to surgery.

- Prior to taking the patient to the operating room, all diagnostic studies should be thoroughly reviewed and the patient appropriately marked on the affected side when appropriate.
- Ensure that the airway is secure and the endotracheal tube is in a stable position. Pre- and postductal oxygen saturation monitoring is maintained in neonates to assess for signs of right-to-left shunting.

OPEN MORGAGNI HERNIA REPAIR

Positioning

- The patient is placed in the supine position on the operating room table (**FIGURE 4**).
- Sterile plastic drapes are used as a barrier over the patient outside of the operative field. A warming blanket is also used to maintain temperature stability.

Incision

- A transverse, subcostal incision is made one to two fingerbreadths below the costal margin. An incision made too close to the costal margin can make for a more difficult repair and subsequent fascial closure. An upper midline incision may also be used.
- The abdominal wall muscle and fascia are divided and the peritoneum entered.

Exposure of the Defect and Hernia Reduction

- The falciform ligament of the liver is taken down off the abdominal wall and the left lateral segment mobilized if needed.
- The liver is carefully retracted away from the diaphragm to expose the posterior and lateral boundary of the diaphragmatic hernia defect (**FIGURE 5**).
- The abdominal contents within the hernia are carefully reduced and returned to the abdomen.
- A hernia sac, when present, is excised with electrocautery.

Repair of the Diaphragm

- An assessment is made to determine the amount of native diaphragm. There is typically no anterior rim of diaphragm and the defect is contiguous with the anterior abdominal wall (**FIGURE 6**).
- If the Morgagni hernia is small enough for primary closure without significant tension, this is preferred. The defect is

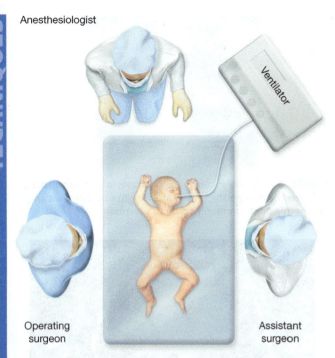

FIGURE 4 • The patient is positioned in a standard fashion in the operating room.

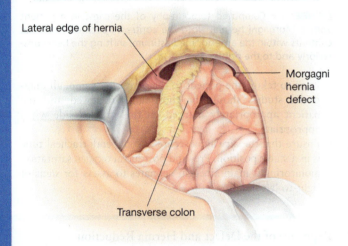

FIGURE 5 • The Morgagni hernia defect is exposed and the hernia contents (transverse colon, omentum) are identified and manually reduced.

to the patch with interrupted sutures using a braided nonabsorbable material. The sutures are left untied initially. Once the posterior wall sutures are all in place, the patch is then parachuted down and the sutures are individually tied secure. Then, before closure of the anterior diaphragmatic defect is initiated, care is taken to ensure hemostasis on the thoracic side of the patch.

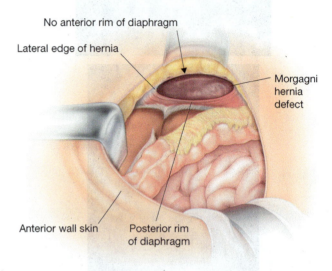

FIGURE 6 • The Morgagni hernia contents have been reduced, providing full exposure of the defect. Note that there is essentially no anterior rim of diaphragm present (*arrow*), and hernia defect is contiguous with the anterior abdominal wall.

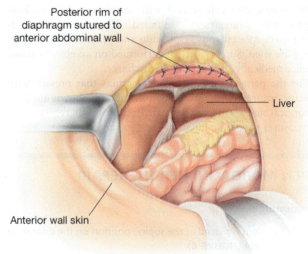

FIGURE 7 • The posterior rim of diaphragm is sutured to the anterior abdominal wall with interrupted nonabsorbable suture for a relatively tension-free primary repair.

repaired with interrupted, simple sutures using nonabsorbable, braided suture material (**FIGURE 7**). Pledgeted mattress sutures may also be used. However, the diaphragmatic muscle is often attenuated, particularly for those well into adulthood. Therefore, an overlay patch to reinforce the repair may be beneficial.

- For those defects that are too large to close primarily, a prosthetic patch is used. Nonbiologic materials, such as polytetrafluoroethylene/expanded polytetrafluoroethylene, or biologic materials are effective. The patch is carefully fashioned so as to maintain the shape of the diaphragm and to have 2 to 3 cm of overlap in neonates, more in larger patients. The posterior wall of the diaphragm is sewn first

- The anterior portion of the patch is then secured to the anterior abdominal wall and posterior rectus sheath with interrupted suture to complete the repair.

Closure

- Once hemostasis and satisfactory repair is assured, the abdominal wall musculature and skin are then closed in layers. A drain is not needed.

MINIMALLY INVASIVE MORGAGNI HERNIA REPAIR

- Both thoracoscopic and laparoscopic approaches have been used for Morgagni hernia repair. They each have their benefits and drawbacks, and the technical aspects of the two approaches are not dissimilar.
- We tend to favor the laparoscopic approach in that it provides excellent visualization of both hemidiaphragms. This minimizes the risk of underestimating or missing a more central or bilateral Morgagni hernia defect.

Positioning

- The patient is positioned in a similar manner as a patient undergoing a laparoscopic fundoplication so that the surgeon may stand at their feet. Infants and young children are supine and frog legged at the end of the operating room table (FIGURE 8). Older children and adults are placed in dorsal lithotomy with their lower extremities in stirrups. The operating surgeon stands between the patient's legs.
- Care is taken to properly pad all pressure points.
- The monitors are positioned over the patient's head.

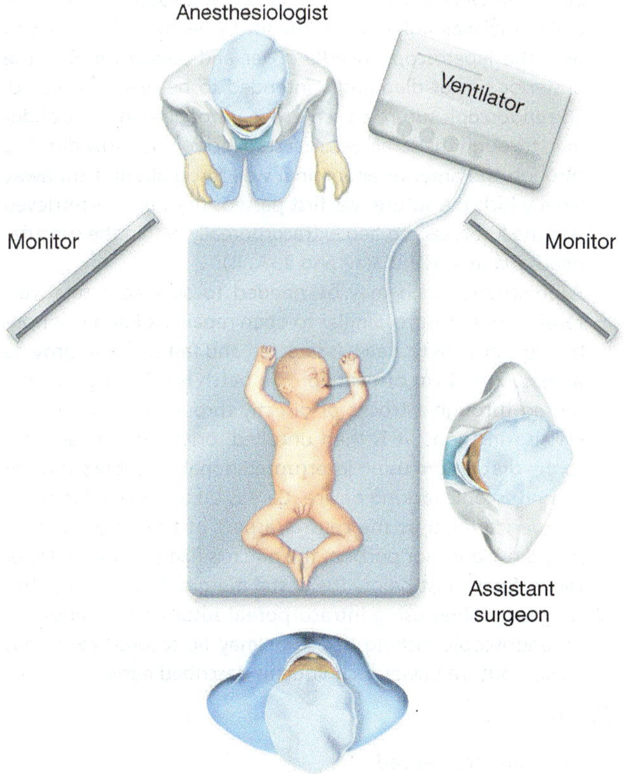

FIGURE 8 • The child is positioned at the end of the operating room table in a "frog-leg" position. The operating surgeon stands at the patient's feet with the monitors placed over the patient's head.

Laparoscopic Morgagni Hernia Repair

Trocar Placement

- A 5-mm trocar is placed in the umbilicus.
- Pneumoperitoneum is initially set between 8 and 15 mmHg depending on the patient's age and size.
- A 5-mm, 30° scope is used for visualization.
- Two additional trocars are placed under direct laparoscopic vision, in the right and left upper quadrants. These will be the primary working ports (FIGURE 9).
- An additional trocar occasionally is needed for retraction.
- A single-incision endosurgical or robotic approach is also feasible.

Reduction of the Morgagni Hernia

- The hernia contents, typically the omentum and abdominal viscera, are carefully reduced with atraumatic graspers (FIGURE 10). Cotton-tipped Endo Kittners are used to help reduce the liver or spleen when present within the hernia.
- To fully expose the native diaphragm, the falciform ligament may be taken down from the abdominal wall (FIGURE 11). This will often lead the surgeon directly to the lateral extent of the Morgagni hernia and allow for adequate overlap with patch placement.
- The hernia sac, if one is present, is carefully excised circumferentially off the diaphragmatic defect using hook cautery or other endoscopic sealing device. However, this may also be left intact when dissection into the mediastinum proves too arduous to avoid the risk of pneumothorax and pneumopericardium.[3] The peritoneum is then taken off the edge of the hernia defect with cautery.

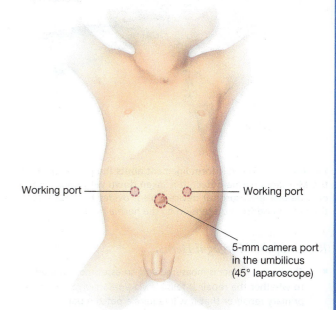

FIGURE 9 • A 5-mm port is placed through the umbilicus. Two additional working ports are typically all that is needed and are positioned to appropriately triangulate the hernia defect.

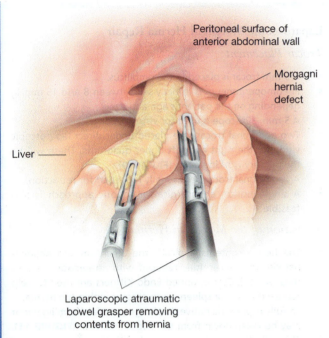

FIGURE 10 • The Morgagni hernia is identified and the hernia contents are reduced back into the abdomen with atraumatic graspers.

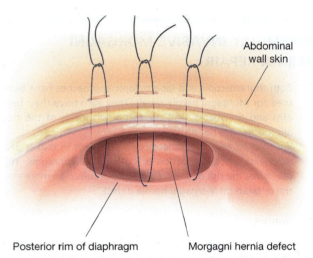

FIGURE 12 • A suture is introduced through the anterior abdominal wall and endoscopically passed through the posterior margin of the diaphragmatic hernia defect. The suture is then passed back out through the anterior abdominal wall and the knots may be tied in the subcutaneous tissue.

- The closure of the defect along the anterior portion of the hernia defect can be challenging but is feasible with intracorporeal suturing techniques. However, we favor a percutaneous technique using an endoscopic suture passer. Small stab incisions are made in the abdominal wall over the central margin of the hernia defect. The suture is percutaneously introduced into the abdomen with an external needle driver through the anterior abdominal wall stab incision. The suture needle is then grasped with the laparoscopic needle driver and passed through the posterior rim of diaphragm intended to be reapproximated. The endoscopic suture passer is then introduced into the abdomen through the same external stab incision but now directed through the anterior abdominal wall fascia about 1 cm away from which the suture was first passed. The suture is retrieved and the knots can be tied extracorporeally within the subcutaneous plane (FIGURES 12 and 13A, B).
- A prosthetic patch may be needed to achieve a relatively tension-free closure. Similar to open repair, a biologic or non-biologic prosthetic patch is selected and fashioned to provide at least 2 to 3 cm of overlap. The patch is rolled tightly and passed through a trocar, or directly through one of the trocar site incisions. It is then unrolled, oriented, and secured to the diaphragm using interrupted nonabsorbable suture or an endoscopic tacking device. Care is taken to avoid injuring the pericardium at the central aspect of the hernia defect. Along the anterior portion, the patch is fixed to the posterior rectus fascia, just below the costal margin (FIGURE 14). This is accomplished using intracorporeal suturing techniques or an endoscopic tacking device or may be secured externally using a suture passer technique as described earlier.

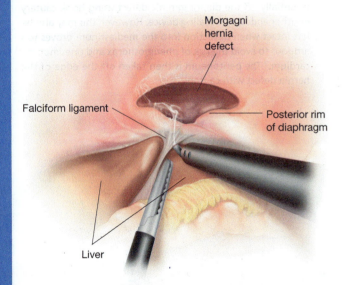

FIGURE 11 • The falciform ligament abuts the posterior rim of the Morgagni hernia defect. It is taken down with hook cautery or a bipolar endosurgical device. This provides full exposure of the defect and frees up tension on the hernia repair.

Repair of the Morgagni Hernia

- The hernia defect is measured and an assessment is made as to whether the repair is feasible via a relatively tension-free primary repair or that it will require a patch repair.
- For a primary repair, the diaphragm is reapproximated using interrupted nonabsorbable sutures. The closure is begun at the most posterior aspect of the hernia and carried up to the anterior abdominal wall.

Closure

- No drains are needed.
- The pneumoperitoneum is released and the liver is allowed to abut the hernia repair.
- The ports are removed in a stepwise fashion.
- The incisions are reapproximated with absorbable suture and skin glue is applied as a dressing.

Chapter 5 REPAIR OF CONGENITAL DEFECTS: MORGAGNI DIAPHRAGMATIC HERNIA

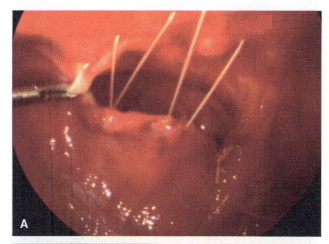

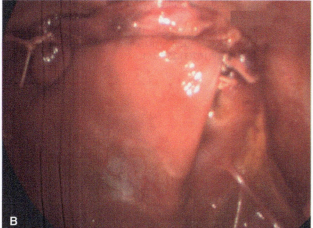

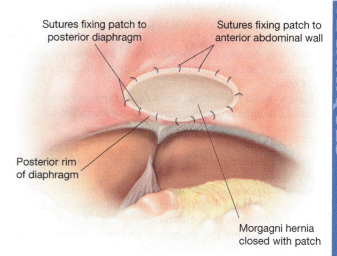

FIGURE 14 • A prosthetic or biologic patch is secured to the diaphragm and anterior abdominal wall with 2 to 3 cm of overlap.

FIGURE 13 • **A,** Percutaneous sutures have been passed through the posterior rim of diaphragm and brought back out through the anterior abdominal wall. **B,** The knots have been tied extracorporeally in the subcutaneous tissue, closing the defect.

PEARLS AND PITFALLS

Preoperative planning	▪ A missed bilateral or more extensive central hernia can be avoided with a transabdominal approach.
Incision	▪ For an open repair, a transverse subcostal incision should be well away from the costal margin so that there is adequate space to close the anterior portion of the diaphragmatic defect.
Hernia reduction	▪ The hernia sac may be left alone to avoid risk of disrupting the pleura or pericardium.
Hernia repair	▪ Multiple stitches may be placed through a single abdominal wall stab incision by dissecting a bit subcutaneously. ▪ Maintain a low threshold for using a prosthetic patch to achieve a tension-free repair.
Laparoscopy	▪ External manual compression of the lower chest and upper abdominal wall can help with suture placement anteriorly.

POSTOPERATIVE CARE

- The majority of patients will be successfully extubated at the completion of the repair.
- They may be admitted postoperatively for observation and, barring other issues, are typically ready for discharge within 24 hours.
- Follow-up PA and lateral chest radiographs are taken at 1 and 12 months postoperatively to assess for recurrence.

OUTCOMES

- Survival is quite good in all age groups and will primarily depend on other comorbidities.
- Meta-analysis in infants and children has demonstrated no difference between laparoscopic and open repair with regard to recurrence rate or complications.[4,5]
- The complication and recurrence rate in adults for laparoscopic or open repair is also fairly low.[6,7]

COMPLICATIONS

- Recurrent hernia
- Patch infection
- Fluid collection in foramen of Morgagni
- Pneumothorax
- Pericardial effusion or pneumopericardium

REFERENCES

1. Al-Salem AH. Congenital hernia of Morgagni in infants and children. *J Ped Surg*. 2007;42(9):1539-1543.
2. Gillory LA, Megison ML, Harmon CM, et al. Laparoscopic surgery in children with congenital heart disease. *J Pediatr Surg*. 2012;47(6):1084-1088.
3. Alkhatrawi T, Elsherbini R, Ouslimane D. Laparoscopic repair of Morgagni diaphragmatic hernia in infants and children: do we need to resect the hernia sac? *Ann Ped Surg*. 2012;8(1):1-4.
4. Lauriti G, Zani-Ruttenstock E, Catania VD, et al. Open versus laparoscopic approach for Morgagni's hernia in infants and children: a systematic review and meta-analysis. *J Laparoendosc Adv Surg Tech*. 2018;28(7):888-893.
5. Tan Y, Banerjee D, Cross KM, et al. Morgagni hernia repair in children over two decades: institutional experience, systematic review, and meta-analysis of 296 patients. *J Pediatr Surg*. 2018;53(10):1883-1889.
6. Horton JD, Hofmann LJ, Hetz SP. Presentation and management of Morgagni hernias in adults: a review of 298 cases. *Surg Endosc*. 2008;22(6):1413-1420.
7. Young MC, Saddoughi SA, Aho JM, et al. Comparison of laparoscopic versus open surgical management of Morgagni hernia. *Ann Thorac Surg*. 2019;107(1):257-261.

Chapter 6 Repair of Congenital Defects: Bochdalek Congenital Diaphragmatic Hernia

Scott A. Anderson and Mike K. Chen

DEFINITION

- A Bochdalek congenital diaphragmatic hernia (CDH) refers to a defect in the posterolateral diaphragm. The abdominal viscera partially translocate through the defect in the thorax and mediastinum shifts to the contralateral side in the developing fetus. This affects the growth and maturation of both lungs. The size of the defect can range from fairly small to complete diaphragmatic agenesis. Affected infants are born with pulmonary hypoplasia, lung immaturity, and pulmonary hypertension, to varying degrees. Successful management of these issues is most critical to a favorable outcome.
- The incidence of CDH is 1 in 2000 to 1 in 5000 births overall. Approximately 80% will occur on the left side; bilateral defects are rare. It continues to be one of the more challenging congenital anomalies in pediatric surgical patients.

DIFFERENTIAL DIAGNOSIS

- Prenatally and postnatally, Bochdalek CDH can be mistaken for a number of other congenital thoracic anomalies. These can include Morgagni CDH, diaphragmatic eventration, congenital cystic lung disease, esophageal hiatal hernia, and primary lung agenesis.
- The various imaging and diagnostic studies used to distinguish among these are discussed in a subsequent section.

PATIENT HISTORY AND PHYSICAL FINDINGS

- Many, but certainly not all, CDH patients are born with the diagnosis already made on prenatal ultrasound. A team of neonatologists, high-risk obstetricians, and pediatric surgeons are involved in their perinatal care to ensure a safe delivery and expeditious treatment. These neonates are immediately resuscitated after delivery with endotracheal intubation and nasogastric decompression. Ventilation with Ambu bag and mask is avoided to minimize gastrointestinal (GI) distention, which can worsen the compression in the thoracic cavity. A strategy of spontaneous respiration and permissive hypercapnia is employed to minimize ventilator-induced lung injury.
- For those without prenatal diagnosis, patients will present shortly after birth with typical signs of respiratory distress, including tachypnea, grunting, and cyanosis. They also will commonly have a scaphoid abdomen, barrel-shaped chest, and diminished or absent breath sounds on the affected side. The heart tones are also shifted toward the contralateral side.
- Ten percent to 50% of CDH patients will have other congenital anomalies, so a thorough physical examination and assessment is indicated. See **TABLE 1**.
- Also, a number of syndromes have been associated with CDH including Frey; Beckwith-Wiedemann; Goldenhar;

Table 1: Associated Congenital Anomalies
Cardiac
VSD
Aortic coarctation
Heart hypoplasia
Outflow tract abnormalities
Musculoskeletal
Tracheobronchial
Genitourinary
Neural tube defects
Chromosomal

VSD, ventricular septal defect.

Fryns; and trisomy 21, 18, and 13. A genetics consult is warranted if any of these are suspected.
- Bochdalek CDH is not commonly seen in adults. The clinical presentation can variably include respiratory or GI symptoms or the patient may be asymptomatic. Adults do not typically have the severe respiratory symptoms seen in neonates due to pulmonary hypoplasia and pulmonary hypertension. Diagnosis is often made by plain radiograph and cross-sectional imaging. Surgical repair is often more elective than neonatal repair though may be urgent if there is associated bowel obstruction or respiratory insufficiency. The operative approach may be either transthoracic or transabdominal and is generally well tolerated.

IMAGING AND OTHER DIAGNOSTIC STUDIES

- Prenatal workup includes ultrasound and/or fetal magnetic resonance imaging (MRI). Evaluation of fetal karyotype via amniocentesis or other methods can provide additional information that aids in properly informing and preparing the parents.
- After birth, a chest radiograph is the primary diagnostic study of choice. For a left-sided CDH, this will classically show multiple gas-filled bowel loops within the left hemithorax and contralateral shift of the mediastinum (**FIGURE 1**). The presence of the liver and/or stomach in the chest on plain film can help estimate the size of the hernia defect. A right-sided CDH may demonstrate only an elevated liver shadow if no other visceral contents have traversed the hernia defect (**FIGURE 2**).
- Computed tomography, MRI, ultrasound, fluoroscopy, and upper GI series with small bowel follow-through may be used as well when the diagnosis is not certain. Diagnostic thoracoscopy or laparoscopy is recommended if the diagnosis remains unclear after appropriate imaging studies.
- An echocardiogram should be obtained as part of the workup for associated congenital anomalies. It can also be useful in quantifying the degree of pulmonary hypertension and then following its treatment. Additionally, intracranial imaging

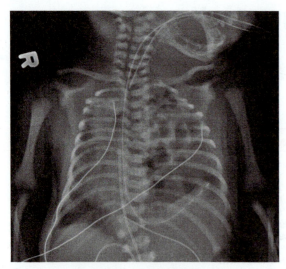

FIGURE 1 • Chest x-ray in neonate demonstrating a left congenital diaphragmatic hernia. Note that the stomach and liver are both transposed into the left chest and the mediastinum is shifted to the right.

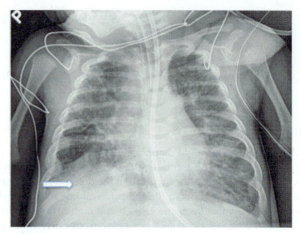

FIGURE 2 • Chest x-ray demonstrating a right congenital diaphragmatic hernia. The *arrow* denotes the elevated liver at the site of the hernia defect.

with a head ultrasound is useful, particularly when perioperative extracorporeal membrane oxygenation (ECMO) is considered as part of the infant's management.

SURGICAL MANAGEMENT

Preoperative Planning

- CDH is a physiologic emergency and not usually a surgical emergency. The careful management of the neonate's pulmonary hypoplasia, lung immaturity, and pulmonary hypertension is most critical to their successful outcome.
- The optimal timing for surgical repair is unclear, although most current strategies include a period of medical stabilization followed by delayed operative repair.
- Both open and minimally invasive techniques can be used for repair. We favor a thoracoscopic repair for a small defect in the stable patient and an open repair in the less stable patient with a larger hernia defect.
- Prior to taking the patient to the operating room, all diagnostic studies should be thoroughly reviewed and the patient should be appropriately marked on the affected side.
- Ensure that the airway is secure and the endotracheal tube in a stable position. Pre- and postductal oxygen saturation monitoring should be maintained.
- Arterial access is ideal for perioperative and intraoperative blood gas monitoring.
- The neonate's own ventilator is preferred over the typical anesthesia circuit.
- If the patient is on ECMO, appropriate perioperative bleeding protocols should be initiated.
- For less stable infants, it may be more appropriate for the surgical repair to take place in their neonatal intensive care unit (NICU) bed space.

OPEN LEFT CDH REPAIR

Positioning

- In the operating room, the infant is placed in the supine position on a shortened bed (**FIGURE 3**).
- Sterile plastic drapes are used as a barrier over the infant outside of the operative field. A warming blanket is also used to maintain temperature stability.
- For operative repairs in the NICU, the infant is brought to the end of their bed at an angle, with their feet directed toward one corner (**FIGURE 4**).
- Both the abdomen and chest are prepared as the operative fields. The umbilical catheters are secured to the patient's lower quadrant, contralateral to the operative side.

Incision

- For a left CDH, an ipsilateral subcostal incision is made. Do not make the incision too close to the costal margin as it may leave little room to work with on the lateral chest wall and it may make closure more difficult. The subcostal incision will need to be extended across midline for larger diaphragmatic hernia defects (**FIGURE 5**).
- The abdominal wall muscle and fascia are divided and the peritoneum entered. The infant's abdominal wall may be gently stretched to help increase domain for the hernia reduction.

Hernia Reduction

- First, the liver needs to be mobilized. The triangular ligament is taken down and the left lateral segment completely freed up. The falciform ligament can usually be left intact.
- The liver is carefully retracted away from the diaphragmatic defect to expose the medial boundary of the diaphragmatic hernia defect (**FIGURE 6**).
- The reduction of the hernia is typically done in a stepwise fashion.

Chapter 6 REPAIR OF CONGENITAL DEFECTS: BOCHDALEK CONGENITAL DIAPHRAGMATIC HERNIA   35

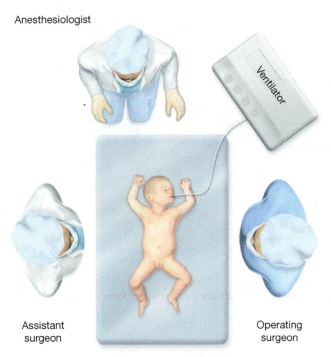

FIGURE 3 • The infant is positioned in the center of a shortened operating room table. The operating surgeon stands on the side of the congenital diaphragmatic hernia with the surgical assistant on the opposite side.

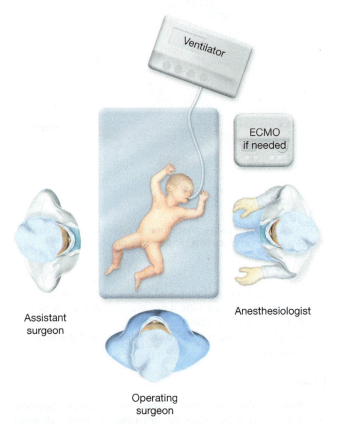

FIGURE 4 • The infant is positioned in their NICU bed at a 45° angle with their feet directed toward one corner. The operating surgeon then stands on the side of the congenital diaphragmatic hernia and the surgical assistant on the opposite side. The ventilator and other equipment are kept at the head of the bed. ECMO, extracorporeal membrane oxygenation.

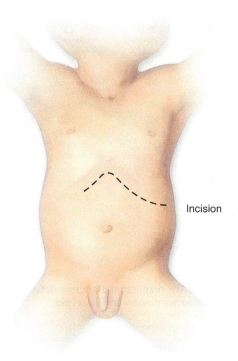

FIGURE 5 • A subcostal incision is made one to two fingerbreadths below the costal margin. It may need to be extended across midline to provide adequate exposure for larger diaphragmatic defects.

- The anterior aspect of the incision is retracted cranially. Next, the liver is very carefully reduced from the hernia (if up) and retracted medially with moist lap pads and soft malleable retractors. Then, the small and large bowels are gently reduced from the hernia. Care is taken to keep the mesentery properly oriented and to avoid trauma to the splenic capsule when reducing the colon. Finally, the stomach and spleen are reduced together. This is best done with the index finger. Special attention is paid to avoid traction on the short gastric vessels. All the abdominal viscera can usually be packed within the abdominal cavity using moistened mini lap pads and malleable retractors. This helps with temperature control and allows some time for the abdominal cavity to begin to accommodate prior to fascial closure. For prolonged procedures, the tightly packed bowel may need to be intermittently unpacked and inspected for ischemia.
- If a hernia sac is present, this is excised.

Repair of the Diaphragm

- An assessment is made to determine the amount of native diaphragm. The posterior aspect of native diaphragm may need to be mobilized and unfolded from the retroperitoneum to fully use it in closure. The anterior diaphragm is then traced medially and the left crus is identified.
- If the diaphragmatic hernia is small enough for primary closure without significant tension, this is preferred. The defect is repaired with interrupted simple sutures using nonabsorbable braided suture material. For those defects that are too large to close primarily, a 1-mm Gore-Tex soft-tissue patch is used. This is carefully fashioned so as to maintain the rounded, dome shape of a normal diaphragm. The posterior wall is sewn first to the patch with interrupted sutures

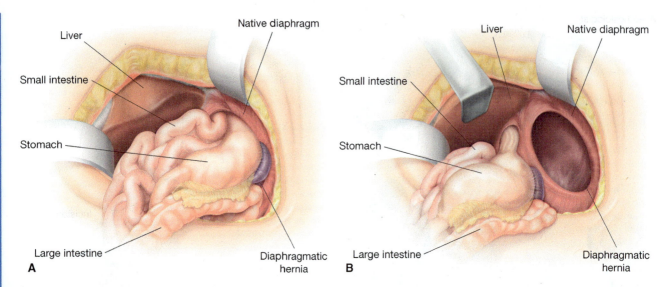

FIGURE 6 • **A,** The diaphragmatic hernia defect is exposed. **B,** The abdominal contents have been reduced from the diaphragmatic hernia and the native diaphragm is assessed.

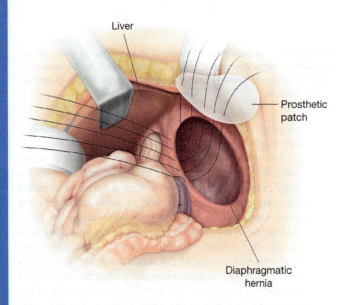

FIGURE 7 • The diaphragmatic patch is first sewn to the posterior diaphragmatic defect or chest wall. The sutures are initially left untied to facilitate adequate placement. Once the posterior row is in place, the patch is parachuted down in place and the sutures are tied. Prior to closing the anterior rim of diaphragm, the thorax is inspected for hemostasis.

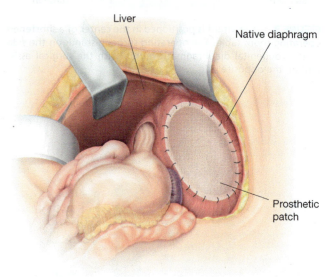

FIGURE 8 • The diaphragmatic hernia repair is completed with the patch sewn in place in a tension-free manner.

using a braided nonabsorbable material. The sutures are left untied initially (**FIGURE 7**). Once all in place, the patch is then parachuted down, and the sutures are individually tied secured (**FIGURE 8**). Then, before closure of the anterior diaphragmatic defect is initiated, care is taken to ensure hemostasis on the thoracic side of the patch.

- For portions of the diaphragmatic defect with no native diaphragm present, the soft-tissue patch is sewn directly to the rib. A thick taper needle is brought in through the superior aspect of the rib and out through the center of the rib to avoid the neurovascular bundle. Once adequate hemostasis is achieved, the anterior wall of the diaphragm is closed (**FIGURE 9**). A chest tube is not placed unless the patient is anticoagulated on ECMO.
- At this time, the retractors are released and the bowel is inspected.

Closure

- Position the abdominal viscera in anatomic position. The spleen is placed in the left upper quadrant abutting the repaired diaphragm. The bowel is positioned to keep the mesentery flat and untwisted. Only if there is little chance for the patient to be anticoagulated, such as for ECMO, are Ladd bands divided. An appendectomy is not routinely performed

Chapter 6 REPAIR OF CONGENITAL DEFECTS: BOCHDALEK CONGENITAL DIAPHRAGMATIC HERNIA   37

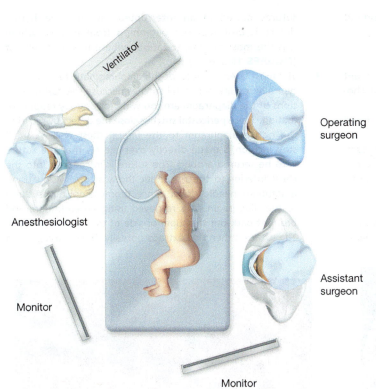

FIGURE 9 • The infant is positioned in lateral decubitus position with the affected side up. The infant is placed at one end of the operating table so that the operating surgeon is able to be positioned at the infant's head and the surgical assistant to their side.

and should be avoided when a prosthetic patch is used. Lastly, the left lateral segment of liver is placed back over the anterior gastric wall.
- The abdominal wall musculature and skin are then closed in layers.

- For some patients, there will be loss of abdominal domain after hernia reduction and primary abdominal closure may not be feasible. If this is the case, a silo or patch may be easily used to avoid potential issues with postoperative abdominal compartment syndrome.

THORACOSCOPIC LEFT CDH REPAIR

Positioning

- The infant is placed in the lateral decubitus position with the affected side up. An axillary roll is placed and care is taken to ensure all pressure points are properly padded.
- The ipsilateral arm is extended anteriorly and superiorly to open the axilla.
- The patient is oriented on the operating room table so that the operating surgeon may stand at the patient's head. The monitor is accordingly positioned over the infant's feet (**FIGURE 9**).

Trocar Placement

- A Veress needle is first introduced followed by a 5-mm radially expanding trocar placed just caudal to the angle of the scapula.
- Pneumothorax is initially set at 4 mm Hg and ventilator changes along with carbon dioxide (CO_2) are closely monitored. Mainstem intubation is typically not needed.
- A 4-mm, 30° scope is used for visualization.
- Two additional 4-mm trocars are placed under direct thoracoscopic vision, anterior and posterior to the first trocar, and one to two rib spaces caudally. These will be the primary working ports (**FIGURE 10**).

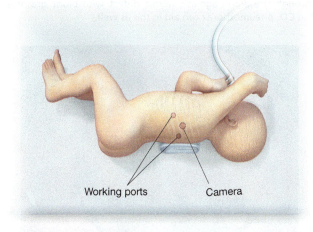

FIGURE 10 • The initial 5-mm port is placed at the angle of the scapula following introduction of pneumothorax via the Veress needle. Two additional 4-mm ports are inserted to the right and left, one to two rib spaces inferiorly. This allows the 4-mm camera to be repositioned when necessary. An additional posterior port may be added if needed.

- An additional trocar may be needed to retract the lung out of the operative field.

Reduction of the Diaphragmatic Hernia

- The abdominal viscera are carefully reduced with blunt graspers and a cotton-tipped Endo Kittner. The pneumothorax will aid in this process (**FIGURES 11** and **12**).
- If the spleen is included in the herniated viscera, this is reduced last, and it may provide an initial "plug" to the defect.
- The hernia sac, if one is present, is carefully excised circumferentially off the diaphragmatic defect using hook cautery. It may be otherwise left attached to any abdominal viscera.

Repair of the CDH

- When a relatively tension-free primary repair is feasible, the defect is reapproximated using braided nonabsorbable sutures placed in an interrupted fashion. The hernia defect is best repaired beginning from medial, where it is the most narrow, to lateral, where it is at its widest (**FIGURES 13** and **14**).
- The most lateral aspects of the diaphragmatic hernia repair typically require pericostal stitches because the costal insertions of the diaphragm are too wide for primary reapproximation. These pericostal stitches close the defect by securing the native diaphragm to the lateral chest wall. A small stab incision is made directly over the rib that the suture is to be secured around. The suture is introduced into the chest inferior to the rib under thoracoscopic vision using a standard needle driver. Once thoracoscopically sutured to the diaphragm, it is retrieved using an endosnare and brought back out the superior side of the rib (**FIGURE 15**). The suture is then tied extracorporeally. The central portion

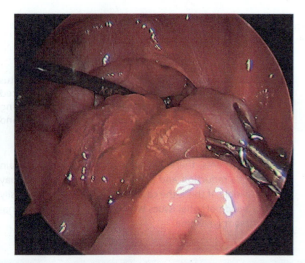

FIGURE 11 • The abdominal viscera are carefully reduced through the diaphragmatic hernia defect with blunt graspers. The CO_2 pneumothorax can aid in this as well.

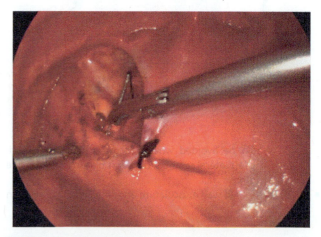

FIGURE 13 • The thoracoscopic hernia repair is begun in a medial to lateral fashion using intracorporeal suturing techniques. The diaphragm is reapproximated using interrupted sutures in a tension-free manner.

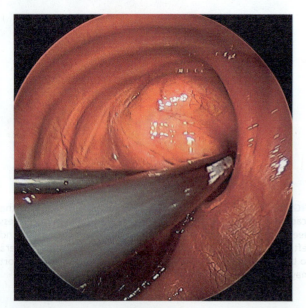

FIGURE 12 • A cotton-tipped Endo Kittner can be particularly helpful with reduction of the spleen.

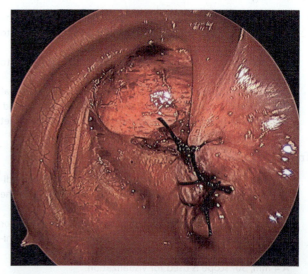

FIGURE 14 • As the repair approaches the lateral chest wall, the defect becomes wider due to the fixed nature of the diaphragm on the chest wall. This will not primarily reapproximate without significant tension.

Chapter 6 REPAIR OF CONGENITAL DEFECTS: BOCHDALEK CONGENITAL DIAPHRAGMATIC HERNIA

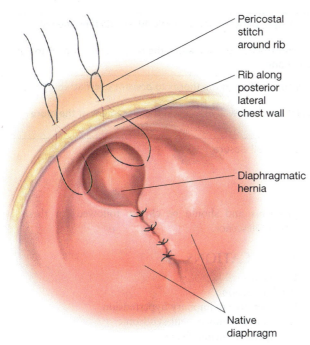

FIGURE 15 • Pericostal stitches are placed through small stab incisions in the patient's lateral chest wall. These both secure the diaphragm repair to the rib and reduce the size of the remaining hernia defect without significant tension.

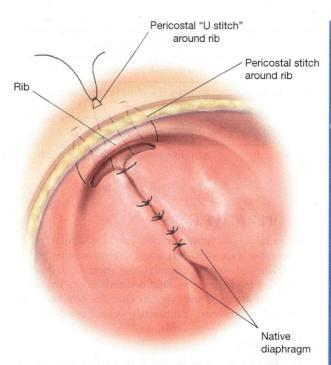

FIGURE 16 • A pericostal U-stitch is used to close the remaining diaphragmatic hernia defect while securing it to the chest wall.

of the diaphragmatic defect usually requires a pericostal "U-stitch" that brings the posterior and lateral rim of the diaphragm together, fixing them to the lateral chest wall (FIGURE 16). This allows complete closure of the hernia defect (FIGURE 17).

- If a patch is needed, this may be secured to the diaphragm in a fashion similar to open repair and to the chest wall using the earlier described pericostal U-stitch technique. Additionally, a synthetic patch may also be used as an onlay for weaker areas of the diaphragmatic repair. Using a thin composite mesh may provide for easier introduction and intracorporeal manipulation.

Closure

- The pneumothorax is released and the lung reexpanded. A chest tube may be placed through the anterior trocar site if deemed necessary.
- The incisions are reapproximated with absorbable suture and skin glue is applied as a dressing.

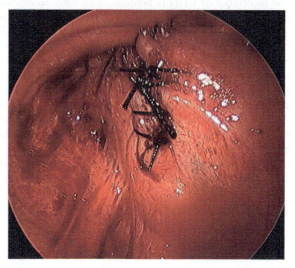

FIGURE 17 • The completed congenital diaphragmatic hernia repair.

PEARLS AND PITFALLS

Incision	■ If perioperative ECMO is likely, use electrocautery as much as safely possible during repair and avoid mobilization of retroperitoneal area.
Hernia reduction	■ Be on the lookout for abnormally draining hepatic veins when mobilizing and reducing the liver. ■ Avoid trauma to the short gastric vessels and splenic capsule.

Hernia repair	▪ The patch may need to be secured to the esophagus, pericardium, or aortic adventitia if no medial diaphragm is present. ▪ Incorporate enough redundancy in the patch construction so as to allow the repaired diaphragm to have a normal, rounded shape instead of a flattened one.
Thoracoscopy	▪ Mark the rib(s) for the pericostal stitches prior to insufflating the thorax to prevent overflattening the diaphragm. ▪ External compression by the assistant on the lateral chest wall may aid in the placement of the more difficult lateral sutures.
Closure	▪ If in question, use a silo or patch to aid abdominal wall closure.

POSTOPERATIVE CARE

- The principles of postoperative care are similar to the preoperative care of CDHs and close monitoring of pulmonary hypertension is critical. Close attention to fluid status is also required as the fluid demands in the immediate postoperative period will typically rise. The ventilator, once stabilized, is slowly and deliberately weaned as tolerated.

OUTCOMES

- The overall survival of infants with CDH varies between 60% and 90%. For the subset of infants that require ECMO, the survival remains at around 50%.[1]
- The recurrence of CDH is bimodal, with early recurrences typically seen within 2 months of surgery and late recurrences at approximately 2 years of age. Data from the CDH registry suggest that the early, in-hospital recurrence rate is significantly higher for thoracoscopic (7.9%) vs open (2.7%) repair.[2]
- Multiple different patch materials have been used. These include nonabsorbable prosthetic, biologic, and native muscle flaps. There is no clear advantage with regard to survival, recurrence, or bowel obstruction among any of these patch materials.[3-5]
- CDH patient survivors are at risk for chronic pulmonary, cardiovascular, neurodevelopmental, GI, and musculoskeletal problems and should be closely followed for these well into adolescence.

COMPLICATIONS

- Recurrence
- Patch infection
- Postoperative pulmonary hypertension
- Abdominal compartment syndrome
- Postoperative hemorrhage
- Bowel obstruction

REFERENCES

1. Hoffman SB, Massaro AN, Gingalewski C, et al. Survival in congenital diaphragmatic hernia: use of predictive equations in the ECMO population. *Neonatology.* 2011;99(4):258-265.
2. Tsao K, Lally PA, Lally KP, et al. Minimally invasive repair of congenital diaphragmatic hernia. *J Pediatr Surg.* 2011;46(6):1158-1164.
3. Gasior AC, St Peter SD. A review of patch options in the repair of congenital diaphragmatic hernia. *Pediatr Surg Int.* 2012;28(4):327-333.
4. Aydin E, Nolan H, Peiro JL, et al. When primary repair is not enough: a comparison of synthetic patch and muscle flap closure in congenital diaphragmatic hernia. *Pediatr Surg Int.* 2020;36(4):485-491.
5. Romao RL, Nasr A, Chiu PP, et al. What is the best prosthetic material for patch repair of congenital diaphragmatic hernia? Comparison and meta-analysis of porcine small intestinal submucosa and polytetrafluoroethylene. *J Pediatr Surg.* 2012;47(8):1496-1500.

SECTION III: Treatment of Paraesophageal Hernias

Chapter 7 — Paraesophageal Hernia Repair: Laparoscopic Technique

Yewande R. Alimi and Mary T. Hawn

DEFINITIONS

- There are four types of hiatal hernias (HHs). Type I, also known as sliding HHs, is where the gastroesophageal junction (GEJ) herniates through the hiatus and the stomach remains positioned below the esophagus. Type I HH accounts for almost 95% of HHs.[1,2] The remainder of the hernia types are encompassed in the category of paraesophageal hernias (PEHs). Type II HH is a true PEH with the GEJ positioned in the abdominal cavity and the stomach herniated through the hiatus adjacent to the esophagus. Type III HH is characterized by a herniated stomach in the paraesophageal position and the GEJ above the hiatus (combination of type I and type II). Finally, type IV HH is characterized by herniation of extragastric organs (**FIGURE 1**).
- The focus of this chapter will be on PEHs, type II to type IV described above. We will focus on the principles of workup and preoperative preparation, surgical repair, and postoperative management. While the focus of this chapter will be primary hernia repair, the tenants and principles can be applied to those performing these procedures in the revisional setting.

PERTINENT HISTORY

- Patients may present with epigastric and/or chest pain, often postprandial, dysphagia, often progressive in nature, weight loss, early satiety, dyspnea, and with anemia in the setting of Cameron ulcers. Patient's symptoms may also be associated symptoms secondary to the resultant gastroesophageal reflux disease. These include heartburn, acid reflux, and dyspepsia.
- Patients may present secondary to the complication of PEH, like gastric volvulus, incarceration, or gastric outlet obstruction. When patients present in the emergent setting, the associated morbidity and mortality are higher than when approached in the elective setting. Data suggest that repair of PEHs in the emergent setting had a demonstrated mortality close to 20%.[3]

IMAGING AND OTHER DIAGNOSTIC STUDIES

- Workup is dependent on the urgency of the clinical setting. In the setting of elective evaluation of a symptomatic PEH, imaging is essential to operative planning. Diagnosis is often with a barium esophagram, endoscopy, or axial imaging.
- Barium esophagram is the diagnostic study of choice in our clinic practice. Barium esophagram provides crucial information in the diagnosis of PEH as well as critical anatomic features to be considered in operative planning. This study is done in the supine and upright positions. The location of the GEJ as it relates to the diaphragm can be determined on this study. Information on esophageal motility as well as the presence of reflux can be noted as well as mucosal-based abnormalities can be detected. Esophageal length can often be approximated with barium esophagram, and the diagnosis of a foreshortened esophagus will need to be considered during surgical approach (**FIGURE 2A** and **B**).
- Esophageal manometry is an important diagnostic study in the preparation of any antireflux procedure. In the setting of PEHs, there may be difficulties with placement of the catheter. However, the study is still warranted to determine the presence of primary esophageal dysmotility, specifically, achalasia, a hypertensive lower esophageal sphincter (LES), diffuse esophageal spasm, and others. Patients with evidence of dysmotility should not undergo a 360° wrap. While nuances exist within manometric studies, we favor avoidance of 360° wraps in patients with overall poor bolus clearance, low distal esophageal pressures, and ineffective esophageal motility.
- Upper endoscopy: All patients should undergo upper endoscopy prior to surgical intervention. Patients with atypical symptoms or concerning features such as microcytic anemia and weight loss, should undergo upper endoscopy to rule out any mucosal-based diseases prior to surgical repair. Regardless, upper endoscopy allows for evaluation of the GEJ, identifying the presence of Cameron's lesions, the presence of esophagitis, and allows for the opportunity for biopsy if abnormalities are present.
- pH testing: While pH testing is not essential in the setting of large PEHs, the results can help guide the extent of fundoplication to be performed.
- Computed tomography (CT): In patients presenting in the emergent or urgent setting, a CT scan is often obtained given the rapidity and easy accessibility of the modality (**FIGURE 3A** and **B**). Many surgeons prefer CT to esophagram; however, it is our experience that it does not change management.

SURGICAL MANAGEMENT

Preoperative Planning

- Imaging and studies should be accessible to the surgeon on the day of surgery. We advocate for establishing the barium esophagram on intraoperative monitors for the preparation of the case. Attention to preoperative manometry is essential in determining the nature of fundoplication to be performed.
    - We advocate for a partial wrap in patients with weak esophageal motility, in patients with demonstrated esophagogastric junction (EGJ) outflow obstruction who fail to normalize on multiple rapid swallows, and in patients

SECTION III TREATMENT OF PARAESOPHAGEAL HERNIAS

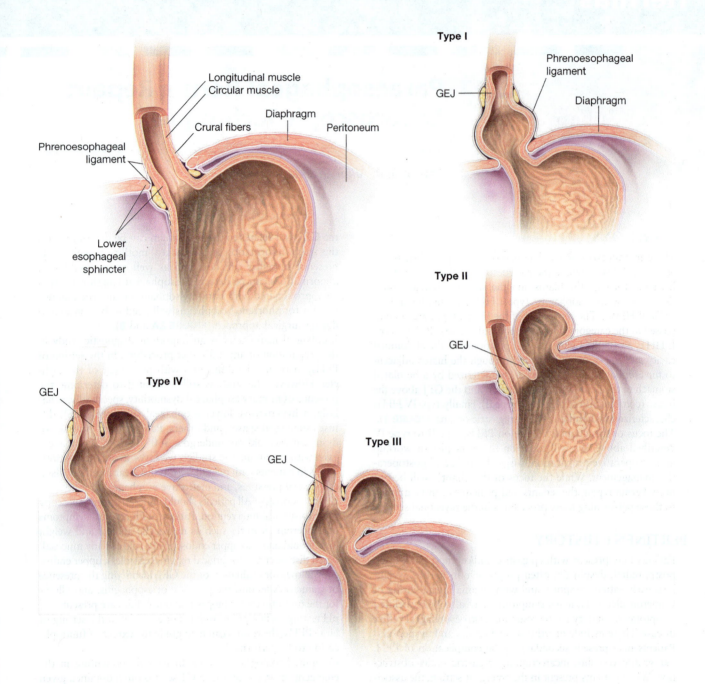

FIGURE 1 • Hiatal hernia types. The four types of hiatal hernia: type I (sliding): gastroesophageal junction (GEJ) translates linearly along the esophageal axis cephalad into the mediastinum; type II (paraesophageal): GEJ resides intra-abdominally with (usually) the gastric fundus or body translating cephalad past the GEJ; type III (combined): GEJ and gastric segments both translate above the diaphragm; and type IV (extragastric): the small bowel, colon, spleen, and even pancreas may translate into the mediastinum and chest.

with large PEH and an inability to obtain good preoperative manometry. A 360° wrap in a patient with a weak esophagus can lead to dysphagia that can be difficult to manage short of surgical revision.
- Patient positioning
  - We perform this procedure in the supine with split leg on a surgical bed with the capabilities of performing steep reverse Trendelenburg. While we routinely perform this with the arms out at 90°, the patient's arms may also be tucked bilaterally. In the case of performing this procedure supine, a foot board is highly recommended.

- Appropriate padding of all pressure points should be attended to.
- Preoperative gastric decompression
  - Placement of an orogastric tube for gastric decompression prior to abdominal entry should be attempted. Caution should be taken if significant resistance is encountered, as a large PEH may preclude additional advancement of the gastric tube.

Abdominal Entry/Port Placement

- Access is obtained to the abdomen in the fashion that is most comfortable to the surgeon. In our practice, this involves

Chapter 7 PARAESOPHAGEAL HERNIA REPAIR: LAPAROSCOPIC TECHNIQUE   43

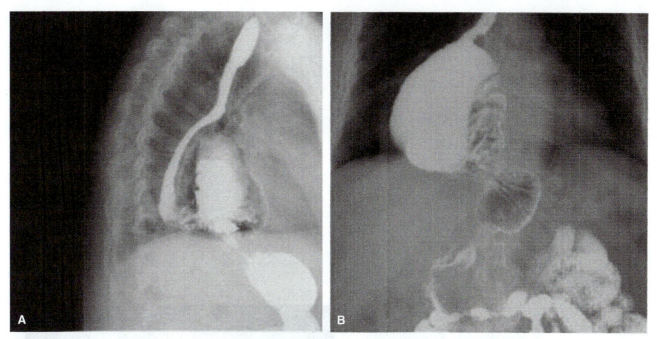

FIGURE 2 • **A,** Lateral view of barium esophagram of type III paraesophageal hernia (PEH). **B,** AP view of barium esophagram of type III PEH.

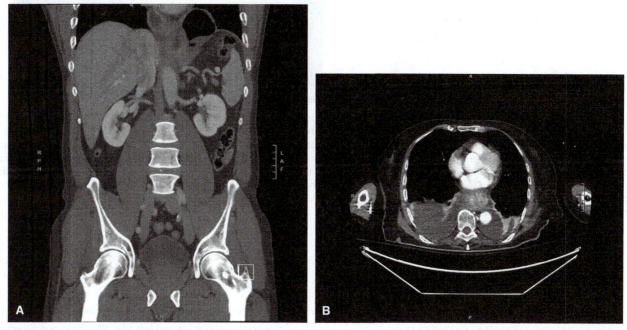

FIGURE 3 • CT scan of paraesophageal hernia repair (PEHR). **A,** Coronal view of slipped Nissen fundoplication. **B,** Axial view of type II PEHR.

access via the Veress needle at Palmer's point that becomes the surgeon's right-hand port. After establishing 15 mm Hg of pneumoperitoneum, a periumbilical camera port is then placed, approximately 14 cm from the xiphoid and 2 cm left of the midline.
- While access is being obtained, the liver retractor setup can be prepared.
- Four additional ports are placed as depicted in **FIGURE 4A** and **B**.
  - An 11-mm trocar is placed on the patient's left side in the subcostal region along the lateral aspect of the midclavicular line.
- Three additional 5 mm ports are placed: one left lateral, right side medial, approximately 30° off of midline, at the level of the left subcostal incision, and a final right lateral port at the horizon of the fat plane and the abdominal wall in the subcostal region.
- A liver retractor is inserted to maintain exposure under the left lateral lobe and at the hiatus via the right lateral port.
  - Alternative placement includes the use of a Nathanson retractor through an epigastric incision.

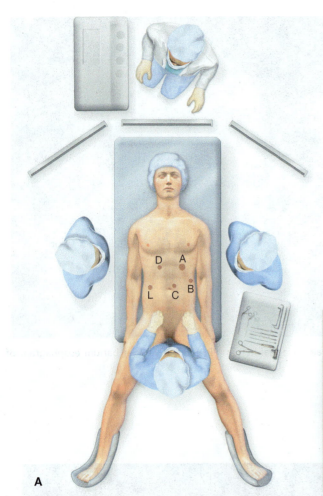
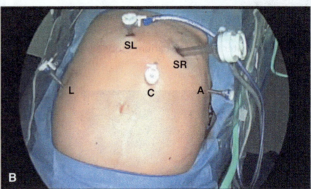

FIGURE 4 • **A,** Illustrated depiction of port placement. **B,** In situ port placement intraoperatively. (C—Camera) A 5-mm supraumbilical camera port, offset just to the left of the midline and 12 cm inferiorly. (SR—Surgeon Right) An 11-mm left upper quadrant port, measured 1 to 2 finger breadths below the costal margin in the midclavicular line. (A—Assistant) An assistant's 5-mm left flank trocar is placed about a palm's width inferiorly and laterally from the 11-mm trocar. (SL—Surgeon Left) A 5-mm right upper quadrant trocar, approximately 30° from the midline drawn from the xiphoid, and 1 to 2 cm inferiorly, for the surgeon's left hand, at the approximate level of port A. This can be placed to the right of the falciform and then through the falciform. (L—Liver) Similarly, a port can be placed at the right flank, symmetrically opposite from the assistant's port for a linear liver retractor. Alternatively, a 5-mm port is placed and removed in the subxiphoid region for the Nathanson liver retractor.

- Consideration in revisional surgery includes the possibility of an extensive adhesiolysis of the liver to the prior fundoplication. When this is encountered, we have an assistant to manually retract the liver as we take down adhesions until the left lateral segment is free to allow placement of the fixed liver retractor.

REDUCTION OF HERNIA CONTENTS

- The hiatus is evaluated and the PEH is assessed. Attempt should be made to reduce all contents intra-abdominally. We begin this by gently reducing the hernia contents along the greater curvature and left crus. We begin our dissection on the left side of the crus as the plane of dissection and the structures of the unreduced PEH are often clearer and it is less likely to result in inadvertent injury to the displaced esophagus (▶ **Video 1: 0:07**).

HIATAL DISSECTION

- Dissection of the hiatus is about dissection and complete reduction of the hernia sac off the crura circumferentially.
- The herniated stomach pushes the esophagus posterior and to the right. As such it is safest to approach the hiatus and hernia sac from the left side and then extend 180° dissection toward the right crus just deep to the peritoneal attachments to the crura (▶ **Video 1: 0:10**). This is key as any deeper can result in injury to the esophagus or vagus nerve. Identifying the right plane and applying traction to the sac will allow the CO_2 to facilitate dissection and reduction of the hernia sac.

Chapter 7 **PARAESOPHAGEAL HERNIA REPAIR: LAPAROSCOPIC TECHNIQUE** 45

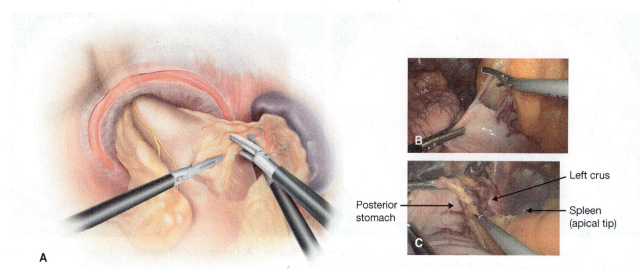

FIGURE 5 • **A–C,** Short gastric vessel ligation. **A** and **B,** Initial dissection begins at a level parallel to the distal splenic tip. **C,** Completion of the short gastric ligation. Note the exposure of the posterior stomach to complete this step.

- In a left crus first approach, early ligation of the short gastric vessels is indicated to get into the lesser sac. The vessels are taken with the ultrasonic dissector close to the stomach and care should be taken to not perform incomplete ligations as these vessels are notorious for immediate retraction.
  - We approach this by presenting the short gastric vessels to the surgeon's right hand in a 90° orientation. This allows for the operator to visualize the structures above the short gastric vessels while completely dividing them.
  - The dissection is continued toward the right crus anteriorly taking down the phrenoesophageal ligament (**FIGURE 5**).
  - As the left crus is approached and we are sufficiently above the spleen, the surgeon's left hand should grasp the hernia sac at the level of the hiatus to retract the hernia sac, continuing this dissection circumferentially (**FIGURE 6**) (▶ Video 1: 0:30).
    - This should be a superficial dissection as the left vagus nerve is often encountered anteriorly at approximately the 1-o'clock position.
- The right crus of the diaphragm is then approached by first entering the pars flaccida to get into the lesser sac.
  - The occurrence of an accessory left hepatic artery in the pars flaccida can occur in up to 11% of patients and should be identified.[4]
  - If encountered, we test clamp the artery and assess hepatic viability. In the absence of decreased perfusion, we doubly clip the artery and then divide it.

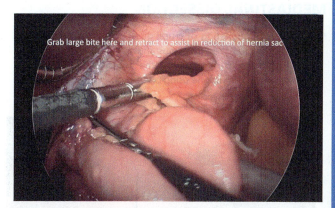

FIGURE 6 • Reduction of the hernia sac.

- The peritoneum overlying the right crus is carefully incised using the ultrasonic dissector and the crural dissection continues circumferentially taking down the phrenoesophageal ligament.
- Reduce the lesser omentum, retracting anterolaterally to continue crural dissection. Of note, the herniated lesser omentum typically contains the left gastric artery (accompanied ▶ Video: 1:14).
- Dissection proceeds from the right crus toward the left crus in a 180° fashion to meet the previous dissection plane.
  - The posterior vagus is often encountered during this dissection at approximately the 7-o'clock position.

POSTERIOR DISSECTION

- To complete the 360° mobilization, the posterior gastric attachments must be taken down. This is done by retracting the stomach anteromedially and distracting the omentum to the left. This exposes the posterior attachments of the splenic vessels to the left gastroepiploic vessel. This can be ligated by the ultrasonic dissector.

- During the posterior dissection, herniated retroperitoneal fat is often encountered (▶ Video 1: 2:32). Reduction of this retroperitoneal fat facilitates completion of the crural dissection (**FIGURE 7A**). As this retroperitoneal fat is reduced, the left crus is able to be visualized from the right side (**FIGURE 7B**).

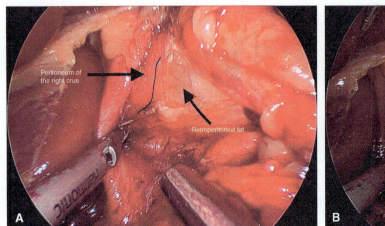
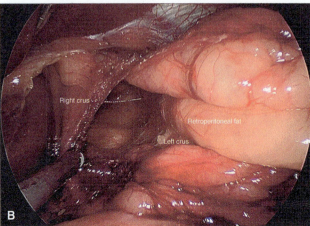

FIGURE 7 • Reduction of retroperitoneal fat, completion of posterior dissection. **A,** Delineation of peritoneal lining of right crus and identification of retroperitoneal fat. **B,** Reduction of retroperitoneal fat and left crus coming into view from right side.

MEDIASTINAL DISSECTION

- After the completion of crural dissection, a Penrose drain is placed around the esophagus and both vagus nerves. With retraction of the esophagus, the mediastinal dissection is completed. This is done using blunt and ultrasonic dissection. It is important that the vagal nerves are identified and protected during this dissection (**FIGURE 8A** and **B**).
- We find this dissection is best carried out by distracting tissue caudally and between two blunt graspers, using energy only when suspected vasculature is encountered to avoid thermal injury to the vagal nerves.

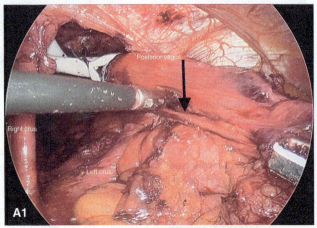
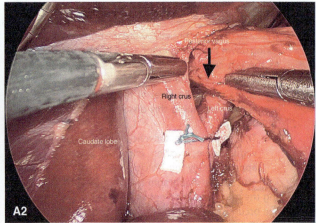
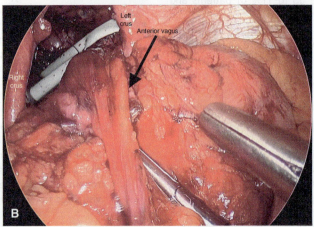

FIGURE 8 • **A1/A2,** Identification of the right vagus nerve (posterior vagus). **B,** Identification of the left vagus nerve (anterior vagus nerve).

ASSESSMENT OF INTRA-ABDOMINAL LENGTH

- In cases with PEH, we routinely perform interoperative endoscopy (esophagogastroduodenoscopy) to evaluate the position of the EGJ. The presence of the redundant hernia sac and distortion of the fundus from chronic herniation can make assessing the location of the GEJ more challenging. The GEJ is identified via endoscopy and we often place a Vicryl stitch on the outside as a marker. A length of 3 cm of intra-abdominal esophagus is desired. If this is not the case, additional mediastinal dissection should be performed. Following a high mediastinal dissection, if there remains less than 3 cm intra-abdominal length, a Collis gastroplasty should be considered (please see Chapter 8).
- During this time, a leak test can be performed to assess for inadvertent injuries.
    - In complex dissections with large PEH, a dilute methylene blue test is performed in the distal esophagus and in the fundus of the stomach, via a retroflexed view.
    - An intra-abdominal sponge can be used in the splenic sulcus to evaluate for any staining with methylene blue to assess for a leak.
    - An alternative to dilute methylene blue is a bubble leak test performed under submerged saline with distal clamping of the stomach. Observation of bubbles submerged in water results in a positive leak test.

EXCISION OF HERNIA SAC

- In an ideal dissection, the hernia sac remains intact and is able to be removed en bloc. We begin this by identifying the anterior vagus nerve, and in layers, dissect the hernia sac away from the stomach lateral to the anterior vagus nerve. If this has been properly performed, this hernia sac is in continuity with the esophageal fat pad. This often requires removal to facilitate fundoplication (▶ Video 1: 3:27).
- Dissection of the hernia sac should proceed a safe distance from the esophagus to prevent thermal injury to the esophagus and the vagal nerves. Mediastinal dissection should also not veer too far from the esophagus as it proceeds on the right and left as this may result in entry into the pleural cavity.
- The redundant herniated retroperitoneal fat pad should be removed carefully to avoid injury to the posterior vagus nerve and the left gastric artery.

POSTERIOR CRUROPLASTY

- After assessment of sufficient intra-abdominal length, using the Penrose drain maintaining lateral retraction on the esophagus, the posterior cruroplasty is performed.
    - Cruroplasty is performed approximately 1 cm apart, 1 cm posterior to the crural edge (▶ Video 1: 3:57).
    - We use a 0-0 ethylene terephthalate braided permanent suture reinforced with a small polytetrafluoroethylene, interrupted suture.
- The number of sutures is often between two and four sutures with the goal to approximate the crura to comfortably accommodate a laparoscopic instrument (**FIGURE 9**). This in general approximates to a diameter of two esophagi.
    - In large defects, the closure may require both posterior and anterior cruroplasty in order to not create a significant acute angle.
    - Reducing the insufflation pressure to 8 to 10 mm Hg facilitates with reapproximation of the crura if the repair is under tension.
    - If anterior sutures are required, these are placed without pledget reinforcement.

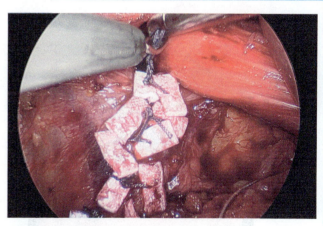

FIGURE 9 • Posterior cruroplasty with pledgeted nonabsorbable braided permanent suture.

MESH REINFORCEMENT

- We do not routinely place mesh reinforcement. In situations in which we are unable to close the hiatus primarily, we advocate for a relaxing incision in the membranous part of the right crus medially, to allow for primary crural closure. These scenarios include undue tension or tearing as the crural closure is completed. After the creation of a relaxing incision, subsequently, mesh fixation occurs to the portion of the right crus that was incised as well as reinforcing the posterior cruroplasty (**FIGURE 10A**). The diaphragmatic defect and the crural closure are then reinforced with a biologic mesh of the surgeon's choice as this is often institution specific (use reference).
- In situations of weak crura and when there is a need for posterior reinforcement, we suggest reinforcement of the cruroplasty with a "U" formation in the setting of no relaxing incision (**FIGURE 10B**).
- Beware about using the tacker anteriorly as this can inadvertently injure the heart.
- Data regarding mesh reinforcement of paraesophageal hernia repairs (PEHRs) have been mixed, though many studies report the safe use of permanent and biologic mesh for this purpose, with acceptable recurrence rates. However, the use of biologic mesh to bridge the defect leads to recurrence.[5]

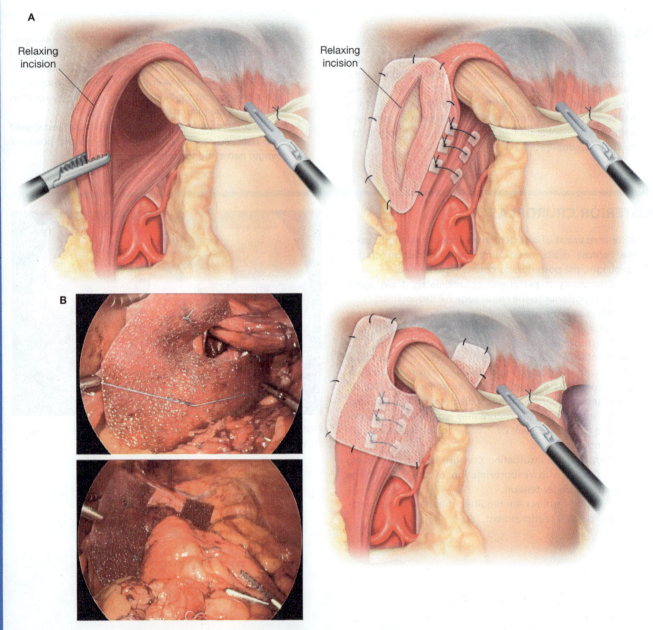

FIGURE 10 • **A,** Placement of mesh following relaxing incision. **B,** Keyhole placement of mesh.

ANTIREFLUX PROCEDURE

- Based on preoperative imaging, an antireflux procedure can be performed. Nissen fundoplications and partial wraps are beyond the scope of this chapter and can be reviewed in Chapters 9 and 10 (**FIGURE 11**); however, their use to reestablish the angle of His and the sphincter mechanism of the LES is indicated in management of PEHs.

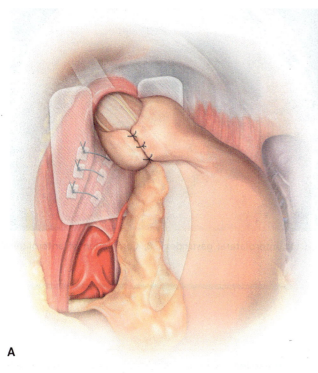

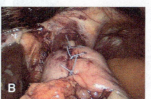

FIGURE 11 • **A**, Nissen fundoplication **B**, Nissen fundoplication in situ.

INTRAOPERATIVE UPPER ENDOSCOPY

- At the conclusion of the creation of the wrap, we do routinely evaluate the fundoplication, the location of the Z line, easy passage of the endoscope without buckling of the mucosa, and the integrity of the wrap. Under retroflexion, the wrap can be seen as a stack of coins following a 360° fundoplication (**FIGURE 12**).

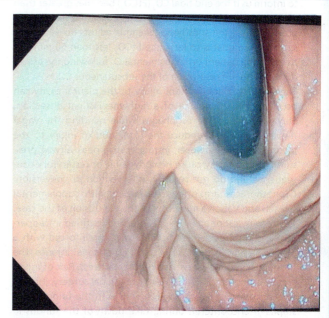

FIGURE 12 • Intraoperative esophagogastroscopy demonstrating 360° (Nissen) fundoplication. A stack of coins is seen following successful 360° wrap around the distal esophagus.

ANTEROLATERAL GASTROPEXY

- An anterolateral gastropexy is performed suturing the greater curve of the fundus (**FIGURE 13A**) to the anterior abdominal wall with a 0-0 ethylene terephthalate braided permanent suture, an additional fixation point to prevent the stomach from repeat herniation into the thoracic cavity[6] (**FIGURE 13B**).

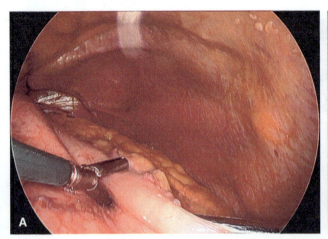 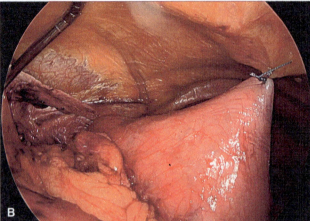

FIGURE 13 • **A,** Anterolateral gastropexy—portion of stomach used for anterolateral gastropexy. **B,** Completion of anterolateral gastropexy.

PEARLS AND PITFALLS

- Pneumomediastinum and hypercapnia: Due to the extensive dissection in the mediastinum, patients can experience hypercapnia. During our time out, we ask our anesthesia colleagues to inform us if the end tidal CO_2 ($EtCO_2$) becomes greater than 40 mm Hg. At this point, we would reduce the insufflation pressure while the anesthesia colleague adjusts the ventilator settings. The goal is to keep the $EtCO_2$ less than 50 mm Hg. Keeping the patient on supplemental O_2 following the procedure assists with resorption of the subcutaneous CO_2.
- Pneumothorax: Inadvertent injury to the pleural cavity can occur during the course of a high mediastinal dissection. Staying close to the esophagus while minding the vagal nerves can help to reduce the likelihood of injury to the pleural cavities. However, intraoperative peak airway pressure changes rarely cause hemodynamic or respiratory consequence and do not result in intervention or conversion. Capnothoraces are often reabsorbed with supplemental oxygen and Valsalva maneuver at the conclusion of the case.
- Gastrotomy/esophageal injury: Injuries identified intraoperatively should be repaired primarily and reinforced with a pleural flap or in the case of distal esophageal injuries, the fundoplication may serve as a natural buttress. Risk of injury can be as high as 20% in cases of revisional surgery. Injuries to the stomach may also be repaired with the firing of the stapler if encountered during take down of the fundus in redo fundoplication.

- Intra-abdominal esophageal length: Failure of an adequate mediastinal dissection resulting in an incomplete intra-abdominal relocation of the esophagus will result in ongoing reflux and results in the formation of a wrap around the stomach, as opposed to the distal esophagus. A complete and high 360° mediastinal dissection allows for a true determination if an esophageal lengthening procedure (Collis) is required. We also advocate for intraoperative evaluation with upper endoscopy to assure that the EGJ lies well within the abdomen.
- A dangerous pitfall is incomplete ligation of the short gastric vessels, which are prone to immediate retraction. Full and complete ligation of these vessels using the ultrasonic dissector on the slow setting should be obtained. Additionally, in revisional cases, additional short gastrics may need to be taken down due to incomplete previous mobilization, which may alter the ability to perform a suitable fundoplication.
- Acute reherniation: PEH repairs are at higher risk of acute reherniation given the extensive mediastinal dissection and laxity of the gastric attachments from chronic herniation. We obtain a barium swallow the morning after surgery. Should acute reherniation be present, the patient should be brought immediately back to the operating room for reduction as the risk of gastric ischemia is higher due to the tight hiatal closure.

POSTOPERATIVE CARE

- Patients are routinely admitted for observation. While a majority of patients with a routine dissection are without significant concern for injury, those patients undergoing a significant adhesiolysis have a higher risk of esophageal injury.
- Regardless of adhesiolysis status, unless there is evidence of a leak or high concern for one postoperatively, we initiate clear liquids immediately postoperatively with smooth advancement to full liquid diet on postoperative day one. They are maintained on antiemetics, as needed.
- In our group, we perform selective postoperative water-soluble esophagrams for type III, type IV, or any revisional PEHs for evaluation of immediate postoperative rehernation and evaluation for esophageal or gastric injury.
- In patients with any concern for pleural violation and capnothorax, we maintain this cohort of patients on supplemental oxygen to facilitate more rapid absorption.
- Patients are advised to crush all tablets or take liquid forms of their home medications. Extended-release formulations are converted to immediate formulations in concert with our in-house pharmacists.
- Patients are advised to avoid carbonated beverages and using straws given the increased risk of air trapping.
- A majority of patients are discharged on postoperative day 1, with a subset of patients who have oral intolerance or medical comorbidities necessitating additional time to convalesce.
- At discharge, patients are maintained on a proton pump inhibitor (PPI) and full liquid diet for 1 to 2 weeks. They are then transitioned to a puree diet for 1 week and then a soft diet for the following week. Patients are seen at 2 and 6 weeks from the date of surgery.

OUTCOMES

- Common complications following laparoscopic PEHR include gas bloating, recurrent GERD, dysphagia, recurrence of PEH, slipped fundoplication, and mesh erosion (if used).
- Outcomes are dependent on the presentation of the patient, with more favorable outcomes in patients who are operated on in the elective setting.
    - Overall morbidity and mortality is low in the elective setting with rates of 0.5% compared to 7.5% in the emergent setting.[7]
- Recurrences: While radiographic recurrences are more common and have been previously reported as high as 50% in some series, symptomatic recurrences are less frequently observed.[7,8] A meta-analysis of 13 retrospective studies reported a clinical recurrence rate of 10.2% (range of 3%-33%), which correlated with a radiographic recurrence rate of 25%. Recurrences were less frequent in patients undergoing a Collis gastroplasty.[9,10] However, symptomatic recurrences requiring reoperation are infrequent, often reported as low as less than 10%,[11] more often attributed to recurrent reflux (2.4%) and dysphagia (2.4%).
- Regardless of approach, patients undergoing PEHR endorse symptomatic relief of heartburn, regurgitation, reflux, dysphagia, and chest pain when evaluating patient-centered outcomes.[12]
- With regard to outcomes of partial vs complete fundoplication, Koch et al in a randomized control trial of 100 patients demonstrated similar outcomes in gastrointestinal quality of life and GERD symptoms.[13] This was recently corroborated in a 2020 systematic review of nine randomized control trials and five observational studies (relative risk (RR) = 0.96, 95% confidence interval (CI): 0.90-1.03, I^2 = 47%, P = .06).[14] However, in patients undergoing 360° wrap, there was a higher occurrence of dysphagia and the inability to belch when compared to those undergoing the partial wrap (270°). In a 2020 systematic review of studies evaluating partial and complete wraps, these data were corroborated though it did not reach statistical significance (RR of dysphagia: 0.73, 95% CI: 0.52-1.02).[14]
- While it not routine practice to use mesh reinforcement, a landmark series by Oelschlager et al in a prospective randomized trial of patients undergoing crural repair with small intestine submucosa (Surgisis, Cook Medical, Bloomington, IN) compared to primary repair showed early promising outcomes of decreased PEH recurrence rate at 6 months (9% Surgisis vs 24% primary repair)[15]; however, in long-term follow-up at 58 months, there was no statistical difference (54% Surgisis, 59% primary repair).[16] Given these data, Inaba et al reviewed their group's selective use of biologic mesh in the repair of PEHs in which they found a low reoperation rate. Selective use includes revisional procedures, patients with poor tissue quality, and perceived high hiatal tension at the time of procedure.[17]

REFERENCES

1. Landreneau RJ, Del Pino M, Santos R. Management of paraesophageal hernias. *Surg Clin*. 2005;85(3):411-432. doi:10.1016/j.suc.2005.01.006
2. Hyun JJ, Bak YT. Clinical significance of hiatal hernia. *Gut Liver*. 2011;5(3):267-277. doi:10.5009/gnl.2011.5.3.267
3. Stylopoulos N, Gazelle GS, Rattner DW. Paraesophageal hernias: operation or observation? *Ann Surg*. 2002;236(4):10.
4. Covey AM, Brody LA, Maluccio MA, Getrajdman GI, Brown KT. Variant hepatic arterial anatomy revisited: digital subtraction angiography performed in 600 patients. *Radiology*. 2002;224(2):542-547. doi:10.1148/radiol.2242011283
5. Crespin OM, Yates RB, Martin AV, Pellegrini CA, Oelschlager BK. The use of crural relaxing incisions with biologic mesh reinforcement during laparoscopic repair of complex hiatal hernias. *Surg Endosc*. 2016;30(6):2179-2185. doi:10.1007/s00464-015-4522-1
6. Malm J, Rosen M, Ponsky J, Fanning A. Anterior gastropexy may reduce the recurrence rate after laparoscopic paraesophageal hernia repair. *Surg Endosc*. 2003;17(7):1036-1041. doi:10.1007/s00464-002-8765-2
7. Luketich JD, Nason KS, Christie NA, et al. Outcomes after a decade of laparoscopic giant paraesophageal hernia repair. *J Thorac Cardiovasc Surg*. 2010;139(2):395-404.e1. doi:10.1016/j.jtcvs.2009.10.005
8. Hashemi M, Peters JH, DeMeester TR, et al. Laparoscopic repair of large type III hiatal hernia: objective followup reveals high recurrence rate. *J Am Coll Surg*. 2000;190(5):8.
9. Mattar SG, Bowers SP, Galloway KD, Hunter JG, Smith CD. Long-term outcome of laparoscopic repair of paraesophageal hernia. *Surg Endosc*. 2002;16(5):745-749. doi:10.1007/s00464-001-8194-7
10. Rathore MA, Andrabi SIH, Bhatti MI, Najfi SMH, McMurray A. Metaanalysis of recurrence after laparoscopic repair of paraesophageal hernia. *JSLS*. 2007;5. Published online.
11. Andujar JJ, Papasavas PK, Birdas T, et al. Laparoscopic repair of large paraesophageal hernia is associated with a low incidence of

recurrence and reoperation. *Surg Endosc.* 2004;18(3):444-447. doi:10.1007/s00464-003-8823-4
12. Hall T, Warnes N, Kuchta K, et al. Patient-centered outcomes after laparoscopic paraesophageal hernia repair. *J Am Coll Surg.* 2018;227(1):106-114. doi:10.1016/j.jamcollsurg.2017.12.054
13. Koch OO, Kaindlstorfer A, Antoniou SA, Asche KU, Granderath FA, Pointner R. Laparoscopic Nissen versus Toupet fundoplication: objective and subjective results of a prospective randomized trial. *Surg Endosc.* 2012;26(2):413-422. doi:10.1007/s00464-011-1889-5
14. McKinley SK, Dirks RC, Walsh D, et al. Surgical treatment of GERD: systematic review and meta-analysis. *Surg Endosc.* 2021;35(8):4095-4123. doi:10.1007/s00464-021-08358-5
15. Oelschlager BK, Pellegrini CA, Hunter J, et al. Biologic prosthesis reduces recurrence after laparoscopic paraesophageal hernia repair: a multicenter, prospective, randomized trial. *Trans Meet Am Surg Assoc.* 2006;124:146-155. doi:10.1097/01.sla.0000237759.42831.03
16. Oelschlager BK, Pellegrini CA, Hunter JG, et al. Biologic prosthesis to prevent recurrence after laparoscopic paraesophageal hernia repair: long-term follow-up from a multicenter, prospective, randomized trial. *J Am Coll Surg.* 2011;213(4):461-468. doi:10.1016/j.jamcollsurg.2011.05.017
17. Inaba CS, Oelschlager BK, Yates RB, Khandelwal S, Chen JY, Wright AS. Characteristics and outcomes of patients undergoing paraesophageal hernia repair with selective use of biologic mesh. *Surg Endosc.* Published online 2021. doi:10.1007/s00464-021-08399-w

Chapter 8 Collis Gastroplasty

Ryland S. Stucke and John G. Hunter

DEFINITION

- Surgical management for gastroesophageal reflux disease (GERD) with hiatal hernia principally requires repositioning of the gastroesophageal junction (GEJ) into the abdomen to achieve adequate outcomes. When a foreshortened esophagus is encountered, esophageal lengthening allows for appropriate location of antireflux procedures below the hiatus. John Leigh Collis first proposed an esophageal lengthening technique via a left thoracotomy in 1957 to address the foreshortened esophagus, therefore avoiding esophageal resection.[1] Collis' technique has subsequently evolved through thoracoscopic and laparoscopic iterations. Our Collis gastroplasty technique involves a fully intraperitoneal laparoscopic approach, whereby a stapled wedge resection of stomach at the angle of His effectively lengthens the distal esophagus about which a fundoplication can be wrapped.[2]

PATIENT HISTORY AND PHYSICAL FINDINGS

- Esophageal foreshortening results from chronic inflammation and fibrotic remodeling of the distal esophagus secondary to advanced GERD (eg, esophagitis, Barrett esophagus, or stricture) and/or a large hiatal hernia.[3] Approximately 10% to 25% of patients with reflux have a shortened esophagus.[4,5] However, the majority of these patients do not require esophageal lengthening as adequate mediastinal dissection typically yields sufficient abdominal esophageal length.[6] Mediastinal dissection can continue as high as is safely feasible, often to the level of the pulmonary veins. Sufficient esophageal length is evidenced by the GEJ lying intra-abdominally without retraction, and a distance between the diaphragmatic hiatus and the GEJ of *at least 2.5 to 3 cm* (approximately the length of a fully opened atraumatic laparoscopic grasper). If 2.5 to 3 cm of intra-abdominal esophageal length cannot be achieved, Collis gastroplasty should be performed.[4] Current series suggest Collis gastroplasty is required in 3% to 25% of reflux operations.

IMAGING AND OTHER DIAGNOSTIC STUDIES

- The preoperative workup for reflux disease includes endoscopy (esophagogastroduodenoscopy [EGD]), esophagram (upper gastrointestinal contrast swallow or esophagram), high-resolution esophageal manometry, and pH probe testing. Ambulatory 48-hour pH testing is not mandated if evidence of reflux disease (eg, esophagitis, Barrett esophagus, or stricture) is identified on endoscopy. Esophageal foreshortening requires intraoperative assessment for diagnosis, but can be suspected based on preoperative testing. Contrast esophagram and endoscopy may suggest esophageal foreshortening when certain findings are present[3,7]:
  - Hiatal hernia of 5 cm or more
  - Giant type III paraesophageal hernia (**FIGURE 1**)
  - Esophagitis, Barrett changes, and/or stricture

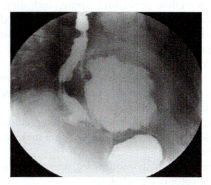

FIGURE 1 • Esophagram demonstrating tortuous esophagus with shortening, distal narrowing or strictures, and a type III paraesophageal hiatal hernia.

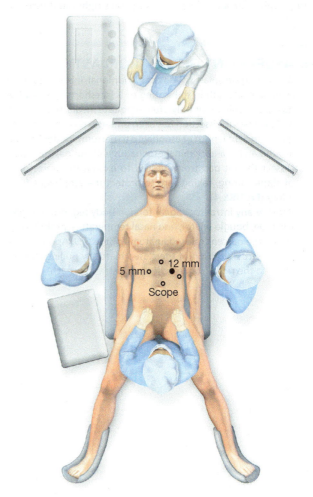

FIGURE 2 • Patient positioning for foregut and antireflux procedures and trocar placement. The left upper quadrant 12-mm port is used for the angulated stapler in the surgeon's right hand.

SURGICAL MANAGEMENT

Preoperative Planning

- Because the Collis gastroplasty is an adjunctive procedure during gastric fundoplication, the principles of a proper antireflux procedure apply, including left and right crural exposure, adequate mediastinal dissection, atraumatic esophageal retraction, and division of the short gastric vessels. Please refer to Chapters 7 and 9 for further details.
- All studies, including esophagram, EGD, manometry, and pH testing should be readily available and reviewed prior to and at the time of surgery.
- Attention to the manometric report should guide fundoplication selection. A Nissen fundoplication may be detrimental in the setting of[8]:
  - Severe esophageal dysmotility (eg, scleroderma esophagus)
  - Heller myotomy for achalasia

Positioning

- Although there are many port placement techniques, the stapled Collis gastroplasty necessitates an endoscopic, angulating stapler introduced with the surgeon's right hand through a 12-mm trocar in the left upper quadrant. Steep reverse Trendelenburg is the position of choice (**FIGURE 2**).
- Assume extensive mediastinal dissection will be required (**FIGURE 3**), increasing the likelihood of inadvertent pleural communication. The sterile skin preparation must be high and wide enough in case tube thoracostomies are necessary from resultant pneumothorax.

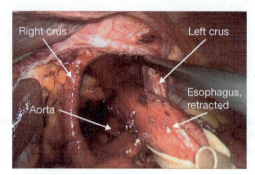

FIGURE 3 • Demonstration of adequate dissection of the mediastinum with clear visibility of the left and right crura, aorta posteriorly, and proximal length achieved of the distal esophagus.

TECHNIQUES

MEASUREMENT OF GASTROPLASTY

- Of note, gastroplasty facilitates additional intra-abdominal esophageal length in the setting of a foreshortened esophagus and should occur only after adequate mediastinal, hiatal, and perigastric dissection has been undertaken in an effort to gain sufficient length of esophagus to perform fundoplication around an intra-abdominal esophagus without gastroplasty.
- Dissect the fat pad from the GEJ to expose the trajectories of stapler firing, taking care to protect the esophagus from injury (**FIGURE 4**).
- Remove any intraesophageal foreign body (eg, oro/nasogastric tube, bougie dilator, and nasal temperature probe) to re-create the nascent relaxed anatomy of the GEJ. Approximate the eventual position of the closed hiatus by pulling the left crura to the right from a posterior gastric approach.

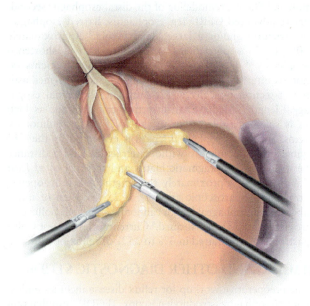

FIGURE 4 • Gastroesophageal junction fat pad dissection. The fat pad is elevated with an atraumatic grasper and resected to define the contours of the gastric wall.

- With an open, premeasured grasper, the intra-abdominal length for the gastroplasty is then estimated (**FIGURE 5**). A distance from the anterior hiatus to the GEJ of less than 2.5 to 3 cm warrants the Collis gastroplasty.
- The gastroplasty landmark is identified by measuring 3 cm distal from the lateral border of the GEJ. A light cautery burn on the serosa 1 cm lateral to this position guides the trajectory of the first perpendicular staple firing.

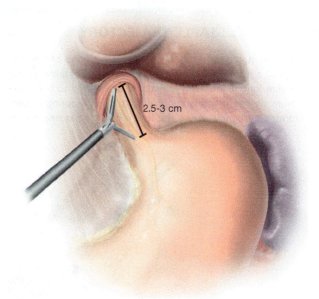

FIGURE 5 • Measurement of intra-abdominal length of esophagus. With a closed crura, the minimum distance between the gastroesophageal junction and the diaphragm should be at least 2.5 cm, or the approximate length of an opened atraumatic grasper.

INTRA-ABDOMINAL RETRACTION AND BOUGIE PLACEMENT

- A 48-Fr dilator is placed transorally (**FIGURE 6**). This serves as the stent about which the Collis gastroplasty is performed.
- The surgeon's left hand elevates the gastric fundus toward the patient's left shoulder while the assistant retracts the greater curve laterally to the left flank.

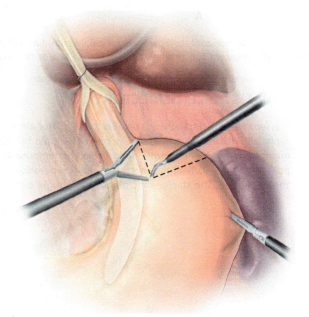

FIGURE 6 • Marking of Collis gastroplasty. With a 48-Fr dilator in place and Penrose drain off tension, measure 2.5 to 3 cm distal to the angle of His and mark a point 1 cm lateral to this position.

HORIZONTAL STAPLE TRAJECTORY

- The first staple trajectory is performed with one or two firings of a rotating and articulating endoscopic stapler using 45 mm long loads. With the stapler articulated to the maximum degree in the surgeon's right hand, stapling is performed perpendicular to the long axis of the stomach and bougie, and up to the body of the bougie dilator just distal to the point predetermined and marked with electrocautery (**FIGURE 7A-C**). Most frequently a second firing of the horizontal staple line is needed to insure that the gastric tube is not too wide. As a "*rule of thumb*," one tries to push the stapler tips around the dilator, and allow the dilator to be pushed out of the stapler jaws as it closes.

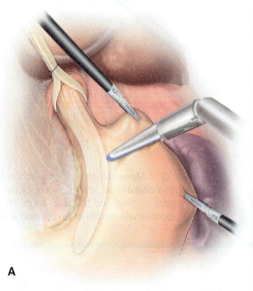
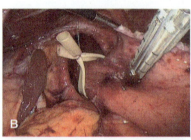
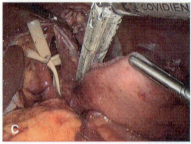

FIGURE 7 • **A,** Horizontal staple trajectory. **B,** Maximal articulation of the stapler to the surgeon's left, aiming toward the previously marked spot adjacent to the dilator. This may take one or two firings to approximate the staple line so it abuts the inserted dilator **(C)**.

VERTICAL STAPLE TRAJECTORY

- The second stapled trajectory is parallel to the dilator aiming cephalad (**FIGURE 8A** and **B**). Again, one or multiple firings might be needed. The Penrose drain should be temporarily positioned proximally in the chest to avoid incorporation in the staple line. The stapler should abut the bougie dilator without placing the tissue on stretch. The proper Collis gastroplasty creates a uniform diameter of the proximal fundus, GEJ, and esophagus (**FIGURE 8C**).
- Remove the wedge of stomach through any means, whether directly through the trocar or via an endoscopic bag. This concludes the Collis gastroplasty portion of the procedure.

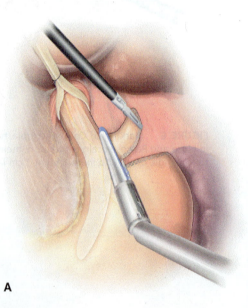
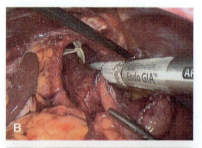
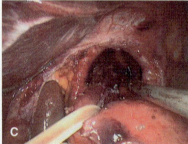

FIGURE 8 • **A,** Vertical staple trajectory. **B,** The vertical staple line is created by firing the stapler parallel and flush against the dilator to create a uniform tube. **C,** The resultant gastric staple line abuts the esophagus.

COMPLETION OF THE FUNDOPLICATION

- Perform the intended complete (Nissen; 360°) or partial (Toupet; 270°) fundoplication as described in other chapters, along with crural closure. The vertical staple line will orient in a posterolateral position, while the horizontal staple line with wrap posteriorly and become the superior edge of the fundoplication (FIGURE 9). The fundoplication should overlap the neoesophagus with the superiormost stitch landing just at the GEJ. Leak test and EGD assessment are routinely performed. We do not routinely place a surgical drain in the operative field.

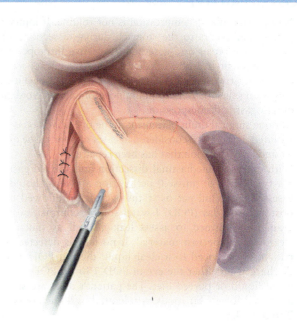

FIGURE 9 • Completion of the antireflux procedure (fundoplication).

PEARLS AND PITFALLS

Inadequate first staple firing	It can be disconcerting to staple onto an endoluminal foreign body (dilator), but it is virtually impossible to staple across a 48-Fr dilator. Failure to staple up to and abutting the dilator will result in a floppy distal esophagus, a wide gastric tube, and decrease in the efficacy of the fundoplication.
Use of short staple loads for first staple firing	The region of the esophageal hiatus is tight quarters. The articulating stapler of 45 mm is preferred over a longer stapler because of the steep angulation needed in these tight spaces. Multiple firings may be needed.
Inaccurate measurement of intra-abdominal length	Key to measuring true intra-abdominal length is the natural lay of the esophagus in the steep reverse Trendelenburg position. Do not insert a dilator, nasogastric, or orogastric tube during this step. Remember to pull the crura together manually and release inferior tension on the esophagus before measuring this length.
Inadequate mediastinal dissection	Inadequate mediastinal dissection results in incomplete abdominal length of the esophagus and may lead to overuse of the Collis gastroplasty. Often the aid of a 0° laparoscope provides better high mediastinal visualization than an angled scope.
Pneumothorax	Prep the bilateral lower chest into the operative field in case percutaneous tube thoracostomy is needed. However, if high peak ventilator pressures from pneumothorax occur, our preferred first step is to place a red rubber catheter through the pleural defect with the opposite end positioned intra-abdominally. Manual bagging and Valsalva maneuvers will often reduce the pneumothorax enough to proceed. An additional step to effectively evacuate pneumothorax, particularly at the case conclusion, is to place one tip of a red rubber catheter through the pleural defect and the opposite end into a bowl of sterile saline (ie, water seal) outside of the patient's abdomen. Evacuation of the pneumothorax with Valsalva maneuvers will be evidenced by bubbles in the water which will eventually cease. A chest tube in not required unless parenchymal injury is suspected or reaccumulation of a pneumothorax occurs.
Ensuring orientation of gastric wedge	The wedge removed should lie on the left lateral aspect along the GEJ encompassing the angle of His, in a plane parallel to the operating table (FIGURE 8A).

POSTOPERATIVE CARE

- Nasogastric tube decompression is not routine. If injury or perforation occurs to the stomach during dissection, adequate tissue repair and a resultant negative intraoperative leak test (methylene blue infusion through the intraoperative oro/nasogastric tube or EGD air insufflation in pooled intracorporeal saline in Trendelenburg position) allow avoidance of nasogastric decompression.
- Routine surgical drain placement in the operative bed is not required, but may be considered in cases of poor tissue quality and/or perforation that has been repaired.
- With extensive mediastinal dissection and stapled gastroplasty, the risk of (missed) perforation and leak should be assessed. Strict nil per os status overnight, followed by a postoperative day (POD) 1 water-soluble contrast esophagram is performed to assess leak as well as functional clearance of contrast material. If no leak is detected, the patient is advanced to a clear liquid diet on POD 1 and discharged on either the eve of POD 1 or on POD 2 with a full liquid or pureed diet. The patient's diets are slowly advanced to regular foods as tolerated over the course of 2 to 3 weeks.
- Temporary use of acid suppression therapy is warranted during the initial recovery period, with ongoing use reassessed based on patient factors and postoperative symptoms.

OUTCOMES

- Collis gastroplasty in addition to hiatal hernia repair and fundoplication does not appear to increase rates of conversion to open approach, leak, stricture, dysphagia, postoperative gastroesophageal reflux symptoms, or hernia recurrence.[9,10] Quality of life, satisfaction with symptom control, and rates of discontinuing antireflux medications are similar between patient who did and did not require Collis gastroplasty during their index procedure.[11]

COMPLICATIONS

- Recurrent hiatal hernia
- "*Slipped*" Nissen
- Postoperative staple line leak
- Leak from extensive mediastinal dissection
- Esophageal stricture

REFERENCES

1. Collis JL. An operation for hiatus hernia with short oesophagus. *Thorax*. 1957;12(3):181-188.
2. Terry ML, Vernon A, Hunter JG. Stapled-wedge Collis gastroplasty for the shortened esophagus. *Am J Surg*. 2004;188(2):195-199.
3. Horvath KD, Swanstrom LL, Jobe BA. The short esophagus: pathophysiology, incidence, presentation, and treatment in the era of laparoscopic antireflux surgery. *Ann Surg*. 2000;232(5):630-640.
4. Johnson AB, Oddsdottir M, Hunter JG. Laparoscopic Collis gastroplasty and Nissen fundoplication. A new technique for the management of esophageal foreshortening. *Surg Endosc*. 1998;12(8):1055-1060.
5. Swanstrom LL, Marcus DR, Galloway GQ. Laparoscopic Collis gastroplasty is the treatment of choice for the shortened esophagus. *Am J Surg*. 1996;171(5):477-481.
6. O'Rourke RW, Khajanchee YS, Urbach DR, et al. Extended transmediastinal dissection: an alternative to gastroplasty for short esophagus. *Arch Surg*. 2003;138(7):735-740.
7. Shouhed D, Patel DC, Shamash K, et al. Patient expectations after collis gastroplasty. *JAMA Surg*. 2020;155(9):888-889.
8. Limpert PA, Naunheim KS. Partial versus complete fundoplication: is there a correct answer? *Surg Clin North Am*. 2005;85(3):399-410.
9. Nason KS, Luketich JD, Awais O, et al. Quality of life after collis gastroplasty for short esophagus in patients with paraesophageal hernia. *Ann Thorac Surg*. 2011;92(5):1854-1860; discussion 1860-1861.
10. Zehetner J, DeMeester SR, Ayazi S, Kilday P, Alicuben ET, DeMeester TR. Laparoscopic wedge fundectomy for collis gastroplasty creation in patients with a foreshortened esophagus. *Ann Surg*. 2014;260(6):1030-1033.
11. Lu R, Addo A, Broda A, et al. Update on the durability and performance of Collis gastroplasty for chronic GERD and hiatal hernia repair at 4-year post-intervention. *J Gastrointest Surg*. 2020;24(2):253-261.

SECTION IV: Treatment of Gastroesophageal Reflux

Chapter 9 | Laparoscopic Nissen Fundoplication

Hope T. Jackson and Brant K. Oelschlager

DEFINITION

- Gastroesophageal reflux disease (GERD), as defined by the Montreal Consensus Group in 2006, is caused by gastric reflux, causing troublesome symptoms and/or complications to the patient that adversely affect their well-being.[1] Symptoms can include heartburn, acid brash, regurgitation, dysphagia, noncardiac chest pain, and pulmonary symptoms such as cough and hoarseness. Complications include esophagitis, Barrett esophagus, esophageal stricture, and aspiration pneumonia.
- GERD results from incompetency or dysfunction of the lower esophageal sphincter (LES). Important factors for adequate LES function include esophageal contraction, gastric cardia sling fibers, diaphragmatic crus, and intra-abdominal position of the LES complex. Hiatal hernias efface the natural valve anatomy, allowing the gastroesophageal (GE) junction to be displaced into the chest, exposing the LES to negative intrathoracic pressure and increased GE reflux. A certain amount of GE reflux is physiologic and not pathologic. However, once symptoms become troublesome to the patient, a diagnosis of GERD can be made.
- GERD can also be due to inadequate esophageal motility resulting in poor clearance of physiologic reflux. Similarly, delayed gastric emptying can lead to GERD due to the increased volume and duration of gastric contents that can potentially reflux into the esophagus.
- A fundoplication is the use of the gastric fundus to recreate the LES valve function. Various fundoplication configurations exist (eg, Nissen, Dor, Toupet) and differ by the number of degrees that encircle the esophagus, the location of the wrap, and the approach used to create the fundoplication.

DIFFERENTIAL DIAGNOSIS

- Peptic ulcer disease
- Esophageal motility disorder (eg, achalasia)
- Malignancy (eg, esophageal or gastric)
- Anatomic abnormality (eg, hiatal hernia)
- Eosinophilic esophagitis
- Coronary artery disease
- Biliary colic
- Pancreatitis
- Functional heartburn
- Hypersensitive esophagus
- Functional dyspepsia
- Other functional bowel diseases (ie, inflammatory bowel syndrome)

PATIENT HISTORY AND PHYSICAL FINDINGS

- The most common GE reflux symptoms reported are heartburn, acid regurgitation, and dysphagia. Atypical presentations are related to laryngeal or pulmonary manifestations such as cough, chest pain, hoarseness, wheezing, globus sensation, and aspiration.[2]
- Patients presenting to a surgeon to discuss GERD treatment have often already trialed acid-reducing therapy in the form of proton pump inhibitors (PPIs). It is important to query the patient's response to these medications. If the patient does not have at least symptomatic improvement to PPI therapy, alternative diagnoses should be considered. Heartburn will almost always improve with PPI therapy, at least partially, within days to a few weeks. Similarly, they will notice worsening of heartburn symptoms with cessation of antacid therapy. Airway symptoms may take longer (2-3 months) and may not respond at all (even when GERD is the etiology).
- Physical examination findings are often limited in a patient with GERD. In all patients with GE complaints, it is important to query about weight loss and hematemesis and to examine for lymphadenopathy, as these could represent an underlying malignancy.

Heartburn

When patients use the term "heartburn," we believe it is very important to ask the patient to actually describe the sensations they are experiencing. Heartburn, as related to GERD, is a retrosternal burning or caustic sensation. Some patients incorrectly use the term heartburn to describe epigastric pain (associated with peptic ulcer disease, gastritis, and functional dyspepsia), right upper quadrant pain (from cholelithiasis or other hepatobiliary diseases), or chest pain (from coronary artery disease). It may also be helpful to ask patients to point on their body as to where they have discomfort when they note that they have heartburn. Classic heartburn does not radiate to the back nor is it usually described as a pressure sensation.

Regurgitation

Regurgitation symptoms can include gastric fluid regurgitation, known as water brash, and/or partially digested food. Regurgitation of food particles can also be associated with esophageal clearance problems such as an esophageal diverticulum or achalasia.

Dysphagia

Dysphagia from a reflux-associated stricture is usually worse with solids than liquids. If both are equally bothersome, a neuromuscular disorder must also be considered. It is important to note that most patients with GERD and dysphagia do *not* have a stricture. Reflux-induced inflammation and local motility effects likely contribute to this sensation of dysphagia.

Airway/Pulmonary Symptoms

Airway-related symptoms (eg, cough, wheezing, voice changes) can be present alone or in conjunction with esophageal symptoms. Disease states that are sometimes related to GERD are idiopathic pulmonary fibrosis (and other interstitial lung diseases), asthma, and recurrent pneumonia.

IMAGING AND OTHER DIAGNOSTIC STUDIES

- Diagnostic testing to confirm objective evidence of abnormal GE reflux is imperative before considering surgical management for GERD[3] Appropriate workup for GERD seeks to establish abnormal esophageal exposure, identify any anatomical and functional abnormalities secondary to reflux, and correlate symptoms to reflux events. The following studies are essential to confirm the diagnosis of GERD and investigate any anatomic considerations necessary for successful operative outcomes:
  - pH monitoring (**FIGURE 1**) assesses distal esophageal pH over a period of time (routinely 24-48 hours) and a composite DeMeester score is calculated. An abnormal DeMeester score is greater than 14.7.[4] Factors contributing to this score include percent total time pH less than 4, percent upright time pH less than 4, percent supine time pH less than 4, number of reflux episodes, number of reflux episodes more than 5 minutes, and longest reflux episode. Proportion of upright and supine reflux and proximal extension can also be important and helpful metrics to assess the extent of pathologic reflux.
  - Upper endoscopy evaluates for esophageal injury and Barrett esophagus secondary to GERD while excluding malignant pathology with biopsies as necessary. Endoscopy allows the surgeon to evaluate for the presence of a hiatal hernia as well as to visually inspect the LES. An added advantage is that a 48-hour wireless pH testing (BRAVO) can also be performed at this time.
  - Esophageal manometry (**FIGURE 2**) assesses LES pressure and relaxation as well as esophageal motility. Patients with esophageal motility disorders can easily be misdiagnosed as having GERD based on symptoms. Understanding a patient's esophageal motility is necessary to plan successful antireflux surgery.
  - An esophagogram evaluates GE anatomy and abnormalities such as a hiatal hernia, stricture, diverticula, or tumors.
- Ancillary tests that may also be useful include laryngoscopy, gastric emptying scintigraphy, and impedance testing.

SURGICAL MANAGEMENT

- There is rarely an absolute indication for antireflux surgery in a patient with GERD. Medical management, including acid suppression therapy and lifestyle modifications (eg, dietary changes, weight loss), is usually sufficient to manage most patients' GERD symptoms. Many factors must be considered in making the decision to proceed with antireflux surgery. These include symptom severity, symptom control with medical therapy, complications of GERD (eg, severe esophagitis, esophageal stricture, Barrett esophagus, chronic respiratory complaints), and the generalized health of the patient.
- Patients best suited for an antireflux procedure are those with documented and confirmed GERD for whom medical and lifestyle changes are not providing adequate quality-of-life improvement. When the quality-of-life impairment justifies accepting the risk of surgery, antireflux surgery is indicated.

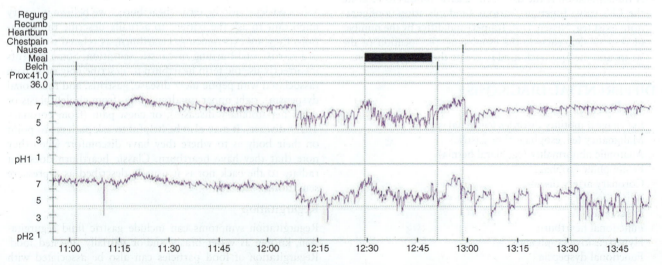

FIGURE 1 • Sample of 24-hour pH tracing demonstrating significant acid reflux with good symptom correlation.

Chapter 9 LAPAROSCOPIC NISSEN FUNDOPLICATION 61

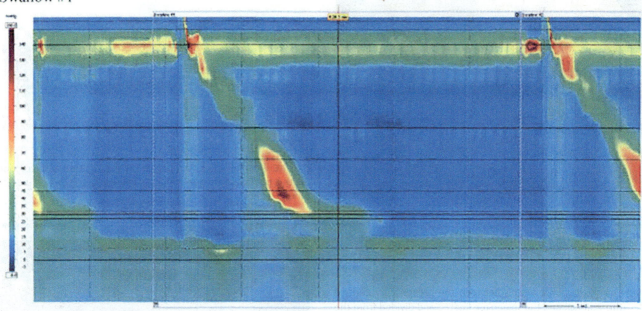

FIGURE 2 • Normal high-resolution manometry.

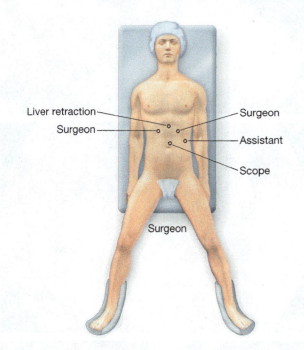

Preoperative Planning

Positioning

- Patient can be positioned in either split leg position or supine position depending on surgeon preference. The split leg position provides superior ergonomics for the surgeon. Both arms should be tucked to not interfere with instrumentation and the patient should be adequately stabilized on the bed to safely accommodate steep reverse Trendelenburg (which allows organs to naturally fall away from the hiatus and left upper quadrant).
- Standard trocar placement includes three working trocars, a fourth trocar for the camera, and a fifth for liver retraction. **FIGURE 3** illustrates standard trocar placement, surgeon, and assistant positioning.
- Elevation of the left lateral lobe of the liver is necessary to visualize the esophageal hiatus. This is most commonly accomplished with a retraction device of the surgeon's choice.

FIGURE 3 • Typical port placement for laparoscopic foregut surgery using a split leg approach.

TAKE DOWN THE LEFT PHRENOGASTRIC LIGAMENT

- After obtaining laparoscopic access to the abdomen and placement of trocars and the liver retractor, the phrenogastric ligament is divided, exposing the left crus. This is most easily accomplished by traction on the GE junction fat pad and the gastric fundus (**FIGURE 4**). Many surgeons start on the right side by dividing the gastrohepatic ligament and right phrenoesophageal ligament. We have found that it is safer to first approach the hiatus from the left, which provides better visualization of both sides of the hiatus, but both approaches are acceptable.

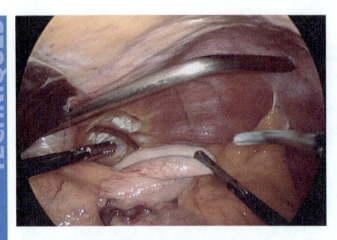

FIGURE 4 • The dissection begins on the left side with traction on the gastroesophageal fat pad caused by retraction of the fundus.

LIGATE AND DIVIDE THE SHORT GASTRIC VESSELS

- The short gastric vessels between the greater curvature of the stomach and the spleen are ligated and divided from the gastric midbody to the angle of His (FIGURE 5). The most superior short gastric vessels can be difficult to expose. Care must be taken to avoid capsule tears to the spleen during this maneuver. We divide the phrenogastric ligament, then make a window medial to the superior most short gastrics, and then take them from medial to lateral in order to avoid traction on these vessels and injury to the spleen. More posterior short gastric vessels and retroperitoneal adhesions must also be released to facilitate full mobilization of the fundus (FIGURE 6).

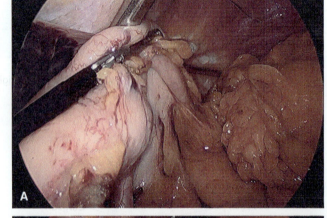

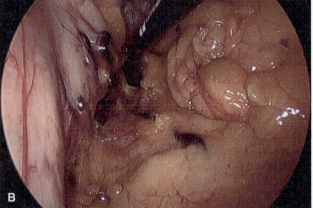

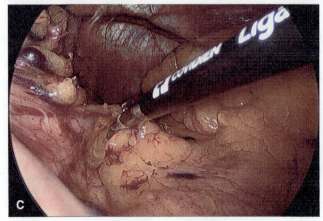

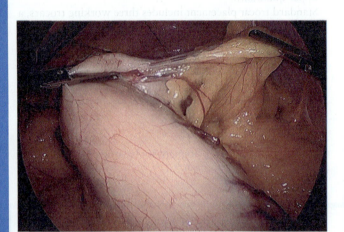

FIGURE 5 • The short gastric vessels are placed on tension to allow for safe division without injury to the stomach. The short gastric vessels are divided close to the greater curve of the stomach.

FIGURE 6 • A-C, The most upper short gastric vessel is posterior and should be divided to free the fundus.

EXPOSE THE ENTIRE LEFT CRUS

- The left phrenoesophageal membrane is opened along its length to expose the left crus (FIGURE 7).

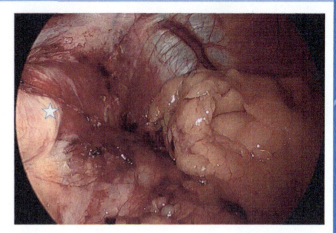

FIGURE 7 • After division of the short gastric vessels, the peritoneal attachments (phrenoesophageal membrane [*star*]) are incised to expose the left crus.

OPEN GASTROHEPATIC LIGAMENT

- The right crus is exposed by opening the gastrohepatic ligament widely, taking care to avoid injury to nerve of Latarjet (FIGURE 8).

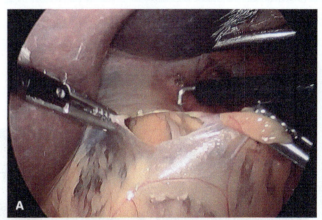

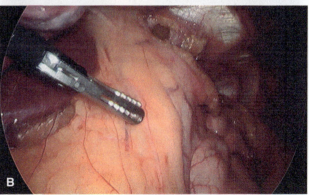

FIGURE 8 • The gastrohepatic ligament is divided with cautery, exposing the caudate lobe of the liver (**A**), taking care to avoid injury to nerve of Latarjet (**B**).

EXPOSE THE RIGHT CRUS

- The right phrenoesophageal membrane is identified overlying the right crus and is divided to expose the crural fibers beneath. The right phrenoesophageal membrane is opened along its length (FIGURE 9).

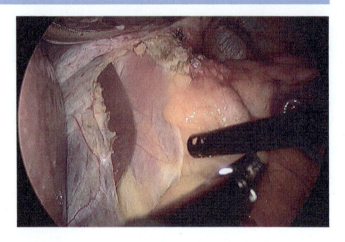

FIGURE 9 • The peritoneal attachments along the right crus are incised.

CONNECT LEFT AND RIGHT HIATAL DISSECTIONS

- The left and right dissections of the phrenoesophageal membrane are connected both anteriorly and posteriorly with caution so as not to injure the anterior and posterior vagus nerves. A Penrose drain is placed around the esophagus to aid in GE junction retraction and esophageal exposure (FIGURE 10).

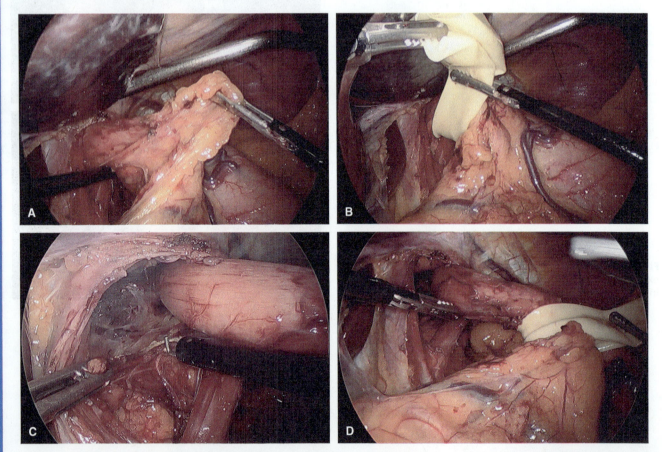

FIGURE 10 • (A) The left and right dissections of the phrenoesophageal membrane are connected both anteriorly and posteriorly (B). A Penrose drain is placed around the esophagus to aid in gastroesophageal junction retraction and esophageal exposure (C). A generous mediastinal dissection is performed with the goal of at least 3 cm of esophagus into the abdominal cavity (D). At least 3 cm of intra-abdominal esophagus is obtained.

ESOPHAGEAL MOBILIZATION

- The areolar connective tissue surrounding the esophagus is exposed and dissected free by retracting the GE junction with the Penrose drain to mobilize adequate intra-abdominal esophageal length (minimum of 3 cm) (**FIGURE 10**). The anterior and posterior vagus nerves as well as the pleura are protected during this dissection.

POSTERIOR CRUS REAPPROXIMATION

- The right and left crura are reapproximated posteriorly with heavy permanent suture (**FIGURE 11**) so that the hiatus comfortably accepts a 52-Fr intraesophageal bougie without any excess room in the hiatus.

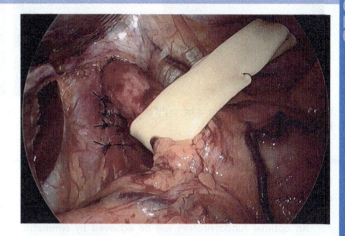

FIGURE 11 • A posterior cruroplasty is performed with permanent sutures (0 silk is our preference shown here).

POSTERIOR STOMACH WALL MARKING STITCH

- Construction of the fundoplication itself is the single critical step where errors are made that affect the short-term and long-term success of the operation. To combat this, we place a loose stitch on the posterior gastric wall to mark the proposed site for the first stitch of the fundoplication. Ideally, this stitch is placed 3 cm distal to the GE junction and 2 cm from the greater curvature (**FIGURE 12**).

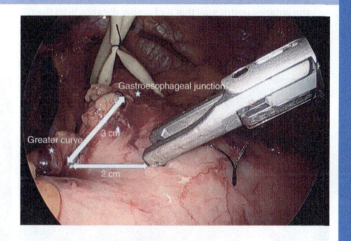

FIGURE 12 • A marking stitch is placed on the posterior gastric wall to identify the portion of the fundus that will be passed posterior to the GE junction.

PASS THE FUNDUS POSTERIOR TO THE GASTROESOPHAGEAL JUNCTION

- The GE junction is then retracted with the Penrose drain and the posterior gastric fundus is grasped and brought posterior to the GE junction (**FIGURE 13**). (Note: If the previously placed marking stitch was well placed, it will become visible as the fundus is passed from the patient's left to the right and will serve to mark the location of the first fundoplication stitch to be placed (**FIGURE 13B**).)

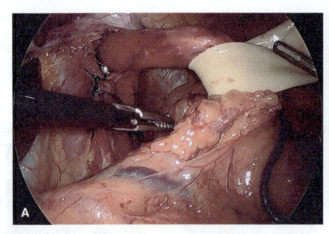
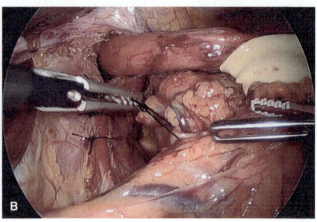

FIGURE 13 • The fundus is brought posterior to the esophagus by retracting the esophagus via the penrose drain (**A**) and using the posterior marking stitch (**B**).

IDENTIFY AND GRASP THE ANTERIOR STOMACH

- An optimal fundoplication will be achieved by symmetric geometry. This is accomplished by identifying the place on the anterior gastric wall that is of similar distance from the GE junction and the greater curvature as the previously placed posterior gastric wall marking stitch (**FIGURE 14A** and **B**).

Once this location is identified, both the anterior and posterior gastric walls are approximated around the distal esophagus at the 10-o'clock position (**FIGURE 14C**). The wrap should be snug without excessive redundancy but not too tight either. The two sites may need to be adjusted slightly to compensate for the size of the esophagus. Contrary to popular belief, making the wrap too floppy can lead to more symptomatic hernias in the case of a recurrent hiatal hernia.

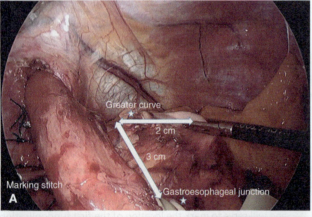
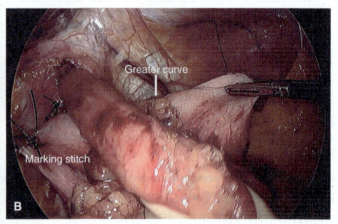
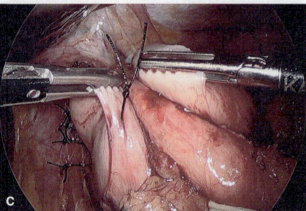

FIGURE 14 • **A-C,** The relationship of the stomach to the esophagus for the fundoplication.

FUNDOPLICATION CREATION

- Once symmetric fundoplication geometry is confirmed, three to four seromuscular permanent sutures are placed from anterior fundus to posterior fundus to secure the fundoplication over a total of 3 cm. Once the first seromuscular stitch is placed (**FIGURE 15A**), the Penrose drain is removed and a 52-Fr intraesophageal bougie is guided into the stomach to aid in fundoplication sizing. To orient the fundal folds appropriately for the second, third, and fourth fundus-to-fundus stitches, grasp the first fundus-to-fundus stitch and retract it cephalad to the right crus (**FIGURE 15B**). This will result in appropriate alignment of the fundal suture line at the 10-o'clock to 11-o'clock positions (**FIGURE 16**).

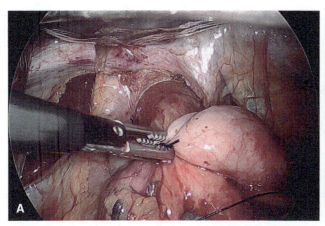 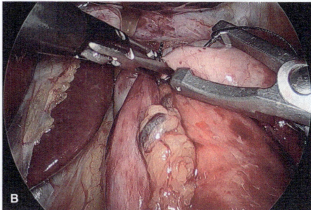

FIGURE 15 • **A** and **B**, The first stitch of the fundoplication is placed most cephalad (**A**). Subsequent sutures are placed by retracting the first fundus-to-fundus stitch cephalad to the right crus (**B**).

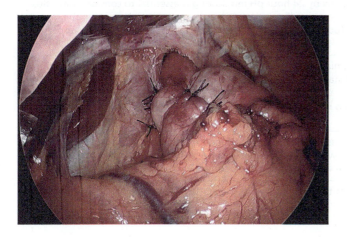

FIGURE 16 • The completed fundoplication with the suture line at the 10-11-o'clock position.

FUNDOPLICATION ANCHORING

- The fundoplication is then anchored with separate stitches to the right and left crura as well as esophagus (fundus-esophagus-crus) to anchor the fundoplication in the abdomen and prevent herniation. Caution must be used so as not to tear the esophageal or crural fibers with these stitches. A final stitch from the posterior fundus to the crural closure can be placed to prevent posterior herniation (the anterior space is protected by the left lateral lobe of the liver) (**FIGURE 17**).

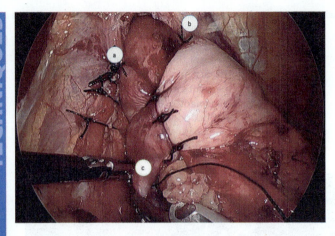

FIGURE 17 • Fundoplication anchoring. Right and left crura are secured to the fundoplication as well as esophagus (fundus-esophagus-crus) (a, b). Posterior fundus to the crural closure to prevent posterior herniation (c).

INTRAOPERATIVE ENDOSCOPY

- Intraoperative endoscopy is used to confirm a well-positioned fundoplication prior to desufflation of the abdomen and removal of trocars.

PEARLS AND PITFALLS

Indications	▪ Objective evidence of abnormal GE reflux by 24-hour pH monitoring is essential to consider antireflux surgery because symptoms alone can be misleading. ▪ Additional mandatory preoperative studies for operative planning: esophageal manometry, upper endoscopy, and esophagogram.
Hiatus dissection	▪ Either a left-to-right or a right-to-left hiatal dissection is acceptable. We prefer starting the dissection on the left as it minimizes the risk of inadvertently tearing short gastric vessels and splenic injury when working from the right. ▪ Mediastinal esophageal mobilization is necessary to gain adequate intra-abdominal esophageal length for proper fundoplication creation.
Fundoplication calibration	▪ A 52-Fr intraesophageal bougie is necessary to calibrate the fundoplication size. ▪ The first fundoplication stitch is easier without the bougie in place. After the first stitch, advancing the bougie into the stomach must be done with caution as the bougie can perforate the GE junction.
Fundoplication orientation	▪ An ideal fundoplication will lay so that the suture line is at the 10- to 11-o'clock positions on the esophagus.

POSTOPERATIVE CARE

- Postoperative dietary modifications: Clear liquids are started postoperatively and are advanced to full liquids the following day. The patient is typically discharged on the first postoperative day. Over 2 weeks, diet is advanced to a soft and then finally a regular diet as the patient's dysphagia resolves.
- Other postoperative instructions: To decrease postoperative bloating, no straws are used and carbonated beverages are avoided. See **FIGURE 18** for a sample Enhanced Recovery After Surgery (ERAS) Protocol.
- Activity restrictions: No lifting greater than 10 to 15 lb or aggressive physical activity is strictly observed for 6 weeks to avoid stress to the diaphragmatic sutures.

OUTCOMES

- Long-term outcomes (median 69-month follow-up) for laparoscopic antireflux surgery reveal 90% of patients have resolved or improved heartburn and regurgitation. Seventy-five percent of patients have resolved or improved dysphagia. Sixty-nine percent of patients have resolved or improved cough and hoarseness.

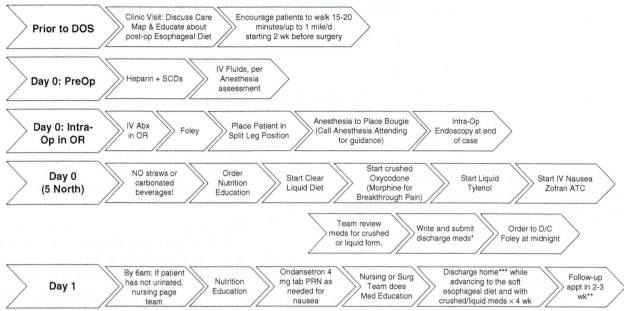

FIGURE 18 • Example of Enhanced Recovery After Surgery (ERAS) fundoplication protocol covering pre-, peri-, and immediate postoperative care.

- Postoperative side effects include new-onset bloating (9%), diarrhea (11%), and dysphagia (2%).
- Ninety percent of patients report that they were happy with their decision to undergo laparoscopic antireflux surgery.[2]

COMPLICATIONS

- Splenic or liver injury
- Hollow viscus perforation
- Dysphagia
- Pneumothorax

REFERENCES

1. Vakil N, van Zanten SV, Kahrilas P, et al. The Montreal definition and classification of gastroesophageal reflux disease: a global evidence-based consensus. *Am J Gastroenterol.* 2006;101:1900-1920.
2. Oelschlager BK, Quiroga E, Parra JD, et al. Long-term outcomes after laparoscopic antireflux surgery. *Am J Gastroenterol.* 2008;103(2):280-287.
3. Bello B, Zoccali M, Gullo R, et al. Gastroesophageal reflux disease and antireflux surgery—what is the proper preoperative work-up? *J Gastrointest Surg.* 2013;17(1):14-20.
4. Johnson LF, DeMeester TR. Twenty-four hour pH monitoring of the distal esophagus. A quantitative measure of gastroesophageal reflux. *Am J Gastroenterol.* 1974;62:325-332.

Chapter 10

Laparoscopic Partial Fundoplication for Gastroesophageal Reflux Disease

Jennifer Colvin and Kyle A. Perry

DEFINITION

- Gastroesophageal reflux disease (GERD) is a chronic condition resulting from the reflux of gastric contents into the esophagus and is associated with a spectrum of symptoms, with or without tissue injury.[1,2]

DIFFERENTIAL DIAGNOSIS

- Several conditions, including irritable bowel syndrome, achalasia, gallbladder disease, coronary artery disease, or psychiatric disorders, can present with heartburn as the main symptom.

PATIENT HISTORY AND PHYSICAL FINDINGS

- Heartburn, regurgitation, and dysphagia are considered *typical* symptoms of GERD.
- GERD can also cause *atypical* symptoms such as cough, wheezing, chest pain, hoarseness, and dental erosions.

IMAGING AND OTHER DIAGNOSTIC STUDIES

- Clinical history, based on *symptoms* only, has a low diagnostic accuracy of GERD in about 30% of patients.[3]
- *Upper endoscopy* is often the first test performed to confirm the diagnosis of GERD. However, about 50% of patients with clinical symptoms of GERD do not have endoscopic sign of esophagitis.[3] In addition, endoscopic evaluation is highly operator dependent, especially in the assessment of low-grade esophagitis.[4] Therefore, the major role of endoscopy is to detect Barrett esophagus (usually present in 1%-5% of patients with GERD) and to exclude gastric and duodenal pathology.
- *Barium swallow* is useful for detecting and characterizing the type and size of a hiatal hernia; for determining the location and size of a stricture; and for evaluating length, diameter, and function of the esophagus. This test, however, is not diagnostic of GERD as a hiatal hernia or reflux of barium can be present in the absence of abnormal reflux or absent in the presence of clinically significant GERD.
- *Esophageal manometry* provides information about the lower esophageal sphincter in terms of resting pressure, length, and relaxation and the amplitude and propagation of esophageal peristaltic waves.
- *48-hour ambulatory pH monitoring* is considered the gold standard for the diagnosis of GERD. Its role is key in the workup as it determines the presence and amount of abnormal reflux and it establishes a temporal correlation between symptoms and episodes of reflux (particularly important when cough or chest pain are present).[5] An abnormal score not only confirms the diagnosis but also is an independent predictor for the successful outcome of antireflux surgery.[6] Finally, pH monitoring is mandatory for the proper evaluation of patients who have recurrent symptoms after antireflux surgery.[7]
- *Combined multichannel intraluminal impedance and pH testing* detects episodes of reflux, regardless of the pH of the refluxate, by identifying changes inducted by the presence of liquids and gas in the esophagus. The episodes are classified as acid, weakly acid, or nonacid on the basis of concomitant pH monitoring. This test is useful in identifying bile reflux and does not require cessation of proton pump inhibitors for testing.

SURGICAL MANAGEMENT

- A laparoscopic fundoplication is currently considered the procedure of choice for the treatment of GERD.
- Even though several eponyms are used to describe different antireflux procedures, we believe that it is more important to focus on the technical elements that make a fundoplication effective and long lasting.
- The type of fundoplication (total vs partial) is tailored to the quality of esophageal peristalsis as documented by the preoperative manometry. In the United States, a partial fundoplication is proposed only to patients with very impaired

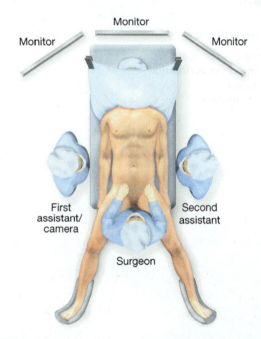

FIGURE 1 • Position of the patient and surgical team in the operating room.

Chapter 10 LAPAROSCOPIC PARTIAL FUNDOPLICATION FOR GASTROESOPHAGEAL REFLUX DISEASE

or absent esophageal peristalsis in order to reduce the risk of postoperative dysphagia.

Preoperative Planning
- A careful symptomatic evaluation is performed in every patient before surgical intervention.

Positioning
- After induction of general endotracheal anesthesia, the patient is positioned in split-leg position with footboards and arms tucked.
- Because increased abdominal pressure from pneumoperitoneum and the steep reverse Trendelenburg position decrease venous return, pneumatic compression stockings are always used as prophylaxis against deep venous thrombosis.
- An orogastric tube is placed to keep the stomach decompressed during the procedure.
- The surgeon stands between the patient's legs. The first and second assistants stand on the right and left side of operative table (**FIGURE 1**).

PLACEMENT OF PORTS

- Five trocars are used for the procedure (see **FIGURE 2B**).
  - Pneumoperitoneum to 15 mm Hg is established using a Veress needle.
  - The abdomen is then marked with the following landmarks: midline and costal margins at steepest points (**FIGURE 2A**).

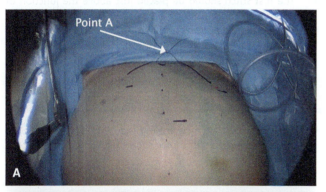
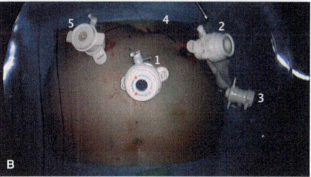

FIGURE 2 • Placement of the ports *(1-5)*. **A,** Anatomical landmarks and measurements for trocar placement. **B,** Final trocar placement for laparoscopic fundoplication.

- **Port 1** (a 10-mm step trocar) is placed 15 cm inferior to the point where lines marking the costal margins transect (see point A in **FIGURE 2A**). This is placed approximately 1 to 2 cm to the left of midline. This is used as the camera port.
- A 30° scope is inserted to inspect the abdomen and the other trocars are inserted under laparoscopic vision.
- **Port 2** (12-mm step trocar) is placed along the left costal margin 12 cm from the point A. This is used for the surgeon's right hand.
- **Port 3** (5 mm step trocar) is placed in the left lateral abdomen at the same level of port 1. It is used by the assistant for traction on the gastroesophageal junction and to take down the short gastric vessels.
- **Port 4** is placed in the epigastrium and is used to place the Nathanson liver retractor to elevate the left lobe of the liver and expose the gastroesophageal junction. The retractor is held in place by a self-retaining system fixed to the operating table.
- **Port 5** is placed along the right costal margin at the same level as port 2. This is used for the surgeon's left hand.
- The instrumentation necessary for laparoscopic partial fundoplication is reported in **TABLE 1**.

Table 1: Instrumentation for Laparoscopic Partial Fundoplication

12-mm trocar, 10-mm trocar, 5-mm trocar × 2
30° scope
Graspers
Needle driver
Scissors
Laparoscopic clip applier
Ultrasonic dissector
Liver retractor
2-0 braided permanent sutures
0 braided permanent sutures
Pledgets
Penrose drain
56 Fr esophageal bougie

DISSECTION OF CRUS (▶ VIDEO 1)

- The gastrohepatic ligament is divided, beginning the dissection above the caudate lobe of the liver, where the ligament is thinner, and continuing toward the diaphragm until the right pillar of the crus is identified.
- The right pillar of the crus is separated from the esophagus by blunt dissection. Dissection is continued anteriorly toward the confluence with the left crus.
- Dissection is carried along the left crus.
- Dissection is then carried inferiorly along the right crus to the confluence with the left crus. The esophagus is separated from the right crus.
- Care should be taken to avoid injury to the vagus nerves during dissection.

DIVISION OF THE SHORT GASTRIC VESSELS

- The short gastric vessels are taken down all the way to the left pillar of the crus, starting at the level of the inferior pole of the spleen (▶ Video 2).

CREATION OF A WINDOW AND PLACEMENT OF A PENROSE DRAIN AROUND THE ESOPHAGUS

- The esophagus is retracted upward and a window is opened by a blunt and sharp dissection under the esophagus, between the gastric fundus, the esophagus, and the left pillar of the crus (▶ Video 3).
- The window is enlarged, and a Penrose drain is passed around the esophagus and secured in place with an Endoloop (▶ Video 3).
- Any hiatal hernia is completely reduced and a minimum of 3 cm of intra-abdominal esophageal length is achieved (▶ Video 4). (See Chapter 8 for short esophagus.)

CLOSURE OF THE CRURA

- Interrupted pledgeted sutures of 0 Ethibond are used to close the diaphragmatic crura (▶ Video 5).
- Retraction of the esophagus upward and toward the patient's left with the Penrose drain provides proper exposure.
- The first stitch should be placed just above the junction of the two pillars.
- Additional stitches are placed 1 cm apart, and a space of about 1 cm is left between the uppermost stitch and the esophagus.

INSERTION OF THE BOUGIE INTO THE ESOPHAGUS AND THROUGH THE ESOPHAGEAL JUNCTION

- The orogastric tube is removed, and a 56 Fr bougie down the esophagus through the esophagogastric junction is inserted.
- The crura must be snug around the esophagus but not too tight: A closed grasper should slide easily between the esophagus and the crura.

PARTIAL FUNDOPLICATION

- *Partial posterior fundoplication*
  - The gastric fundus is gently pulled under the esophagus with two graspers, taking care to grasp the greater curve. The portion of fundus that will be used for the right side of the wrap is carefully chosen and the top portion of the right side of the wrap is grasped with the left hand. The greater curve is then grasped with the right hand and a shoe-shine maneuver is performed to ensure proper orientation and that there is no redundant fundus. Once this is done, the left hand does not let go of its position on the fundus (▶ Video 6).
  - A 2-0 Ethibond suture is placed between the muscular layer of the esophageal wall and the gastric fundus. A second suture of 2-0 Ethibond is placed inferior to the first stitch on the right side of the wrap. When taking the esophageal bites, care is taken to avoid injury to the anterior vagus nerve (▶ Video 7).
  - The greater curve on the patient's left side is again grasped and the proper location for the top stitch on the left side of the wrap is confirmed. Once this is done, a suture of 2-0 Ethibond is placed between the gastric fundus and the muscular layer of the esophagus, again taking care to avoid injury to the anterior vagus nerve. An additional suture is placed inferior to this stitch on the left side of the wrap (▶ Video 8).
  - A third suture is placed inferiorly on each side of the wrap (▶ Video 9).
  - The resulting wrap measures about 270° (FIGURE 3).
- *Partial anterior fundoplication* (See Chapter 16 for more details.)
  - It is a 180° anterior fundoplication.
  - Two rows of sutures (2-0 silk) are used. The first row is on the left side of the esophagus and has three stitches. The top stitch incorporates the fundus of the stomach, the muscular layer of the left side of the esophagus, and the left pillar of the crus.
  - The second and third stitches incorporate the gastric fundus and the muscular layer of the left side of the esophagus.

Chapter 10 LAPAROSCOPIC PARTIAL FUNDOPLICATION FOR GASTROESOPHAGEAL REFLUX DISEASE

- The fundus is then folded over the esophagus so that the greater curvature of the stomach is next to the right pillar of the crus.
- The second row of sutures on the right side of the esophagus consists of three stitches between the fundus and the right pillar of the crus.
- Finally, two additional stitches are placed between the fundus and the rim of the esophageal hiatus to eliminate any tension from the fundoplication.

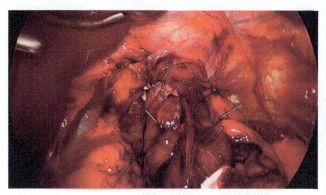

FIGURE 3 • Completed Toupet fundoplication.

PEARLS AND PITFALLS

Indications	■ A careful evaluation, including manometry, pH monitoring, upper endoscopy, and barium swallow must be done.
Placement of ports	■ Extreme care must be taken when positioning port 1 because the site of insertion is just above the aorta. ■ If port 4 (liver retractor) is too low, the left lateral segment of the liver will not be properly retracted, resulting in inadequate exposure of the esophagogastric junction. ■ Port 1 (camera port) should be placed slightly to the left of midline to give adequate visualization of the gastroesophageal junction and hiatus. If this port is placed too low, it can make the hiatal and mediastinal dissection difficult. ■ If ports 2 and 5 (surgeon left and right hands) are too low, the dissection at the beginning of the procedure and the suturing at the end will be challenging. It will also be difficult to do a proper mediastinal dissection.
Dissection	■ An accessory left hepatic artery originating from the left gastric artery is frequently present in the gastrohepatic ligament. The vessel should be saved if possible. Placing the Penrose drain superior to the vessel can aid in exposure. If this vessel greatly limits the exposure, it can be divided. ■ The electrocautery should be used with extreme caution. Because of the lateral spread of the monopolar current, vagus nerves may be damaged even without direct contact. A bipolar instrument represents a safer alternative.
Short gastric vessels division	■ Bleeding, either from the short gastric vessels or from the spleen, and damage to the gastric wall are possible complications. ■ Excessive traction and division of a vessel not completely coagulated are usually the main causes of bleeding. ■ A burn caused during dissection of the short gastric vessels or traction applied with the graspers are the most common mechanisms of damage to the gastric wall.
Creation of a window and placement of a Penrose drain around the esophagus	■ Left pneumothorax and perforation of the gastric fundus are two main complications that can occur during this step of the procedure. ■ Left pneumothorax is usually created when the dissection is performed in the mediastinum above the left pillar of the crus rather than between the crus and the gastric fundus. ■ Proper identification and dissection of the left pillar of the crus are crucial. ■ Perforation of the gastric fundus is usually caused by pushing a blunt instrument under the esophagus or by using monopolar electrocautery for dissection.
Closure of the crura	■ The bougie is not placed inside the esophagus during this step of the procedure in order to have proper exposure for suturing.
Insertion of the bougie into esophagus and through esophageal junction	■ The most serious complication during this step is an esophageal perforation. ■ Lubrication of the bougie and instruction to the anesthesiologist to advance the bougie slowly and to stop if any resistance is encountered help to prevent this complication. ■ All instruments must be removed from the esophagogastric junction and the Penrose drain must be opened. In this way, the creation of an angle between the stomach and the esophagus, which increases the risk of perforation, is prevented.
Partial fundoplication	■ Atraumatic graspers must be used to reduce the risk of injury to the gastric wall.

POSTOPERATIVE CARE

- Patients are usually discharged on postoperative day 1.
- Patients start clear liquids on the day of surgery and are discharged home on a full liquid diet.
- Diet is advanced to soft solids after 1 week. Patients are instructed to avoid meat, bread, and carbonated beverages.
- The time to full recovery ranges between 4 and 6 weeks.

OUTCOMES

- Long-term studies conducted in United States have reported less effective control of GERD with a partial fundoplication rather than a total fundoplication.[8-10]
- At 5-year follow-up, recurrence of GERD confirmed by pH monitoring is reported in more than 50% of patients after partial fundoplication.[8]

COMPLICATIONS

- Esophageal or gastric perforation can be caused either by traction or by an inadvertent electrocautery burn during any step of the dissection.
- A leak usually manifests itself during the first 48 hours.
- Peritoneal signs will be present if the spillage is limited to the abdomen; shortness of breath and a pleural effusion will be noted if spillage also occurs in the chest.
- The site of the leak must always be confirmed by a contrast study using a water-soluble contrast agent.
- Optimal management of a leak consists of a reoperation and direct repair. An esophagectomy may be indicated in case of a too extensive damage or when the extent of the inflammatory reaction makes the direct repair impossible. Wide drainage, feeding jejunostomy tube placement, and use of a covered esophageal stent may also assist in healing the injury when it cannot be directly repaired.
- Acute gastroesophageal junction and wrap slippage into the chest rarely occurs when the crura are properly closed.[11] The main symptoms of recurrence are dysphagia and regurgitation. A barium swallow confirms the diagnosis.
- The incidence of paraesophageal hernia may be increased if the closure of the crura is not performed or if it is too loose.[11,12]

ACKNOWLEDGEMENT

We gratefully acknowledge the contributions of Marco E. Allaix and Marco G. Patti as portions of their chapter were retained in this revision.

REFERENCES

1. Moraes-Filho J, Cecconello I, Gama-Rodrigues J, et al. Brazilian consensus on gastroesophageal reflux disease: proposals for assessment, classification, and management. *Am J Gastroenterol.* 2002;97:241-248.
2. Vakil N, van Zanten SV, Kahrilas P, et al. The Montreal definition and classification of gastroesophageal reflux disease: a global evidence-based consensus. *Am J Gatreoenterol.* 2006;101:1900-1920.
3. Patti MG, Diener U, Tamburini A, et al. Role of esophageal function tests in the diagnosis of gastroesophageal reflux disease. *Dig Dis Sci.* 2001;46:597-602.
4. Amano Y, Ishimura N, Furuta K, et al. Interobserver agreement on classifying endoscopic diagnoses of nonerosive esophagitis. *Endoscopy.* 2006;38:1032-1035.
5. Patti MG, Arcerito M, Tamburini A, et al. Effect of laparoscopic fundoplication on gastroesophageal reflux disease-induced respiratory symptoms. *J Gastrointest Surg.* 2000;4:143-149.
6. Campos GM, Peters JH, DeMeester TR, et al. Multivariate analysis of factors predicting outcome after laparoscopic Nissen fundoplication. *J Gastrointest Surg.* 1999;3:292-300.
7. Galvani C, Fisichella PM, Gorodner MV, et al. Symptoms are a poor indicator of reflux status after fundoplication for gastroesophageal reflux disease: role of esophageal function tests. *Arch Surg.* 2003;138:514-518.
8. Horvath KD, Jobe BA, Herron DM, et al. Laparoscopic Toupet fundoplication is an inadequate procedure for patients with severe reflux disease. *J Gastrointest Surg.* 1999;3:583-591.
9. Oleynikov D, Eubanks TR, Oelschlager BK, et al. Total fundoplication is the operation of choice for patients with gastroesophageal reflux and defective peristalsis. *Surg Endosc.* 2002;16:909-913.
10. Patti MG, Robinson T, Galvani C, et al. Total fundoplication is superior to partial fundoplication even when esophageal peristalsis is weak. *J Am Coll Surg.* 2004;198:863-869.
11. Patti MG, Arcerito M, Feo CV, et al. An analysis of operations for gastroesophageal reflux disease. Identifying the important technical elements. *Arch Surg.* 1998;133:600-606.
12. Patterson EJ, Herron DM, Hansen PD, et al. Effect of an esophageal bougie on the incidence of dysphagia following Nissen fundoplication: a prospective, blinded, randomized clinical trial. *Arch Surg.* 2000;135:1055-1061.

Chapter 11: The Endoscopic Approach to Gastroesophageal Reflux Disease

W. Scott Melvin and Luke M. Funk

DEFINITION
- Endoscopic therapies for gastroesophageal reflux disease (GERD) include transoral incisionless fundoplication (TIF) and the application of radiofrequency energy to the lower esophageal sphincter (LES). These therapies are designed to reduce GERD symptoms by minimizing the reflux of gastric contents into the esophagus and are alternatives to traditional surgical fundoplication techniques.

DIFFERENTIAL DIAGNOSIS
- Typical GERD symptoms
  - Achalasia
  - Biliary colic/cholecystitis
  - Delayed gastric emptying
  - Esophageal cancer, esophagitis, and esophageal motility disorders
  - Gastritis
  - Hiatal hernia
  - *Helicobacter pylori* infection
  - Irritable bowel syndrome
- Atypical GERD symptoms
  - Coronary artery disease
  - Asthma
  - Bronchogenic carcinoma

PATIENT HISTORY AND PHYSICAL FINDINGS
- History taking should focus on identifying both typical and atypical symptoms associated with GERD.
  - Typical symptoms include heartburn, regurgitation, water brash (salty taste related to salivary secretion), and dysphagia.
  - Atypical symptoms include dyspnea, cough, wheezing, chest pain, recurrent pneumonias, hoarseness, and dental erosions.
- Response to antireflux medications, such as proton pump inhibitors and H_2 blockers is important to illicit, as the majority of patients with typical GERD symptoms will respond to these medications. Failure to respond to these medications should heighten the surgeon's concern that the patient's symptoms may be unrelated to GERD.
- Once the diagnosis of GERD is confirmed with objective testing, several key points should be discussed with the patient:
  - Medical therapy, including lifestyle modifications (ie, diet modification, weight loss, smoking cessation) and antireflux medications, should control typical GERD symptoms for most patients. Surgical intervention is indicated for GERD patients who (1) cannot take antireflux medications due to side effects, (2) would prefer not to take antireflux medications due to cost or lifestyle impact, or (3) continue to experience symptoms despite antireflux medications.
  - Laparoscopic gastric fundoplication (ie, Nissen fundoplication) is considered to be the gold standard surgical therapy for the treatment of GERD. Endoscopic therapies should probably be reserved for GERD patients who are candidates for surgical intervention who (1) would prefer a less invasive option than laparoscopic fundoplication surgery or (2) would be considered too high risk for laparoscopic fundoplication due to comorbidities or previous abdominal surgery, including prior laparoscopic fundoplication.
- Of the two procedures discussed in this chapter, only TIF involves general anesthesia in the vast majority of cases. Conscious sedation is usually adequate for radiofrequency therapy. Thus, poor candidates for general anesthesia (ie, those with cardiopulmonary conditions such as severe chronic obstructive pulmonary disease or congestive heart failure) may be better candidates for radiofrequency therapy. The presence of these comorbid conditions should be sought out in the history. Additional contraindications for these procedures are listed in **TABLE 1**.
- Because there are few physical exam findings associated with GERD, the physical exam should focus on conditions that might suggest an alternative explanation for the patient's symptoms. These include recent weight loss or progressive inability to tolerate solids and liquids (malignancy), atypical symptoms associated with exertion (coronary artery disease or asthma), or diarrhea (irritable bowel syndrome).

IMAGING AND OTHER DIAGNOSTIC STUDIES
- Establishing GERD as the etiology of the patient's symptoms is critical before proceeding with any intervention. Patients may have subjective complaints of heartburn or dysphagia that are unrelated to their reflux disease. The four diagnostic tests that are most commonly used to establish a diagnosis are upper endoscopy, barium esophagogram, pH testing, and manometry.
- Upper endoscopy (esophagogastroduodenoscopy [EGD])

Table 1: Contraindications for Undergoing Treatment

For both procedures
Barrett esophagus (relative)
Dysphagia (ie, multiple times per week)
Esophageal dysmotility, strictures, and varices
Esophagitis (grade C or D esophagitis according to the Los Angeles classification)
Hiatal hernia (>2-3 cm)
Obesity (BMI > 35)

Specific to transoral incisionless fundoplication
Inability to tolerate general anesthesia

BMI, body mass index.

- All patients undergoing an antireflux procedure should have an EGD.
- EGDs can identify the presence of hiatal hernias and rule out other pathology, which may be contributing to the patient's symptoms, such as peptic ulcer disease or malignancy.
- GERD-related complications such as esophagitis, Barrett esophagus, and esophageal strictures can also be identified (**FIGURE 1**).
- Ambulatory pH testing
  - This is considered to be the gold standard test for diagnosing the presence of symptomatic GERD.
  - Patients should typically not be taking their antireflux medications when the study is performed.
  - pH testing can be performed via catheter-based systems (ie, 24-hour pH probe testing) or wireless systems (ie, 48-hour Bravo testing).
  - Both catheter-based and wireless systems allow for the quantification of six variables including total/upright/supine time that the pH is <4, number of reflux episodes, number of episodes longer than 5 minutes, and longest episode. These variables can be combined to calculate the "DeMeester score," which is used by many surgeons as definitive evidence for the presence of GERD.[1]
- Barium esophagogram
  - This is a dynamic fluoroscopic study that characterizes both anatomic and functional aspects of the esophagus. It involves multiple swallows of barium and barium-coated solid food.
  - The two most important things to characterize with a barium esophagogram are the position of the GE junction relative to the diaphragmatic hiatus and overall esophageal motility. The presence of a large hiatal hernia (**FIGURE 2**) or significant esophageal dysmotility is a contraindication for any of the three procedures.[2]
  - Esophagograms can also identify the presence of reflux that is characterized by the spontaneous reflux of barium back into the esophagus. However, they are less sensitive than pH studies and thus a negative finding here does not rule out GERD.
- Video recording of this study is crucial because it allows the surgeon to actively assess esophageal peristalsis and the functional significance of hiatal hernias.
- Manometry
  - Esophageal manometry uses pressure transducers within a transnasal catheter to provide data regarding the LES resting pressure, LES abdominal and total length, and adequacy of LES relaxation. It also characterizes esophageal motility by quantifying the amplitude, duration, and propagation of each contraction.
  - The presence of significant esophageal dysmotility is a contraindication for both procedures.
- Multichannel impedance testing and gastric emptying studies are also used on occasion to identify nonacidic GERD and assess gastric functionality, respectively.

SURGICAL MANAGEMENT

Preoperative Planning

Transoral Incisionless Fundoplication

- At our institution, general anesthesia is administered and the procedure is performed in the operating room.
- Nasotracheal intubation is performed so the oropharynx can be used entirely for the EsophyX device. A bite block is placed to protect the teeth from the device and scope.
- Commonly two physicians perform the procedure. One manipulates the endoscope while the other controls the device.

Radiofrequency Energy Application to the Lower Esophageal Sphincter

- Conscious sedation is usually adequate for use of the Stretta system. At our institution, Stretta is usually performed in the endoscopy suite as opposed to the operating room.

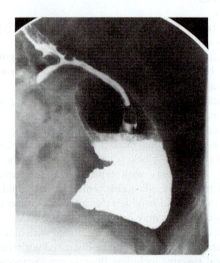

FIGURE 2 • A lateral view of a barium esophagram. A large hiatal hernia is present with a significant portion of the stomach herniated into the chest. A small distal esophageal diverticulum is seen. All three procedures would be contraindicated in the presence of this hernia.

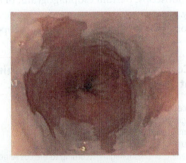

FIGURE 1 • The presence of Barrett esophagus is a contraindication to TIF, radiofrequency energy application, and laparoscopic LES augmentation surgery.

Chapter 11 **THE ENDOSCOPIC APPROACH TO GASTROESOPHAGEAL REFLUX DISEASE**

- Only one physician is typically needed to perform the procedure.

Positioning

Transoral Incisionless Fundoplication

- After intubation, the patient is placed into the left lateral decubitus position with the head elevated slightly (**FIGURE 3**).
- Prophylactic antibiotics are administered before the procedure begins because transluminal fasteners are placed, which may increase the risk of postoperative infections.

Radiofrequency Energy Application to the Lower Esophageal Sphincter

- After administration of conscious sedation medications, the patient is placed into the left lateral decubitus position and a bite block is placed.

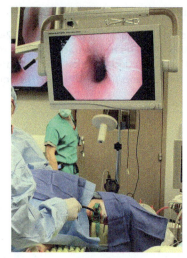

FIGURE 3 • With the patient in the left lateral decubitus position and a nasotracheal tube present, a bite block is placed to facilitate passage of the endoscope and subsequently the EsophyX device.

TRANSORAL INCISIONLESS FUNDOPLICATION

- Approved by the U.S. Food and Drug Administration (FDA) in 2007, the only TIF device that is currently available for use in the United States is the EsophyX device (EndoGastric Solutions, Redmond, WA).
- EsophyX re-creates the LES by plicating the distal esophagus and the gastric cardia together, thus creating an antireflux valve similar to that of a laparoscopic Nissen fundoplication.
- The device consists of a handle, an 18-mm diameter shaft, a tissue invaginator composed of holes in the side of the device (which are connected to a suction device), an articulating arm, which approximates gastric and esophageal tissue and deploys the tissue fasteners, a helical screw, two stylets, and 20 polypropylene H-fasteners (10 plication sets) (**FIGURE 4**).

Placement of the Transoral Incisionless Fundoplication Device into the Stomach

- Preprocedure endoscopy is performed to verify anatomic landmarks.
- A 56-Fr bougie is inserted into the esophagus and then removed to facilitate subsequent passage of the EsophyX device (**FIGURE 5**).
- The EsophyX device is lubricated and a standard endoscope is threaded through the device (**FIGURE 6**). Both are placed through a bite block and advanced through the esophagus into the stomach.
- The scope is advanced into the gastric lumen and then retroflexed to examine the GE junction. Using a standard, high-flow insufflator, the stomach is insufflated with carbon dioxide to a pressure of 15 mm Hg via the working channel of the endoscope. Once the articulating arm is visualized

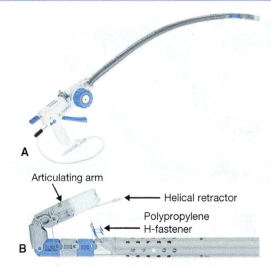

FIGURE 4 • **A,** EsophyX device with the articulating arm fully extended. **B,** Articulating arm is flexed with the H-fasteners visible between the shaft and the distal end of the articulating arm. The helical retractor is visible as well. (Images © 2017 EndoGastric Solutions, Inc.)

within the stomach, the scope is withdrawn into the device, the articulating arm is flexed, and the scope is then advanced back into the retroflexed position within the gastric lumen (**FIGURE 7**).

- The exact positioning of the fasteners has evolved for optimal outcomes over time. Most commonly, using the retroflexed view, the GE junction is envisioned as a clock face with the 12-o'clock position located at the lesser curvature, the 6-o'clock position at the greater curvature, and the 9-o'clock position located along the posterior gastric wall (**FIGURE 8**).[3]

Anterior Rotational Plication Fasteners

- The closed articulating arm is placed at the 12-o'clock position (**FIGURE 9A**). The helix retractor portion of the device is also at the 12-o'clock position and advanced into the squamocolumnar junction (**FIGURE 9B**). The entire device is then advanced distally a couple of centimeters and rotated clockwise on the screen. This allows the articulating arm to be opened and the helical retractor disengaged from the articulating arm.
- The articulating arm is then rotated back to the 6-o'clock position, partially closed, and pulled back 1 to 2 cm (**FIGURE 9C**). The GE junction is advanced caudally by applying tension to the helical retractor.
- The stomach is then desufflated and the articulating arm is rotated toward the 1-o'clock position. This maneuver rotates the fundus anteriorly around the esophagus thereby initiating the fundoplication. Externally, the handle of the device is rotated approximately 180° (**FIGURE 10**). This has been described in the literature as the "Bell Roll maneuver."[3]
- The helical retractor and articulating arm are secured in place and the suction is applied.
- The first H-fastener set is then deployed.
- The stomach is then reinsufflated to visualize deployment of a pair of H-fasteners. Two sets of additional H-fasteners are subsequently placed at varying distances from the GE junction.
- This will result in the placement of six fasteners 1 to 3 cm above the squamocolumnar junction.

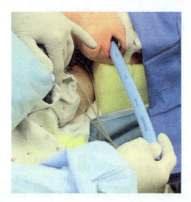

FIGURE 5 • Passage of a large bougie after diagnostic endoscopy facilitates advancement of the EsophyX device into the stomach and minimizes the likelihood of esophageal injury during passage of the device.

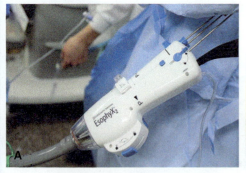
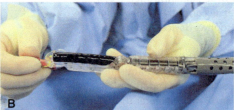

FIGURE 6 • **A,** The endoscope is passed through the handle of the EsophyX device and can be seen exiting the distal end of the device (**B**). The articulating arm is fully extended in this image. Once the scope and device are advanced into the stomach, the scope is withdrawn into the body of the device and the articulating arm is flexed. The scope is advanced back into the stomach and retroflexed to obtain a view of the GE junction.

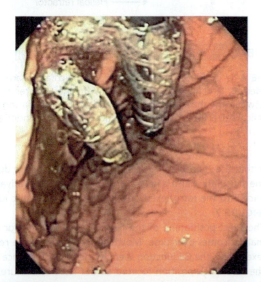

FIGURE 7 • The articulating arm of the device is flexed within the gastric lumen. The arm will subsequently be rotated into the 12-o'clock position at the lesser curve to facilitate placement of the helix retractor.

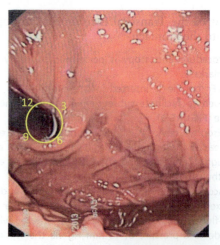

FIGURE 8 • Using a clock face to describe the anatomy of the GE junction in a retroflexed view, the lesser curvature is at 12 o'clock while the greater curvature is at 6 o'clock.

Chapter 11 THE ENDOSCOPIC APPROACH TO GASTROESOPHAGEAL REFLUX DISEASE

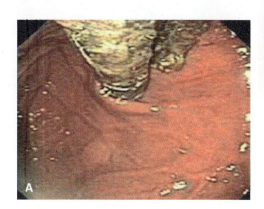
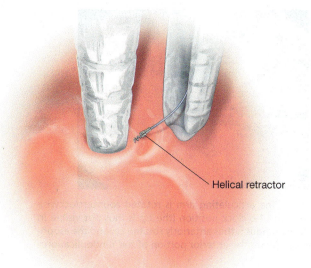
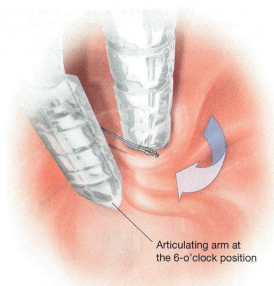

FIGURE 9 • **A,** With the articulating arm at 12 o'clock, the helix retractor is placed into the squamocolumnar junction. **B,** The helix retractor can be seen as a thin, horizontally oriented wire entering the gastric lumen. The device is then advanced distally into the stomach and rotated clockwise on the screen so that the articulating arm is at 6 o'clock **(C)**.

Posterior Rotational Plication Fasteners

- The helix retractor portion of the device is maintained at the 12-o'clock position.
- The articulating arm is rotated counterclockwise through the lesser curve to the 8-o'clock position, partially closed, and pulled back 1 to 2 cm. The GE junction is advanced caudally by applying tension to the helical retractor.
- The "Bell Roll" maneuver is again performed, but this time in the clockwise direction (clockwise on the screen). The stomach is desufflated and the articulating arm is rotated clockwise to the 11-o'clock position. This maneuver rotates the fundus posteriorly around the esophagus (**FIGURE 11**).

- The first set of posterior rotational plication fasteners is then deployed.
- The process is then repeated to place two additional sets of H-fasteners at varying distances from the GE junction.

Anterior Corner Longitudinal Plication

- To address a gap in the anterior component of the plication that is often appreciated only after the anterior and posterior sets have been placed, an anterior corner plication set is often placed.
- The articulating arm is rotated counterclockwise through the lesser curve toward the 1-o'clock position.

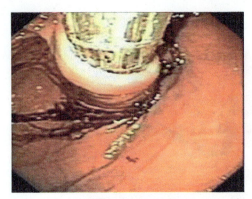

FIGURE 10 • The articulating arm is rotated counterclockwise back toward the 1-o'clock position (the tip is thus not visible in this view). The fundus is thus anteriorly rotated around the esophagus. This completes the anterior portion of the fundoplication.

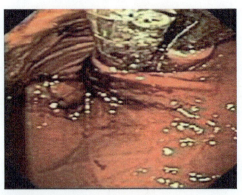

FIGURE 11 • To perform the posterior component of the fundoplication, the articulating arm is rotated clockwise to the 11-o'clock position. This maneuver is a mirror image of the maneuver used to create the anterior component of the fundoplication.

- Tension is applied to the helical retractor caudally and the approximating arm is pulled proximally while desufflating the stomach.
- Two additional sets of H-fasteners are deployed around the 1-o'clock position.

Greater Curve Deep Plication

- The purpose of this maneuver is to fixate the greater curvature slightly more proximally on the esophagus. This lengthens the antireflux valve.
- The helix retractor is disengaged from the 12-o'clock position and re-engaged at the squamocolumnar junction at the 6-o'clock position.
- The reticulating arm is moved into the 5-o'clock position and one or two sets of fasteners are 2 to 4 cm proximal to the squamocolumnar junction (**FIGURE 12**).
- The newly constructed antireflux valve should be 200° to 300° in circumference.

Inspection of the Newly Created Antireflux Valve

- The device and endoscope are withdrawn together and then the endoscope is removed from the EsophyX device.
- The endoscope is then advanced back into the stomach to allow inspection of the antireflux valve and to assess

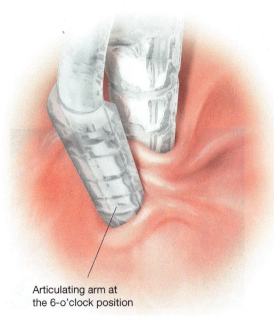

FIGURE 12 • The shaft of the device has been pulled back into the esophagus 3 to 4 cm. This allows placement of the greater curve plication sutures with the articulating arm near the 6-o'clock position. This move adds length to the antireflux valve.

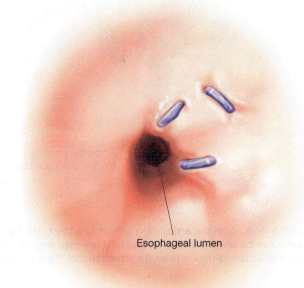

FIGURE 13 • Multiple purple polypropylene fasteners are visualized with the distal esophagus after TIF is completed. These fasteners are not typically seen when retroflexing from within the stomach.

for any bleeding or injuries to the esophagus and stomach. The fasteners are visualized in the distal esophagus (**FIGURE 13**).
- The fundoplication created by the EsophyX device should have a similar endoscopic appearance as one created by a laparoscopic Nissen fundoplication.

Chapter 11 THE ENDOSCOPIC APPROACH TO GASTROESOPHAGEAL REFLUX DISEASE

RADIOFREQUENCY ENERGY APPLICATION TO THE LOWER ESOPHAGEAL SPHINCTER

- Approved by the FDA in 2000, the Stretta system (Restech, Houston TX, USA) is currently the only device on the market that uses radiofrequency energy for the treatment of GERD.[4]
- The application of radiofrequency energy to the GE junction results in thermal injury and subsequent scarring, which reduces LES compliance, decreases the number of transient LES relaxations, and thereby decreases the incidence of reflux symptoms.
- The Stretta system is composed of two main components: a radiofrequency generator and a catheter system that connects to the generator. The catheter system is composed of an outer sheath, a 30-Fr bougie tip, and four nickel-titanium 22-gauge needle electrodes surrounding a balloon. The system also includes a channel for suction and another for irrigation (FIGURE 14).

Placement of the Stretta Device Into the Distal Esophagus

- A standard endoscope is advanced down to the GE junction. The distance from the patient's lips to the squamocolumnar junction is measured.
- A guidewire is inserted through the working channel of the endoscope and the endoscope is removed.
- Under fluoroscopic guidance, the catheter system is then passed over the guidewire into the stomach. The catheter tip is then positioned 1 cm above the squamocolumnar junction based on measurements obtained from the endoscopic evaluation.

Application of Radiofrequency Energy

- The balloon is inflated to a pressure of 2 lb/in.²
- The electrodes are then deployed through the mucosa and into the muscularis propria. Suction and irrigation are initiated through their respective working channels.
- The generator is activated and radiofrequency energy is applied for approximately 90 seconds per application. During this process, the muscularis propria is heated to a temperature of 85 °C, whereas the esophageal mucosa is maintained below 50 °C via cold water that is instilled through the catheter system. This creates four ablation sites that are distributed 90° apart from each other.
- After the 90-second interval is complete, the catheter system is rotated 45° and another cycle of radiofrequency energy is delivered for 90 seconds. Following this cycle, eight lesions approximately 45° apart are created in a circumferential fashion at that level.
- The catheter system is advanced approximately 5 mm and the process is repeated to create another eight sites of ablation. In total, this process is performed at six levels (from 1 cm proximal to the squamocolumnar junction to the proximal gastric cardia), creating 48 ablation sites (FIGURE 15).
- The Stretta system is then removed.

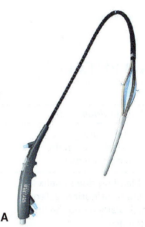

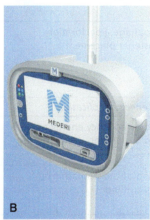

FIGURE 14 • **A**, Schematic representation of the Stretta catheter system. The distal end is composed of a 30-Fr bougie tip. The nickel-titanium needle electrodes can be seen pointing outward surrounding the balloon. **B**, Radiofrequency generator. (Images © 2022 Respiratory Technology Corporation.)

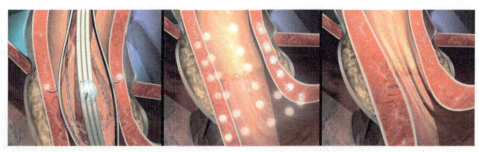

FIGURE 15 • Coronal section through the esophagus with the electrodes positioned 1 cm proximal to the squamocolumnar junction. Two electrodes can be seen entering the muscularis propria. After the non-ablative radio frequency has been applied at six levels (indicated by white dots), the thermal effect stimulates the myofibroblasts resulting in the formation of strong collagen 1 fibers. The net effect is that muscle tissue in and surrounding the lower esophageal sphincter is remodeled, becoming thicker, stronger, and longer. (Images © 2022 Respiratory Technology Corporation.)

Inspection of the Gastroesophageal Junction

- The endoscope is advanced back down to the GE junction to allow inspection of the radiofrequency energy application site (**FIGURE 16**).

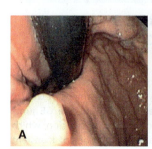 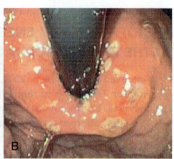

FIGURE 16 • Retroflexed views of the GE junction immediately before **(A)** and after **(B)** use of the Stretta device.

PEARLS AND PITFALLS

Pitfall	Pearl
Transoral incisionless fundoplication	
Cervical esophageal injury during placement of the device given the relatively large size of the device	Dilation of the esophagus with a large bougie (ie, 56 Fr) and generous application of lubricant to the device will minimize the likelihood of esophageal injury. Nasotracheal intubation will help clear the oropharynx for EsophyX device insertion.
Postoperative bleeding due to helix retractor placement or during fastener placement, particularly along the lesser curve of the stomach	Minimize the number of times that the helix retractor is deployed (once at the 12-o'clock position and once at the 6-o'clock position should be enough). Minimize fastener placement along the lesser curvature. Postprocedural EGD will identify early bleeding that may occur during these steps; if identified, endoclips can be placed.
Gastric or esophageal perforation related to fastener placement	Avoid placement of the fasteners through the diaphragmatic crura by ensuring that the fasteners are deployed below the point where the crura cross the esophageal wall. Administer antiemetics aggressively to avoid significant postoperative retching, which may pull on the fasteners.
Radiofrequency energy application	
Imprecise radiofrequency energy application due to patient movement during the procedure	Adequate amounts of anxiolytic and narcotic medications will help minimize patient movement; if necessary, general anesthesia can be administered.
Overdistention of the stomach from excess irrigation fluid	Monitor the suction return closely to prevent the stomach from filling up with irrigant; there should be essentially a 1:1 correlation between irrigation and suction fluid.
Uneven energy application via the four-needle electrodes due to asymmetry of the GE junction (ie, if a small hiatal hernia is present)	More than two device rotations per level may be necessary to ensure that the radiofrequency energy is applied at numerous points throughout the circumference of the esophagus.

POSTOPERATIVE CARE

- TIF—Patients are admitted postoperatively for overnight observation. A liquid diet is initiated following the procedure and advanced to a soft solid diet within the next several weeks. Antiemetics are administered liberally to minimize postoperative retching. Routine postoperative imaging is not obtained.
- Radiofrequency energy application—Patients are discharged home on the day of the procedure. They are kept on a liquid diet for the first several weeks and are subsequently advanced to a soft solid diet. Routine postoperative imaging is not obtained.

OUTCOMES

- TIF—With the earliest case series being published in 2008,[5] truly long-term data regarding TIF are lacking. In 2012, Trad and colleagues[6] published their data, which involved 28 patients and a median follow-up of 14 months. Eighty-two

percent of patients remained off their daily antireflux medications, whereas 68% were satisfied with the results of the procedure.[6] Heartburn and regurgitation symptoms were eliminated in 65% and 80% of patients, respectively.
- Radiofrequency energy application—In the earliest multicenter trial conducted in the United States (involving 47 patients), 87% of patients had discontinued their antireflux medications at 6 months while quality of life improved and esophageal exposure to acid (pH < 4.0) decreased by over 50% (11.7%-4.8% of the total time).[7] Four-year follow-up data from a study published in 2007 found that, along with sustained improvements in quality of life scores, 85% of patients remained off proton pump inhibitors or had decreased their use by half.[8]
- TIF
  - Esophageal laceration/perforation
  - Postoperative bleeding
  - Gastric leak, mediastinal abscess
  - Early fundoplication failure
- Radiofrequency energy application
  - Bloating, dyspepsia
  - Esophageal ulceration/bleeding
  - Esophageal perforation

REFERENCES

1. Herbella AM, Peters JH. Anatomic and physiologic tests of esophageal function. In: Soper NJ, Swanström LL, Eubanks WS, eds. *Mastery of Endoscopic and Laparoscopic Surgery*. Lippincott Williams & Wilkins; 2009:68-82.
2. Howard D, Richards R. Endoluminal therapy for gastroesophageal reflux disease. In: Murayama KM, Chand B, Kothari SN, et al. eds. *Evidence-Based Approach to Minimally Invasive Surgery*. Cine-Med; 2012:29-38.
3. Bell RC, Cadière GB. Transoral rotational esophagogastric fundoplication: technical, anatomical, and safety considerations. *Surg Endosc*. 2011;25:2387-2399.
4. Nikfarjam M, Ponsky JL. Endoluminal approaches to gastroesophageal reflux disease. In: Cameron JL, Cameron AM, eds. *Current Surgical Therapy*. 10th ed. Elsevier; 2010:19-21.
5. Bergman S, Mikami DJ, Hazey JW, et al. Endolumenal fundoplication with EsophyX: the initial North American experience. *Surg Innov*. 2008;15(3):166-170.
6. Trad KS, Turgeon DG, Deljkich E. Long-term outcomes after transoral incisionless fundoplication in patients with GERD and LPR symptoms. *Surg Endosc*. 2012;26:650-660.
7. Triadafilopoulos G, Dibaise JK, Nostrant TT, et al. Radiofrequency energy delivery to the gastroesophageal junction for the treatment of GERD. *Gastrointest Endosc*. 2001;53(4):407-415.
8. Noar MD, Lotfi-Emran S. Sustained improvement in symptoms of GERD and antisecretory drug use: 4-year follow-up of the Stretta procedure. *Gastrointest Endosc*. 2007;65(3):367-372.

Chapter 12
Magnetic Sphincter Augmentation for GERD

William Richards and Richard Rieske

DEFINITION

- Minimally invasive surgical procedures for the treatment of medically refractive gastroesophageal reflux disease (GERD) continue to progress.
- Magnetic sphincter augmentation (MSA) surgery involves the laparoscopic placement of a strand of magnetic beads (**FIGURE 1**) around the esophagus designed to:
  - augment the antireflux barrier of the LES.
  - decrease reflux of gastric contents into the esophagus.[1]
- MSA has been demonstrated safe and effective in controlling GERD symptoms, reducing proton pump inhibitor (PPI) use, and reducing esophagitis, for at least 5 years after surgery.[2]
- This therapy is emerging as an important alternative to traditional Nissen fundoplication because:
  - MSA results in similar objective control of GERD, symptom improvement, but with improved quality of life.
  - Compared with Nissen fundoplication, MSA creates a more physiologic antireflux barrier associated with reduced bloating and reduced flatulence and facilitates belching.
  - In contrast to MSA, Nissen fundoplication rearranges the anatomy of the gastroesophageal junction (GEJ) to create an enhanced valve mechanism but impairs the ability to belch and vomit, which causes many disabling symptoms.[3-5]

DIFFERENTIAL DIAGNOSIS

- Achalasia
- Gastroparesis
- Esophagogastric junction outlet obstruction
- Esophageal motility disorders
- Esophageal malignancy
- Eosinophilic esophagitis
- Candida esophagitis
- Pill-induced esophagitis/ulcer

PATIENT HISTORY AND PHYSICAL FINDINGS

- Patient history centers on typical and atypical GERD symptoms.
  - Typical symptoms include dyspepsia, heartburn, regurgitation, mild dysphagia, and increased salivation associated with foul taste.
  - Atypical symptoms include hoarseness of voice, chest pain, persistent cough, dyspnea, recurrent pneumonias, moderate to severe dysphagia, and dental erosions.
- Adjuncts to oral history taking include objective symptom questionnaires. These surveys help diagnose and quantify patients' individual symptoms. One helpful questionnaire is the GERD Health Related Quality of Life (GERD-HRQL).[6]
  - This is a self-administered, 10-question survey, which tracks individual symptoms using a 5-point scoring scale.
  - A score of 0 represents no symptoms, and a score of 5 represents incapacitating symptoms that render the patient unable to perform daily activities.

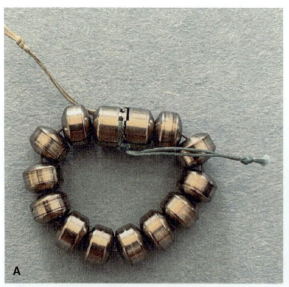
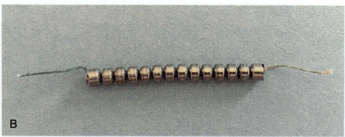

FIGURE 1 • Magnetic sphincter augmentation device. **A,** MSA device as it is clasped in place around esophagus. **B,** Device as it is inserted and placed around esophagus.

- The survey tracks recent medication use with PPI therapy or H2 blockers in relation to symptoms severity.
- The questionnaire highlights the most severe symptoms for the individual patient and can allow the surgeon better insight into symptom management over time when administered across multiple visits.
- Consistent use of acid suppression medications and lifestyle modifications are the mainstay of medical treatment for reflux.
- A patient's response to medication including H2 antagonists and PPIs should be obtained during the interview. Heartburn symptoms typically respond at first to medical therapy but over time lose some of the effectiveness particularly for symptoms of regurgitation.
- If patients report no clinical response to medical therapies, then other causes not related to reflux should be considered. Surgery is reserved for patients who:
  - have persistent symptoms on reflux medications
  - are unable to take medications due to poor tolerance
  - prefer to avoid long-term medication use due to lifestyle factors
- The Caliber study randomized controlled trial of MSA vs escalation of medical therapy convincingly showed that MSA is far superior in symptom control, reduction of esophageal acid exposure, and patient satisfaction compared with escalation of PPI therapy.[7]
- The Caliber study results demonstrate the fallacy of the old adage that, if patients did not respond to PPI therapy, they should not be subjected to antireflux surgery and in fact bolsters the approach of offering MSA to patients who have symptoms of regurgitation while on PPI therapy as the preferred approach.
- The surgeon should specifically ask about a history of allergies to titanium, stainless steel, nickel, or ferrous materials, and these are a contraindication to implantation.
- History of vomiting and suspicion of gastroparesis should be studied with Tc-99 solid phase gastric emptying, and if gastroparesis is identified, it provides a relative contraindication to MSA.
- Postoperative diet for patients with MSA is fundamentally different from a post-Nissen diet in that patients are instructed to eat solid foods frequently (six times/day) or three regular meals with snacks in-between to exercise the LINX beads to prevent scarring around the beads that prevents normal functioning of the beads. Thus, patients who are unable to comply with postoperative diet instructions or who have unusual eating disorders (eating once per day) are not appropriate candidates for MSA shown in **TABLE 1**.

- The surgeon should have a conversation with the patients regarding limitation of MRI scanning after implantation. Current technology of the LINX MSA beads allows the patients to undergo MRI scanning in machines that deliver 1.5 T or less.
- Patients need to notify the physician and radiology staff that they have an implant that will be damaged with a 3-T MRI. Should patients require a 3.0-T MRI they should be advised that this will demagnetize the MSA beads and make the device ineffective.
- After symptom evaluation, objective testing should confirm the clinical diagnosis of GERD, provide an anatomic roadmap of the esophagus and the presence and size of the hiatal hernia, and determine the ability of the esophagus to overcome increased pressure at the lower esophageal sphincter prior to surgical intervention.
- Preoperative patient counseling is an important part of surgical preparation, and the surgeon should emphasize the indications for reflux surgery, the postop diet, and the need to avoid MRI scans >1.5 T.

IMAGING AND OTHER DIAGNOSTIC STUDIES

- All efforts to confirm reflux disease as the cause of the patient's symptoms should be taken prior to surgery. Misdiagnosis of reflux with other diseases that have similar presenting symptoms can lead to patient dissatisfaction and persistence of symptoms after surgery.
- The standard workup for reflux prior to surgical intervention includes high-resolution esophageal manometry (HRM), upper gastrointestinal endoscopy, barium swallow, and 24-hour esophageal pH monitoring.
- In certain cases, use of Technetium-99 scrambled egg gastric emptying study is needed to identify patients with delayed gastric emptying, which needs to be addressed prior to MSA.

High-Resolution Esophageal Manometry

- Manometry is a mainstay in evaluating esophageal motility. New advances have improved the technology to include a high-resolution transnasal catheter, which can detect and transmit intraluminal pressure data into a visual display along the length of the esophagus at 1-cm intervals. This dynamically quantifies esophageal contractions and relaxation of the lower esophageal sphincter over time.
- Disorders of esophageal motility such as achalasia, scleroderma, esophagogastric junction outlet obstruction, <80% peristaltic contractions of the smooth muscle portion of the esophagus, and ineffective esophageal motility are contraindications for MSA.
- HRM also allows measurement of the strength of the esophageal contractions. Vigorous esophageal contractility is identified by an elevated distal contractile integral (DCI). Patients with a DCI greater than 40,000 mm Hg cm/s had a progressive increase in persistent dysphagia with 42.9% of the patients with a DCI greater than 7000 having progressive persistent dysphagia post MSA.
- The surgeon should be alert to the nuances of the HRM study to identify patients with severe vigorous esophageal contractions and offer a partial fundoplication (Toupet, Dor) in place of MSA.

Table 1: Contraindications to Magnetic Sphincter Augmentation

Known or suspected allergy to titanium, stainless steel, nickel, or ferrous materials
Patients who will need to undergo MRI > 1.5 T studies
Inability or unwillingness to adhere to postop diet of 6-7 small solid food meals or solid snacks every 2 h between meals for 8 wk postop
Ineffective esophageal motility

Endoscopic Functional Lumen Imaging Probe

- There is a small cohort of patients who will not tolerate placement of nasal manometry probe to perform HRM.
- The endoscopic functional lumen imaging probe (EndoFLIP) system:
  - investigates geometric data at the GEJ
  - determines the distensibility of the lower esophageal sphincter and the esophagogastric junction
  - measures the cross-sectional area of the GEJ
  - can be performed under conscious sedation in the endoscopy lab while endoscopy is being performed.
- The EndoFLIP can rule out the presence of achalasia or esophagogastric junction outlet obstruction, which are two major contraindications to performance of MSA.[8]

Esophagogastroduodenoscopy

- Upper gastrointestinal endoscopy is necessary in all patients being considered for MSA.
- Esophagogastroduodenoscopy with thorough inspection of the esophagus/stomach and biopsy for identification of Barrett esophagus (using narrow band imaging), concentric furrows consistent with eosinophilic esophagitis (biopsies of distal and mid esophagus), erosive esophagitis, and stricture should be performed.
- The stomach is inspected for ulceration, malignancy, and grading of the gastroesophageal valve to determine the Hill classification and identification of hiatal hernia.

Barium Esophagram

- The barium esophagram utilizes radiographic images with oral contrast to assess the esophagus from a structural perspective.
- The study also provides a functional assessment of motility as motion is recorded across multiple swallows.
- Dysmotility and size and type of hiatal hernia must be assessed to determine suitability for MSA.

Twenty-Four-Hour Esophageal pH Monitoring

- Multichannel 24-hour pH probe testing serves as the gold standard for diagnosing pathologic acid reflux. The probe assesses both the chemical and physical properties of reflux.
- The acidity can be measured, and composition of reflux as liquid, gaseous, or mixed material is determined.
- Several variables are measured including total time that pH is less than 4 by position upright vs supine, the number or reflux episode longer than 5 minutes, and the time of the longest episode.
- These can then be utilized to calculate the DeMeester score. The reflux events are then correlated to clinical symptoms.
- Testing is performed off PPI therapy for 7 days, to confirm the pathophysiologic mechanism of acid reflux that is responsible for the patient's symptoms.

SURGICAL MANAGEMENT

Laparoscopic Magnetic Sphincter Augmentation Minimal Hiatal Dissection

- The original operative approach for MSA was to perform it only in patients who had a hiatal hernia less than 3 cm in size.
- The operative approach was a minimal dissection of the esophageal hiatus with a small 2-cm window made at the medial border of the left crus, then dissection of the right crus, identification of the posterior vagus, and creation of a window between the posterior vagus and the esophagus through which the esophageal sizing instrument is used to measure the proper size of the MSA beads.
- The MSA beads are passed through the window between esophagus and posterior vagus and securely fastened on the esophagus.
- The operative procedure was completed without circumferential dissection of the phrenoesophageal membrane and was only performed on patients with less than 3 cm hiatal hernia.
- A cruroplasty using nonabsorbable 0 suture was performed selectively per surgeon discretion. This minimally invasive approach focused on minimal dissection of the esophageal hiatus with placement of the magnetic beads around the lower esophagus and had good results but was not considered for patients with larger hiatal hernias.
- Recurrence of GERD symptoms after MSA using the minimal hiatal dissection (MHD) was found to be associated with a higher number of post-MSA hiatal hernias, with migration of the MSA beads into the mediastinum, which was thought to be related to failure to repair the hiatal hernia.[9]

Rationale for Complete Dissection of the Gastroesophageal Junction and Repair of Hiatal Hernia With MSA

- In patients with a hiatal hernia and GERD the crural diaphragm is thinner than normal and is associated with decreased lower esophageal sphincter pressure and lower integrated LES relaxation pressures.[10]
- Other studies demonstrate the antireflux barrier of the lower esophageal sphincter is determined by the hiatal hernia crural closure and by the Nissen fundoplication.[11]
- Several surgical groups found that patients with a greater-than-3-cm hiatal hernia could undergo repair of the hiatal hernia and MSA safely with excellent results.[12-14]
- Tatum and colleagues[9] compared MHD, that is, the original surgical strategy of just augmenting the LES with minimal dissection to obligatory dissection (OD) of the diaphragmatic hiatus with obligatory closure of the diaphragmatic hiatus posteriorly with suture.
- The OD of the hiatus with crural closure resulted in reduction in reflux symptoms and reduction in recurrence of hiatal hernia despite a greater proportion of patients with large, more complex hiatal hernias in the OD group.
- The recognition that the diaphragm is an important aspect of the normal antireflux barrier and repair of the hiatal hernia concomitantly to MSA is paramount to understanding the evolution of MSA procedure from MHD to OD as the standard operative approach.

PREOPERATIVE PLANNING

- The operation requires general anesthesia. Prophylactic antibiotics should be administered to reduce risk for postoperative infection.

POSITIONING

- The patient is positioned supine ensuring to apply padding to all pressure points, similar to positioning for laparoscopic Nissen fundoplication.
- Patients may also be placed in the split leg or supine position based on surgeon preference.
- Sequential compression devices are applied.

PORT PLACEMENT

- Standard techniques are used to obtain initial CO_2 pneumoperitoneum, and a 5-mm optical trocar is inserted into the left upper quadrant. The abdominal cavity is then inspected.
- Additional 5-mm trocars are placed in the left flank, the supraumbilical mid abdomen, and the right flank.
- One 10-mm trocar is placed in the right mid abdomen to allow placement of the magnetic beads and use of the 10-mm suturing devices into the abdominal cavity.
- A Nathanson liver retractor is placed to elevate the liver and expose the crura and GEJ.

DISSECTION OF THE GASTROESOPHAGEAL JUNCTION

Original Concept MSA Minimal Hiatal Dissection (▶ Video 1)

- **Step 1.** The fundus of the stomach is dissected of the left crus, and 3 cm of the anterior edge of the inferior medial border of the left crus is freed from the esophagus.
- **Step 2.** The pars flaccida region of the gastrohepatic ligament is opened using the harmonic scalpel, and the medial border of the right crus is identified.
- **Step 3.** The space anterior to the right crus is incised, and blunt dissection is used to dissect behind the esophagus in order to develop the retroesophageal space behind the esophagus and over to the space developed on the left crus.
- **Step 4.** The posterior vagal trunk is identified and allows passage of a 5-mm grasper between the esophagus and the posterior vagus nerve. The grasper coming from the right subcostal position is passed between the posterior vagus nerve and the esophagus so that the vagus is excluded from the augmentation device once placed. A ¼-in Penrose drain is passed into the tunnel between the vagus and esophagus.
- **Step 5.** Remove any tubes (NG < OG) from the esophagus. Use the MSA sizing tool through the far-right side subcostal trocar to measure the diameter of the esophagus through which the esophageal sizer and ultimately the MSA beads can be placed.
- **Step 6.** Insert the correct size MSA beads into the 10-mm trocar and clasp the device securely together. Sutures attached to the magnetic beads are removed, and the procedure is completed.

MSA With Obligatory Dissection of the GEJ and Repair of Hiatal Hernia:

- Port placement and use of the Nathanson liver retractor is identical to the MSA procedure without hiatal hernia repair.
- First the pars flaccida portion of the gastrohepatic membrane is divided using the harmonic scalpel or electrocautery.
- The hepatic branch to the anterior vagus is preserved and the gastrohepatic membrane is divided superior to the hepatic branch of the vagus exposing the right crus.
- The phrenoesophageal membrane or hernia sac is divided using the harmonic scalpel and dissection of the right crus is taken down to the arcuate ligament and the left crus of the diaphragm.
- A retroesophageal tunnel is made bluntly using two graspers or harmonic scalpel to pass posterior to the esophagus and the Penrose drain is placed in position as shown in **FIGURE 2**.
- Then attention is directed to the left crus, which is dissected out dividing the phrenoesophageal membrane down to the

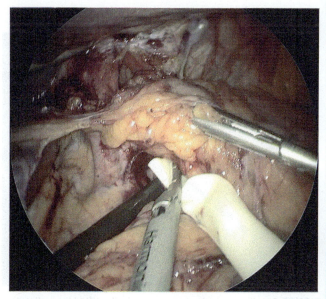

FIGURE 2 • Creation of the retroesophageal tunnel and complete dissection of the phrenoesophageal membrane circumferentially.

position of the Penrose drain, which is then used to retract the esophagus and further divide the phrenoesophageal membrane attachments from the left and right crus to the esophagus using the harmonic scalpel.
- At this time, both the anterior and posterior vagal trunks should be visible and preserved. With blunt dissection and judicious use of the harmonic scalpel, the esophagus is mobilized so that at least 3 cm of lower esophagus is replaced back within the abdominal cavity.
- The esophageal hiatus is closed using interrupted figure-of-eight 0 braided polyester sutures using either intracorporeal or extracorporeal techniques of knot tying to securely close the diaphragmatic hiatus. This is closed to allow a 5-mm grasper to be placed between the right crus and the esophagus without tension as shown in **FIGURE 3**. This is performed without any bougies or nasogastric tubes within the body of the esophagus.

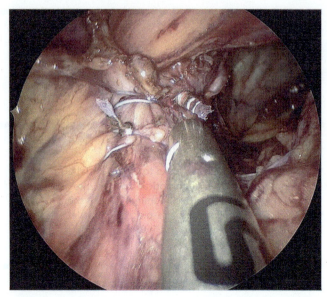

FIGURE 3 • Closure of the esophageal hiatus using 0 polyester braided figure-of-eight sutures posterior to the esophagus. This is closed to fit snuggly around the esophagus so as to allow a closed 5-mm grasper to fit in-between the esophagus and right crus.

DEVICE SELECTION AND PLACEMENT

- The posterior vagus is identified and retracted posteriorly while a Maryland clamp or 5-mm grasper is utilized to dissect the plane between the posterior vagus and the esophagus just above the GEJ as shown in **FIGURE 4**.
- With the esophagus now exposed, a Penrose drain is placed into the upper abdomen and pulled through the space between the posterior vagus and the esophagus just cephalad to the GEJ. This facilitates placement of the sizing device.
- The sizing device is then placed with the surgeon's left hand through the 5-mm port placed laterally almost to the anterior axillary line just inferior to the rib cage behind the esophagus through the retroesophageal plane. The white portion of the sizing device is deployed and tightened around the esophagus ensuring to be cephalad to the hepatic branch of the anterior vagus.

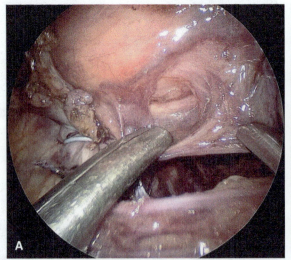 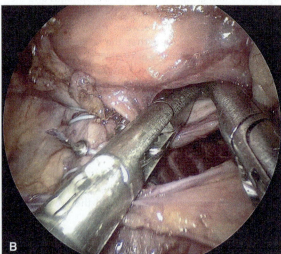

FIGURE 4 • The posterior vagus nerve is identified immediately cephalad to the GE junction in **(A)**. In **(B)** a tunnel between the esophagus and posterior vagus nerve is made bluntly with a Maryland clamp.

Chapter 12 MAGNETIC SPHINCTER AUGMENTATION FOR GERD

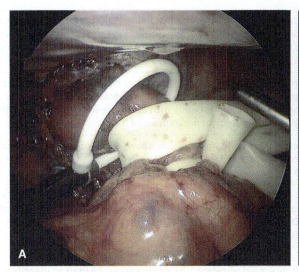
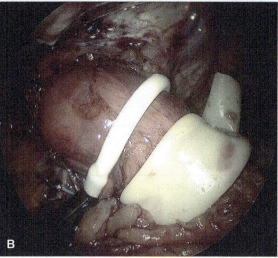

FIGURE 5 • After passing a Penrose drain through the tunnel between the esophagus and posterior vagus, the MSA sizing device is passed from the far right trocar through the tunnel between esophagus and vagus in **(A)**. **B**, The sizing device is used to size the esophagus without any tubes inside. The sizing device should fit loosely around the esophagus and not compress it.

- The sizing tool is closed until it is in circumferential contact with the esophagus but does not compress the esophagus. The appropriate size is indicated on the device, and the sizing device should fit loosely around the esophagus as shown in **FIGURE 5**.[15]
- Another method to size the esophagus measures three beads from the point of release of the magnetic sizing device; for example, if the sizing tool releases at 14, a size 17 LINX device would be chosen.[16] The MSA device is then placed within the abdomen taking care to use minimal handling of the device with laparoscopic instruments and brought through the posterior esophageal space.
- The magnetic clasps are then approximated with manipulation. This is best facilitated by holding the suture in the left hand with a grasper anteriorly while the right hand pulls the other suture posteriorly, and through manipulation the clasp comes together securely.
- While holding the left-hand suture anteriorly the right hand is used to push the clasp securely together. Once the clasp is securely closed, the sutures are removed from the MSA device as shown in **FIGURE 6**. The abdomen is desufflated, the ports are removed, and the skin incisions are then closed.

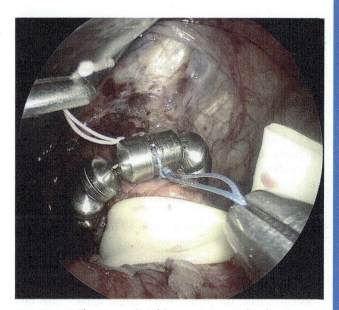

FIGURE 6 • The Magnetic Sphincter Augmentation beads are in place around the esophagus. The MSA beads fit in the small tunnel between the posterior vagus and esophagus.

PEARLS AND PITFALLS

MSA placement using minimal dissection of the crura without complete dissection of the phrenoesophageal membrane left small hiatal hernias undiagnosed and unrepaired.	■ Complete circumferential dissection of the hiatus and closure of the crura posteriorly with figure-of-eight 0 braided sutures reduced recurrent hiatal hernias with migration of the MSA beads into the mediastinum and GERD.[9]
Closure of the esophageal hiatus is not performed. This leads to a high rate of migration of the MSA beads into the mediastinum and GERD.	■ The hiatal closure should be closed securely so that a 5-mm grasper can fit between the crus and the esophagus.

Smaller MSA devices are associated with a higher rate of early and late postoperative dysphagia.	▪ Proper sizing of the MSA device is one of the most important parts of the procedure that will reduce dysphagia. Sizing of the esophagus is done so that there is no compression/indentation of the MSA beads on the esophagus. Most patients will do well with 15-, 16-, or 17-sized MSA device.[16]
Postoperative dysphagia 2-8 wk postop	▪ Postoperative diet (ingestion of solid food 6-7 times per day or with snacks ingested every 2 hours) is essential to provide effective physical therapy to the esophagus and prevent encapsulation of the magnetic beads with inflexible scar. The diet is instituted the day after surgery and continued for a minimum of 8 wk.
More severe postop dysphagia 2-8 wk postop	▪ Institution of oral steroids is helpful and typically allows resumption of regular solid food within 48 h. A treatment regimen that works is Prednisone 10 mg BID for 1 wk, Prednisone 5 mg BID for 1 wk, and Prednisone 5 mg Q Day for 1 wk.
Esophageal spasm 1-8 wk postop	▪ Dietary counseling is important during this early period and many patients find ingestion of cold liquids causes esophageal spasm and dysphagia, which can be alleviated with warm liquids PO and in severe cases Baclofen 10 mg PO TID or course of steroids. Endoscopic dilation is contraindicated until 8 weeks postop.[17]
Dysphagia >8 wk postop not responding to diet or steroids	▪ Endoscopic dilation under fluoroscopy is done with 15 mm diameter endoscopic balloon dilator under direct visualization.[17] Fluoroscopy can be used to identify proper opening and location of the magnetic beads. A course of steroids is administered post dilation along with re-education on eating solid food 6-7 times per day.

POSTOPERATIVE CARE

- Postoperatively, the patient should be placed on multimodal pain therapy to minimize opioid narcotic use. Early recovery after surgery protocols are employed to encourage ambulation, pulmonary toilet, and bowel motility.
- Particular attention is given to the postoperative diet. An MSA postoperative diet consisting of solid foods with small portions administered every 2 hours increases the frequency of swallowing. Through frequent exercise, the motion of the mechanical beads on the MSA device prevents the formation of tight scar bands and minimizes the risk of postprocedural dysphagia.
- Patient education emphasizes the need to continue this diet in the postoperative period for 8 weeks. Adherence to the prescribed MSA diet is imperative for quality outcomes.
- Once the patient has met goals for safe discharge including diet tolerance, adequate oral hydration, and control of postoperative pain, the patient is discharged home. Usual discharge is anticipated on the afternoon of surgery or on the first postoperative day.

OUTCOMES

MSA With Minimal Hiatal Dissection

- Originally the concept of MSA was to perform an MHD of the esophageal hiatus and augment the lower esophageal sphincter with the magnetic beads.
- The exclusion criterion for patients was a greater-than-3-cm hiatal hernia, and occasionally surgeons would perform a posterior cruroplasty based only on the posterior dissection, which again remained minimal.
- The 3-year results were first reported in 2013 and identified that the primary outcome of normalization of esophageal acid exposure or 50% reduction in acid exposure at 1 year was obtained in 64% of the patients. Ninety-three percent of the patients had at least 50% reduction in use of PPIs.[18]
- Long-term results at 5 years revealed that MSA provided a significant and sustained control of gastroesophageal reflux with minimal side effects. There was sustained reduction in median GERD–health-related quality of life (GERD-HRQL) scores from baseline and patients' use of PPIs decreased to only 15.3% at 5 years post implantation. Moderate or severe regurgitation occurred in 57% of patients at baseline, but only 1.2% suffered from regurgitation 5 years after implantation.
- Dysphagia was present in 5% of patients at baseline and only 6% after 5 years. Similarly, gas bloat was present in 52% of patients at baseline but decreased to only 8.3% of patients 5 years after implantation. These 5-year reports results show that MSA provides significant and durable control of GERD with minimal side effects or complications.
- Most of the durability of MSA can be attributed to the fact that the rare earth magnets used in the MSA beads are considered permanent magnets with minimal deterioration after hundreds of years. Of importance, outside of the early postop window no new safety events emerged over the 5 years of follow-up.[2]

MSA With Obligatory Dissection and Hiatal Hernia Repair

- The original procedure was performed in patients without a hiatal hernia using minimal dissection of the esophageal hiatus and placement of the MSA device around the esophagus. The procedure has evolved to a complete, circumferential esophageal and hiatal dissection with posterior repair of the hiatus hernia in patients who have demonstrable hiatal hernias.
- The studies show that patients undergoing concomitant MSA and hiatal hernia repair had nearly equivalent results to patients undergoing only MSA. Eighty-nine percent of the patients undergoing combined MSA/hiatal hernia repair remained off PPIs and 97% of the patients reported resolution or improvement of GERD symptoms.[13,14]

Table 2: Results of MSA vs BID PPI in Caliber Trial[19]

	Baseline	1-y MSA (%)	PPI BID
GERD HRQL >50% improvement		96	0%
Control of regurgitation	0%	96	19%
Dysphagia	15%	7	15%
Bloating	55%	25	55%
PPI use	100%	9	100%
Esophageal acid exposure time %	10.7%	1.3	N/A

- A comparison of outcomes was made between OD of the esophageal hiatus with closure of the hiatus and MHD with no hiatal hernia was repaired. Recurrent GERD was found more frequently after MHD than after OD (16.3% vs 3.6%).
- Dysphagia was more common in the MHD group compared with the OD group (8.6% vs 1.2%), and recurrent hiatal hernia did not occur in the OD group as it did 11.5% of the time in the MHD group. The authors conclude that OD of the esophageal hiatus recognizes and repairs more hiatal hernias as well as yields much better postoperative results.[9]

Medical Therapy vs MSA

- The Caliber study randomized 152 patients with moderate to severe regurgitation symptoms despite once daily PPI use to twice daily PPI therapy or to MSA. MSA was much better than BID PPI in controlling regurgitation symptoms (89% vs 10%, $P < .001$) at 6 months. Furthermore, 91% of the patients with MSA were off PPI therapy, and there were no significant safety issues in the patients with MSA.[7]
- The follow-up at 1 year revealed that MSA was able to reduce regurgitation in 95% of the patients. They concluded that MSA is superior to twice daily PPI therapy in reducing regurgitation symptoms that was sustained over a 12-month period. In addition, 81% of the patients undergoing MSA had improvements in GERD-HRQL greater than 50%, and 91% of the patient's discontinued daily PPI use. It is important to note that the patients with dysphagia decreased from 15% baseline to 7%, as well as bloating decreased from 55% to 25% and esophageal acid exposure time decreased from 10.7% to 1.3% at baseline to 1 year after MSA; shown in **TABLE 2**.

MSA vs Nissen

- Comparisons of laparoscopic Nissen fundoplication (LNF) with MSA have shown that patient satisfaction and GERD-HRQL scores improve when compared with patient's preoperative symptoms while using PPI medications. Furthermore, patients after MSA had much less negative side effects such as gas bloat, inability to belch, and inability to vomit, which were commonly associated with LNF as shown in **TABLE 3**.[3-5]

COMPLICATIONS

Postoperative Dysphagia

- Transient dysphagia in the postoperative period has been very common in large series. Typically, 50% of the patients required endoscopic dilation during the early experience of MSA circa 2013 to 2014. The high rate of dysphagia was

Table 3: Matched Pair Analysis MSA vs LNF at 1-y Postop[4]

	MSA	LNF
PPI use	17%	8.5%
Severe bloating	0%	10.6%
GERD-HRQL	4.2	4.3
Inability to vomit	4.3%	21.3%
Inability to belch	8.5%	25.5%

reduced by the institution of the dietary exercise, that is, eating solid food frequently either with three standard meals with in-between snacks or eating six to seven small meals of solid food per day.
- By 2017 it was found that early dilation prior to 8 weeks post implant created more inflammation with no improvement in symptoms, so a recommendation was made to dilate only after 8 weeks.
- Finally, a change in device sizing was instituted in 2018. Prior to this time sizing was indicated by encircling the esophagus at the GEJ and sizing the implant two beads above the size where the magnetic sizing device released completely.
- In 2018, sizing was changed to three beads larger than the size identified by complete release of the sizing device. The change in the device sizing protocol reduced necessity for endoscopic dilation down to only 18%, and it also reduces the prevalence of immediate dysphagia occurring within the first month after implantation from above 65% down to 36%.[16]

Early Dysphagia First 8 Weeks Postoperative

- Physical exercise for the esophagus, that is, frequent[6,7] small meals of solid food or snacking every 2 hours with solid food in-between meals.
- Avoid cold liquids, and drinking warm liquids such as tea or coffee before meal may relax the esophagus around the device and prevent spasm.
- Avoid endoscopic dilation in the first 8 weeks.
- Baclofen 10 mg p.o. 3 times daily to help control esophageal spasm has been helpful in many patients.
- Use of steroids for more severe dysphagia. One regimen used is prednisone 5 mg tablets, 2 twice daily for 1 week, 1 twice daily for 1 week, 1 daily for 1 week has been very successful in many patients with early dysphagia.
- A few patients develop such severe dysphagia that they are unable to swallow saliva. In this case, they need admission to hospital, intravenous (IV) fluids, and IV steroids; typically, Solumedrol 30 mg Q6h breaks the cycle of inflammation, spasm, and dysphagia. Regular diet is then instituted, and oral steroids are started.

Late Dysphagia After 8 Weeks

- Endoscopic dilation under fluoroscopy is done with 15-mm-diameter endoscopic balloon dilator under direct visualization. Fluoroscopy is extremely useful during the first dilation to identify proper placement, proper opening of the magnetic beads, and closure of the beads.
- A course of steroids is administered post dilation along with reeducation on eating solid food six to seven times per day or even eating solid food snack every 2 hours. Consideration for explanation of the implant should be entertained with

continued dysphagia after three endoscopic dilations have failed to alleviate the dysphagia.
- It has been found that small MSA devices should be avoided secondary to the risk of refractory dysphagia. The antireflux effect of MSA is related to the inhibition of sphincter effacement from gastric distention with the magnetic beads in place. Larger devices sizes 15 to 17 beads appear to offer excellent reflux control with less dysphagia.

Device Migration

- Worldwide there were 9453 devices implanted from February 2007 through July 2017. There have been 29 reported cases of erosions of which the majority (62%) came with the 12-bead-sized device (4.93% erosion rate). Since it was associated with such a high incidence of erosion it is no longer on the market.
- Undersizing the magnetic sphincter device is the most likely contributory factor in the development of erosions of the device. The device functions to resist opening of the LES, which thereby increases the gastric yield pressure. In this additional resting tension of the device compressing on the LES does not increase efficacy. There has been only one erosion among 4399 devices sized 15, 16, or 17 for a 0.02% erosion rate.[20]
- Thus, it is recommended that larger device sizes be used for treatment. Typically, erosions occur more than 1 year after implantation with average median time to erosion of 26 months. Patients present with dysphagia or chest pain, and diagnosis is made with endoscopy.
- Endoscopic removal of the magnetic beads eroded into the esophagus is usually performed first followed by delayed laparoscopic approach to remove the magnetic beads not removed endoscopically. After removal of the magnetic beads laparoscopically, a leak test using endoscopic insufflation of CO_2 while submerging the esophagus and upper stomach under saline is performed.
- The technique for removal of the MSA device requires placement of one 10-mm trocar to remove the beads and three 5-mm trocars and a Nathanson liver retractor to expose the GEJ.
- Monopolar cautery is used with L hook or scissors to use cautery on the capsule right on the magnetic beads. Once the capsule is opened the beads can be pulled up and more capsule divided to allow eventual extraction of the MSA beads. The MSA beads are connected to the adjacent beads with an individual posted wire between each pair; therefore, when a wire is cut, only the two beads immediately adjacent will separate and the device can be extracted with all the beads connected.
- Once the beads are extracted the number of beads must be counted and compared with the number of beads placed in the original operative note to ensure complete extraction of all the foreign bodies. The capsule between the MSA beads and the esophagus is left intact. If the MSA beads are removed for treatment of dysphagia, it is recommended not to perform repeat placement of magnetic beads or antireflux procedures.[21]

Device Malfunction

- Disruption of the ring of magnetic beads has been seen in a very small number of cases. The patient notices recurrence of GERD symptoms, and plain radiographs of the abdomen are diagnostic of disruption of the device. Treatment is extraction with replacement of similarly sized magnetic beads.

REFERENCES

1. Louie BE, Smith CD, Smith CC, et al. Objective evidence of reflux control after magnetic sphincter augmentation: one year results from a post approval study. *Ann Surg*. 2019;270(2):302-308.
2. Ganz RA, Edmundowicz SA, Taiganides PA, et al. Long-term outcomes of patients receiving a magnetic sphincter augmentation device for gastroesophageal reflux. *Clin Gastroenterol Hepatol*. 2016;14(5):671-677.
3. Louie BE, Farivar AS, Shultz D, Brennan C, Vallieres E, Aye RW. Short-term outcomes using magnetic sphincter augmentation versus Nissen fundoplication for medically resistant gastroesophageal reflux disease. *Ann Thorac Surg*. 2014;98(2):498-504; discussion 505.
4. Reynolds JL, Zehetner J, Wu P, Shah S, Bildzukewicz N, Lipham JC. Laparoscopic magnetic sphincter augmentation vs laparoscopic Nissen fundoplication: a matched-pair analysis of 100 patients. *J Am Coll Surg*. 2015;221(1):123-128.
5. Richards WO, McRae C. Comparative analysis of laparoscopic fundoplication and magnetic sphincter augmentation for the treatment of medically refractory GERD. *Am Surg*. 2018;84(11):1762-1767.
6. Velanovich V, Vallance SR, Gusz JR, Tapia FV, Harkabus MA. Quality of life scale for gastroesophageal reflux disease. *J Am Coll Surg*. 1996;183(3):217-224.
7. Bell R, Lipham J, Louie B, et al. Laparoscopic magnetic sphincter augmentation versus double-dose proton pump inhibitors for management of moderate-to-severe regurgitation in GERD: a randomized controlled trial. *Gastrointest Endosc*. 2019;89(1):14-22 e1.
8. Desprez C, Roman S, Leroi AM, Gourcerol G. The use of impedance planimetry (Endoscopic Functional Lumen Imaging Probe, EndoFLIP(R)) in the gastrointestinal tract: a systematic review. *Neuro Gastroenterol Motil*. 2020;32(9):e13980.
9. Tatum JM, Alicuben E, Bildzukewicz N, Samakar K, Houghton CC, Lipham JC. Minimal versus obligatory dissection of the diaphragmatic hiatus during magnetic sphincter augmentation surgery. *Surg Endosc*. 2019;33(3):782-788.
10. E Souza MÂ, Nobre RA, Bezerra PC, Dos Santos AA, Sifrim D. Anatomical and functional deficiencies of the crural diaphragm in patients with esophagitis. *Neurogastroenterol Motil*. 2017;29(1):12899-12900.
11. Louie BE, Kapur S, Blitz M, Farivar AS, Vallieres E, Aye RW. Length and pressure of the reconstructed lower esophageal sphincter is determined by both crural closure and Nissen fundoplication. *J Gastrointest Surg*. 2013;17(2):236-243.
12. Buckley FPIIIrd, Bell RCW, Freeman K, Doggett S, Heidrick R. Favorable results from a prospective evaluation of 200 patients with large hiatal hernias undergoing LINX magnetic sphincter augmentation. *Surg Endosc*. 2018;32(4):1762-1768.
13. Rona KA, Reynolds J, Schwameis K, et al. Efficacy of magnetic sphincter augmentation in patients with large hiatal hernias. *Surg Endosc*. 2017;31(5):2096-2102.
14. Rona KA, Tatum JM, Zehetner J, et al. Hiatal hernia recurrence following magnetic sphincter augmentation and posterior cruroplasty: intermediate-term outcomes. *Surg Endosc*. 2018;32(7):3374-3379.
15. Ethicon. *Steps to Use Esophagus Sizing Tool in a LINX Reflux Management System | Ethicon*.youTube2020; 2020.
16. Ayazi S, Zheng P, Zaidi AH, et al. Magnetic sphincter augmentation and postoperative dysphagia: characterization, clinical risk factors, and management. *J Gastrointest Surg*. 2020;24(1):39-49.
17. Fletcher R, Dunst CM, Abdelmoaty WF, et al. Safety and efficacy of magnetic sphincter augmentation dilation. *Surg Endosc*. 2021;35(7):3861-3864.
18. Ganz RA, Peters JH, Horgan S, et al. Esophageal sphincter device for gastroesophageal reflux disease. *N Engl J Med*. 2013;368(8):719-727.
19. Bell R, Lipham J, Louie BE, et al. Magnetic sphincter augmentation superior to proton pump inhibitors for regurgitation in a 1-year randomized trial. *Clin Gastroenterol Hepatol*. 2020;18(8):1736-1743 e2.
20. Alicuben ET, Bell RCW, Jobe BA, et al. Worldwide experience with erosion of the magnetic sphincter augmentation device. *J Gastrointest Surg*. 2018;22(8):1442-1447.
21. Tatum JM, Alicuben E, Bildzukewicz N, Samakar K, Houghton CC, Lipham JC. Removing the magnetic sphincter augmentation device: operative management and outcomes. *Surg Endosc*. 2019;33(8):2663-2669.

Chapter 13 Redo Fundoplication

C. Daniel Smith

DEFINITION

- A variety of fundoplication procedures are used today (**TABLE 1**), primarily to treat gastroesophageal reflux disease (GERD).
- The 360° fundoplication (Nissen fundoplication) is the most popular of the various fundoplication techniques.
- Although fundoplication, when done by an experienced surgeon, results in control of GERD and significant improvement in quality of life in the majority of patients, this operation does fail, necessitating further surgery or a redo fundoplication.[1-3]
- Broadly speaking, there are three reasons that an operation will fail to control a patient's symptoms and/or GERD:
  - Errors in workup or patient selection
  - Errors in operative management
  - Natural history of the particular antireflux operation or condition being treated

DIFFERENTIAL DIAGNOSIS

- Fundoplication failure is defined as either recurrence of the condition or symptoms that necessitated the fundoplication (eg, recurrent GERD or recurrent hiatal hernia) or the development of new symptoms not present preoperatively (eg, dysphagia, nausea, or regurgitation).
- One typically sees failure of a fundoplication in a few distinct patterns.[4-6] These are outlined in **TABLE 2** and **FIGURES 1** and **2**.
- When considering these reasons for failure, hiatal hernia is the most common cause (44% of cases). Wrap disruption or breakdown is the next leading cause, accounting for 16% of failures. Slipped wraps account for 11.7% of failure, and finally, wraps improperly positioned at the time of their initial construction is found in 3.9% of cases.[7]
- Wrap or crural stenosis is a rare cause of failure and often times hard to determine as a primary etiology of failure.
- If mesh was used at the initial operation, a distinctly different pattern of failure and management strategy is needed.[8]

Table 1: Fundoplication Procedures

360° fundoplication (Nissen fundoplication)
270° posterior fundoplication (Toupet fundoplication)
180° anterior fundoplication (Dor fundoplication)
Posterior gastropexy (Hill procedure)
Transthoracic posterior plication (Belsey procedure)
Endoscopic valvuloplasty (transabdominal modified Belsey)

Table 2: Patterns of Fundoplication Failure

- Wrap disruption or loosening
- Wrap migration or slip
- Hiatal hernia or recurrent hiatal hernia
- Wrap or crural stenosis
- Wrap too loose/tight or misplaced at the initial operation

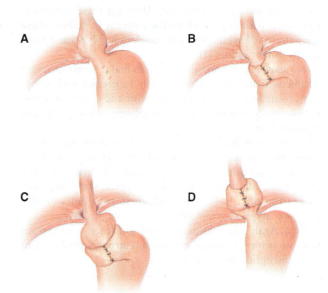

FIGURE 1 • Common anatomic patterns of antireflux surgery failure. **A**, Fundoplication disruption, **B**, tight fundoplication or crural stenosis, **C**, slipped fundoplication, and **D**, hiatal herniation.

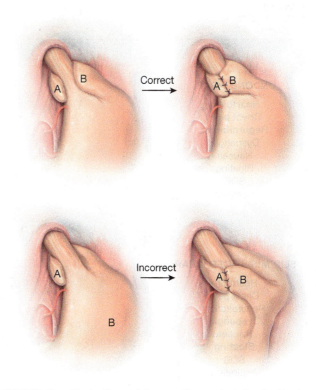

FIGURE 2 • Illustration of incorrectly created fundoplication compared to correct creation.

PATIENT HISTORY AND PHYSICAL FINDINGS

- Common symptoms of failure of fundoplication are outlined in **TABLE 3**.
- Recurrent GERD is the most common (59%) and dysphagia (31%) the next most common. Although these symptoms can occur with any or all of the patterns of failure, there are patterns of symptoms that correlate highly with a given mechanism of failure (**FIGURE 3**).
- Gross anatomic abnormalities such as hiatal hernia or severe wrap/crural stenosis are more likely to present with symptoms related to poor esophageal transit and emptying. These symptoms commonly include dysphagia, chest pain, and regurgitation.
- The wrap that has loosened or come undone more commonly presents with recurrent GERD symptoms, often identical to those being experienced before the first antireflux procedure. Commonly, this includes typical symptoms such as heartburn, regurgitation, and chest pain but can also be more atypical symptoms such as cough, laryngitis, or asthma. Again, the relationship and similarity of symptoms to those before the initial operation is strongly predictive of wrap disruption or loosening.
- A slipped wrap will often have a broad constellation of symptoms with more prevalence of nausea and epigastric pain than the other presentations.
- A favorable response to antisecretories and postural regurgitation predicts wrap loosening or incompetence, whereas poor tolerance of heavy dense foods or weight loss predicts hiatal herniation or esophageal outlet issues. Improvement with dilation supports esophageal outlet restriction. Failure of symptoms to respond to any intervention is more likely with wrap slippage.
- A confusing presentation is the patient with early postprandial bloating or meal-induced diarrhea. With this symptom constellation, one should be suspicious of vagal nerve injury or inflammation (dysfunctional gastric emptying). This symptom complex in the absence of an obvious anatomic abnormality or a positive pH test should lead one to pursue further workup rather than a redo antireflux operation.

IMAGING AND OTHER DIAGNOSTIC STUDIES

- Testing for suspected fundoplication failure falls into testing to secure a diagnosis or reason for failure and testing for operative planning. An algorithm for the workup of patients suspected to have failed a prior fundoplication is shown in **FIGURE 4**.

Establishing the Diagnosis

- In pursuit of a diagnosis of failure, the workup should start with an anatomic assessment. This usually includes an upper endoscopy (esophagogastroduodenoscopy [EGD]) and contrast esophagram.
- Often, a contrast esophagram is all that is needed to identify the pattern of failure. **FIGURE 5** depicts the esophagram findings corresponding to the various patterns of failure.
- Alternatively, an EGD may clearly show an anatomic abnormality. The common endoscopic findings of failure are outlined in **TABLE 4**.

Table 3: Common Symptoms of Fundoplication Failure

- Heartburn
- Chest pain
- Regurgitation
- Dysphagia
- Nausea
- Bloating
- Shortness of breath
- Aspiration

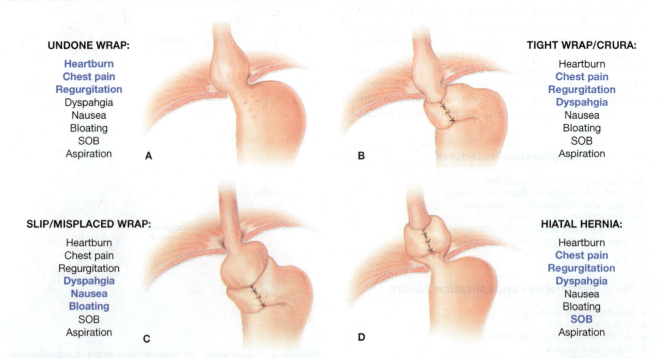

FIGURE 3 • A–D, Symptoms of antireflux surgery failure correlated with anatomic pattern of failure. SOB, shortness of breath.

Chapter 13 REDO FUNDOPLICATION

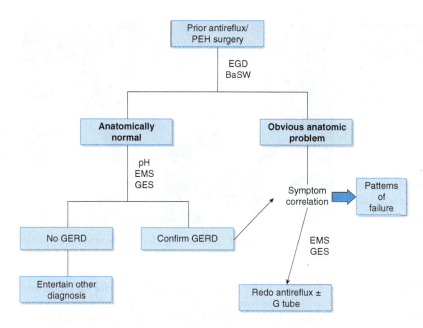

FIGURE 4 • Flowchart of workup for possible antireflux surgery failure. *EMS*, esophageal motility study; *GERD*, gastroesophageal reflux disease; *GES*, gastric emptying study; *PEH*, paraesophageal hernia.

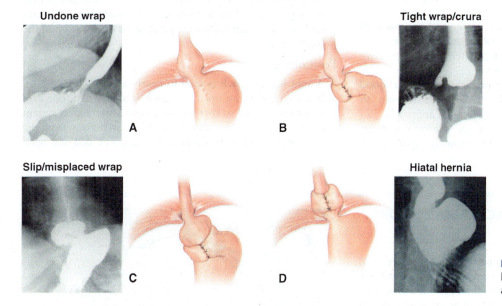

FIGURE 5 • A-D, Contrast swallow examples for each common anatomic pattern of failure.

Table 4: Endoscopic Findings of Failed Fundoplication

Viewing location	Findings (pattern of failure)
Retroflex view of distal esophagus	• Gastric folds extending into wrap (slipped/misplaced fundoplication) • Esophagogastric junction does not hug scope (loose or undone fundoplication) • Gastric mucosa extending above hiatal indentation (hiatal hernia)
Forward view of distal esophagus	• Narrowing that does not accept scope (tight wrap or crural stenosis) • Esophagitis/esophageal ulcers (loose or undone fundoplication) • Constriction on proximal stomach below constriction of wrap (hiatal hernia) • Constriction of wrap distal to esophagogastric junction (slipped or misplaced wrap)

- In many cases, if the presenting symptoms correlate with findings on an esophagram or EGD, this is all that is needed to diagnose failure and the need for reoperation.
- If recurrent GERD is the dominant presentation, then pH testing should be obtained.

Planning for Operative Management

- With a diagnosis of fundoplication failure secured, further testing may be indicated to help plan the most effective reoperative strategy.
- The most common conditions associated with failure that need to be investigated are esophageal motility problems and impairment in gastric emptying. All patients should undergo an esophageal motility study and a gastric emptying study before redo surgery.
- Impairment in esophageal motility may indicate the need for a partial 270° fundoplication rather than a 360° fundoplication.

Classically, a partial fundoplication should be considered if normal esophageal peristalsis is present in less than 70% of swallows or esophageal body pressure is less than 30 mm Hg.
- Delayed gastric emptying may require the addition of a gastrostomy tube to provide gastric decompression in the early postoperative period, thereby preventing gastric distension–induced crural or wrap disruption.

SURGICAL MANAGEMENT

- Redo fundoplication can be both rewarding and challenging. Although the right diagnosis and proper preparation are important, they are no substitute for experience with all manner of foregut surgery. Redo fundoplication should not be undertaken by a general surgeon who occasionally performs elective fundoplication.

Preoperative Planning

- For a skilled laparoscopic surgeon, almost all redos can be approached laparoscopically. Early conversion to an open approach is more likely in the following situations:
  - Multiple prior foregut procedures, especially prior open repairs
  - Hiatal hernia with a significant amount of the stomach incarcerated in the chest, especially if mesh was used
  - Prior operations that were complicated by postoperative leak, fistula, or early reoperation
- In these situations where one may predict a higher likelihood of conversion, it is prudent to be prepared for not only an open approach but also a thoracoabdominal approach.
- Thoracoscopy can be used to mobilize a herniated wrap incarcerated in the chest, thereby allowing laparoscopic reduction and repair.

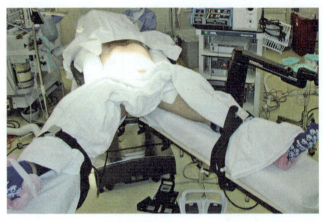

FIGURE 6 • Patient positioning for reoperative antireflux operation.

- EGD should be available intraoperatively for all redos, and an EGD performed by the surgeon before scrubbing provides valuable firsthand anatomic information that is useful intraoperatively. Leaving the scope in the stomach allows intraoperative identification of key anatomic structures such as the squamocolumnar junction or the location of the fundoplication.

Positioning

- A split-leg approach is used in nearly all cases (**FIGURE 6**). If conversion to an open approach is anticipated, one arm should be tucked so that a table-mounted retraction system can be secured at the patient's shoulder, well away from the surgeons' standing position at the patient's side for open access.

TECHNIQUES

GAINING ABDOMINAL ACCESS AND PORT PLACEMENT

- If the prior fundoplication was performed laparoscopically, it is reasonable to attempt abdominal access by passing a Veress needle through an area in the upper abdomen free of prior incisions. The safest means of access is a visualized access using an open technique.
- A five-trocar technique as depicted in **FIGURE 7** is used.

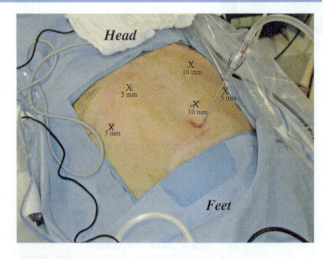

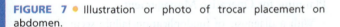

FIGURE 7 • Illustration or photo of trocar placement on abdomen.

IDENTIFY AND EXPOSE HIATAL ANATOMY

- The dissection commences by approaching the esophageal hiatus from the left. The greater curve of the stomach is found and followed upward toward the angle of His while using a tissue-sealing device to divide any remaining short gastric vessels or vascularized scar tissue (**TABLE 5**).

- Once the base of the left crus is found, the left crus is cleared of adhesions up to and around the crural arch as far as possible (**FIGURE 8**). Often, the left lobe of the liver is fused to the fundus starting along the crural arch limiting how much crural arch can be exposed at this point in the operation.
- The mediastinum is entered from the left as far posterior as possible. Usually, this opens a plane just anterior to the aorta

Chapter 13 REDO FUNDOPLICATION

Table 5: Sequence for Successful Hiatal Dissection

- Start along greater curve of the stomach.
- Divide any remaining short gastric vessels (ideally none are encountered).
- Expose the left crus from base through arch.
- Enter the mediastinum from left and posterior to hiatal content.
- Dissect further proximal into the mediastinum and from left to right along the plane anterior to the aorta until over the spine.
- Leave left side of the hiatus and develop the plane between anterior surface of the stomach and undersurface of the liver to find caudate lobe of the liver.
- Following lower edge of caudate lobe of the liver, expose the right crus from base to arch (often need to free wrap adhesions to the right crus).
- Enter the mediastinum from right and complete retroesophageal window.
- Encircle the esophagus with Penrose drain to manipulate and control the esophagus during rest of mediastinal dissection and esophageal mobilization.
- After the hiatus is completely dissected and esophagus mobilized, take down prior wrap by releasing fusion/sutures and dissect wrap from the esophagus.
- Intraoperative endoscopy to identify the location of squamocolumnar junction (adequate esophageal length) and wrap has been completely taken down (retroflexed view).

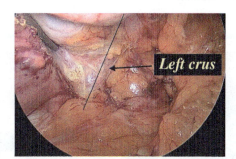

FIGURE 8 • Photo of left crus exposure.

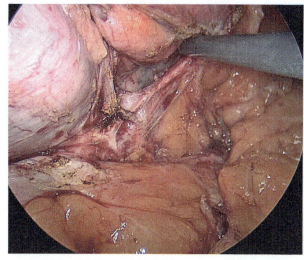

FIGURE 9 • Posterior mediastinum opened from left.

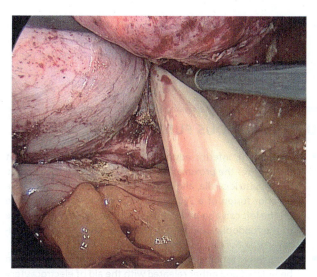

FIGURE 10 • Penrose drain left in mediastinum from left.

and behind the esophagus (FIGURE 9). This plane is often very friendly, allowing the posterior mediastinum to be cleared proximally and to the right, over the top of the aorta toward the spine. A 1/2-in Penrose drain cut 6-in long can be left in the posterior mediastinum (FIGURE 10) to be found later when the mediastinum is entered from the right posteriorly.

- With at least half of the esophageal hiatus exposed from the left, the more complicated dissection of the right crus can be undertaken more safely with some awareness of the esophageal hiatus relationship to the scar plate that tends to envelop the right side of the hiatus.
- Starting distal along the lesser curve of the stomach and well below the adhesions of the left lobe of the liver to the anterior surface of the stomach will often reveal a friendly dissection plane, leading under the caudate lobe of the liver and to the base of the right crus (FIGURE 11).
- Once the base of the right crus is exposed, the mediastinum is entered from the right and the Penrose drain left in the mediastinum from the right is retrieved (FIGURE 12). At this point, the Penrose drain can be brought around the entire hiatal contents and used as a retractor to facilitate the remainder of the hiatal dissection.

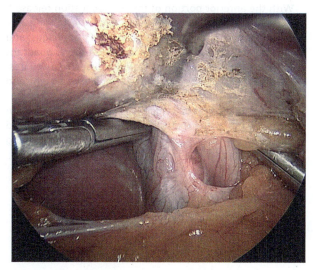

FIGURE 11 • Approaching the base of right crus along caudate lobe of the liver.

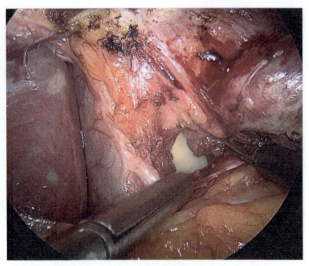

FIGURE 12 • Penrose drain retrieved from right.

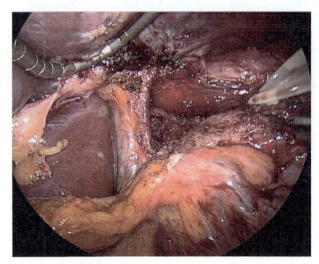

FIGURE 13 • Completed hiatal dissection.

- This technique of starting on the left and using the crura as the edges of dissection assures safe isolation of hiatal content, thereby minimizing the risk of esophagogastric perforation or vagal nerve injury (**FIGURE 13**).

- At this point, an EGD is useful to confirm anatomy, assess for any unsuspected perforation, and help localize the fundoplication in preparation for undoing the fundoplication.

UNDO PREVIOUS FUNDOPLICATION

- Finding the inferior edges of the fundoplication where it drapes over the proximal stomach, especially on the left side of the gastric cardia, allows the edge to be traced toward the anterior fusion of a 360° fundoplication. A similar exposure on the left can also be accomplished, but the left lower edge of the fundoplication tends to be more fused along the neurovascular bundles of the lesser curve.
- Once the anterior fusion of the fundoplication is found, it can be isolated and either released with the aid of electrocautery or separated by firing a linear cutting stapler between the two limbs (**FIGURE 14**).
- With the anterior portion of the fundoplication released, the right limb is dissected away from the lesser curve of the stomach and right side of the esophagus and returned to its normal location in the left upper quadrant (**FIGURE 15**). As the fundoplication is dissected away posteriorly, the posterior vagus nerve should be sought and protected.
- With the fundoplication completely undone, an EGD is again performed to assure that the wrap is completely mobilized and assess for any perforation. This is done by submerging

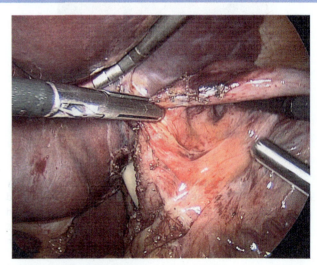

FIGURE 14 • Exposed anterior fusion of wrap.

the area of the gastroesophageal junction (GEJ) under saline while inflating the lumen of the esophagus and stomach with air and looking for an air leak externally.

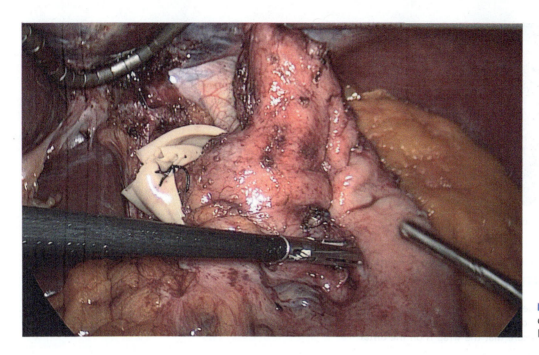

FIGURE 15 • Gastric fundus returned to normal location.

RECONSTRUCT ESOPHAGEAL HIATUS

- The esophageal hiatus is reconstructed using permanent sutures to approximate the crura posteriorly. Pledgets can be used to limit the sawing effect of the suture over time (**FIGURE 16**).
- If the hiatal defect is large, the intra-abdominal pressure is decreased to 10 to 12 mm Hg, thereby unloading the pressure on the diaphragm and crural repair.
- Several anterior crural sutures may be needed if the defect is large and the posterior-only closure is creating an angle at the GEJ.
- The crural reconstruction should result in the crura effacing the esophagus circumferentially without impinging.

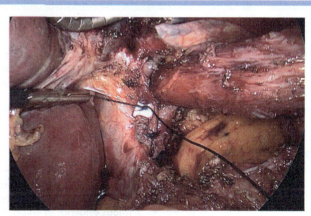

FIGURE 16 • Hiatal reconstruction.

REDO FUNDOPLICATION

- A standard technique for fundoplication can be used.[9,10] This entails a 360° fundoplication if there is adequate fundus and the preoperative esophageal motility is adequate (peristalsis in 70% or more of swallows or esophageal body pressure of 30 mm Hg or greater). A 270° fundoplication should be used if these criteria are not met (**TABLE 6**).
- Fundoplication should be calibrated by completing the wrap around a 56 to 60 Fr dilator placed across the GEJ (**FIGURE 17**).

Table 6: Options for Redo Fundoplication

Reconstruction option	Uses
360° fundoplication	Adequate fundus and normal esophageal motility
270° fundoplication	Poor esophageal motility or inadequate fundus for 360° fundoplication
No fundoplication	Tight wrap or hiatal stenosis with inadequate fundus for any fundoplication
Proximal divided gastroplasty/gastrectomy with Roux-en-Y gastrojejunostomy	Recurrent GERD following multiple prior antireflux operations and/or no fundus for redo fundoplication with/without injury to gastric cardia/fundus during redo
Esophagogastric myotomy with/without partial fundoplication	Pseudoachalasia
Esophagectomy with gastric pull-up or colon interposition	Severe pseudoachalasia with massive esophageal dilation
Roux-en-Y esophagojejunostomy	Recurrent GERD following multiple prior antireflux operations and injury to gastric cardia or distal esophagus during redo
LINX placement	Gastric fundus is not suitable for a repeat fundoplication and periesophageal scar and dissection trauma are limited

GERD, gastroesophageal reflux disease.

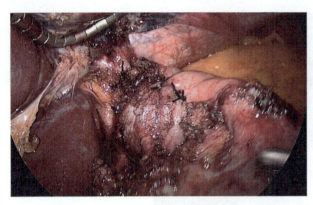

FIGURE 17 • Completed redo fundoplication.

- It is best if the fundus is positioned for the fundoplication, but not sutured, before this dilator is placed; otherwise, the wrap can be very difficult to bring around the esophagus posteriorly with the dilator in place.
- Two to three permanent sutures that include the anterior esophagus are placed to produce a 2-cm-long fundoplication.

ASSESS FOR POTENTIAL COMPLICATIONS

- One final EGD is recommended to assess the location of the wrap and look for any potential complications. A retroflex view is very helpful to assure that the wrap is on the distal esophagus and not the proximal stomach (the appearance of gastric folds extending up and into the wrap suggests a wrap that is too low).

CONSIDER ADJUNCTS

- If the hiatal dissection or undoing the wrap was particularly difficult, a gastrostomy tube can be used to allow gastric decompression and possible gastric feeds while waiting for proximal gastrointestinal (GI) function to return and normalize.

PEARLS AND PITFALLS

Indications for surgery and diagnosis of failure	■ Functional reasons for symptoms after fundoplication (eg, misdiagnosed GERD, other GI problems) *cannot* be corrected with surgery. ■ Without evidence of an obvious anatomic failure or confirmation of recurrent GERD by pH testing, surgery should be avoided.
Preoperative testing	■ Preoperative tests are intended to assure that correct redo technique is performed (eg, total vs partial fundoplication). ■ Skipping testing may compromise redo success.
Identify and expose hiatal anatomy, mobilize wrap	■ Injury to the liver, lesser curve of the stomach, the wrap, and the esophagus is more likely if dissection is started on the right. ■ Starting on the left allows exposure of the hiatus before working in the more anatomically congested right side. ■ Careful wrap mobilization posteriorly is critical to avoiding injury to the posterior vagus nerve.
Intraoperative testing	■ Liberal use of intraoperative endoscopy to guide dissection by frequently assessing anatomy. ■ Assess for potential luminal injury penetration.
Surgical technique	■ A standardized technique adhering to key technical principles will help assure successful outcomes (TABLE 7). ■ Only surgeons routinely performing antireflux surgery and experienced with diagnosis and surgical technique of reoperative foregut surgery should undertake redo fundoplication.
Postoperative care	■ Managing nausea to prevent retching starts in the operating and recovery room and is critical to minimizing early postoperative trauma that could disrupt the redo. ■ Gastric decompression avoids gastric distension that could disrupt a wrap or cruroplasty. ■ Tube access to the stomach may allow nonoperative management of a small leak found postoperatively.

Table 7: Standard Technique for Redo Fundoplication Success

- Full hiatal dissection (reduce and resect any hiatal hernia sac).
- Adequate esophageal mobilization—3-4 cm of esophagus below the diaphragm.
- Divide all short gastric vessels (be sure to mobilize fundus posteriorly to find and divide any high posterior vessel[s]).
- Resect any epiphrenic fat (careful to not undermine the anterior vagus).
- Determine esophageal length and location of EGJ (use endoscopy if unsure).
- Careful handling of crura during dissection and closure.
- Decrease pneumoperitoneum to unload the diaphragm during closure.
- Anterior crural stitch if large hiatal defect.
- Calibrate wrap (assure the fundus is in contact with the esophagus circumferentially—you can make a wrap too loose).
- Use gastrostomy tube for gastric decompression if large hiatal hernia or excessive manipulation of the stomach/area of vagal nerves.
- Avoid postoperative nausea (use preemptive antiemetics).

EGJ, esophagogastric junction.

Table 8: Outcomes of Redo Fundoplication

Author	Date	No. of patients	Mortality	Morbidity (%)	Success (%)	Follow-up (mon)
Vignal	2012	47	0	4.3	78	24
Musunuru	2012	38	0	18.4	63	35
Frantzides	2009	68	0	5.9	86	27
Smith	2005	259	0	15.4	89	14
Khajachee	2007	176	0	9.8	75	9
Byrne	2005	118	0	1.7	84	12
Légner	2011	106	0	35.8	90	22
Dalleagne	2011	129	0	7	83	75

POSTOPERATIVE CARE

- Postoperative management after reoperative antireflux surgery mirrors the care of any foregut surgery patient. A one- to two-night stay is pretty typical if the redo is laparoscopic, extra days if open. Key aspects of postoperative care are oral intake and return to activity.
- A preventable cause of antireflux surgery failure is early postoperative retching. The two most common reasons for early postoperative retching are nausea and dietary indiscretion.
- Patients should receive preemptive nausea control and antiemetics and be counseled carefully about maintaining a liquid and soft food diet for at least 1 month after surgery.
- Instructing patients to ingest only pourable liquids for the first week after surgery provides a simple rule to follow, and then providing a detailed menu of acceptable soft foods for another 3 weeks will help effect compliance with the postoperative diet.
- Too rapid advancement to activity that will result in increased intra-abdominal pressure can put sutures and the reconstructed anatomy at risk. A full 30 days of limiting lifting to no more than 30 lb and no vigorous exercise during this time provides simple guidelines for patients to follow.
- Setting appropriate expectations for patients with regard to their overall recovery, diet progression, and resolution of preoperative symptoms is important. Dysphagia may linger for more than 4 weeks after a redo and preparing patients for this likelihood will allow them to accept this more readily.
- Early dilation may improve the dysphagia, but it also increases the risk of recurrent GERD and therefore should be avoided if possible. We reserve dilation within the first 3 months after any antireflux operation for only those patients whose difficulty swallowing makes it hard to handle their own saliva or maintain hydration.
- It can take from 6 to 12 months before all healing and scar remodeling is complete and the full outcome of a redo is known. Again, setting patient's expectations is critical to long-term success.

OUTCOMES

- The outcomes of redo fundoplication can be comparable to primary antireflux surgery, and in patients suffering with significant and debilitating symptoms, the operations can return patients to a nearly normal quality of life with low morbidity and virtually no mortality[11,12] (TABLE 8).
- The patient requiring multiple reoperations for failed fundoplication is a special situation that deserves special mention. When undertaking a fourth redo, the failure rate jumps from around 7% to over 17%.[7] We will rarely simply undertake a redo after three prior attempts. A divided gastroplasty and Roux-en-Y reconstruction for recurrent severe GERD, an esophagogastric myotomy for pseudoachalasia or esophagectomy for severe pseudoachalasia with massively dilated esophagus, or an esophagojejunostomy for poor esophageal emptying with severe GEJ distortion is instead advised.

COMPLICATIONS

- Complications can best be understood, identified, and managed considering their occurrence.

Intraoperative

- Bleeding
- Liver injury
- Esophagogastric perforation
- Pneumothorax
- Vagal nerve injury

Postoperative—Short Term
- Pneumonia
- Esophageal obstruction (edema) with inability to swallow
- Delayed gastric emptying
- Atelectasis and hypoxemia

Postoperative—Long Term
- Sticture—recurrent GERD, scar
- Vagal nerve injury—gastroparesis, dumping
- Poor esophageal emptying—pseudoachalasia

REFERENCES

1. Dallemagne B, Perretta S. Twenty years of laparoscopic fundoplication for GERD. *World J Surg.* 2011;35:1428-1435.
2. Morgenthal CB, Lin E, Shane MD, et al. Who will fail laparoscopic Nissen fundoplication?Preoperative prediction of long-term outcomes. *Surg Endosc.* 2007;21:1978-1984.
3. Oelschlager BK, Ma KC, Soares RV, et al. A broad assessment of clinical outcomes after laparoscopic antireflux surgery. *Ann Surg.* 2012;256:87-94.
4. Broeders JA, Roks DJ, Draaisma WA, et al. Predictors of objectively identified recurrent reflux after primary Nissen fundoplication. *Br J Surg.* 2011;98:673-679.
5. Engström C, Cai W, Irvine T, et al. Twenty years of experience with laparoscopic antireflux surgery. *Br J Surg.* 2012;99:1415-1421.
6. Salminen P, Hurme S, Ovaska J. Fifteen-year outcome of laparoscopic and open Nissen fundoplication: a randomized clinical trial. *Ann Thorac Surg.* 2012;93:228-233.
7. Smith CD, McClusky DA, Rajad MA, et al. When fundoplication fails: redo? *Ann Surg.* 2005;241:861-869; discussion 869-871.
8. Parker M, Bowers SP, Bray JM, et al. Hiatal mesh is associated with major resection at revisional operation. *Surg Endosc.* 2010;24:3095-3101.
9. Dallemagne B, Arenas Sanchez M, Francart D, et al. Long-term results after laparoscopic reoperation for failed antireflux procedures. *Br J Surg.* 2011;98:1581-1587.
10. Légner A, Tsuboi K, Bathla L, et al. Reoperative antireflux surgery for dysphagia. *Surg Endosc.* 2011;25:1160-1167.
11. van Beek DB, Auyang ED, Soper NJ. A comprehensive review of laparoscopic redo fundoplication. *Surg Endosc.* 2011;25:706-712.
12. Chlottmann F, Laxague F, Angeramo CA, et al. Outcomes of laparoscopic redo fundoplication in patients with failed antireflux surgrey: a systemic review and meta-analysis. *Ann Surg.* 2021;274:78-85.

Chapter 14

Roux-en-Y (Roux Limb Reconstruction) for Recurrent Hiatal Hernia

Joseph Adam Sujka and Christopher DuCoin

DEFINITION

- Hiatal hernias are broken down into four subtypes, 1 through 4. Type 1 (95%) is also known as a sliding hiatal hernia. Type 2 paraesophageal hernias have the gastroesophageal junction in the normal anatomic position; however, a portion of the fundus herniates adjacent to the esophagus into the thorax. Type 3 paraesophageal hernias are a combination of type 1 and 2 with both the fundus and gastroesophageal junction herniating through the hiatus. Type 4 is a paraesophageal hernia that contains another organ in addition to a hiatal hernia. Among the paraesophageal hernia types, type 3 is the most common, making up 90%, and type 2 is the least common[1-4] (**FIGURE 1**).
- A more nebulously defined type of hiatal hernia is the "giant" paraesophageal hernia. Some have advocated for giant hiatal hernias to be defined as type 3 or 4 paraesophageal hernias (**FIGURE 2**), while others suggest that the amount of stomach contained in the chest, half the stomach or more, be used to define this type of hiatal hernia. It is the opinion of the authors that a giant hiatal hernia is simply a large paraesophageal hernia requiring more mediastinal dissection than typically required for hiatal hernia repair.[5-7]
- The final type of hiatal hernia is a recurrent hiatal hernia. Defining a recurrence begins with radiologic proof; however, clinical symptoms may not always accompany radiologic findings. While there is no strict definition of what constitutes a radiologic recurrence, some define it as a recurrence only when it is 2 cm in length.[8-11] Larger hiatal hernias and patients with medical comorbidities may have an increased chance of recurrence. With each recurrence the chance of needing Roux reconstruction increases.

DIFFERENTIAL DIAGNOSIS

- The diagnosis of a hiatal hernia can be completed through various radiologic tests. Once the diagnosis of a hiatal hernia has been completed no further testing is required for operative repair if the patient is symptomatic.
- Other diagnoses outside of hiatal hernia are unlikely given radiologic findings; however, other processes of the esophagus such as achalasia, postobesity esophageal dysfunction,[12] and esophagogastric junction outflow obstruction should be ruled out.
- Patients who may benefit from a Roux limb reconstruction are those who have had multiple hiatal surgeries in the past, present with emergent gastric volvulus, or have an elevated body mass index (BMI).

PATIENT HISTORY AND PHYSICAL FINDINGS

- Patient symptoms vary based on the size and type of their hiatal hernia but can include nausea, vomiting, gastroesophageal reflux disease, dysphagia, regurgitation, abdominal pain, and even complete obstruction.

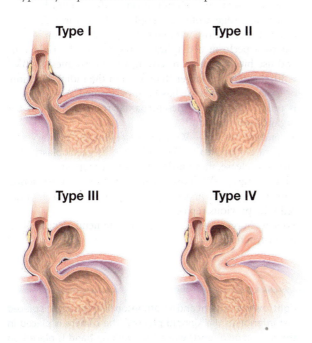

FIGURE 1 • Subtypes of hiatal hernias.

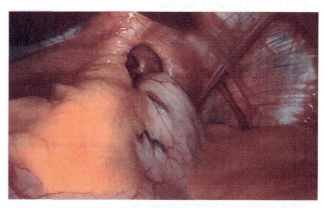

FIGURE 2 • "Giant" paraesophageal hernia.

- Careful discussion should occur prior to taking the patient for elective revisional surgery, including normal perioperative risks. If there is a high suspicion of needing partial or total gastrectomy the accompanying risks and reconstruction types (this includes Roux-en-Y, jejunum, colon, tube grafts,[13] etc) should also be discussed in detail.[14,15]
- The patient's previous operative records should be obtained to determine their anatomy and the presence or previous mesh placement. The patient's abdomen should also be carefully examined for surgical scars to guide the conversation on the ability to successfully perform open, laparoscopic, or robotic interventions.

IMAGING AND OTHER DIAGNOSTIC STUDIES

- Many preoperative imaging studies can be utilized prior to revisional hiatal hernia repair including chest x-ray, upper gastrointestinal series (UGI), and computed tomography (CT) scans. In addition, functional studies such as manometry and pH Bravo studies may be utilized but are less useful.
- Multislice CT scans with coronal, sagittal, and 3D reformatted images have been shown to increase the sensitivity of CT scans for diagnosis of hiatal hernias.[16]
- The most useful study preoperatively is a CT angiogram (CTA) of the chest, abdomen, and pelvis. CTA of the chest, abdomen, and pelvis is useful not only to delineate preoperative anatomy but also to determine what vessels continue perfusing the stomach. With this information, attempts to avoid these feeding vessels can be made intraoperatively to potentially avoid total gastrectomy.

SURGICAL MANAGEMENT

- Nutritional optimization should be performed prior to operative intervention. If patients are unable to maintain their nutrition, they may benefit from preoperative total parenteral nutrition or additional interventions.
- Other specialists, such as colorectal surgeons and plastic surgeons, should be made aware of the case preoperatively if they are needed for creation of a colonic or tube graft conduit, but this is rarely needed.
- Patients are placed supine in all types of surgical intervention. If laparoscopic repair is attempted the patient should be placed in stirrups and split leg.
- Indocyanine green (ICG) is a useful adjunct intraoperatively to determine perfusion of the stomach as well as to determine the course of surrounding vessels.
- With each surgical procedure the risk of partial of total gastric resection of the stomach increases. This is due to the complexity of these cases and possible devascularization of the stomach.
- A *Partial Gastrectomy* is commonly utilized when the fundoplication is undone, leaving a devascularized portion of the stomach, specifically the fundus. This area of tissue can usually be resected with little consequence. ICG may be employed to confirm poor blood flow to this region.
- A *Total Gastrectomy (near total)* is rarely needed but should be considered in the setting of severe gastroparesis or if there is pathology that would affect the remanent stomach. Another indication for total gastrectomy is when there is damage to the left gastric artery. This can occur during the primary surgery or during the redo operation. Prior to the redo operation, it is our practice to obtain a CTA of the abdomen to evaluate the left gastric artery. We also perform intraoperative ICG to confirm the viability of the left gastric artery. If there is damage to this artery, we will elect to perform a near total gastrectomy as the left gastric artery is the blood supply to the gastric pouch. Our reconstruction of choice is to bring up a Roux limb.
- Our operative mindset varies depending on the number or previous operations the patient has undergone. Utilization of Roux reconstruction with partial vs near total gastrectomy in elective benign surgery specifically on the topic of recurrent hiatal hernia is as follows.
    - Primary Surgery—Ensure 3 cm of intra-abdominal esophagus is present after mobilization; if this cannot be done ensure a wedge Collis gastroplasty is performed. Next, ensure the crus close with no tension and if tension is present then perform a diaphragm release on the right crus and use biologic mesh to cover. Also utilize mesh if BMI > 30, the defect is larger than 5 cm in the radial direction, or a diaphragm release has been performed. A gastropexy is utilized if there is mesentroaxial rotation but not for organoaxial rotation.
    - Secondary Surgery—We will not repeat the primary surgery, rather add to it. We add a Collis gastroplasty, diaphragm release, mesh utilization, or gastropexy.
    - Third Surgery—We now consider a Roux reconstruction with partial or near total gastrectomy, but will at times redo the previous repair.
    - Fourth Surgery—We always recommend Roux limb reconstruction.

ROUX LIMB RECONSTRUCTION

- Typically, we perform our redo hiatal hernia repairs utilizing the robotic platform; however, this can also be done laparoscopically. Regardless of the platform, we always utilize a minimally invasive approach first as this provides excellent exposure of the hiatus. For our robotic setup, four ports are placed just superior to the umbilicus in a horizontal fashion across the abdomen. These are two 8-mm ports and two 12-mm ports. In addition, an assist port is placed in the patient's right lower quadrant and a Nathanson liver retractor is placed just inferior to the xiphoid process. The camera is placed in the most medial port, while the working hand is placed on the patient's left. The most lateral port is a grasper, and the medial port (next to the camera) is the energy source. The port on the patient's right is also a bipolar grasper and allows for an additional source of energy.
- We begin the case by dissecting out the pars flaccida or the adhesive tissue present in this area. We separate the hernia sac from the right crus and carry this plane from 9 o'clock

Chapter 14 ROUX-EN-Y (ROUX LIMB RECONSTRUCTION) FOR RECURRENT HIATAL HERNIA   105

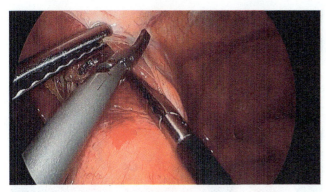

FIGURE 3 • Dissection of the pars flaccida or the adhesive tissue present.

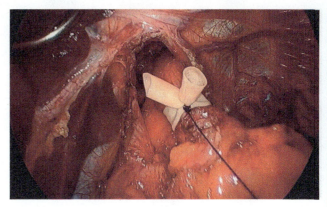

FIGURE 5 • Intraoperative observation and indocyanine green to decide next steps.

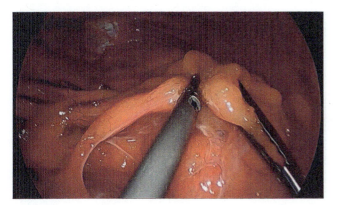

FIGURE 4 • Dissection along the greater curve up to the left crus.

clockwise to approximately 2 o'clock on the left crus. We then separate the hernia sac from the right crus with gentle parallel force between the esophagus and right crus combined with small amount of electrocautery (FIGURE 3).
- If the above is not possible as lesser curve of the stomach and right crus have no safe surgical plane we will move to the greater curve. Usually, the short gastrics can be divided and a surgical plane that has not been previously dissected can be identified. We carry the dissection along the greater curve up to the left crus (FIGURE 4).
- If the right crus has now been dissected we will then turn our attention to the greater curve. We enter the lesser sac and carry our dissection to the left crus. Once here, we separate the hernia sac from the left crus and connect this dissection plane to the previously developed hernia sac plane that came to the 2-o'clock position.
- Usually, a plane that has not been dissected previously can be found. The higher you dissect into the chest the more likely this novel dissection plane is to be found. The most challenging portion of this case will be reducing the stomach from the chest.
- This dissection is continued until the stomach has been fully reduced into the abdomen. A Penrose drain can be placed posterior to the stomach and used for traction. The hernia sac is removed, and the stomach is evaluated. Utilizing intraoperative observation and ICG we decide on the next steps (FIGURE 5).

- Our utilization of ICG has increased, and we prefer to use 2.5 mg/mL, which is prepared by diluting 25 mg in 10 mL. This will allow the surgeon to test for arterial supply, namely, the left gastric artery and perfusion of the tissue, that is, the undone fundoplication. This is ordered and given by anesthesia at the request of the surgeon.
- If there is no issue with perfusion of either the stomach and/or the left gastric then we continue in the fashion of a standard Roux-en-Y gastric bypass (see Chapter 46).
- If there is a perfusion issue to the undone fundoplication or remnant gastric fundus, we will then perform a wedge resection of this portion of stomach. Again, we follow the normal steps of a Roux-en-Y gastric bypass, but the devascularized portion of remnant stomach will be resected.
- If there is an issue with the left gastric artery or perfusion of the gastric pouch, or the patient has a severe history of gastroparesis, then we prefer a near total gastrectomy. A description of this can be found elsewhere.
- The key to a near total gastrectomy is to leave a small portion of stomach in place just distal to the esophagogastric (EG) junction as a gastric jejunal anastomosis has a much lower leak rate then an EG anastomosis.
- The following steps are unique to a near total gastrectomy.
- In short, the fundoplication is taken down, the greater curve and short gastrics are transected, and the left gastric artery is isolated and transected as it is in the resected field (FIGURE 6). The proximal portion of the stomach is transected at the EG junction (or just distal leaving a small cuff of proximal stomach) under endoscopic visualization (FIGURE 7). The right gastric artery is then identified and transected; the right gastroepiploic is identified and transected. The dissection is carried down to the pylorus, and the first portion of the duodenum is transected. This completes the gastrectomy for benign disease.
- For esophagojejunostomy we utilize an end-to-side anastomosis utilizing an OrVil stapler device with a 25 mm diameter. If the OrVil cannot be placed then we suture in the standard 25-mm anvil. We recommend against the 21-mm anvil as this is prone to anastomotic stricture formation.
- Silk stay sutures are placed in the distal esophagus for traction at 3 and 9 o'clock as the esophagus is prone to retract. The OrVil device is passed through the patient's mouth and guided through the esophagus till it reaches the blind end of the esophagus.

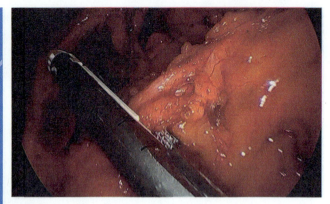

FIGURE 6 • Left gastric artery is isolated and transected as it is in the resected field.

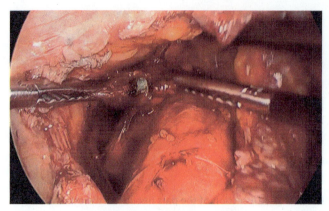

FIGURE 8 • Small esophagotomy.

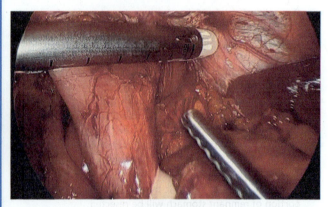

FIGURE 7 • The proximal portion of the stomach is transected at the EG junction (or just distal leaving a small cuff of proximal stomach) under endoscopic visualization.

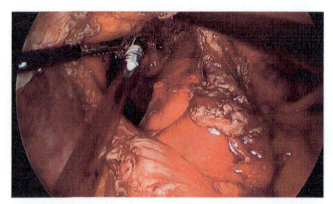

FIGURE 9 • Tip of the OrVil device passed through small esophagotomy.

- A small esophagotomy is created (**FIGURE 8**) and the tip of the OrVil device passed through it (**FIGURE 9**). Care should be taken as overvigorous manipulation of the distal esophagus can lead to tearing or malposition of the device. If the OrVil is not used a standard end-to-end anastomosis (EEA) 25-mm anvil is used and sutured in place using a purse string approach with a 2-0 Prolene.
- Next, we divide the omentum. This done from the most caudal region to the transverse colon, and in line with the esophageal hiatus. Thus, if the small bowel is brought up in an antecolic fashion, the bulky omentum will no longer apply tension on the Roux limb and somewhat decreases the distance the small bowel needs to travel to the hiatus.
- Once the anastomotic device of choice is in position the ligament of Treitz is identified at the base of the transverse mesocolon. The inferior mesenteric vein must be visualized to confirm the beginning of the jejunum.
- Upon elevating the small bowel to the esophagus you want to ensure the Roux limb will have enough length to reach the distal esophagus. We bring this up in the omega 'Ω' technique wherein the biliopancreatic (BP) limb is kept on the patient's left and the Roux limb will be to the patient's right. If more length is needed, try to rotate the small bowel to the patient's left feeding the Roux limb toward the BP limb. If there is still a length issue, you can fenestrate the mesentery if it is shortened and/or you can use a retrocolic approach.

- To fenestrate the small bowel use the scissors or hook cautery to divide the single layer of peritoneum over the mesentery without injuring the vasculature below. To locate the area of tension pull the omega loop cranial toward the esophagus and locate the point of tension on the mesentery. Make multiple cuts in a fashion that is parallel to the small bowel on the mesentery just dividing the peritoneum. These are usually 5 cm in length and 1 cm apart from each other. This should release the area of tension and provide additional length on the small bowel.
- If a retrocolic window is used this will reduce the travel distance of the small bowel to the hiatus as it will not need to travel over the omentum and transverse colon. Elevate the transverse colon and identify the middle colic artery. Again, this is a good time to use ICG if needed. There is an avascular window that is located to the patient's left of the middle colic artery, just above the ligament of Treitz, and right below the hiatus. This will drastically reduce the distance the small bowel needs to traverse to reach the hiatus.
- If length is still an issue, give 1 amp of glucagon as a smooth muscle relaxant. This will cause the esophageal muscles to relax and provide additional length. Roughly 2 to 3 cm of additional esophageal length can be achieved in this manner.
- At the site where the small bowel reaches the EG junction divide the bowel more on the BP side. This will now separate the BP limb away from the Roux limb while leaving redundant Roux limb that will be used to place the EEA. The BP limb will now fall away to the patient's left side.

Chapter 14 ROUX-EN-Y (ROUX LIMB RECONSTRUCTION) FOR RECURRENT HIATAL HERNIA

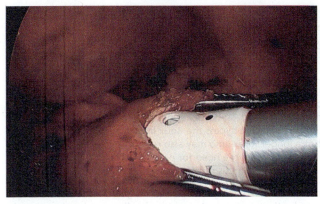

FIGURE 10 • EEA stapler to abdomen and through the opened Roux limb in a retrograde fashion.

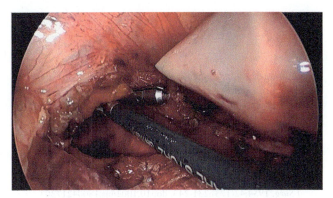

FIGURE 11 • Spike through the Roux limb.

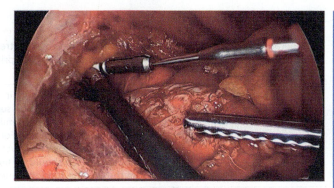

FIGURE 12 • Anvil device fully passed through the esophagus.

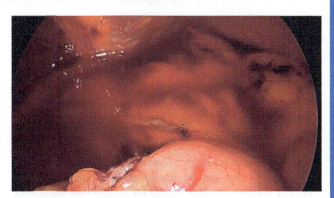

FIGURE 13 • Leak test.

- Using the redundant Roux limb, coming from the patient's left side, cut away the staple line. Now pass the EEA stapler into the abdomen and through the opened Roux limb in a retrograde fashion (FIGURE 10). Select an appropriate site on the jejunum on the antimesenteric side of the Roux limb. An appropriate site is one that reaches the esophageal stump without tension.
- Once the position is confirmed pass the spike through the Roux limb (FIGURE 11). Make sure that the spike is fully deployed; usually there is a color indicator (orange) showing that the anvil device is also fully passed through the esophagus (FIGURE 12).
- Progressively advance the EEA stapler to the anvil device. Line up the two ends and push them together until a click is felt.
- The device and spike are now connected and can be fired. Prior to firing make sure that nothing is caught between the two ends of the stapler.
- Fire the stapler and close the open end of the jejunum with either stapler or sutures.
- Perform a leak test (FIGURE 13).
- We then perform our stapled jejunojejunostomy.
- The Roux limb is counted 75 cm from the esophagojejunostomy. Then a 2-0 Vicryl is used to approximate the Roux limb and the BP limb. Enterotomies are made in both bowel limbs below the Vicryl suture.
- A linear stapler is passed into both lumens of small bowel and a common channel created. Then either a stapled or suture closure can be performed. We utilize a 2-0 Vicryl to place four sutures across the common channel. We lift upward on the most medial and lateral sutures and then fire a stapler across the lumen to close it.
- Mesenteric defects are then closed with barbed sutures.
- A nasogastric tube (NGT) is placed across the esophagojejunostomy under direct visualization prior to closure.
- A 19 French Blake drain is placed at the esophagojejunal anastomosis.
- We do not routinely place a small bowel feeding tube for this case.

PEARLS AND PITFALLS

Preoperative planning	▪ It is rarely needed, but if a total gastrectomy is planned to be performed, reconstruction should be discussed in detail with the patient prior to operative intervention. NGT should be placed at the time of operation.
Operative pearls	▪ CTA prior to redo hiatal hernia repair is crucial not only to define the anatomy of the revisional surgery but also to reveal the current blood supply of the stomach. ▪ Method of Roux reconstruction is similar to a gastric bypass; however, the Roux limb length is shorter at 75 cm as this is not for weight loss. For Roux-en-Y gastric bypass the Roux limb is on the order of 100-150 cm. Some authors argue, however, that a longer Roux limb may also reduce reflux. ▪ Use of intraoperative ICG should be liberal to determine the need for partial gastric resection; this is usually from the undone fundoplication or remaining fundus of the stomach.
Postoperative care	▪ Routine postoperative UGI should be performed in the setting of revisional surgery to rule out an early post operative leak. Other longer-term complications such as a stenosis can be diagnosed and managed endoscopically.

POSTOPERATIVE CARE

- UGI should be considered sometime between postoperative day (POD) 1 and POD 3 to rule out an anastomotic leak. If NG tube output is low, it is removed at this time.
- Clear liquid diet can be started after negative UGI. The patient remains on clear liquids for 3 days, full liquids for 4 days, a soft diet for 2 weeks, follow by a mechanical soft diet for 4 weeks. At this point the patient can usually be moved to a regular diet.
- Care should be taken to follow aspiration precautions such as head of bed elevation to prevent aspiration, etc.
- Postoperative ileus is not uncommon. If this is suspected and an NGT is warranted after initial removal, it may be preferable to place this endoscopically through the anastomosis.

COMPLICATIONS

- Typical complications from a hiatal hernia repair such as pneumothorax, mediastinal air, and mediastinal abscess are always a possibility.
- Postoperative dysphagia can be normal. However, intolerance to saliva or liquids is concerning for dysphagia and will require intervention. Causes of dysphagia can be postoperative swelling, anastomotic stenosis, or an overly tight crural repair.
- Immediate recurrence with transdiaphragmatic herniation of the new anastomosis is possible. This can lead to ischemia and perforation. No specific incidence is known for esophagojejunostomy but in those with fundoplication wrap migration can range from 7% to 20%.[17,18]
- Anastomotic leak is the most dreaded complication with esophagojejunostomy. It can present with a variety of findings from tachycardia up to hypotension and sepsis. UGI or CT scan with oral contrast are effective first-line tests. These tests should be used to differentiate between a pseudoleak, contained leak, and free perforation. If there is any question of the location or severity of the leak and the patient is stable they can be taken to fluoroscopy to evaluate the leak in real time, but typically patients should undergo emergent surgical repair with any suspicion of a leak.[19,20] Leaks can be managed endoscopically through the scope clip, over the scope clip, or more commonly with an esophageal stent or endo vac system (please see Chapter 51). If the patient is unstable, they are taken urgently to the operating room for washout, drainage, and usually on omental patch.

REFERENCES

1. Barrett NR. Hiatus hernia: a review of some controversial points. *Br J Surg*. 1954;42(173):231-243. doi:10.1002/bjs.18004217303
2. Kavic SM, Segan RD, George IM, Turner PL, Roth JS, Park A. Classification of hiatal hernias using dynamic three-dimensional reconstruction. *Surg Innovat*. 2006;13(1):49-52. doi:10.1177/155335060601300108
3. Kohn GP, Price RR, DeMeester SR, et al. Guidelines for the management of hiatal hernia. *Surg Endosc*. 2013;27(12):4409-4428. doi:10.1007/s00464-013-3173-3
4. Ahmed SK, Bright T, Watson DI. Natural history of endoscopically detected hiatus herniae at late follow-up. *ANZ J Surg*. 2018;88(6):E544-E547. doi:10.1111/ans.14180
5. Awais O, Luketich JD. Management of giant paraesophageal hernia. *Minerva Chir*. 2009;64(2):159-168.
6. Litle VR, Buenaventura PO, Luketich JD. Laparoscopic repair of giant paraesophageal hernia. *Adv Surg*. 2001;35:21-38.
7. Mitiek MO, Andrade RS. Giant hiatal hernia. *Ann Thorac Surg*. 2010;89(6):S2168-S2173. doi:10.1016/j.athoracsur.2010.03.022
8. Hazebroek EJ, Koak Y, Berry H, Leibman S, Smith GS. Critical evaluation of a novel DualMesh repair for large hiatal hernias. *Surg Endosc*. 2009;23(1):193-196. doi:10.1007/s00464-008-9772-8
9. White BC, Jeansonne LO, Morgenthal CB, et al. Do recurrences after paraesophageal hernia repair matter?: ten-year follow-up after laparoscopic repair. *Surg Endosc*. 2008;22(4):1107-1111. doi:10.1007/s00464-007-9649-2
10. Parameswaran R, Ali A, Velmurugan S, Adjepong SE, Sigurdsson A. Laparoscopic repair of large paraesophageal hiatus hernia: quality of life and durability. *Surg Endosc*. 2006;20(8):1221-1224. doi:10.1007/s00464-005-0691-7
11. Oelschlager BK, Pellegrini CA, Hunter J, et al. Biologic prosthesis reduces recurrence after laparoscopic paraesophageal hernia repair: a multicenter, prospective, randomized trial. *Ann Surg*. 2006;244(4):481-490. doi:10.1097/01.sla.0000237759.42831.03
12. Miller AT, Matar R, Abu Dayyeh BK, et al. Postobesity surgery esophageal dysfunction: a combined cross-sectional prevalence study and retrospective analysis. *Am J Gastroenterol*. 2020;115(10):1669-1680. doi:10.14309/ajg.0000000000000733

13. LoGiudice JA, Wyler von Ballmoos MC, Gasparri MG, Lao WW. When the gastrointestinal conduit for total esophageal reconstruction is not an option: review of the role of skin flaps and report of salvage with a single-stage tubed anterolateral thigh flap. *Ann Plast Surg.* 2016;76(4):463-467. doi:10.1097/SAP.0000000000000389
14. Coevoet D, Van Daele E, Willaert W, et al. Quality of life of patients with a colonic interposition postoesophagectomy. *Eur J Cardio-Thorac Surg Off J Eur Assoc Cardio-Thorac Surg.* 2019;55(6):1113-1120. doi:10.1093/ejcts/ezy398
15. Urschel JD. Late dysphagia after presternal colon interposition. *Dysphagia.* 1996;11(1):75-77. doi:10.1007/BF00385803
16. Eren S, Ciriş F. Diaphragmatic hernia: diagnostic approaches with review of the literature. *Eur J Radiol.* 2005;54(3):448-459. doi:10.1016/j.ejrad.2004.09.008
17. O'Boyle CJ, Heer K, Smith A, Sedman PC, Brough WA, Royston CM. Iatrogenic thoracic migration of the stomach complicating laparoscopic nissen fundoplication. *Surg Endosc.* 2000;14(6):540-542. doi:10.1007/s004640000102
18. Watson DI, de Beaux AC. Complications of laparoscopic antireflux surgery. *Surg Endosc.* 2001;15(4):344-352. doi:10.1007/s004640000346
19. Yoo C, Levine MS, Redfern RO, Laufer I, Buyske J. Laparoscopic Heller myotomy and fundoplication: findings and predictive value of early postoperative radiographic studies. *Abdom Imaging.* 2004;29(6):643-647. doi:10.1007/s00261-004-0182-7
20. Singhal T, Balakrishnan S, Hussain A, Grandy-Smith S, Paix A, El-Hasani S. Management of complications after laparoscopic Nissen's fundoplication: a surgeon's perspective. *Ann Surg Innov Res.* 2009;3(1):1. doi:10.1186/1750-1164-3-1

SECTION V: Treatment of Esophageal Cancer

Chapter 15: Esophagectomy: Transhiatal and Reconstruction

Robert E. Glasgow

DEFINITION

- Transhiatal esophagectomy (THE) or esophagectomy without thoracotomy is defined as removal of the esophagus and upper stomach using an incision in the left anterior neck for purposes of dissection of the upper third of the esophagus and anastomosis via the thoracic inlet, and an upper midline abdominal incision for purposes of dissection of the stomach and lower two-thirds of the esophagus and creation of a conduit for esophageal reconstruction (stomach, colon).
- Although THE is usually applied for purposes of treating esophageal and gastroesophageal (GE) junction carcinoma, THE may also be used for treatment of benign esophageal conditions including end-stage achalasia and medically/endoscopically recalcitrant esophageal stricture from caustic injection or end-stage reflux disease and acute perforation.
- The remainder of this discussion will focus on the use of THE in the treatment of malignant disease. Most aspects of the diagnostic workup and operative techniques also apply to the evaluation and treatment of benign conditions for which THE is being considered.

DIFFERENTIAL DIAGNOSIS

- THE is most commonly used in treatment of esophageal cancer. In particular, adenocarcinomas of lower third of the esophagus and Siewert types I and II GE junction adenocarcinoma (**FIGURE 1**; **TABLE 1**) are optimally suited for this approach.
- Squamous cell carcinomas (SCCs) of the lower third of the esophagus may also be approached via THE, whereas tumors of the middle and upper third of the esophagus usually require

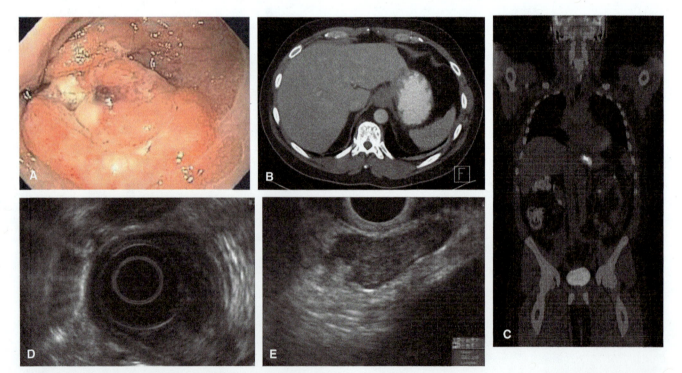

FIGURE 1 • Imaging and diagnostic evaluation of a patient with a localized T3, N1, M0 Siewert type II gastroesophageal junction adenocarcinoma undergoing consideration for transhiatal esophagectomy. **A**, Upper endoscopy showing ulcerated mass in the lower third of the esophagus. **B**, Computed tomography (CT) showing an enlarged mass at the lower third of the esophagus. **C**, Positron emission tomography–CT. **D**, Endoscopic ultrasound showing mucosal-based mass invading into the adventitia of the esophagus. **E**, Endoscopic ultrasound showing enlarged lymph node fine-needle aspiration biopsy confirming adenocarcinoma.

Chapter 15 ESOPHAGECTOMY: TRANSHIATAL AND RECONSTRUCTION

> **Table 1: Siewert Classification for Gastroesophageal Junction Adenocarcinoma**
>
> Type I: Adenocarcinoma of the lower esophagus with the center located within 1 to 5 cm above the anatomic EGJ.
> Type II: True carcinoma of the cardia with the tumor center within 1 cm above and 2 cm below the EGJ.
> Type III: Subcardial carcinoma with the tumor center between 2 and 5 cm below EGJ, which infiltrates the EGJ and lower esophagus from below.
>
> EGJ, esophagogastric junction.
>
> Reprinted with permission from Rüdiger Siewert J, Feith M, Werner M, et al. Adenocarcinoma of the esophagogastric junction: results of surgical therapy based on anatomical/topographic classification in 1,002 consecutive patients. Ann Surg. 2000;232(3):353-361.

transthoracic esophagectomy (TTE) to allow for direct visualization of the dissection of the involved esophagus, at-risk lymph nodes, and surrounding mediastinal structures.

PATIENT HISTORY AND PHYSICAL FINDINGS

- All patients should undergo a comprehensive medical history with emphasis on not only clinical history pertinent to the primary indication for consideration of THE but also the pertinent comorbid conditions that would influence treatment planning. Included in this history is a comprehensive past medical, surgical, and social history. An evaluation and plan for mitigation of all comorbid medical conditions that may impact perioperative risk must be done. This includes careful consideration of cardiac, respiratory, renal, and metabolic comorbidities. This also includes careful examination of patient smoking history and physical function. Smoking cessation and optimization of preoperative nutritional and physical function is imperative. Prior surgical history is important as well. Prior fundoplication will make dissection of the esophageal hiatus more difficult. Patients with a prior history of gastric resection, for example, may not be candidates for use of the stomach as a conduit for reconstruction because of inadequate length or blood supply. Finally, if the colon is to be considered for use for reconstruction, the influence of prior colectomy on anatomy and blood supply should be very carefully considered. Review of recent and up-to-date colonoscopy is important.
- Whether it be for benign or malignant disease, the principal symptom at the time of presentation for a patient who would undergo THE is dysphagia. Often, these patients have significant nutritional impairment, most notably, weight loss.
- In patients with adenocarcinoma of the esophagus and GE junction, a history of GE reflux disease should be elicited as well as a careful history of prior endoscopic and radiographic evaluations. In patients with SCC, a prior and current history of tobacco and alcohol use should be elicited.
- A comprehensive physical examination should be performed with special attention to the cervical and supraclavicular areas for enlarged lymph nodes, chest examination for possible effusions, and abdominal examination for palpable masses and periumbilical lymph nodes (Sister Mary Joseph nodule).

IMAGING AND OTHER DIAGNOSTIC STUDIES

Upper Endoscopy With Biopsy

- All patients presenting with dysphagia should undergo upper gastrointestinal endoscopy and biopsy, with the goal of making a diagnosis and localizing the site of obstruction (FIGURE 1).
  - Multiple biopsies of suspicious areas (nodules, ulceration, stricture, possible Barrett) should be obtained.
  - Endoscopic mucosal resection of focal nodules should be performed to provide accurate T staging and to evaluate degree of differentiation and vascular and/or lymphatic invasion.
  - For cancer, the location of the tumor as measured from the incisors and GE junction and extent of tumor length, circumferential involvement, and degree of obstruction should be documented.

Computed Tomography of the Chest and Abdomen

- Once a diagnosis of cancer is made, a computed tomography (CT) of the chest and abdomen with oral and intravenous contrast is done.
- Tumor location, locoregional involvement or invasion, regional and extraregional lymph node involvement, and metastatic disease should be evaluated and recorded.
- If metastasis is suspected, biopsy of concerning lesions should be undertaken to confirm stage and direct palliative treatment.

Positron Emission Tomography–CT

- In patients in whom a standard CT of the chest and abdomen is unremarkable, a positron emission tomography–CT should be performed to confirm primary tumor location and extent, evaluate regional and extraregional nodal involvement, and exclude occult metastases.

Endoscopic Ultrasound

- In patients without metastatic disease (stage 4), an endoscopic ultrasound is done to document depth of invasion of the tumor (T stage) and evaluate mediastinal and perigastric/celiac lymph node involvement (N stage). Biopsy of suspicious lymph nodes is indicated.
- All patients should then be assigned a pretreatment TNM stage to guide treatment planning discussions, preferably under the direction of a multidisciplinary treatment planning conference attended by surgical, medical, and radiation oncology.[1] The National Comprehensive Cancer Network (NCCN) defines optimal treatment planning algorithms.[2]
- In considering options for reconstruction, the two most common conduits are the stomach and colon. Although variations in stomach blood supply are very rare, variations in colonic blood supply are common enough to justify preoperative evaluation of arterial anatomy and collateral circulation by visceral angiography in planning choice of conduit.
  - For purposes of using the stomach as a conduit for esophageal reconstruction, an intact right gastric and, more importantly, right gastroepiploic artery is imperative (FIGURE 2).
  - For purposes of the colon as a conduit for esophageal reconstruction following a THE, an adequate collateral blood supply via an intact marginal artery is required (FIGURE 3). A colonoscopy to exclude and/or treat colonic pathology must be done prior to use of the colon.

SURGICAL MANAGEMENT

- As THE is a technically complex operation with a high degree of associated morbidity and mortality, this operation should be done by surgical teams experienced in

SECTION V TREATMENT OF ESOPHAGEAL CANCER

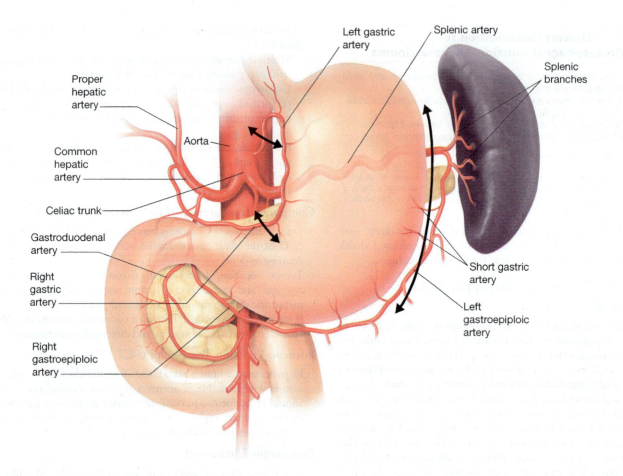

FIGURE 2 • Stomach blood supply for purposes of using the stomach as a conduit for reconstruction following transhiatal esophagectomy. *Arrows* show lines of division including the short gastric arteries, left gastroepiploic artery, left gastric artery, and ligation of the right gastric artery at the incisura angularis at the point of origin of the gastric conduit staple line.

the perioperative management of these patients.[3-5] This includes experienced operating room personnel and anesthesiologists.

Preoperative Planning
- Patients should undergo preoperative evaluation by the surgical and anesthesia team for purposes of mitigating perioperative risks in the area of cardiac, pulmonary, and renal comorbidities.
- A discussion should be done with the patient as to how pain will be measured and managed following surgery. Regional anesthetics such as an epidural catheter are very helpful in alleviating pain, thereby allowing the patient to be more engaged in early mobilization and physical therapy.
- Perioperative antibiotics should be administered within 60 minutes of skin incision and redosed in a timely manner during the operation. Cefazolin, dosed to weight specifications and redosed every 4 hours, is recommended. Cefoxitin can also be used and redosed every 3 hours. For patients with a beta-lactam allergy, clindamycin or vancomycin and aminoglycoside or aztreonam or fluoroquinolone are used. All prophylactic antibiotics are not necessary beyond surgery completion.[6]
- Perioperative monitoring with an arterial line is helpful especially during blunt mediastinal esophagus dissection where transient hypotension is common because of decreased venous return and compression on the heart. Rarely is a central line indicated.
- Appropriate deep venous thrombosis prophylaxis is required. Intermittent sequential compression devices should be placed prior to induction of anesthesia and continued after surgery. Chemical prophylaxis should be instituted postoperatively once clinically indicated.
- Urinary catheters are placed following induction of anesthesia and discontinued within 24 hours of surgery.

Positioning
- Patients undergoing THE are positioned supine on the operating room table (**FIGURE 4**).
- Both arms are tucked and pressure points padded to prevent injury during the course of the operation.
- A towel or medium gel roll is placed behind the shoulders to allow for mild extension of the neck. This is of particular importance in obese, short-necked patients.
- The head is rotated 30° to the right to open exposure to the left neck.

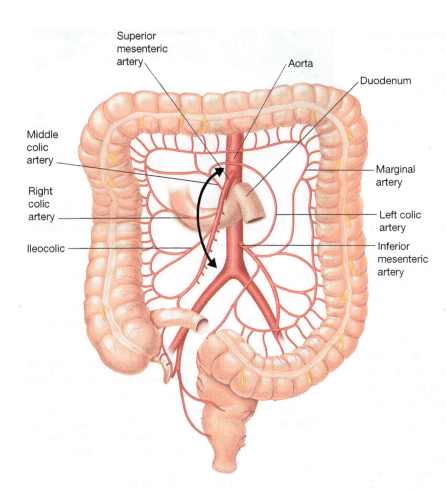

FIGURE 3 • Colon blood supply for purposes of using the colon as a conduit for reconstruction following transhiatal esophagectomy. *Arrow* shows line of division of mesentery to include ileocolic, right colic, and, if necessary for conduit length, the middle colic artery.

Placement of Surgical Incisions

- A midline laparotomy from the xiphoid process to the umbilicus is made (**FIGURE 4**).
- After verifying the patient to be a candidate for resection and verifying that THE can proceed, a 5-cm incision is made overlying the anterior border of the left sternocleidomastoid muscle with the inferior extent at the head of the clavicle. Contraindications to THE include difficult mediastinal blunt dissection of the esophagus because of tumor or treatment effect, excessive mediastinal bleeding with blunt dissection, and inadequate conduit length for reconstruction.

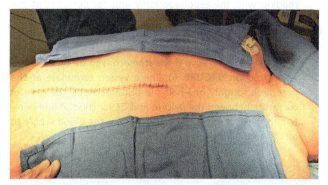

FIGURE 4 • Supine position with location of surgical incisions for transhiatal esophagectomy.

TRANSHIATAL ESOPHAGECTOMY

Abdominal Exploration to Exclude Metastatic Disease

- Upon entering the abdomen, visceral and parietal peritoneal surfaces are palpated to exclude occult peritoneal carcinomatosis. This should include inspection of the lesser sac by opening through the gastrocolic omentum.
- The liver is palpated for suspicious nodules and biopsy performed. Intraoperative ultrasound can be a useful adjunct in this step. If indeterminate lesions are noted on preoperative imaging, ultrasound-guided biopsy is indicated.
- Metastatic disease is an absolute contraindication to proceeding with surgical resection.

Exploration of the Esophageal Hiatus to Determine Local Resectability

- Prior to proceeding with dissection of the stomach, the esophageal hiatus is explored to make sure the distal esophagus and GE junction can be dissected free of the esophageal

hiatus and surrounding abdominal and mediastinal structures. If so, and in the absence of metastatic disease, resection can proceed.
- This dissection and subsequent dissections are facilitated by use of an electrosurgical device such as an ultrasonic or bipolar scalpel.
- The pars flaccida is opened, including division of an accessory or replaced left hepatic artery, if necessary.
- The peritoneum and phrenoesophageal membrane overlying the junction of the right crus of the diaphragm and esophagus are incised, allowing the esophagus to be dissected off the right crus.
- The phrenoesophageal membrane just cephalad to the GE fat pad is divided as is the peritoneal reflection overlying the angle of His.
- The esophagus is dissected off the left crus of the diaphragm and esophagus encircled with a 1-in Penrose drain (**FIGURE 5**).
- The esophagus and GE junction are then dissected free of the crural confluence of the esophageal hiatus, and esophagus with associated periesophageal fatty tissue and lymph nodes dissected free of the esophageal hiatus and underlying aorta.
- If the esophagus and GE junction are free of surrounding structures, resection can proceed. If adherent to or invading the pleura, pericardium, or diaphragm (T4a), resection of these structures can be performed. If adherent to the aorta, vertebral body, or trachea (T4b), resection should be aborted.

Mobilization of the Stomach and Duodenum

- Once it is determined that resection can proceed, the stomach and duodenum are mobilized. Most often, the stomach is used as the conduit for reconstruction following THE. Therefore, mobilization of the stomach for purposes of proceeding with the esophagectomy and for purposes of the creation of the gastric conduit occur simultaneously.
- The right gastroepiploic artery and vein are identified along the greater curvature of the stomach. An adequate pulse in this vessel is imperative if the stomach is to be used for the reconstruction (**FIGURE 6**). These vessels terminate at the bare area roughly one-half the distance along the greater curvature between the pylorus and GE junction. It is imperative to preserve these vessels as they are the blood supply to and from the conduit.

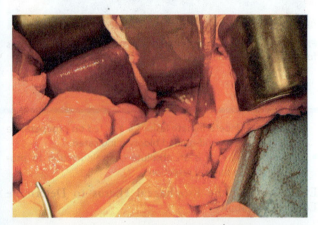

FIGURE 5 • Dissection of the gastroesophageal junction and encirclement with a Penrose drain to facilitate manipulation.

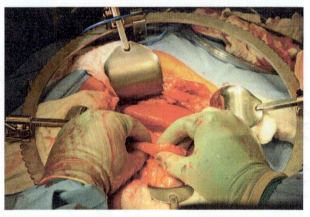

FIGURE 6 • Palpation of the right gastroepiploic pedicle along the greater curvature of the stomach to ensure an adequate pulse to permit use of the stomach as a conduit for reconstruction.

- Once these vessels are identified, the gastrocolic ligament is entered several centimeters from the bare area entering the lesser sac.
- Using an electrosurgery device, the gastrosplenic ligament and short gastric vessels are divided proceeding along the greater curvature toward the esophageal hiatus. Placing a surgical clip on the distal ends of larger vessels, including the left gastroepiploic artery, can ensure ongoing hemostasis of these vessels. The posterior leaflet of the gastrosplenic ligament is likewise divided as are the congenital adhesions of the stomach to the anterior surface of the pancreas. This frees the greater curvature.
- Division of the gastrocolic ligament then proceeds distally, paying careful attention to stay at least a few centimeters away from the right gastroepiploic vessels (**FIGURE 7**). Careful attention should be paid to not placing traction or trauma to these vessels while freeing the stomach from the colon. This is especially true as one frees the stomach from the anterior surface of the pancreas and approaches the origin of these vessels from under the duodenal bulb. Traction of the vein, in particular, can traumatize these vessels resulting in impaired venous outflow and conduit venous congestion.
- After freeing the stomach from the colon, a Kocher maneuver is performed to permit mobilization of the duodenum. An adequate Kocher maneuver permits mobilization of the pylorus to reach the esophageal hiatus (**FIGURE 8**).
- At this point, the remainder of the gastrohepatic ligament is divided and left gastric pedicle is identified.
- The lymph nodes along the left gastric pedicle and celiac axis and surrounding aorta are dissected free of the origin of the left gastric artery and included in the surgical specimen. The left gastric artery and vein are then divided with either a vascular load of a surgical stapler or suture ligated.
- The stomach is now free of its upper attachments and vasculature. If a colon conduit is preferred, preparation of the colon should proceed. If a gastric conduit is preferred, the gastric conduit is created to avoid trauma to the conduit during retraction of the stomach necessary for the inferior mediastinal dissection. This also allows verification of the adequacy of the blood supply to the apex of the conduit and

Chapter 15 ESOPHAGECTOMY: TRANSHIATAL AND RECONSTRUCTION   115

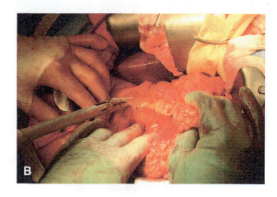

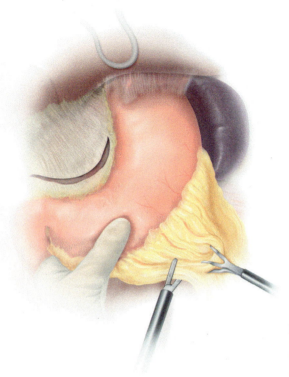

FIGURE 7 • **A** and **B,** Mobilization of the greater curvature of the stomach by dividing the gastrosplenic and gastrocolic ligament being careful to not injure the gastroepiploic pedicle.

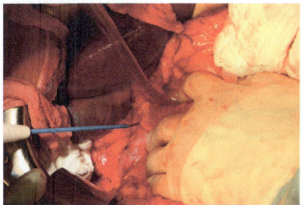

FIGURE 8 • Kocher maneuver to ensure adequate mobility of the pylorus. This is ensured if the pylorus can freely reach to the hiatus without tension.

length of the conduit prior to proceeding with the transhiatal dissection. This will be discussed in the following text. For this discussion, the mediastinal dissection will be described.
- With a Penrose drain around the GE junction for caudal retraction of the stomach and lower esophagus, associated lymphatic tissue is dissected under direct visualization from the lower mediastinum. This dissection is facilitated by a medium handheld malleable retractor and the use of an electrosurgical device. Approximately 5 to 10 cm of mediastinal esophagus can be dissected under direct visualization by this technique. Mobility of the mediastinal esophagus to ensure feasibility and safety of a transhiatal blunt dissection is verified.
- After the limits of direct visualization are reached, blunt mediastinal dissection can proceed. To ensure proper tactile orientation of the esophagus during blunt dissection, a 44 Fr bougie dilator or equivalent is placed in the esophagus.
- The hand is then first advanced posterior to the esophagus, between the esophagus and aorta. The surgeon's fingers are then advanced up this plane with pressure on the bougie containing esophagus to ensure proper tissue plane dissection (**FIGURE 9**).
- The same dissection is then performed anterior to the esophagus.
- If vagal nerve sparing is planned, the vagus nerves are elevated off the esophagus by hooking the nerves with the index finger and bluntly dissecting them down and off the esophagus where they are then dissected free from the GE junction and stomach. As this operation is most often performed for malignancy, division of the vagal nerves is required to ensure proper oncologic dissection. The nerves are then divided at the level of the hiatus with the electrosurgery device.
- This completes the abdominal stomach and esophagus mobilization.

SECTION V TREATMENT OF ESOPHAGEAL CANCER

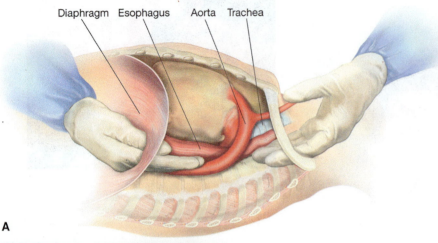

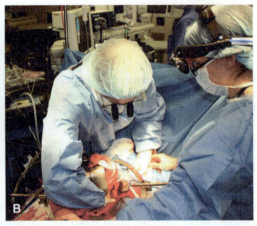

FIGURE 9 • **A** and **B,** Mediastinal mobilization of the esophagus with a hand placed through the esophageal hiatus from the abdominal incision and finger placed through the cervical incision.

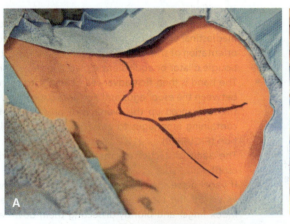

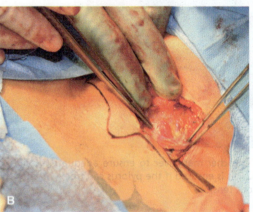

FIGURE 10 • Cervical skin incision and dissection. **A,** Location of cervical skin incision. **B,** Dissection through platysma.

Cervical and Upper Mediastinal Esophageal Mobilization

- The cervical esophagus is approached through a 5-cm incision anterior to the left sternocleidomastoid muscle. The skin, subcutaneous tissues, and platysma are divided with electrocautery (**FIGURE 10**).
- The thin fascial layer surrounding the anterior border of the sternocleidomastoid muscle is incised with cautery.
- The dissection is carried medial and deep to the sternocleidomastoid muscle. The omohyoid muscle is identified and divided with cautery. The inferior thyroid artery and middle thyroid vein, if identified, are ligated with fine silk or absorbable suture.
- Dissection is carried medial to the carotid sheath with gentle lateral traction on the sternocleidomastoid and carotid sheath and medial traction on the trachea and thyroid. The recurrent laryngeal nerve (RLN) is identified and preserved

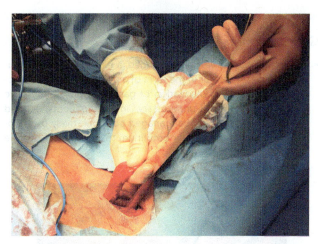

FIGURE 11 • Dissection of the cervical esophagus is facilitated by placement of a Penrose drain around the esophagus after sharply dissecting the esophagus free of other vital cervical structures, including the recurrent laryngeal nerve.

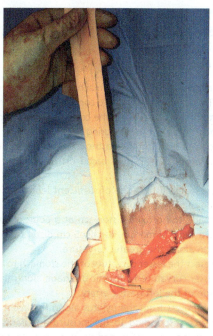

FIGURE 12 • Removal of the esophagectomy specimen through the abdominal incision after attaching a Penrose drain to the cut distal end of the esophagus to guide advancement of the reconstruction conduit back up through the esophageal bed in the posterior mediastinum.

- adherent to the tracheoesophageal groove. Dissection is carried down to the prevertebral fascia allowing the surgeon to then pass the index finger between the prevertebral fascia and esophagus.
- The cervical esophagus is then sharply dissected from trachea, being careful to neither dissect free nor injure the RLN. Once free of the trachea, a blunt right-angle clamp placed between the trachea and esophagus rotated and advanced to the prevertebral fascia facilitates placement of a Penrose drain around the esophagus (**FIGURE 11**).
- Upward traction is placed on the cervical esophagus and blunt mediastinal dissection of the upper and middle third of the esophagus can ensue (**FIGURE 9**). The surgeon maintains contact between the volar aspect of the first two fingers and the esophagus at all times to the proper tissue plane of dissection. Again, a small-caliber bougie dilator placed in the esophagus facilitates tactile feedback of the esophagus.
- With anterior and upward traction of the cervical esophagus and caudal retraction on the stomach, a hand is inserted through the hiatus posterior to the esophagus and is met by fingers inserted through the neck incision down the prevertebral plane. Loose areolar attachments are divided until fingers meet.
- The same dissection is then performed anterior to the esophagus. When performing this dissection, the surgeon must maintain constant pressure on the esophagus to avoid injury to the membranous trachea. Both the anterior and posterior planes can usually be dissected relatively easily.
- Having freed the esophagus from its anterior and posterior attachments, the lateral attachments are then divided. This is often done with a combination of direct downward pressure on these attachments with the index finger from above or by placing the inferior index finger above the attachment pulling down along the insertion of the attachment into the esophagus.
- Alternatively, the bougie can be removed from the esophagus and the lateral attachments divided under direct visualization as the esophagus is retracted anteriorly out the cervical incision. Usually, some sort of bimanual dissection in the posterior mediastinum is required.
- At any point where this dissection proves difficult because of difficult adhesions; fused tissue planes especially in the vicinity of the membranous trachea, carina, and azygous vein; lack of mobility of the esophagus; or excessive bleeding, the blunt dissection should be abandoned and dissection under direct visualization performed via an incision in the right chest.

Removal of the Esophagus

- After complete mobilization of the esophagus, the cervical esophagus is delivered into the next for several centimeters and divided leaving approximately 20 cm of length to the esophagus. The remaining esophagus can subsequently be divided further at the time of anastomosis.
- A 1-in Penrose is affixed to the distal esophagus and the stomach and esophagus drawn down through the hiatus dragging the Penrose thru the esophageal bed into the abdomen. This will allow the reconstruction conduit to be attached to the Penrose and delivered cephalad up into the cervical incision for subsequent anastomosis to the cervical esophagus (**FIGURE 12**).

RECONSTRUCTION: GASTRIC CONDUIT

Creation of Gastric Conduit

- After mobilization of the stomach, the gastric conduit is created. This is best done prior to completion of the mediastinal dissection so as to protect the conduit from trauma due to manipulation of stomach during dissection.
- The goals of creating the gastric conduit are as follows:
  - Create a gastric tube based on the greater curvature blood supply.
  - Create a gastric tube of sufficient length to reach into the cervical incision.
  - Divide the proximal stomach at a point assuring negative surgical margin, usually 5 cm distal to the GE junction along the greater curvature.
  - Resect the lesser curvature of the stomach to include the lesser curvature lymphatic drainage along the distribution of the left gastric artery.
- Six centimeters from the pylorus along the lesser curvature, roughly corresponding to the incisura angularis, the lesser curvature neurovascular pedicle is suture ligated. Careful attention is directed at preserving the integrity of the right gastric artery.
- Using a surgical stapling device, the stomach is divided from this point along the lesser curvature parallel to the greater curvature creating a 5-cm wide gastric tube (FIGURE 13). The division of the stomach is completed 5 cm from the GE junction along the greater curvature (FIGURE 14). For this step, a "thick" load of the stapling device is recommended.
- Length of the conduit is inspected by delivering the conduit over the patient's torso (FIGURE 15). The apex should reach to the sternal notch to be of sufficient length to reach into the cervical incision once brought through the esophageal bed.
- The conduit should be inspected for viability. If the viability is in question, removal of some of the apex of the stomach may result in insufficient length forcing conversion to a transthoracic approach where gastric conduit length is less of a concern.

Gastric Drainage Procedure

- As the vagus nerves will be divided, a gastric drainage is usually necessary either in the form of a pyloromyotomy or pyloroplasty. With tubularization of gastric conduit, some have omitted this step as unnecessary.[7] In these patients, delayed gastric emptying can be managed postoperatively by endoscopic balloon dilation or botulinum toxin injection into the pylorus.

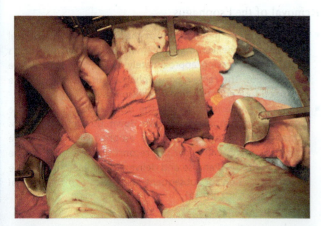

FIGURE 13 • The gastric conduit is begun by ligating the lesser curvature neurovascular pedicle and then starting the conduit staple line at the incisura angularis.

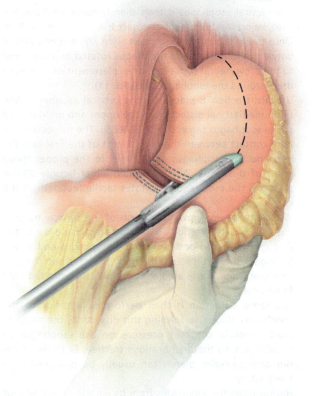

FIGURE 14 • **A** and **B**, The staple line proceeds cephalad toward the hiatus giving rise to a 5-cm wide gastric conduit while removing the lesser curvature of the stomach and straightening the natural curvature of the stomach to optimize conduit length. The gastric staple line terminates 5 cm from the gastroesophageal junction along the greater curvature of the stomach.

Chapter 15 ESOPHAGECTOMY: TRANSHIATAL AND RECONSTRUCTION

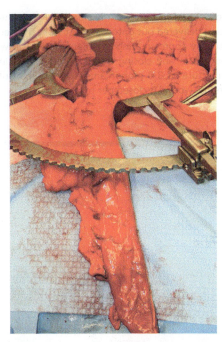

FIGURE 15 • The completed gastric conduit.

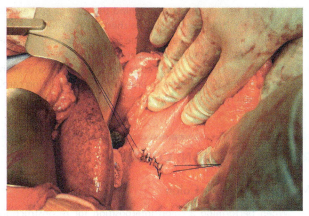

FIGURE 16 • A Heineke-Mikulicz pyloroplasty is made by making a 4-cm longitudinal incision centered at the pylorus. This full-thickness incision is closed transversely with interrupted 3-0 silk sutures using a full-thickness bite.

- For pyloromyotomy, an incision measuring 1.5 cm along the stomach extending 1 cm along the anterior surface of the duodenum across the pylorus is made using the needle tip cautery. With a fine mosquito clamp, the pyloric muscle fibers are divided. An omental patch can be used to patch the exposed submucosa using a Graham patch technique.
- For pyloroplasty, a 4-cm full-thickness longitudinal incision is made beginning 2 cm proximal to the pylorus on the anterior stomach. This full-thickness incision is then closed transversely with interrupted full-thickness 3-0 silk suture (FIGURE 16).

Esophagogastrostomy

- The apex of the gastric conduit is then sutured to the end of the Penrose drain. The Penrose is then drawn up and out the cervical incision delivering the stomach into the neck. Typically, the stomach reaches with excess length permitting trimming of further stomach off the apex of the conduit. Similarly, the esophagus can be further trimmed and both additional specimens marked and sent for final proximal and distal margin analysis.
- The cervical anastomosis can be accomplished either by a handsewn or stapled approach.[8,9]
- For handsewn approach, two-layer anastomosis is performed with an outer layer of interrupted 3-0 silk suture in a seromuscular fashion and inner layer of running full-thickness monofilament absorbable suture. Others have described a single-layer anastomosis using monofilament absorbable running suture.
- For a stapled anastomosis, a stay suture of 2-0 silk is placed at the 6-o'clock position of the cervical esophagus. A 2-cm long longitudinal gastrotomy is made on the anterior surface of the gastric conduit close to the greater curvature. The 2-0 silk is then placed at the apex of this gastrotomy and tied to serve as stay suture holding orientation of cervical esophagus and gastric conduit for application of the stapler. A 45-mm

stapler is advanced with one arm in the esophagus and the other in the stomach. The stapler is directed toward the right ear with the anastomosis placed along the greater curvature of the stomach. The remaining common enterotomy is closed in two layers with an inner layer of running full-thickness, 3-0 monofilament suture and an outer layer of interrupted 3-0 silk suture in a seromuscular fashion (FIGURE 17).
- After completion of the anastomosis, careful caudal traction of the stomach at the hiatus is applied as the anastomosis is

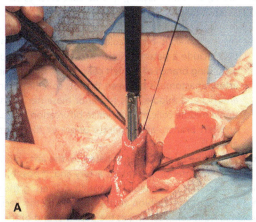

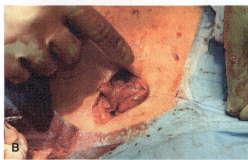

FIGURE 17 • A, Linear stapled esophagogastrostomy using a 45-mm line stapler in a side-to-side fashion. B, Suture closure of the anterior portion of the anastomosis or common enterotomy of the esophagogastrostomy.

- delivered back into the neck behind the trachea and excess redundancy of the conduit in the chest is straightened out.
- Either a nasojejunal feeding tube is placed or surgical jejunostomy tube placed for postoperative nutrition.
- The gastric conduit is anchored to the arch of the hiatus with interrupted 3-0 silk suture to prevent herniation being careful to avoid the gastroepiploic pedicle.
- The soft closed suction drain is placed through the thoracic inlet and delivered out onto the chest wall. The neck wound is closed by approximating the platysma muscle with interrupted suture and closing the skin with a running subcuticular suture of 3-0 monofilament absorbable suture. The abdominal wound is closed per routine.

RECONSTRUCTION: COLON CONDUIT

Mobilization of the Colon

- When performing a colon interposition for reconstruction following THE, the stomach is preserved other than the portion removed to ensure adequate distal margins. This would include preservation of the left gastric artery. To facilitate the use of the colon, however, complete gastric mobilization as discussed earlier is necessary as the preferred route for the colon is retrogastric to decrease tension on the conduit and blood supply.
- Complete colonic mobilization is required including mobilization of both the splenic and hepatic flexures. This often entails extension of the surgical incision below the umbilicus.
- Once mobilization is complete, verification of adequacy of blood supply for the subsequent conduit is needed even in the setting of preoperative angiography. This can be accomplished by serial ligation of the ileocolic artery, then right colic artery, and, if necessary, middle colic arteries with bulldog clamps (FIGURE 3).
    - Angiographic arterial anatomy requirements for a successful left colic–based colon interposition reconstruction include a patent inferior mesenteric artery, patent ascending branch of the left colic artery, intact marginal artery anastomosis between the left colic (inferior mesenteric) and middle colic (superior mesenteric) arteries, single middle colic trunk prior to bifurcation into a right and left branch, and separate origin of the right colic artery.[10]
- To reach to the neck, a conduit based on the left colic artery branch of the inferior mesenteric artery and, if possible, middle colic arteries is needed. This entails delivering the colon in an isoperistaltic fashion to the neck with the cecum or proximal right colon serving as the proximal end of the colon conduit (FIGURE 18).
- If the blood supply is adequate for a left colic vascular–based conduit, the ileocolic artery is ligated as low in the mesentery as possible, as is the right colic artery. The mesentery of the ascending colon is likewise divided to the level of the middle colic arteries.
- The terminal ileum is divided with a surgical stapler.
- The cecum is rotated up to the neck to verify adequate conduit length. If not, the middle colic branches can be divided as well (FIGURE 19).

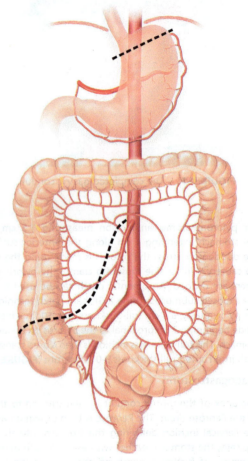

FIGURE 18 • Creation of the colon conduit based on the left colic artery.

Delivery of Colon

- Once the colon is mobilized, the colon is delivered through the hiatus in a fashion similar to the gastric conduit as discussed earlier. To decrease demands on conduit length, it is optimal to deliver the colon to the hiatus behind the stomach in a retrogastric position. Alternatively, the colon can be delivered through a retrosternal pathway if the posterior mediastinum is no longer a viable option. The disadvantage of this route is increased demand on conduit and blood supply length.

Chapter 15 ESOPHAGECTOMY: TRANSHIATAL AND RECONSTRUCTION

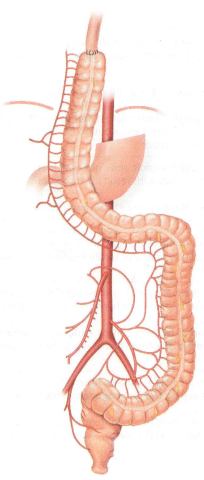

FIGURE 19 • Delivery of the colon through the mediastinum by rotating the cecum up through the esophageal bed and out the cervical incision.

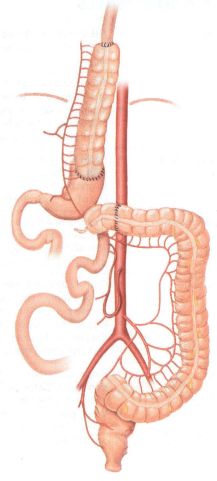

FIGURE 20 • The completed reconstruction with both esophageal-to-colon and colon-to-stomach anastomoses.

- As there is typically adequate length to the colon conduit, the proximal end of the colon can be amputated back, usually removing the cecum. This has the advantage of decreasing the size differential between the cervical esophagus and colon as the colon narrows in luminal diameter and becomes thicker and more muscular. Also, as one moves distally on the colon, the reliance on mesenteric arcades for blood supply decreases.

Anastomoses

- The esophagus-to-colon anastomosis is accomplished in a similar fashion as described in the section on the use of the stomach as a conduit for reconstruction. This can be stapled using a linear stapler or hand sewn in either a one- or two-layer technique. Although circular staplers can be used, conduit length is often inadequate, making this awkward (**FIGURE 20**).

- The cervical anastomosis is drawn back in the neck by careful caudal traction on the colon at the hiatus.
- The colon is then divided at a point along the posterior stomach to permit a subsequent colon-to-stomach anastomosis. This is optimally done using a linear stapler joining the colon and stomach in a side-to-side fashion and closing the common enterotomy with an additional stapler load or handsewn closure.
- In manipulating the colon for this anastomosis, it is imperative to not disturb the mesentery of the colon out of concern for disrupting the mesenteric vessels.
- Enteric continuity is restored by completing the small bowel-to-colon anastomosis using surgical staplers in a standard fashion.
- A jejunostomy feeding tube is placed for nutritional support as is a cervical closed suction drain.
- A gastric drainage procedure is done if vagotomy was performed during the course of esophageal resection.

PEARLS AND PITFALLS

Indications	- THE should only be performed for curative intent when treating malignancy. - NCCN guidelines should be followed as to preoperative evaluation, staging, and treatment algorithms.
Approach	- THE should only be considered for patients with appropriate pathology (middle, lower third of the esophagus, and GE junction tumors). - In patients with unfavorable prior surgical history (prior gastric surgery rendering the gastric conduit inadequate) or locally advanced tumors that require a direct visualization of mediastinal dissection, a THE is contraindicated in favor of a transthoracic approach.
Gastric mobilization	- Avoid any traction or direct trauma to the right gastroepiploic and right gastric artery pedicles so as to avoid disrupting these vessels or causing venous injury with resultant thrombosis as this will lead to graft failure. - Use of an electrosurgical device greatly improves efficiency and effectiveness of gastric mobilization.
Esophageal dissection	- If excessive adhesions are encountered secondary to tumor extension or treatment effect or excessive bleeding is encountered with blunt dissection of the esophagus, a TTE should be performed. - A small-caliber bougie dilator (44 Fr) in the esophagus facilitates tactile localization of the esophagus during blunt mediastinal dissection.
Reconstruction	- Graft failure and anastomotic leak result from ischemia, which is a consequence of inadequate blood supply, venous congestion, tension on the anastomosis, or hypoperfusion in the early postoperative period. These factors should be avoided. - Proper orientation of the conduit with prevention of twisting is made easier by drawing parallel lines on the Penrose drain and making sure the drain does not twist as it is pulled out through the neck delivering the conduit to the cervical incision.
Anastomosis	- Proper orientation of the cervical anastomotic staple lines should be maintained to maximize perfusion of the gastric wall. This is accomplished by keeping the esophagogastrostomy staple line as far away from the conduit lesser curvature staple line. - When placing the anastomosis back in the neck, it should be straightened by reducing redundancy of the conduit by caudal traction on the conduit at the hiatus. Avoid placing tension on the anastomosis.

POSTOPERATIVE CARE

- Patients recover in the intensive care unit until acute cardiac, respiratory, and volume status issues are resolved.
- As hypoxia and hypotension can lead to hypoperfusion of the reconstruction with anastomotic leak or, in the worst scenario, conduit necrosis, this should be avoided and quickly remedied if clinically encountered.
- As respiratory failure and pneumonia are the most common complications encountered, aggressive pulmonary care is required. Early ambulation is mandatory.
- Fluid overload can lead to hypoxia, pulmonary edema, and dysrhythmia (most often atrial fibrillation).
- Enteric nutrition is begun slowly on postoperative day 1.
- Patients should be carefully followed for signs of postoperative complications (see the following text) and evaluation and mitigation strategies employed at the first sign of such issues.
- If the patient is medically stable to consider oral intake, a water-soluble contrast study followed by barium is done on the fourth postoperative day to make sure there is no significant anastomotic leak and the conduit empties adequately into the small intestine.
- If ok, a liquid diet is started and continued for 2 weeks at which time the patient is transitioned to a soft diet for an additional 2 weeks prior to resuming a normal diet. The rationale for this approach is to avoid food impaction during the critical period of anastomotic healing. The surgical drain is removed after a negative study and no evidence of oral fluids in the drain within 48 hours of oral liquid intake.
- The feeding tube is discontinued when the patient is able to take adequate oral intake, usually within the first to second week following surgery.
- Patients should be counseled as to how to optimize their fluid and nutritional intake during this period of transition to regular diet and manage dumping symptoms with dietary and lifestyle modification.
- Patients should be advised as to the early signs of anastomotic stricture and need for esophageal dilation.

OUTCOMES

- THE is a very morbid, high-risk procedure with very high associated operative morbidity and mortality (see the following text).
- Regarding functional outcome, the best data available are reviews from patients who underwent this procedure for benign indications and early stage cancer given the longer survival in these patients compared to patients with cancer.[11,12]
- Symptoms of physical impairment, including GE reflux, dumping, and dysphagia, are very common after surgery but show gradual improvement toward baseline over the first year, not quite reaching baseline. Long-term physical impairment is less common after THE compared to TTE.

- Overall health-related quality of life (ability to work, social interaction, daily activities, emotional function, perception of health, energy level, and mental health) decreases after surgery but returns to baseline national norms within 1 year of surgery.
- Regarding cancer-specific outcome, long-term survival is a function of the underlying biology and stage of the tumor rather than surgical approach.[13,14]

COMPLICATIONS

- Perioperative complications occur in 40% to 50% of patients and fall into specific categories depending on the point of time in which they appear following surgery. Reported overall 30-day mortality for THE ranges from 1% in select single-center reports to 10% in nonselective administrative database reports.[13,15,16]
- Early postoperative period (0-2 days)
  - Technical complications
    - Bleeding
    - RLN injury with resultant hoarseness (unilateral) and airway obstruction (bilateral)
    - Pleural violation with pneumothorax or pleural effusion
    - Conduit necrosis requiring removal of conduit and cervical esophagostomy
  - Medical complications
    - Respiratory complications (respiratory failure, pneumonia)
    - Cardiac complications (dysrhythmia, myocardial infarction, heart failure)
    - Urinary tract complications (renal failure or insufficiency)
- Intermediate postoperative period (2-14 days)
  - Technical complications
    - Anastomotic leak manifests as cervical wound infection and drainage or drainage of oral secretions via closed suction drain
    - Conduit necrosis requiring removal of conduit and cervical esophagostomy
    - Thoracic duct injury with chyle leak usually manifests by pleural effusion at onset of enteric or oral nutrition
  - Medical complications
    - Respiratory complications (respiratory failure, pneumonia)
    - Cardiac complications (dysrhythmia, myocardial infarction, heart failure)
    - Urinary tract complications (renal failure/insufficiency, urinary tract infection)
    - Infectious complications (line infection, organ space infection, wound infection)
- Late postoperative period (after 14 days)
  - Technical complications
    - Anastomotic stricture
    - Delayed gastric emptying
    - Dumping syndrome
  - Medical complications
    - Malnutrition
    - Cancer recurrence

REFERENCES

1. Amin MB, Edge S, Greene F, et al, eds. *AJCC Cancer Staging Manual.* 8th ed. Springer International Publishing: American Joint Commission on Cancer; 2017 [cited 2021 Dec 24].
2. Ajani JA, D'Amico TA, Bentrem DJ, et al. Esophageal and esophagogastric junction cancers. *J Natl Compr Canc Netw.* 2019;17(7):855-883.
3. Birkmeyer NJ, Goodney PP, Stukel TA, et al. Do cancer centers designated by the National Cancer Institute have better surgical outcomes? *Cancer.* 2005;103(3):435-441.
4. Dimick JB, Wainess RM, Upchurch GR Jr, et al. National trends in outcomes for esophageal resection. *Ann Thorac Surg.* 2005;79(1):212-216; discussion 217-218.
5. Voeten DM, Gisbertz SS, Ruurda JP, et al. Overall volume trends in esophageal cancer surgery results from the Dutch upper gastrointestinal cancer audit. *Ann Surg.* 2021;274(3):449-458.
6. Cataife G, Weinberg DA, Wong HH, et al. The effect of Surgical Care Improvement Project (SCIP) compliance on surgical site infections (SSI). *Med Care.* 2014;52(2 suppl 1):S66-S73.
7. Arya S, Markar SR, Karthikesalingam A, Hanna GB. The impact of pyloric drainage on clinical outcome following esophagectomy: a systematic review. *Dis Esophagus.* 2015;28(4):326-335.
8. Honda M, Kuriyama A, Noma H, et al. Hand-sewn versus mechanical esophagogastric anastomosis after esophagectomy: a systematic review and meta-analysis. *Ann Surg.* 2013;257(2):238-248.
9. Price TN, Nichols FC, Harmsen WS, et al. A comprehensive review of anastomotic technique in 432 esophagectomies. *Ann Thorac Surg.* 2013;95(4):1154-1160; discussion 1160-1161.
10. Peters JH, Kronson JW, Katz M, et al. Arterial anatomic considerations in colon interposition for esophageal replacement. *Arch Surg.* 1995;130(8):858-862; discussion 862-863.
11. de Boer AG, van Lanschot JJ, van Sandick JW, et al. Quality of life after transhiatal compared with extended transthoracic resection for adenocarcinoma of the esophagus. *J Clin Oncol.* 2004;22(20):4202-4208.
12. Darling GE. Quality of life in patients with esophageal cancer. *Thorac Surg Clin.* 2013;23(4):569-575.
13. Chang AC, Ji H, Birkmeyer NJ, et al. Outcomes after transhiatal and transthoracic esophagectomy for cancer. *Ann Thorac Surg.* 2008;85(2):424-429.
14. Hulscher JB, van Sandick JW, de Boer AG, et al. Extended transthoracic resection compared with limited transhiatal resection for adenocarcinoma of the esophagus. *N Engl J Med.* 2002;347(21):1662-1669.
15. Orringer MB, Marshall B, Chang AC, et al. Two thousand transhiatal esophagectomies: changing trends, lessons learned. *Ann Surg.* 2007;246(3):363-372; discussion 372-374.
16. Mertens AC, Kalff MC, Eshuis WJ, et al. Transthoracic versus transhiatal esophagectomy for esophageal cancer: a nationwide propensity score-matched cohort analysis. *Ann Surg Oncol.* 2021;28(1):175-183.

Chapter 16 | Ivor Lewis Esophagectomy

Robert E. Merritt

DEFINITION
- An Ivor Lewis esophagectomy is defined as a resection of the esophageal tumor using a laparotomy incision and a right thoracotomy. The Ivor Lewis operation can also be performed with a minimally invasive esophagectomy approach, which involves right video-assisted thoracoscopy and laparoscopy. The esophagogastric anastomosis is performed in the right thoracic cavity. The Ivor Lewis technique is appropriate for patients with resectable tumors in the middle and distal third of the esophagus as well as the gastroesophageal junction.

PATIENT HISTORY AND PHYSICAL FINDINGS
- Patients who present with esophageal carcinoma should undergo a complete history and physical examination.
- Patients often complain of dysphagia to solid food and liquids. This symptom is related to esophageal obstruction from a bulky tumor.
- Barrett intestinal metaplasia or gastroesophageal reflux disease may precede the diagnosis of esophageal cancer.
- Significant weight loss is a common symptom of patients with esophageal cancer. The weight loss may be secondary to poor oral intake related to dysphagia or cancer cachexia.
- The cervical lymph nodes and supraclavicular lymph nodes should be thoroughly examined during physical examination. The cervical and supraclavicular lymph nodes are a common site for metastatic spread from esophageal carcinoma.

IMAGING AND OTHER DIAGNOSTIC STUDIES
- An esophagogastroduodenoscopy should be performed on every patient with esophageal carcinoma (**FIGURE 1**). Upper endoscopy allows access to the tumor for diagnosis and determination of the histologic subtype (adenocarcinoma vs squamous cell carcinoma). The location of the tumor is also important to determine whether an Ivor Lewis esophagectomy would be feasible. Esophageal tumors in the proximal third of the esophagus would require a transhiatal or three-field esophagectomy with a cervical esophagogastrostomy anastomosis.
- Endoscopic ultrasound (EUS) is a critical staging technique for esophageal cancer (**FIGURE 2**). The EUS determines the depth of invasion of the tumor into the esophageal wall (T stage). Esophageal tumors that penetrate through the esophageal wall are considered locally advanced and have a high propensity to metastasize to locoregional lymph nodes. Periesophageal lymph nodes that are enlarged can be visualized with EUS and fine-needle aspiration biopsy can be

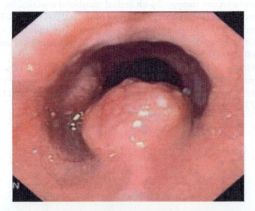

FIGURE 1 • An upper endoscopy demonstrating a large distal esophageal carcinoma. An endoscopic biopsy was consistent with a moderately differentiated adenocarcinoma.

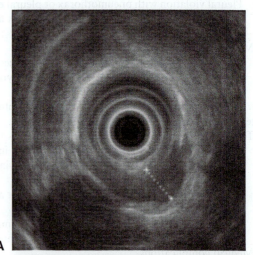

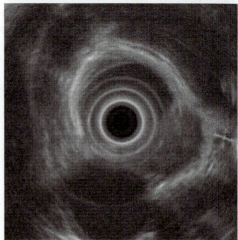

FIGURE 2 • **A,** An endoscopic ultrasound image demonstrating a T3 esophageal carcinoma with extension into the adventitia. **B,** Demonstration of a peritumoral lymph node.

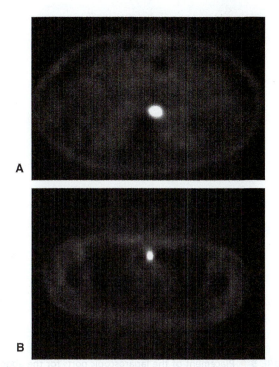

FIGURE 3 • **A,** The first positron emission tomography (PET) image demonstrates a hypermetabolic esophageal carcinoma located in the distal third of the esophagus. **B,** The second PET image demonstrates a hypermetabolic cervical lymph node that represents distal metastatic disease.

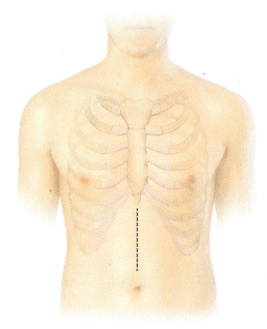

FIGURE 4 • A midline laparotomy incision is located between the xiphoid and the umbilicus.

performed to determine locoregional lymph node involvement. Patients with biopsy-proven lymph node involvement will typically be referred for preoperative chemotherapy or combined chemoradiation.
- All patients who are being considered for esophagectomy should undergo a computed tomography (CT) scan of the chest, abdomen, and pelvis to evaluate the primary tumor in the esophagus and the locoregional lymph nodes. The liver, celiac lymph nodes, bone, and adrenal glands are common sites for metastatic disease secondary to esophageal carcinoma. Positron emission tomography (PET) is an essential staging technique for esophageal carcinoma (**FIGURE 3**). PET scans can detect occult metastatic disease that was not identified on standard CT scans in about 10% to 15% of cases. This detection of occult metastatic disease will prevent patients with stage IV esophageal carcinoma from undergoing an unnecessary esophageal resection.

SURGICAL MANAGEMENT

Preoperative Planning
- Any patient who is being evaluated for an Ivor Lewis esophagectomy should undergo a complete and thorough cardiopulmonary evaluation prior to the operation. Cardiac disease and respiratory compromise should be identified in the preoperative period to properly access perioperative risk of complications and mortality.
- Pulmonary function tests should be obtained to measure the forced expiratory volume in 1 second (FEV_1) and diffusion capacity. Patients with a history of chronic obstructive pulmonary disease will have diminished values for FEV_1 and diffusing capacity of lung for carbon monoxide; therefore, they will be at increased risk for perioperative respiratory complications.
- A transthoracic echocardiogram is obtained to assess the left ventricular ejection fraction and left ventricular wall motion. A treadmill stress test should be obtained when the echocardiogram findings are abnormal.
- Prior to surgical resection, a patient's nutritional status should be optimized. A preoperative feeding access for enteral nutrition may be necessary in cases of severe malnutrition. A prealbumin level can be measured to further assess the patient's nutritional status.
- Perioperative antibiotics should be given within 30 minutes of the first incision. Compression boots are placed on the lower extremities and subcutaneous unfractionated heparin is given to minimize the risk of postoperative deep venous thrombosis (DVT).
- An arterial line and central venous catheter should be placed for intraoperative hemodynamic monitoring.
- An epidural catheter should be placed for postoperative pain management. Epidural infusion of local anesthetic minimizes postthoracotomy pain and allows patients to participate in pulmonary toilet exercises.

Positioning
- The Ivor Lewis esophagectomy technique uses two incisions. Patients are positioned in the supine position first for the midline laparotomy incision (**FIGURE 4**) or with multiple laparoscopy incisions (**FIGURE 5**). The second portion of the operation is performed through a right posterior lateral thoracotomy (**FIGURE 6**) or multiple thoracoscopic incisions (**FIGURE 7**). Patients are positioned in the left lateral decubitus position. A beanbag is used to help hold patients into position. The operating room bed is flexed to open the rib spaces.

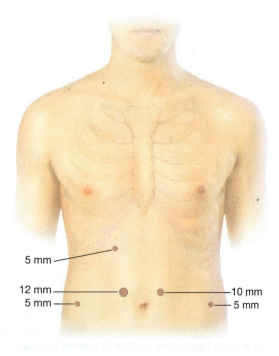

FIGURE 5 • Placement of the laparoscopic ports for the abdominal phase of minimally invasive esophagectomy.

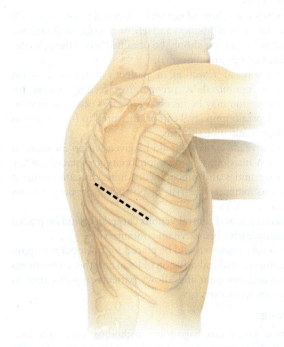

FIGURE 6 • A standard posterior lateral thoracotomy incision provides excellent exposure of the intrathoracic esophagus.

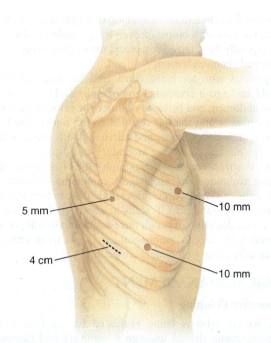

FIGURE 7 • Placement for the thoracoscopic ports for the thoracic phase of minimally invasive esophagectomy.

MOBILIZATION OF THE GASTRIC CONDUIT

- The patient is positioned supine on the operating table. A double-lumen endotracheal tube is placed for single lung isolation. An arterial line, central venous catheter, and epidural catheter are placed by the anesthesia team. Compression boots and subcutaneous heparin are given for DVT prophylaxis.
- A midline laparotomy incision is performed from the xiphoid down to the umbilicus for the open approach. A full inspection of the abdominal cavity is performed to rule out tumor dissemination on peritoneal surfaces or liver metastasis. A Bookwalter retractor is used to provide exposure. The triangular ligament of the left lobe of the liver is divided and the left lateral segment is retracted cephalad to expose the esophageal hiatus.
- The dissection of the gastric conduit begins by entering the lesser sac along the great curvature of the stomach. The right gastroepiploic artery should be identified and preserved. The greater omentum is divided along the greater curvature of the stomach with an ultrasonic dissector by divided branches of the right gastroepiploic arcade and carefully preserving the gastroepiploic trunk (**FIGURE 8**).
- The gastrocolic omentum is divided toward the duodenum. The stomach is retracted upward and any adhesions between the stomach and pancreas should be carefully divided (**FIGURE 9**). The duodenum is then mobilized with the Kocher maneuver.
- The short gastric vessels are ligated using the ultrasonic dissector. The short gastric vessels should be ligated close to the spleen to avoid thermal injury to the stomach.
- The lesser omentum is then divided toward the esophageal hiatus. A replaced left hepatic artery should be identified and preserved if present. The right gastric artery can be preserved in most cases when the anastomosis is performed in the right thorax.
- The left gastric pedicle is identified along the lesser curvature of the stomach. The left gastric pedicle is divided at the origin from the celiac axis using an Endo GIA linear stapler. The surrounding adipose tissue and lymph nodes should be swept upward prior to ligation of the left gastric pedicle (**FIGURE 10**).
- The crura of the diaphragm are identified and the distal esophagus should be visualized. The phrenoesophageal membrane is then divided to facilitate mobilization of the esophagus around the esophageal hiatus (**FIGURE 11**). The right crus of the diaphragm is divided if necessary to permit four fingers to fit into the opened esophageal hiatus. This prevents compression of the esophageal conduit and possible ischemia.

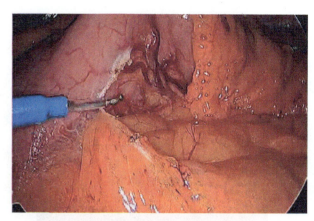

FIGURE 9 • Mobilization of the stomach.

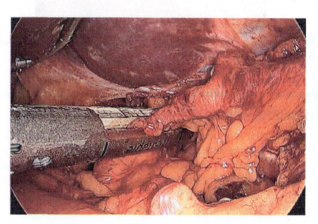

FIGURE 10 • Division of the left gastric artery.

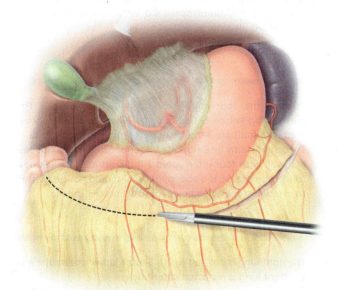

FIGURE 8 • The division of the gastrocolic ligament along the great curvature of the stomach. The right gastroepiploic artery is preserved.

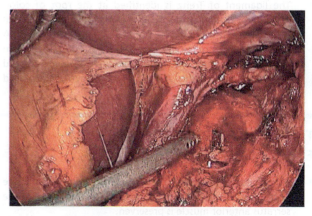

FIGURE 11 • Dissection of the hiatus.

FORMATION OF THE GASTRIC CONDUIT

- The Endo GIA linear stapler is used to divide the stomach along the lesser curvature. The staple line is started along the lesser curvature just proximal to the right gastric artery (FIGURE 12). The staple line should end between the cardia and the fundus. The staple line is oversewn with multiple interrupted 3-0 silk sutures to cover the staple line with serosa. The gastric tube should be 4 to 5 cm in width.
- The gastric tube is secured to the remnant of the gastric cardia with two interrupted 0 silk sutures. This will allow the gastric conduit to be pulled into the chest along with the esophagogastric specimen.

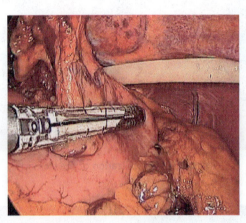
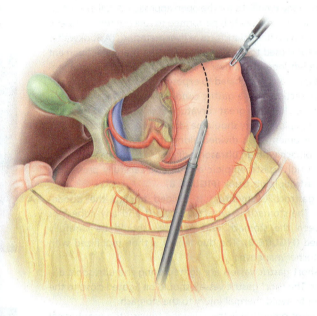

FIGURE 12 • Left and Right, The formation of the gastric conduit using a linear endoscopic stapler. The gastric conduit should be 5 to 6 cm in diameter.

HEINEKE-MIKULICZ PYLOROPLASTY

- The pylorus muscle is identified with direct palpation at the border of the antrum of the stomach and the first portion of the duodenum. The pylorus muscle is incised longitudinally using the cautery and ultrasonic dissector. The incision is carried through the mucosal layer. The incision is then closed transversely with interrupted 4-0 Vicryl sutures and second layer of 3-0 silk sutures.

JEJUNOSTOMY FEEDING TUBE

- The ligament of Treitz is identified at the root of colon mesentery. The jejunostomy tube is placed in the proximal jejunum about 30 to 40 cm from the ligament of Treitz. A purse-string suture is placed on the serosa of the jejunum using a 4-0 chromic suture. A small enterotomy is created within the purse string. A 10 Fr jejunostomy tube is placed through the abdominal wall and into the jejunum. The purse-string suture is tied and the jejunostomy site is covered with multiple 3-0 silk sutures to imbricate the serosa.
- The jejunostomy insertion site is then secured to the abdominal wall with four interrupted 2-0 silk sutures. The jejunostomy tube site on the abdominal wall should not be twisted to avoid postoperative bowel obstruction or ischemia.

THORACIC MOBILIZATION OF THE ESOPHAGUS

- A right posterior lateral thoracotomy is performed and the right chest is entered through the fifth intercostal space. The serratus anterior muscle is preserved.
- The right lung is isolated with a double lumen chest tube and the right lung is retracted anteriorly.
- The inferior pulmonary ligament is incised with cautery and the level 9 lymph nodes are harvested. The mediastinal pleura along the anterior esophagus is incised with the

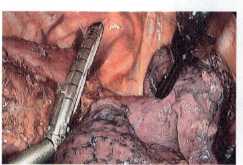
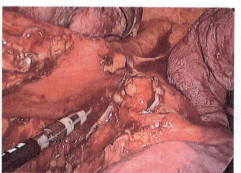

FIGURE 13 • Dissection (left) and mobilization (right) of the esophagus.

cautery. The distal esophagus is dissected from the pericardium and the aorta posteriorly (FIGURE 13). The esophagus is then encircled with a 1-in Penrose drain.

- The esophagus is mobilized from the esophageal hiatus to the azygous vein (FIGURE 14). The ultrasonic dissector or LigaSure device can be used to divide small vessels and lymphatics. The thoracic duct should be suture ligated if the structure is injured during the esophageal dissection. The thoracic duct enters the right thorax through the aortic hiatus and is usually located between the azygous vein and the aorta. The thoracic duct crosses over to the left side at T4-T5 and passes behind the aortic arch. The thoracic duct passes posteriorly to the left carotid sheath and drains into the junction of the left jugular and subclavian vein.
- The azygous vein is routinely dissected and divided with an Endo GIA linear stapler. The esophagogastric anastomosis is usually performed at the level of the azygous vein. In cases where the esophageal tumor is located in midesophagus, the esophageal dissection may have to be carried more proximally toward the thoracic inlet.

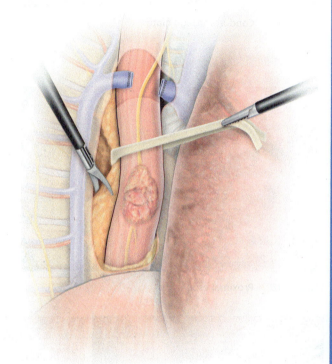

FIGURE 14 • The mobilization of the intrathoracic esophagus using an ultrasonic dissector. The azygous vein is routinely divided. The esophagogastric anastomosis is usually performed at the level of the azygous vein.

ESOPHAGOGASTRIC ANASTOMOSIS

- The gastric conduit is pulled into the right chest and the sutures attaching to the esophagogastrectomy specimen are divided (FIGURE 15). The esophagus is divided 2 cm above the azygous vein with an Endo GIA linear stapler (FIGURE 16). The proximal esophageal margin and distal gastric margin are evaluated with frozen section.
- The 2-0 Prolene purse-string suture is placed through the mucosa and muscular layers of the esophagus. A 25- or 28-mm anvil is placed in the esophageal lumen and the purse-string suture is tied around the shaft of the anvil. A second purse-string suture is placed as well.
- A gastrotomy is performed along the proximal lesser curvature of the gastric conduit. An end-to-end anastomosis (EEA) circular stapler is inserted through the gastrotomy and the pin is deployed proximally along the great curvature. The anvil and EEA stapler are connected and the stapler is deployed (FIGURES 17 and 18).
- The esophagogastric anastomosis should be inspected and checked for completeness (FIGURE 19). The "doughnuts" should be complete to ensure esophageal and gastric mucosal apposition. A nasogastric tube is then passed under direct vision.

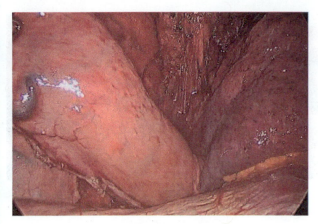

FIGURE 15 • Conduit through hiatus.

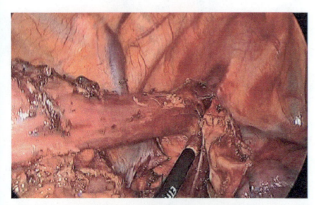

FIGURE 16 • Proximal esophagus.

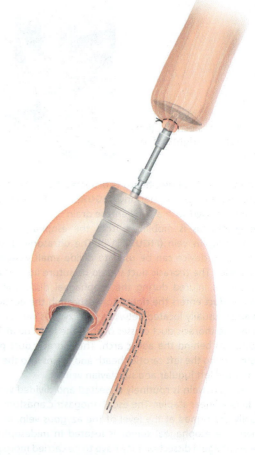

FIGURE 17 • The formation of the esophagogastric anastomosis using a circular end-to-end anastomosis stapler.

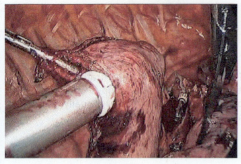
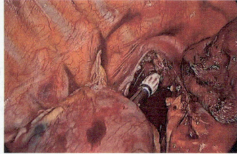

FIGURE 18 • End-to-end anastomosis in conduit (left) with anvil in esophagus (right).

- The gastrotomy site is resected with one to two applications of the Endo GIA stapler (**FIGURE 20**). The staple line is oversewn with interrupted 3-0 silk sutures.
- The anastomosis is reinforced with 3-0 silk sutures placed between the muscular layer of the esophagus and the serosa of the gastric conduit.
- A pleural flap is harvested and used to wrap the esophagogastric anastomosis. Omentum or intercostal muscle flaps could be used as alternatives for coverage of the esophagogastric anastomosis.

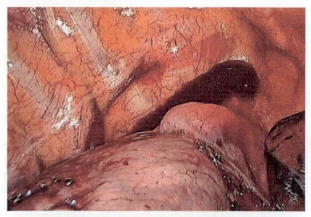

FIGURE 19 • Anastomosis.

Chapter 16 IVOR LEWIS ESOPHAGECTOMY   131

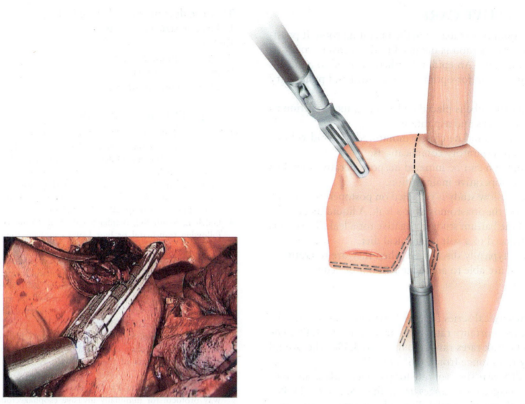

FIGURE 20 • The completion of the esophagogastric anastomosis with resection of the gastrotomy site (left) with a linear endoscopic stapler (right).

PEARLS AND PITFALLS

Preoperative evaluation	▪ Preoperative staging should include a PET/CT scan and EUS. Patients with transmural tumors and nodal disease benefit from preoperative chemotherapy and radiation. ▪ Patients with a history of previous gastric surgery may require the use of a colonic or jejunal conduit. ▪ Patients should undergo pulmonary function tests and echocardiography to assess perioperative risk.
Mobilization of the stomach	▪ The right gastroepiploic artery and vein must not be injured. The primary blood supply to gastric conduit is derived from this vascular arcade. ▪ The gastric conduit should be 4-5 cm in diameter. ▪ The gastric conduit tip could be ischemic and should be resected if there is necrosis detected.
Esophagogastric anastomosis	▪ The anastomosis should be covered with a vascularized pedicle, such as omentum, pleura, or intercostal muscle. An anastomotic leak within the thorax could result in life-threatening mediastinitis. ▪ A two-layer anastomosis should be performed regardless of the technique.
Postoperative care	▪ Postoperative barium esophagram should be obtained 5-7 d after the procedure to evaluate the integrity of the esophagogastric anastomosis. Contained leaks can be managed with bowel rest and antibiotics. Large leaks typically require operative repair.

POSTOPERATIVE CARE

- Patients should be extubated in the operating room if possible. A chest radiograph is obtained in the recovery room or intensive care unit. An epidural catheter is used to administer local anesthesia for optimal pain control and pulmonary toilet.
- The nasogastric tube is placed on low continuous suction to avoid gastric stasis and aspiration.
- Fluid balance should be closely monitored to avoid volume overload and respiratory complications.
- Enteral nutrition can be initiated on postoperative day 3 to minimize perioperative malnutrition.
- A barium swallow study is obtained on postoperative days 5 to 7 to assess the anastomosis for a leak. A liquid diet can be initiated if the barium study is negative for a leak. The diet is slowly advanced to a soft mechanical diet.
- Patients are typically discharged when they are tolerating a soft diet and are able to ambulate without difficulty.

OUTCOMES

- In modern surgical series for Ivor Lewis esophagectomy, the perioperative mortality rates range from 1.4% to 4.4%. The anastomotic leak rates range from 0% to 3.5%. The overall morbidity rates range from 26.6% to 45%.
- The overall 5-year survival rate for patients undergoing Ivor Lewis esophagectomy ranges from the 25.2% to 33.3%. Patients with positive nodal disease have a worse prognosis compared to patients with negative nodal disease.
- Minimally invasive Ivor Lewis has demonstrated fewer respiratory complications and a shorter hospital length of stay compared to the open approach.

COMPLICATIONS

- Pneumonia
- Anastomotic leak
- Thoracic duct injury and chyle leak
- Delayed gastric emptying
- Reflux
- Aspiration pneumonitis
- Pulmonary embolism
- Acute myocardial infarction

SUGGESTED READINGS

1. Cerfolio RJ, Bryant AS, Bass CS, et al. Fast tracking after Ivor Lewis esophagogastrectomy. *Chest.* 2004;126:1187-1194.
2. Visbal AL, Allen MS, Miller DL, et al. Ivor Lewis esophagogastrectomy for esophageal cancer. *Ann Thorac Surg.* 2001;71:1803-1808.
3. Karl RC, Schreiber R, Boulware D, et al. Factors affecting morbidity, mortality, and survival in patients undergoing Ivor Lewis esophagogastrectomy. *Ann Surg.* 2000;231:635-643.
4. Gulch L, Smith RC, Bambach CP, et al. Comparison of outcomes following transhiatal or Ivor Lewis esophagectomy for esophageal carcinoma. *World J Surg.* 1999;23:271-275.
5. Griffin SM, Shaw IH, Dresener SM. Early complications after Ivor Lewis subtotal esophagectomy with two-field lymphadenectomy: risk factors and management. *J Am Coll Surg.* 2002;194:285-297.
6. Van Hagen P, Hulshof MC, Van Lanshot JB, et al. Preoperative chemoradiotherapy for esophageal or junctional cancer. *N Engl J Med.* 2012;366:2074-2084.
7. Hulscher JB, Van Sandick JW, De Boer GEM, et al. Extended transthoracic resection compared with limited transhiatal resection for adenocarcinoma of the esophagus. *N Engl J Med.* 2002;347:1662-1669.
8. Merritt RE, Kneuertz PJ, D'Souza DM, et al. A successful pathway protocol for minimally invasive esophagectomy. *Surg Endosc.* 2020;34(4):1969-1703.
9. Merritt RE, Kneuertz PJ, D'Souza DM, et al. An analysis of outcomes after transition from open to minimally invasive Ivor Lewis Esophagectomy. *Ann Thorac Surg.* 2021;11(4):1174-1181.
10. Merritt RE, Kneuertz PJ, D'Souza DM, Perry KA. Total laparoscopic and thoracoscopic Ivor Lewis esophagectomy after neoadjuvant chemoradiation with minimal overall and anastomotic complications. *J Cardiothorac Surg.* 2019;14(1):123.

Chapter 17 | Minimally Invasive Esophagectomy

Jordan A. Wilkerson, Thomas J. Birdas, and DuyKhanh P. Ceppa

DEFINITION

- Minimally invasive esophagectomy (MIE) involves the resection of all or part of the esophagus utilizing a combination of laparoscopy and/or thoracoscopy with the intent of minimizing the morbidity associated with traditional open approaches without compromising the oncologic outcome.
- The majority of the traditional surgical approaches to esophageal resection may be performed minimally invasively. However, if any portion is done through an open incision, the term "hybrid MIE" is more accurate.
- While MIE is most commonly performed in the setting of esophageal cancer, it may also be utilized in the treatment of benign esophageal conditions necessitating resection, such as esophageal stricture or end-stage achalasia.
- Although the location of the primary tumor or esophageal pathology ultimately dictates the preferred surgical approach, the remainder of this chapter focuses on the minimally invasive Ivor Lewis esophagectomy technique.

DIFFERENTIAL DIAGNOSIS

- The differential diagnosis is rather broad for patients presenting with symptoms of dysphagia, as both structural and functional esophageal abnormalities must be considered. Esophageal malignancy must always be considered in the adult patient with new or progressive symptoms.
- Other potential etiologies of dysphagia include esophageal motility disorders (achalasia, diffuse esophageal spasm), esophageal stricture, hiatal hernia, external compression (vascular abnormalities, fibrosis), and eosinophilic esophagitis.

PATIENT HISTORY AND PHYSICAL FINDINGS

- A thorough history and physical should be obtained on all patients presenting for evaluation with the objective of identifying any symptoms or risk factors that may suggest a specific etiology or extent of disease. Additionally, a thorough history and physical examination will assist in assessing the patient's overall surgical candidacy.
- Patients with esophageal malignancy classically present with symptoms of progressive dysphagia and weight loss. A minority of asymptomatic patients may be diagnosed at an early stage through screening and surveillance endoscopy.
- A history of gastroesophageal reflux disease and Barrett esophagus should be sought in patients given the strong correlation with esophageal adenocarcinoma. In contrast, heavy tobacco and alcohol use is more commonly associated with squamous cell carcinoma.
- Symptoms of odynophagia, neurological changes, hemoptysis, melena, and hoarseness should be ascertained, though these tend to be less common and suggest more advanced disease.
- Physical examination is often unremarkable in the setting of esophageal cancer. Evaluation for supraclavicular and cervical lymphadenopathy should be undertaken given the proclivity of advanced esophageal cancer to spread to these locations. Evidence of distant disease (ascites, effusion) and malnutrition may also be apparent. Lastly, prior surgical scars should be noted and further questioned, as this may affect the feasibility of a minimally invasive technique.

IMAGING AND OTHER DIAGNOSTIC STUDIES

Esophagogastroduodenoscopy

- All patients should undergo upper GI endoscopic evaluation with biopsy of any suspicious lesions to allow for tissue diagnosis via histologic examination. Upper endoscopy also provides for direct assessment of any lesions as well as determining the location, degree of obstruction, and extent of the involved esophagus.

Computed Tomography of the Chest/Abdomen

- Contrast-enhanced computed tomography (CT) imaging should be obtained as part of the initial workup of any esophageal malignancy once the diagnosis has been established as it allows for clinical evaluation of the local extent of the primary tumor and its relationship to adjacent structures, assisting with determining resectability. CT imaging may also identify the presence of metastatic disease.

Endoscopic Ultrasound

- An essential component in the locoregional staging of esophageal cancer, endoscopic ultrasound assesses the depth of tumor invasion (T stage) as well as nodal involvement (N stage). The addition of a fine-needle aspirate allows for the sampling of any suspicious nodes. There is an increased likelihood of nodal metastasis associated with deeper tumor penetration.

Positron Emission Tomography/CT

- Integrated positron emission tomography (PET)/CT imaging remains the preferred modality to evaluate for occult metastatic disease in esophageal cancer given better spatial resolution and improved sensitivity when compared to PET or CT imaging alone, respectively. Unexpected suspicious distant lesions identified on PET/CT should prompt biopsy for tissue confirmation.

Additional Studies

- Further studies may be indicated to assist with staging a newly diagnosed esophageal cancer in certain clinical situations. Bronchoscopy should be considered for all tumors located at or above the carina given the potential for airway invasion. Endoscopic mucosal resection may be performed in early-stage lesions that are confined to the mucosa only (T1a).

SURGICAL MANAGEMENT

Preoperative Planning

- All patients being considered for esophagectomy should be optimized nutritionally prior to undergoing such major surgery. If they are unable to tolerate sufficient oral intake, a preoperatively placed jejunostomy tube should be considered to establish enteral access. While not prohibitory, gastrostomy tube placement should be avoided if possible given the increased risk of compromising the future gastric conduit.
- Perioperative pain control is an important aspect in patient recovery and, thus, should be optimized. A multimodal approach is utilized with a patient-controlled analgesia (PCA) in the early postoperative period, though thoracic epidural placement can be considered. A thorough intercostal nerve block at the time of surgery is also strongly encouraged.
- Patients undergoing esophagectomy for underlying malignancy are considered high risk for venous thromboembolism and, thus, require aggressive perioperative deep vein thrombosis (DVT) prophylaxis. Postoperative patients should be routinely discharged on 4 weeks of DVT chemoprophylaxis to mitigate the potential morbidity associated with thrombosis. Consideration can be given to starting chemoprophylaxis as early as 2 hours preoperatively.

Positioning

- A minimally invasive Ivor Lewis esophagectomy entails a two-stage approach. Starting with the abdominal portion, the patient is positioned supine with both arms tucked. A double-lumen endotracheal tube is placed for single lung ventilation during the thoracic portion of the procedure. A nasogastric (NG) tube is advanced into the stomach for gastric decompression; the NG tube will need to be withdrawn prior to dividing the stomach. An arterial line and Foley catheter should also be placed.
- Following completion of the abdominal portion, the patient is then placed in left lateral decubitus with the right side up in anticipation for the thoracoscopic approach. The bed is appropriately flexed to allow for opening of the intercostal spaces.

TECHNIQUES

ABDOMINAL

Port Placement, Instrumentation (FIGURE 1)

- An initial supraumbilical right paramedian incision is made through which a 12-mm trocar is introduced into the peritoneal cavity to allow for insufflation. This port is no more than 12 to 15 cm inferior to the xiphoid process. Upon establishment of pneumoperitoneum, the laparoscope is inserted and the abdomen is thoroughly inspected to confirm no evidence of distant disease prior to proceeding. Any suspicious lesions should be biopsied and sent for pathologic review.
- Additional port placement includes a 12-mm port at the same level to the left paramedian, and bilateral 5-mm subcostal ports. The surgeon stands to the patient's right and the assistant stands on the patient's left; each uses the ports on their respective sides.
- The patient is then placed in reverse Trendelenburg and an epigastric 5-mm port serves as an access point for the liver retractor. We prefer the Nathanson liver retractor, but a snake liver retractor is also commonly used. Exposure of the hiatus is facilitated by reflecting the left lobe of the liver superiorly.

Hiatal Dissection (▶ Video 1)

- The dissection is initiated by dividing the gastrohepatic ligament along the lesser curve with a laparoscopic energy device to expose the hiatal structures. One must be cognizant of a potential aberrant left hepatic artery during this dissection, which should be preserved if identified.
- Beginning along the right crus just lateral to the esophagus, the phrenoesophageal membrane is divided and the dissection is continued circumferentially around the esophageal hiatus and along the left crus. Attention should then focus on creating a retroesophageal window through which a Penrose drain can be passed and used for retraction.
- With the assistant providing downward traction on the Penrose, the distal esophagus is mobilized in the chest

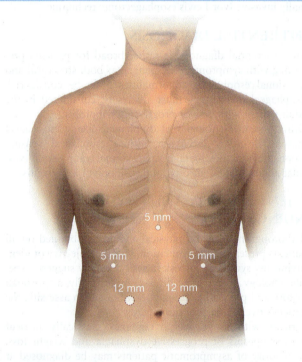

FIGURE 1 • Port placement for the abdominal portion of the minimally invasive esophagectomy.

through mediastinal dissection. Such dissection will simplify the thoracoscopic esophageal mobilization.

Gastric Mobilization (▶ Video 2)

- Utilizing atraumatic bowel graspers, the stomach is carefully reflected toward the patient's right with the assistant providing countertraction on the omentum, thus exposing the greater curvature. The lesser sac is then entered and the dissection is continued cephalad by dividing the gastrosplenic ligament. The short gastric vessels are encountered and ligated in series using the laparoscopic energy device or laparoscopic clip applier.
- Continuing along the greater curve distally, the gastrocolic ligament is divided to mobilize the stomach from the transverse mesocolon. The right gastroepiploic vascular pedicle must be identified and preserved throughout this dissection. In general, a 2 to 3 cm margin is advised to prevent any inadvertent thermal injury to the artery, which may compromise the conduit.
- Full mobilization of the stomach to the pylorus is critical to achieving tension-free delivery of the conduit into the hemithorax and assuring sufficient conduit length.

Lymph Node Dissection (▶ Video 3)

- During the dissection of the lesser curvature of the stomach, the left gastric artery pedicle is identified and can be traced back to its origin from the celiac axis. A complete D2 lymph node dissection is performed by gently sweeping the celiac lymph nodes and adipose tissue upward to be included with the resected specimen. The left gastric artery is fully exposed and divided at its base with an endovascular stapler utilizing a vascular load.

Conduit Formation (▶ Video 4)

- Adequacy of the gastric mobilization can be assessed by ensuring that the pylorus can reach to the level of the esophageal hiatus without any undue tension.
- Starting two vascular arcades distal to the ligated left gastric artery, the creation of the gastric conduit is initiated by utilizing an Endo GIA stapler with a vascular load along the lesser curve, dividing any vascular structures.
- Gastric tubularization continues with a series of green, purple, or black staple loads—depending on the thickness of the stomach—on the Endo GIA stapler. Progressing toward the fundus, each successive staple fire should be oriented parallel to the greater curve while maintaining a conduit width of approximately 4 to 5 cm.
- Prior to completing the conduit, the remaining several centimeters near the fundus are left undivided, thus leaving the specimen and conduit attached. Delaying this final staple fire will assist with delivery of the conduit into the hemithorax. A securing/tension stitch can be placed between the specimen and conduit.
- The specimen and attached gastric conduit can be advanced into the lower mediastinum, along with the Penrose, to assist with esophageal mobilization during the thoracic portion of the case. The hiatus is then inspected and crural stitches can be placed if the hiatal defect is felt to be large and at risk for paraconduit herniation.
- A chemical pyloroplasty can be performed using botulinum toxin injected on the anterior pyloric surface. Alternatively, this can also be accomplished surgically.

J-Tube Placement

- We routinely place a jejunostomy tube at the time of esophagectomy for enteral access during the postoperative period.
- After identifying the ligament of Treitz, a site on the jejunum approximately 25 cm distally is identified and the antimesenteric border is sutured to the abdominal wall.
- The Seldinger technique is employed to advance an introducer needle and guidewire transabdominally into the jejunal lumen, followed by a dilator through which a 12 to 14 French jejunostomy tube can be advanced into the bowel distally. Additional tacking sutures as well as a purse-string suture can then be placed once the feeding tube has been appropriately advanced.

THORACIC

Port Placement, Instrumentation (FIGURE 2)

- With the patient placed into the left lateral decubitus position, the right lung is isolated and the right chest is initially entered in the ninth intercostal space along the posterior axillary line. An angled thoracoscope is introduced and the right pleural space is inspected. Additional thoracoscopic ports include one at the fifth intercostal space along the anterior axillary line. An access incision at the seventh intercostal space in the anterior axillary line is used for specimen retrieval and introduction of staplers.
- A wide intercostal nerve block is performed for postoperative pain management.

Esophageal Mobilization (▶ Video 5)

- With the right lung isolated and deflated, the inferior pulmonary ligament is divided and any level 9 lymph nodes can be harvested at this time. If the diaphragm is obstructing one's view during this step, consideration can be given to placing a stitch through the central tendon to allow for retraction of the diaphragm inferiorly and facilitate better exposure of the distal esophagus.
- The mediastinal pleura is incised utilizing electrocautery or an energy device beginning at the diaphragm and continuing up to the level of the azygous vein. Further mobilization of the esophagus is achieved by dissecting pericardial or aortic attachments and ligating small aortic arterial branches with an energy device.
- The thoracic duct, which commonly courses between the aorta and azygous vein, is at risk for injury during the esophageal mobilization and mediastinal dissection. Any small

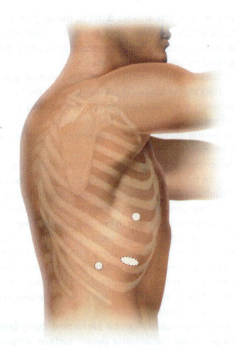

FIGURE 2 • Port placement for the thoracic portion of the minimally invasive esophagectomy.

lymphatic branches requiring division should be clipped to prevent a chyle leak. Alternatively, prophylactic thoracic duct ligation can be considered.
- The azygous vein is divided using an endovascular stapler.

Lymph Node Dissection

- A thorough mediastinal lymphadenectomy is performed once the esophagus has been adequately mobilized. The paraesophageal level 8 lymph nodes may be included with the esophageal specimen. The level 7 subcarinal lymph node packet should be fully dissected and removed.

Delivery of Conduit

- With the thoracic esophagus fully mobilized up to the level of the azygous vein, the conduit is delivered into the right pleural cavity through the esophageal hiatus by applying gentle tension on the esophageal specimen. Following complete delivery, any sutures attaching the two structures can be divided and the final Endo GIA stapler can be employed to fully separate the conduit and specimen.
- The gastric conduit should be inspected at this time to ensure it is viable and properly orientated with the staple line directed laterally.
- The esophagus is sharply divided proximally. The specimen is placed in a specimen bag and retrieved through the access incision.
- Frozen section is performed to confirm negative margins prior to proceeding with the anastomosis.

Anastomosis (▶ Video 6)

- After properly positioning the conduit in the posterior mediastinum, it is important to confirm that there is adequate conduit length to complete the anastomosis without tension and that there is no axial rotation that may have occurred during conduit delivery.
- The esophagogastric anastomosis is created by first placing a purse-string suture in the open end of the esophagus. Upon completion of the purse-string suture, an end-to-end anastomosis (EEA) stapler anvil is inserted. We prefer a 29-mm EEA. The purse-string suture is secured around the anvil shaft. A second purse string can be placed to doubly secure the anvil. We often use an Endoloop of polydioxanone as a secondary purse-string suture.
- A gastrotomy is created at the tip of the conduit. The EEA stapler is introduced via the access incision and inserted into the conduit. The spike is advanced several centimeters distal to the tip at the appropriate conduit length. The stapler and anvil were engaged and the stapler deployed. The anastomotic rings should be evaluated to confirm they are complete. The gastrotomy is then closed with an Endo GIA stapler and an air leak test may be performed with endoscopy.
- With the anastomosis complete, an NG tube may be advanced into the conduit under direct visualization. Drainage tubes are placed.

PEARLS AND PITFALLS

- Full mobilizing the stomach to the pylorus is critical to achieving tension-free delivery of the conduit into the hemithorax.
- Mediastinal dissection of the lower esophagus performed during the laparoscopic portion of the operation will greatly facilitate esophageal mobilization during the intrathoracic portion. It will also obviate the need for diaphragm retracting maneuvers as the distal portion of the esophagus will already be mobilized.
- Be extremely cautious if using energy devices while completing the esophageal mobilization and lymph node dissection by the carina. Thermal spread of energy can cause an airway injury.

POSTOPERATIVE CARE

- Patients are managed in a protocolized fashion following MIE. They are routinely extubated in the operating room and admitted to the intensive care unit (ICU) postoperatively. Alternatively, patients can be admitted immediately postoperatively to a stepdown unit, depending on the institution. Our institutional postoperative care algorithm is given below.

POD 0-1

- PCA utilized for analgesia
- Maintenance intravenous fluids are initiated at a rate of 84 mL/h
- The right-sided chest tube is left to water seal
- Use of an NG tube for conduit decompression is optional
- Patients are transferred to stepdown surgical unit (if in the ICU POD0)

POD 2-3

- The intravenous fluids are decreased to a rate of 42 mL/h
- Trickle tube feeds (10 mL/h) are initiated via the jejunostomy tube

POD 4-5

- Tube feeds are advanced to goal with return of bowel function
- Esophagram obtained (POD 4-5) to ensure integrity of anastomosis
- Sips of clears/ice chips permitted if the esophagram is negative

POD 6-9

- Diet advanced from clear to full liquids
- Chest tubes removed if output appropriate
- Discharge to home on full liquid diet and goal tube feeds

COMPLICATIONS

- Despite overall improved outcomes in recent years, esophagectomy continues to be associated with a relatively high rate of morbidity. Pulmonary complications remain the most common morbidity postoperatively with pneumonia occurring approximately 10% of the time; however, a minimally invasive thoracic approach helps mitigate pulmonary risks. Anastomotic leak remains the most feared complication seen 10% of the time. Additionally, atrial fibrillation is seen in 5% to 10% of patients. Chyle leaks (6.5%), sepsis (4%), myocardial infarction (2%), and DVT (2%) are rare.

SUGGESTED READINGS

1. Ajani JA, D'Amico TA, Bentrem DJ, et al. Esophageal and esophagogastric junction cancers, version 2.2019, NCCN clinical practice guidelines in oncology. *J Natl Compr Cancer Netw*. 2019;17(7):855-883.
2. Antoch G, Saoudi N, Kuehl H, et al. Accuracy of whole-body dual-modality fluorine-12-2-fluoro-2-deoxy-D-glucose positron emission tomography and computed tomography (FDG-PET/CT) for tumor staging in solid tumors: comparison with CT and PET. *J Clin Oncol*. 2004;22(21):4357-4368.
3. Biere SS, van Berge Henegouwen MI, Maas KW, et al. Minimally invasive versus open oesophagectomy for patients with oesophageal cancer: a multicentre, open-label, randomised controlled trial. *Lancet*. 2012;379:1887-1892.
4. Cerfolio RJ, Laliberte AS, Blackmon S, et al. Minimally invasive esophagectomy: a consensus statement. *Ann Thorac Surg*. 2020;110(4):1417-1426.
5. Gottlieb-Vedi E, Kauppila JH, Malietzis G, et al. Long-term survival in esophageal cancer after minimally invasive compared to open esophagectomy: a systematic review and meta-analysis. *Ann Surg*. 2019;270:1005-1017.
6. Mariette C, Markar SR, Dabakuyo-Yonli TS, et al. Hybrid minimally invasive esophagectomy for esophageal cancer. *N Engl J Med*. 2019;380:152-162.
7. Meyers BF, Downey RJ, Decker PA, et al. The utility of positron emission tomography in staging of potentially operable carcinoma of the thoracic esophagus: results of the American College of Surgeons Oncology Group Z0060 trial. *J Thorac Cardiovasc Surg*. 2007;133(3):738-745.
8. Naffouje SA, Salloum RH, Khalaf Z, Salti GI. Outcomes of open versus minimally invasive ivor-Lewis esophagectomy for cancer: a propensity-score matched analysis of NSQIP database. *Ann Surg Oncol*. 2019;26(7):2001-2010.
9. van Vliet EP, Heijenbrok-Kal MH, Hunink MG, Kuipers EJ, Siersema PD. Staging investigations for oesophageal cancer: a meta-analysis. *Br J Cancer*. 2008;98(3):547-557.

SECTION VI: Treatment of Esophageal Perforation

Chapter 18 | Treatment of Esophageal Perforation: Cervical, Thoracic, and Abdominal

Roslyn Alexander, Abigail Gotsch, Aanuoluwapo Obisesan, Andrew M. Brown, and Meredith A. Harrison

DEFINITION
- An esophageal perforation is defined as a defect in all layers of the esophagus—mucosa, submucosa, and muscularis propria. The esophagus lacks a strong serosa, therefore making it more susceptible to perforation. It is instead covered in adventitia, a thin layer of connective tissue that contains nerves, small blood vessels, and lymphatic channels.

DIFFERENTIAL DIAGNOSIS
- Presentation of esophageal perforation can vary widely, from a patient who is asymptomatic to one who is in florid septic shock and sometimes even multisystem organ failure. Patients can present with pain or discomfort in the neck, chest, or abdomen, which can mimic other conditions including coronary artery disease, myocardial infarction, aortic dissection, pneumothorax, gastroesophageal reflux disease, or esophageal dysmotility. These must all be considered and ruled out during workup.

PATIENT HISTORY AND PHYSICAL FINDINGS
- Etiology can vary but can generally be traumatic (iatrogenic or noniatrogenic) vs spontaneous. Iatrogenic traumatic injury is typically secondary to trauma from endoscopy, while noniatrogenic traumatic injury is secondary to blunt/penetrating injury or caustic/foreign body ingestion. Spontaneous perforation (Boerhaave syndrome) is typically related to a sudden and drastic rise of intraesophageal pressure through the lower esophageal sphincter, commonly during forceful vomiting. This intraluminal pressure will lead to a perforation, most commonly, of the left posterolateral wall just proximal to the gastroesophageal junction, where there is an inherent weakness in the longitudinal muscle fibers from the esophagus as they taper out onto the wall of the stomach.[1]
- Symptomatology depends on the area of perforation. The presenting symptoms of a cervical perforation are often neck pain or stiffness, as well as dysphonia and dysphagia. An abdominal perforation will often present as abdominal pain or generalized peritonitis. The onset of symptoms from a thoracic perforation may be more insidious. Patients with thoracic esophageal perforations present with chest pain, dysphagia, or crepitus in the chest.
- Patients with esophageal perforation may report an acute onset of pain (neck, chest, or abdominal pain) that radiates to the back or left shoulder.[2] Mackler triad, which includes subcutaneous emphysema, chest pain, and vomiting, is a pathognomonic sign for esophageal rupture, which can be observed in approximately 50% of patients.[1] Other symptoms can include dysphagia, dysphonia, hoarseness, and fevers. Interestingly hematemesis or melena are rarely found in patients who present with this problem.
- Findings on physical examination can include crepitus or swelling in the neck or chest and/or signs of SIRS (systemic inflammatory response syndrome), such as tachycardia, tachypnea, or fevers. These may be mild at presentation but can quickly progress to septic shock with hypotension and end-organ failure.

IMAGING AND OTHER DIAGNOSTIC STUDIES
- Early diagnosis for esophageal perforation is essential, as mortality rates are significantly higher in those with delayed diagnosis, 9% mortality for early (≤24 hours) vs 29% for late (>24 hours) diagnosis.[3] Having a high index of suspicion, particularly in those who have had recent instrumentation of the esophagus or who have a clinical story consistent with perforation, is essential for early diagnosis and subsequent treatment.[4]
- The simplest imaging study to start with is a plain film radiograph (posteroanterior, lateral, and upright views). This may rule in or rule out some of the conditions in the differential diagnosis, although an x-ray performed immediately after a suspected injury may be completely normal. In a patient with esophageal perforation, expected findings would be subcutaneous emphysema along the neck or chest and pneumomediastinum (**FIGURE 1**). A lateral view may also demonstrate air in the prevertebral space. Other associated findings that may be seen in these patients are pleural effusion, pneumothorax, hydropneumothorax, or pneumoperitoneum.
- Contrast esophagography is also an essential tool. Plain film radiographs may be negative up to 12% of the time in a patient with a perforated esophagus.[5] Although water-soluble contrast (Gastrografin) is preferred as the initial contrast choice for esophagography, if a water-soluble contrast study is negative and there is still a high suspicion for perforation, it

Chapter 18 TREATMENT OF ESOPHAGEAL PERFORATION: CERVICAL, THORACIC, AND ABDOMINAL

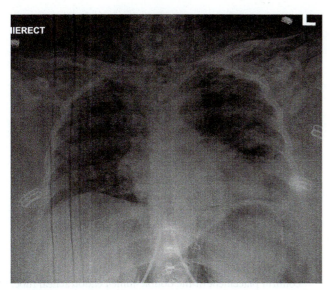

FIGURE 1 • Chest x-ray demonstrating extensive subcutaneous emphysema tracking up to the neck bilaterally.

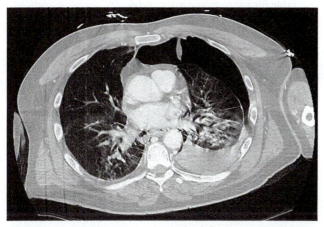

FIGURE 2 • Axial cut CT scan demonstrating classic findings of an esophageal perforation including a pneumothorax, pneumomediastinum, and a left pleural effusion.

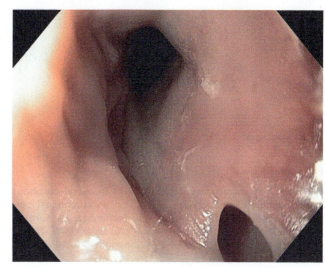

FIGURE 3 • Esophagogastroscopy showing an esophageal perforation in the bottom right corner. The esophageal lumen is seen in the upper left corner. Note the clear margins of the perforation and the absence of mucosal necrosis.

should be followed by a barium swallow. A barium swallow is more sensitive, but barium itself does have the propensity to perpetuate an inflammatory response and leads to fibrosing mediastinitis.[6-8] However, if a patient truly does have a perforation, the barium will likely be washed out of the mediastinum when they undergo surgical intervention, and therefore the benefits of the study outweigh the risks.

- Cervical and thoracic computed tomography (CT) with oral contrast can be performed to evaluate a patient for esophageal defects in addition to other diagnoses. It is important to be aware that there can be false positives for esophageal perforation on CT scans; if a CT is positive, it should be immediately followed by a contrast esophagram. A CT in a patient with a perforated esophagus can demonstrate oral contrast extravasation into the prevertebral or pleural spaces, subcutaneous emphysema, a pleural effusion, or pneumomediastinum (FIGURE 2). The benefits of CT also include a comprehensive view of the entire cervical or thoracic cavity for operative planning.

- Patients may also require endoscopy during the diagnostic workup (FIGURE 3). Direct visualization of the esophagus can identify the anatomic location and size of a perforation, in addition to any other coexisting diseases of the esophagus such as Barrett esophagus, achalasia, or esophageal cancer. It can also be used for interventional planning to determine if a perforation can be treated with an esophageal stent. Of course, endoscopy and its associated insufflation can worsen a preexisting perforation, so the endoscopist—whether they be a trained advanced gastroenterologist or an experienced surgeon—should proceed with caution. Endoscopy should also always be performed intraoperatively during any intervention for esophageal perforation.

SURGICAL MANAGEMENT
Preoperative Planning

- Initial management of esophageal perforation is the same for all zones of perforation (cervical, thoracic, abdominal) and is centered around prompt diagnosis and treatment. The patient should be made strict NPO (nil per os). Adequate peripheral access should be established for fluid resuscitation. Broad-spectrum antibiotics should be administered intravenously. Piperacillin-tazobactam, ampicillin-sulbactam, or a carbapenem are appropriate options. Antifungal coverage is important to include, such as fluconazole. The patient should be placed in an intensive care unit for close hemodynamic monitoring and for appropriate fluid resuscitation. Preparation for operative management including appropriate laboratory tests (complete blood count, coagulation studies, type, and screen) is also important.[9-11] There should be no delay in expeditiously transporting these patients to the operating room for surgical intervention.

- An esophagogastroduodenoscopy should be done prior to patient positioning to identify the location and extent of the injury as well as identify any associated pathology such as distal obstruction (achalasia, malignancy). This is important as it may convert the operative plan to a resection or a diversion.

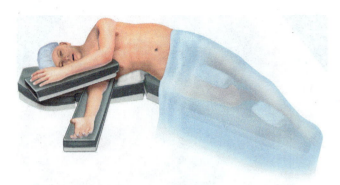

FIGURE 4 • A correctly positioned patient in lateral decubitus in preparation for a thoracic approach to an esophageal perforation. (Redrawn from Sancheti MS, Fernandez. FG Surgical management of esophageal perforation. *Oper Tech Thorac Cardiovasc Surg*. 2015;20(3):234-250. Copyright © 2016 Elsevier. With permission. Figure 3.)

Positioning

- Cervical
  - The patient should be placed in the supine position, with the neck hyperextended and rotated toward the right side. A bump can be placed behind the scapula to help accentuate neck hyperextension. The endotracheal tube should be fastened to the right side of the mouth, as to not disrupt the surgical field. The incision should be placed along the anteromedial border of the left sternocleidomastoid muscle.
- Thoracic
  - The left lateral decubitus position is preferred for perforations involving the upper two-thirds of the esophagus, while the right lateral decubitus position is appropriate for lower one-third injuries.
  - The patient should be placed in lateral decubitus such that flexion of the bed will open the intercostal spaces. Care should be taken to pad all pressure points and consideration of axillary roll placement should be given to prevent a brachial plexus injury. The dependent arm is flexed as is the superior arm ("praying position"); this prevents shoulder and brachial plexus injury (**FIGURE 4**).
  - A flexible bronchoscopy may be performed at this point to confirm placement of the double-lumen endotracheal tube.
- Abdominal
  - Patient should be positioned supine with both arms extended to provide enough room on either side of the table for surgeon and assistant(s).

CERVICAL PERFORATION AND REPAIR TECHNIQUE

- The treatment of cervical esophageal perforations is usually more straightforward and easier to accomplish than thoracic or intra-abdominal esophageal perforations. This is, in part, due to the anatomy of the structures in the neck. The tissue planes in the neck make it so that there is limited space for the spread of contamination, making extraluminal contamination confined and infection easier to control. The attachments of the esophagus to the prevertebral fascia limit the spread of contamination of the esophageal flora. This makes drainage of the perforation an adequate mechanism to control leakage and enhance healing.[12]
- Drainage alone is reserved for cervical esophageal perforations when the perforation site is not able to be visualized. This technique is contraindicated in esophageal perforations located in the thorax or abdomen. In the case of an unstable patient and/or a large cervical esophageal perforation, surgical management is necessary.
- An incision along the left lower third of the sternocleidomastoid muscle should be made. A right sided incision is reserved for a right-sided esophageal perforation. The sternocleidomastoid muscle is retracted laterally (**FIGURE 5**).
- Visualization and identification of anatomic structures at this point is very important. The carotid sheath is exposed, left intact, and retracted laterally. It is occasionally necessary to ligate the middle thyroid vein and divide the omohyoid muscle in order expose the trachea and larynx. Once these structures are exposed, they are retracted to the right. Care must be taken to avoid injury to these structures, especially the left recurrent laryngeal nerve, as this lies in the tracheoesophageal groove. Once the prevertebral plane is entered, the esophagus is then displaced anteriorly. This retropharyngeal plane is bluntly dissected cranially and caudally down to the level of the carina. Anterior and posterior planes are bluntly dissected around the esophagus, down to the mediastinum, posterior to the esophagus and anterior to the prevertebral fascia. This helps assure adequate drainage (**FIGURE 6**).
- If the perforation is visualized, primary repair should be performed. Primary repair should always start with debridement of the devitalized tissue and extension of the opening in the muscularis propria to expose the hole in the mucosa. The opening in the mucosa is oftentimes larger than the opening in the muscularis propria, making this an important step. After the entire length of the perforation is exposed, single interrupted absorbable sutures

Chapter 18 **TREATMENT OF ESOPHAGEAL PERFORATION: CERVICAL, THORACIC, AND ABDOMINAL**

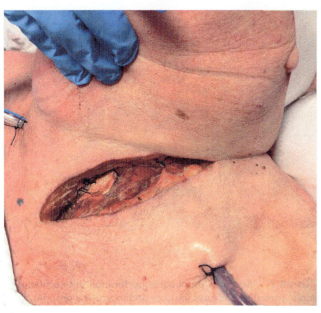

FIGURE 5 • Slight hyperextension of the neck allows easy access for neck dissection. Incision along the medial border of the sternocleidomastoid muscle.

should be placed on the mucosal layer followed by nonabsorbable suture on the muscularis layer. Identification of both layers is sometimes skewed secondary to surrounding inflammation. In this instance, a single-layer repair using single interrupted absorbable suture is appropriate. Care is taken to avoid significant narrowing of the esophagus by placement of a bougie orally. The authors will often repair a defect over an endoscope in order to prevent narrowing.

- A vascularized flap placement over the repair can potentially decrease the rate of leaks from primary esophageal perforation repairs. This can be achieved with a sternocleidomastoid flap. The sternal head of the sternocleidomastoid is detached from the sternum and it is rotated over the site of perforation following primary repair. Multiple interrupted sutures should be placed around the repair to secure the muscle in place. Important principles in any vascularized flap still hold true in this instance. It is important for the muscle to be tightly opposed to the repair site. It is also important that the muscle flap cover the site in its entirety. If the trachea is also injured, the muscle flap should be positioned between the repaired esophagus and the repaired trachea. This helps to avoid formation of a tracheoesophageal fistula.
- Once primary repair and flap placement are complete, the prevertebral fascia should be copiously irrigated. Wide drainage is an important part of contamination control in esophageal perforations. Drains should be placed in this area and brought out through separate skin incisions.
- The wound is then closed in layers, with reapproximation of the platysma using absorbable sutures. The skin should be closed loosely with staples.

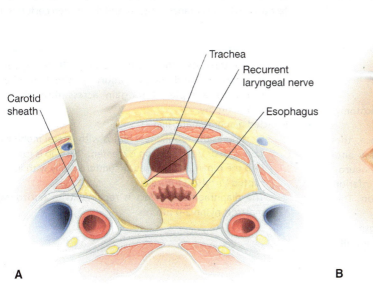
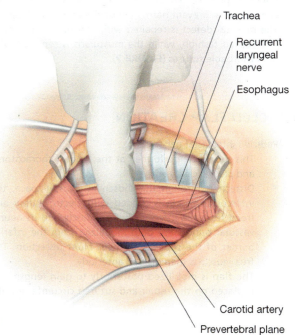

FIGURE 6 • **A**, Transverse section showing the prevertebral space. Dissection is carried medially to the carotid sheath. The recurrent laryngeal nerve is protected within the tracheoesophageal groove. **B**, Lateral view of the dissected prevertebral space with trachea, esophagus, and recurrent laryngeal nerve retracted anteriorly.

THORACIC PERFORATION AND REPAIR TECHNIQUE

- An upper endoscopy following induction of general anesthesia is invaluable in localizing the esophageal defect.
- Standard access to the esophagus is via a posterolateral thoracotomy. The tip of the scapula is marked, and the incision is started 2 to 4 cm below the scapula tip, depending on how distal the esophageal defect is.
- The incision is curved posteriorly and superiorly coursing between the posterior midline and the medial border of the scapula. The serratus anterior should be preserved if possible (retract anteriorly) or be divided inferiorly to limit denervation. The incision is carried down with electrocautery. Thought should be given to preserving an intercostal muscle flap while entering the chest to provide additional buttress to a repair of the esophagus.
- The intercostal flap, if chosen for repair reinforcement, should be prepared (discussed below) during this stage of the operation. A Finochietto-type rib retractor is inserted with the large blade placed superiorly to retract the scapula. Food, gastric contents, and other debris are suctioned upon mediastinal entry and fluid can be sent for cultures. The inferior pulmonary ligament is divided with electrocautery and the lung is gently retracted cephalad with moist gauze sponges.
- The mediastinal pleura over the site of the perforation is opened widely and thoroughly debrided. The esophagus can be circumferentially mobilized and encircled with a Penrose drain if necessary. However, if the defect is clearly visible, circumferential mobilization may not be necessary. A longitudinal myotomy is performed until the entire mucosal defect is seen. Repair over a bougie or over an endoscope should be considered to prevent narrowing of the esophageal lumen. The mucosal defect is repaired with absorbable sutures in interrupted fashion, while the muscularis is repaired with nonabsorbable sutures (**FIGURE 7**).

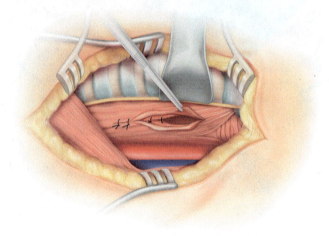

FIGURE 7 • Repair of esophageal perforation in two planes of single interrupted sutures (mucosa and muscularis propria).

- The repair is then buttressed with a pedicled intercostal flap.
- After repair, a nasogastric tube should be placed under direct visualization distal to the repair. A leak test may also be performed at this point with gentle air insufflation of the esophagus with the scope. The pleural cavity and mediastinum are both thoroughly irrigated with normal saline and both are drained. Multiple drains should be placed to provide adequate drainage for a contaminated field.
- The ribs are reapproximated with Vicryl 2 sutures in figure-of-8 fashion tying down the sutures only after the lung has been reinflated under direct visualization. Layered closure of the fascia, muscle, subcutaneous tissue, and skin is then performed.

PEDICLED FLAP CREATION

- Pedicled intercostal flap
  - This should be performed at the time of thoracotomy and pleural cavity entry.
  - Dissecting through the chosen intercostal space, the intercostal muscle is divided with electrocautery and freed from the inferior rib. The muscle and its neurovascular bundle are both mobilized from the inferior border of the superior rib with blunt dissection. The free muscle is then divided anteriorly.
  - The flap is mobilized posteriorly to gain length and is placed on the repair and sutured circumferentially with interrupted Vicryl 3-0 sutures (**FIGURE 8**). Care is taken to avoid traction injury on the flap when retractors are placed to gain access through the thoracotomy.
- Pedicled diaphragmatic flap
  - Starting at the esophageal hiatus with lateral mobilization, a U- or V-shaped flap is created. This flap is rotated into the repair and sutured circumferentially with interrupted Vicryl 2-0 sutures.
  - The diaphragmatic defect is repaired with horizontal mattress nylon 2-0 sutures.

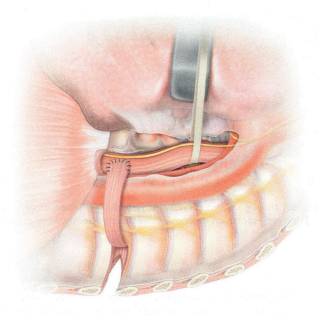

FIGURE 8 • Placement of an intercostal muscle flap over a primary esophageal defect repair. (Redrawn from Sancheti MS, Fernandez FG. Surgical management of esophageal perforation. *Oper Tech Thorac Cardiovasc Surg*. 2015;20(3):234-250. Copyright © 2016 Elsevier. With permission. Figure 8.)

ABDOMINAL PERFORATION AND REPAIR TECHNIQUE

- A midline laparotomy in the upper abdomen from xiphoid to umbilicus is made and carried down through skin and subcutaneous tissues until the fascia can be divided and the peritoneal cavity entered.
- The gastroesophageal junction is exposed by circumferentially mobilizing the esophagus from the crura of the diaphragm while taking care to protect both vagus nerves. The short gastric vessels are carefully ligated.
- Just as in cervical and thoracic perforations, visualizing the full extent of the mucosal injury is paramount to an appropriate primary repair. After the injury is fully exposed, necrotic tissue should be debrided followed by a primary repair in two layers with absorbable suture. Either a fundoplication or an omental flap should be performed to buttress the repair. Of note, if there is any concern for achalasia, a Nissen fundoplication should not be performed.
- The abdomen should be irrigated extensively and the area surrounding the esophageal repair should be drained widely.
- Closure is accomplished with running or interrupted figure-of-8 polydioxanone suture to reapproximate the fascial layer. Skin should be loosely reapproximated with staples given concern for contamination to allow for continued drainage.

ESOPHAGEAL DIVERSION

- The salvage procedure of exclusion and diversion should be considered for the most critically ill patients, especially those who present in multisystem organ failure or late in the disease process (over 24 hours after perforation). This procedure involves division of the esophagus in the neck and abdomen, cervical esophagostomy, tube gastrostomy, feeding jejunostomy, and wide drainage. Esophagectomy can be performed if the benefit of a prolonged procedure outweighs the risk of mediastinal contamination from the remaining esophageal segment.
- Esophageal exclusion can be performed using either a transthoracic approach or a transhiatal approach. The esophagus should be stapled at the gastroesophageal junction, followed by a standard tube gastrostomy and feeding jejunostomy. Either the entirety of the esophagus or the diverted portion should be brought out through a left cervical incision; an end or loop esophagostomy can then be performed (**FIGURE 9A**).
- The stoma should be matured using 2-0 or 3-0 Vicryl suture in an interrupted fashion to the skin. A stoma appliance can then be applied in the standard fashion (**FIGURE 9B**). Should the patient improve clinically, the surgeon can consider esophagostomy reversal. Esophageal continuity can be restored with either a gastric conduit or colonic interposition graft.

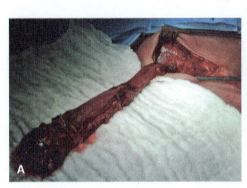
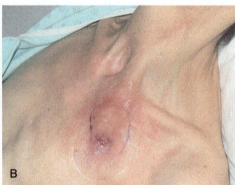

FIGURE 9 • **A,** Thoracoabdominal esophagus dissected and brought out through a left cervical incision. **B,** End result of cervical esophagostomy with enterostomal appliance removed. Note that the conserved esophagus extends below the clavicle, showing preservation of a maximum length of tissue above the site of perforation.

CONSERVATIVE MANAGEMENT

- Conservative management, which includes nasogastric tube drainage, intravenous fluids and antibiotics, parenteral nutrition, and serial imaging, can be employed in a certain population of patients. These patients should be hemodynamically stable without severe sepsis, with either an isolated cervical perforation or a thoracic perforation with a contained collection or abscess on imaging or contrast study. A conservative approach can also be considered in patients with severe comorbidities that would preclude aggressive operative intervention.
- Image-guided percutaneous drainage with chest tubes can also be utilized to successfully treat this select group of patients conservatively.[13]
- If attempting conservative management, the patient should be closely observed for any fevers, tachycardia, leukocytosis, or other signs of sepsis that would indicate failure of nonoperative management. These patients should be taken to the operating room as soon as possible and their management should then follow the principles as stated above.

PEARLS AND PITFALLS

- Symptomatology depends on the area of perforation.
- Early diagnosis is essential to reduce morbidity and mortality associated with acute esophageal perforation. Having a high index of suspicion is necessary, especially in patients with recent instrumentation.
- Direct visualization of the entire extent of the mucosal injury is crucial in repair of an acute esophageal perforation. Failure to do so can result in persistent perforation, ongoing contamination, sepsis, and ultimately unnecessary morbidity and mortality.
- It is essential to ensure that there is no distal obstruction when repairing an esophageal perforation or the repair will fail. If the perforation is in the setting of an esophageal cancer, esophagectomy may be the best option for the patient.
- Esophageal diversion and exclusion procedures carry significant long-term morbidity and therefore should be reserved for critically ill patients in multisystem organ failure or patients who present late in the disease process.

POSTOPERATIVE CARE

- Patients should be continued to be monitored closely in the intensive care unit postoperatively. They should remain strictly NPO with a nasogastric tube in place to protect the area of repair. IV antibiotics/antifungals, in addition to IV proton pump inhibitors, should be continued in the immediate postoperative period for at least 7 days. If a distal enteral feeding tube was inserted, enteral feeding should be initiated and gradually advanced to the goal. Drains inserted should be monitored for volume and characteristics of the output.
- After at least 5 days, the repair should be assessed with an oral contrast imaging study (ideally barium swallow). If no leak is seen and there is no clinical suspicion for leak, the nasogastric tube can be removed, and the patient may begin a clear liquid diet. The diet may be advanced as the patient tolerates, and drains can be removed.

OUTCOMES

- Outcomes can vary widely depending on the area of perforation, size of said perforation, hemodynamic status at the time of presentation, patient's age and/or comorbidities,

and—perhaps most importantly—the timing from patient's symptoms to diagnosis. If diagnosis, and thus treatment, was delayed more than 24 hours from the patient's initial presentation, mortality can increase by as much as a factor of 2.[4]
- Mortality is reported as varying from 2% to 27%; likewise, morbidity from 53% to 81%.[13-16]

COMPLICATIONS
- Leak
- Tracheoesophageal fistula
- Wound infection
- Mediastinitis
- Pleural effusion/empyema
- Abscess
- Esophageal stricture
- Sepsis
- Respiratory failure
- Death

REFERENCES

1. Wu JT, Mattox KL, Wall MJ Jr. Esophageal perforations: new perspectives and treatment paradigms. *J Trauma*. 2007;63(5):1173-1184.
2. Soreide JA, Viste A. Esophageal perforation: diagnostic work-up and clinical decision-making in the first 24 hours. *Scand J Trauma Resusc Emerg Med*. 2011;19:66.
3. Reeder LB, DeFilippi VJ, Ferguson MK. Current results of therapy for esophageal perforation. *Am J Surg*. 1995;169(6):615-617.
4. Brinster CJ, Singhal S, Lee L, et al. Evolving options in the management of esophageal perforation. *Ann Thorac Surg*. 2004;77(4):1475-1483.
5. Han SY, McElvein RB, Aldrete JS, Tishler JM. Perforation of the esophagus: correlation of site and cause with plain film findings. *Am J Roentgenol*. 1985;145(3):537-540.
6. Ginai AZ, ten Kate FJ, ten Berg GM, Hoornstra K. Experimental evaluation of various available contrast agents for use in the upper gastrointestinal tract in case of suspected leakage: effects on mediastinum. *Br J Radiol*. 1985;58(691):585-592.
7. Wu CH, Chen CM, Chen CC, et al. Esophagography after pneumomediastinum without CT findings of esophageal perforation: is it necessary? *Am J Roentgenol*. 2013;201(5):977-984.
8. Lang MH, Bruns DH, Schmitz B, et al. Esophageal perforation: principles of diagnosis and surgical management. *Surg Today*. 2006;36:332-340.
9. Sharma P, Kozarek R. Practice Parameters Committee of American College of Gastroenterology. Role of esophageal stents in benign and malignant diseases. *Am J Gastroenterol*. 2010;105(2):258-273; quiz 274. doi:10.1038/ajg.2009.684
10. Raff LA, Schinnerer EA, Maine RG, et al. Contemporary management of traumatic cervical and thoracic esophageal perforation: the results of an Eastern Association for the Surgery of Trauma multi-institutional study. *J Trauma Acute Care Surg*. 2020;89(4):691-697. doi:10.1097/TA.0000000000002841. PMID: 32590561.
11. Qadeer MA, Dumot JA, Vargo JJ, et al. Endoscopic clips for closing esophageal perforations: case report and pooled analysis. *Gastrointest Endosc*. 2007;66(3):605-611. doi:10.1016/j.gie.2007.03.1028. PMID: 17725956.
12. McGovern M, Egerton MJ. Spontaneous perforation of the cervical oesophagus. *Med J Aust*. 1991;154(4):277-278.
13. Vogel SB, Rout WR, Martin TD, Abbitt PL. Esophageal perforation in adults: aggressive, conservative treatment lowers morbidity and mortality. *Ann Surg*. 2005;241(6):1016.
14. Eroglu A, Turkyilmaz A, Aydin Y, et al. Current management of esophageal perforation: 20 years experience. *Dis Esophagus*. 2009;22:374-380.
15. Cooke DT, Lau CL. Primary repair of esophageal perforation. *Operat Tech Thorac Cardiovasc Surg*. 2008;13(2):126-137.
16. Liu HT, Luo Q, Zhang J, et al. Analysis in diagnosis and treatment of 29 cases of cervical esophageal perforation. *Zhonghua Er Bi Yan Hou Tou Jing Wai Ke Za Zhi*. 2019;54(8):610-613.

Chapter 19: Endoscopic Management of Esophageal Perforation

John M. Campbell and Salvatore Docimo Jr.

DEFINITION
- Esophageal perforation is defined as a full-thickness rupture of the mucosa and muscularis propria layers of the esophagus with the majority occurring in the thoracic esophagus[1] (**FIGURE 1**).

DIFFERENTIAL DIAGNOSIS
- Though dependent on location, the most common complaint is pain, often within the chest or neck area. The most common cause of esophageal perforation is iatrogenic, related to a recent esophageal procedure. Other etiologies include Boerhaave syndrome, trauma, ingestion of a caustic or foreign body, or underlying malignancy. Often, the diagnosis of esophageal perforation can be delayed considering clinical presentation and can be attributed to myocardial infraction, pulmonary embolism, gastroesophageal reflux disease, esophageal spasms, aortic dissection, or aneurysm rupture.

PATIENT HISTORY AND PHYSICAL FINDINGS
- Patient symptoms are dependent on the anatomic location of the perforation, time from the inciting event to clinical presentation, and underlying comorbidities.[1] Patients presenting with esophageal perforation may report recent bouts of forceful emesis, blunt chest or abdominal trauma, endoscopy, and ingestion of caustic or blunt substances. Patient may also have an underlying esophageal pathology such as achalasia or malignancy.
- The most common presenting symptoms is chest pain. The pain is usually acute with radiation to the back or left shoulder. They may also have shortness of breath or dysphonia. Patient may have subcutaneous emphysema with crepitus and can be in distress. They may be febrile with tachycardia and a leukocytosis. Severe cases may have accompanied hypotension.
- A history of previous esophageal pathology, such as achalasia or malignancy, may alter management. Previous surgery or radiation within the mediastinum or abdomen is also critical to determine a treatment algorithm. Cardiac and pulmonary conditions will need to be evaluated and optimized if time permits.

IMAGING AND OTHER DIAGNOSTIC STUDIES
- As part of the standard workup for chest pain, a chest x-ray will often be the first imaging obtained. On chest x-ray, pneumomediastinum and subcutaneous emphysema around the neck and chest wall may be noted. Other findings can include pleural effusion, pneumothorax, hydrothorax, or pneumoperitoneum (**FIGURE 2**)
- The next imaging study often obtained is a computed tomography (CT) of the chest and abdomen. When CT is

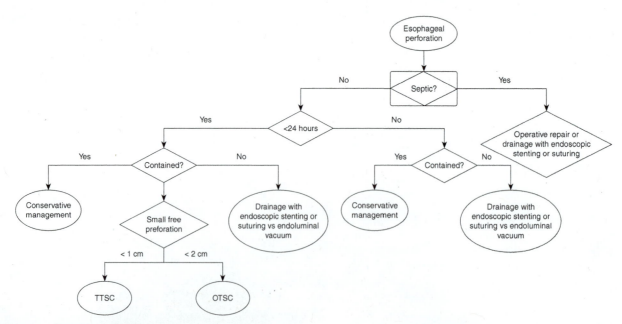

FIGURE 1 • Flowchart depicting when various treatment modalities are appropriate for esophageal perforation. OTSC, over-the-scope clip; TTSC, through-the-scope clip.

Chapter 19 ENDOSCOPIC MANAGEMENT OF ESOPHAGEAL PERFORATION   147

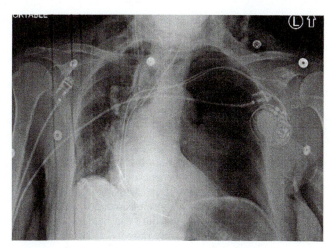

FIGURE 2 • This is a chest x-ray of a patient with a pneumothorax after an esophageal perforation. The patient perforated then went into respiratory distress requiring intubation.

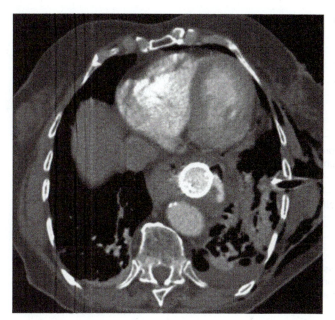

FIGURE 3 • CT scan of a patient with a thoracic esophageal perforation. A left pleural effusion can be seen with extraluminal contrast.

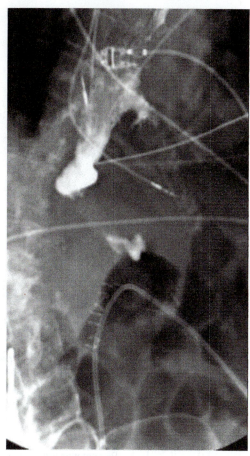

FIGURE 4 • Example of an esophagogram. There is a contained extravasation of contrast from the thoracic esophagus.

- Endoscopy is often done shortly after presentation for definitive diagnosis. Not only can endoscopy diagnose a perforation, it also provides important information such as the extent of the perforation, distal obstruction, and tissue quality, which aid in management. Esophagoscopy can also provide a means of treatment. It should be done by an experienced endoscopist under minimal insufflation using CO_2 gas (**FIGURE 5**).

SURGICAL MANAGEMENT

- Over the last few decades, endoscopy has started to take more of a role in the management of esophageal perforation. There are now various techniques and tools available to the endoscopist in the treatment of esophageal perforation. It has been proven to be an effective treatment and can have higher success rates than surgical treatment in some situations[2] (**FIGURE 6**).

Perioperative Planning

- As previously discussed, the area of perforation should be asserted with imaging, either CT or esophagogram, or with endoscopy. Management begins with making the patient nil per os and initiating intravenous fluids. All management begins with antibiotics. Antibiotics should be broad

pursued, it should be done with oral contrast. In a patient with esophageal perforation, contrast extravasation will be seen into either the cervical, thoracic, or abdominal region (**FIGURE 3**). CT can also aid in evaluating of the neck, mediastinum, abdomen, and pleural space, which aids in operative planning.

- Depending on patient stability and availability of other imaging modalities, an esophagogram study may be pursued. Gastrografin is first done considering it is water soluble; however, it lacks the sensitivity of barium, which should be done if the gastrografin swallow is negative and a perforation is suspected (**FIGURE 4**).

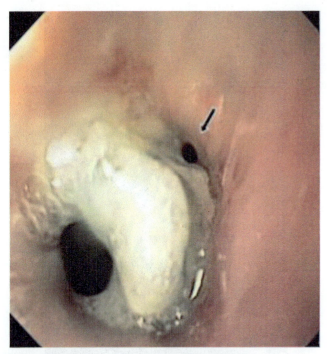

FIGURE 5 • Endoscopic view of a cervical esophageal perforation. The *black arrow* shows the perforation into the mediastinum.

spectrum and cover for upper respiratory as well as gastrointestinal (GI) organisms. Any esophageal perforation should also be managed with antifungal agents. Proton pump inhibitors should also be used. Total parenteral nutrition should also be initiated if indicated.[3] All preoperative imaging should be readily available in the operating room and endoscopic equipment on the ready.

Patient Positioning

- For endoscopic procedures, most patients are intubated with the patient in a supine position. It can be done under conscious sedation, which is beneficial for those with comorbidities. Patients are often placed with the head of the bed elevated roughly 45° when conscious sedation is used. If the patient is intubated, the procedure can be done completely supine or with the head slightly raised.

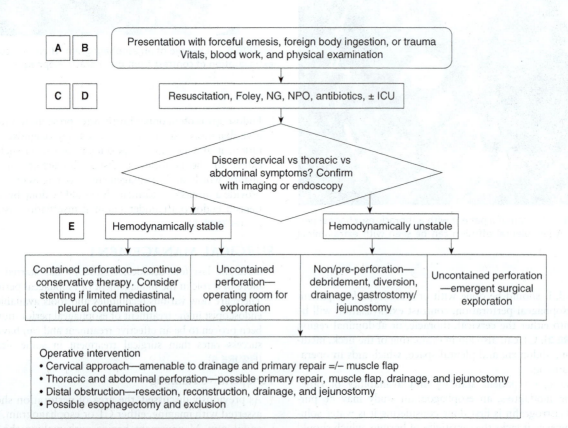

FIGURE 6 • Diagram demonstrates a working algorithm on how to approach esophageal perforations. This is a common way many may still approach perforation. However, as endoscopy advances and becomes more commonplace, there will likely be more emphasis placed on it. (Reprinted from Möschler O, Nies C, Mueller MK. Endoscopic vacuum therapy for esophageal perforations and leakages. *Endosc Int Open.* 2015;3(6):E554-E558. Copyright © 2015 Georg Thieme Verlag KG.)

ENDOSCOPIC MANAGEMENT

Clips

- For mucosal defects smaller than 1 cm with healthy edges around the defect, through-the-scope endoscopic clips (TTSCs) can be utilized. Clips are placed through the endoscope in a distal to proximal direction, so the scope does not dislodge them. Care must be taken to align the edges of the mucosa for proper healing (**FIGURE 7**).
- Currently, it is the authors' preference to utilize over-the-scope clips (OTSCs) for acute perforations. The OTSC is made from magnetic resonance imaging–compatible nitinol and delivered via a plastic applicator cap that is mounted at the end of the endoscope. Hemostatic clips or TTSCs have a width of less than 11 cm, while OTSC has a width of up to 14 cm.[4] As the defect size increases, additional clips may be needed.[5] Prior to the placement of an OTSC, the authors encourage the use of contrast injection with fluoroscopy to localize the perforation. All foreign bodies, if present, should be removed. Once the clip/cap is localized over the perforation, aggressive suction is utilized to draw in the edges of the perforation and then the OTSC is deployed (**FIGURE 8**). In cases with thickened and friable mucosa, an accessory device (OTSC Anchor or OTSC Twin Grasper, Ovesco Endoscopy) would be used as an adjunct to aggressive suction.[6] The defect edge can be grasped with forceps and pulled into the lumen of cap prior to deploying the OTSC (**FIGURE 9**). OTSCs have three available teeth options: type a (blunt, primarily for compression), type t (small spikes, compression and anchoring effect), and type gc (elongated teeth with spikes, closure of gastric wall). Type t is typically utilized for closure of esophageal perforations (**FIGURES 10-12**).

Nasomediastinal Drainage

- For patients who present with delayed perforation, often their mediastinal infection or abscess will be a more pressing issue than the perforation repair itself. In a certain cohort of patients who may not be surgical candidates acutely, nasomediastinal drainage is an option. A nasogastric (NG) tube is endoscopically grasped and mobilized through the esophageal defect into the abscess cavity. The tube can then be placed to suction and periodically flushed to assist with drainage.

Stents

- Stents have become a durable and viable option for esophageal perforation. Compared with surgery, they have shown shorter length of stay, earlier feeding, and better quality of life.[7] They also can be utilized in a variety of situations.[8]
- First, the perforation is identified with the endoscope. A guidewire is then threaded through the scope into the stomach or duodenum well beyond the perforation, usually with fluoroscopic guidance. The guidewire has radiopaque markers for length. Fluoroscopy is then used to the measure the length of stent needed (**FIGURE 13**). A covered self-expanding stent

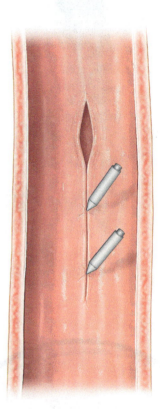

FIGURE 7 • This illustration demonstrates how endoscopic clips are utilized for esophageal perforations. Clips are placed from an inferior to superior direction. (Redrawn by permission from Springer: Gurwara S, Clayton S. Esophageal perforations: an endoscopic approach to management. *Curr Gastroenterol Rep*. 2019;21(11):57.)

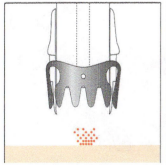 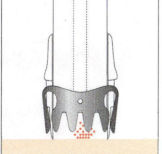 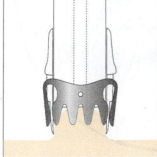 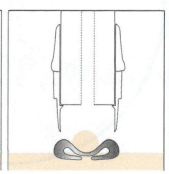

FIGURE 8 • The pictures demonstrate how suction can be used to draw the defect into the over-the-scope clip grasp to allow for deployment. (Used with permission from OVESCO Endoscopy AG.)

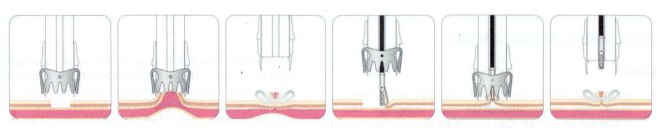

FIGURE 9 • When the mucosa is too thickened and friable or the defect does not come together well with suction, an accessory device with forceps can be used to grasp and pull the defect into the lumen of cap. (Used with permission from OVESCO Endoscopy AG.)

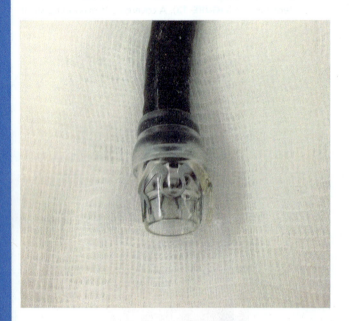

FIGURE 10 • An over-the-scope clip can be seen mounted onto the endoscope. (Reprinted with permission from Fischer JE. *Fischer's Mastery of Surgery*. 7th ed. Wolters Kluwer; 2019. Figure 79.4.)

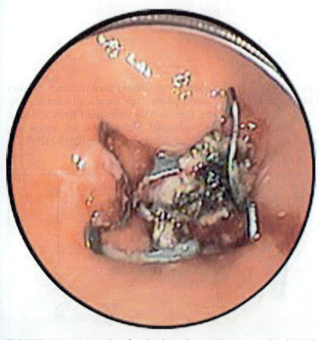

FIGURE 11 • Example of a deployed over-the-scope clip (OTSC) used to close perforations. Closure of persistent percutaneous endoscopic gastrostomy fistula using the OTSC Anchor. (Used with permission from OVESCO Endoscopy AG.)

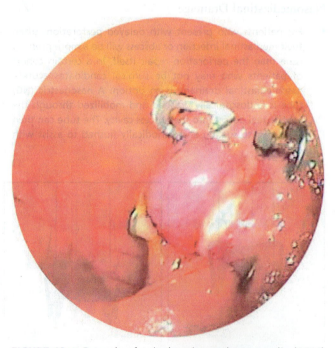

FIGURE 12 • Example of a deployed over-the-scope clip (OTSC) used to close perforations. Perforation closure in the colon with OTSC Twin Grasper. (Used with permission from OVESCO Endoscopy AG.)

Chapter 19 ENDOSCOPIC MANAGEMENT OF ESOPHAGEAL PERFORATION 151

can be used as they allow for easier retrieval but have higher rates of migration. A partially covered stent has less migration risk but can pose difficulties during retrieval (FIGURE 14). Fully covered stents have been shown to have better seal rates than partially covered stents.[7] There are many stents available. Fully covered stents come in lengths ranging from 120 to 230 mm. Partially covered stents can come in various sizes as well but the most common is 150 mm. Plastic stents are not as widely studied but can be utilized. They are more difficult to deploy and have high migration rates but are easier to retrieve.

- The stent should be placed to ensure adequate coverage over the area of perforation. Stents deployed too distal or proximally can be adjusted endoscopically following deployment. In practice, it is easier to pull a deployed stent back into proper position rather than mobilizing a stent distally after it is has been deployed too proximal. In some instances, a partially deployed stent can be resheathed to adjust placement prior to deployment. However, the ability to resheath a partially deployed stent is variable and manufacturing specifics should be reviewed prior to use.
- An alternative to fluoroscopic guided deployment uses endoscopic guidance. After the guidewire is inserted under endoscopic guidance, it was withdrawn and the stent deploying

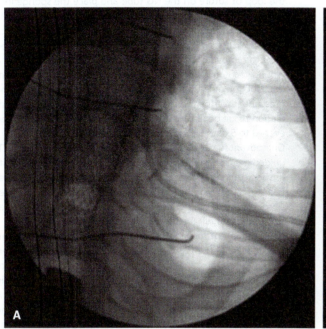
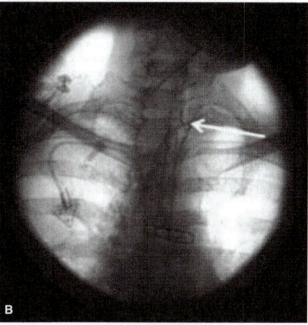

FIGURE 13 • A, This image demonstrates the radiographic makers that are used for measuring the length. B, This image shows the tip of a deployed stent (*white arrow*) with a paper clip at the distal end. (Reprinted by permission from Springer: Ross AS, Kozarek RA. Esophageal stents: indications and placement techniques. In: Kozarek R, Baron T, Song HY, eds. *Self-expandable Stents in the Gastrointestinal Tract*. Springer; 2013:129-140.)

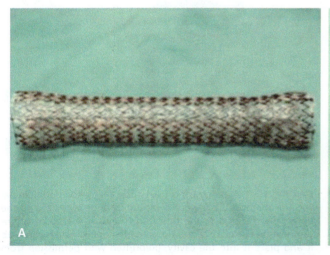
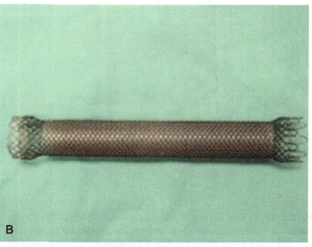

FIGURE 14 • A, Example of a fully covered stent. B, A partially covered stent, WallFlex esophageal stent. (Reprinted by permission from Springer: Docimo S, Pryor AD. Management of leaks with endoluminal stents. In: Chand B, ed. *Endoscopy in Obesity Management*. Springer; 2018.)

device is placed on the guidewire. The scope can then be reinserted. The stent can then be deployed while being visualized with the endoscope. Postoperative chest films can be periodically completed if the question of migration arises.

Endoscopic Suturing

- For larger defects, endoscopic suturing can be utilized. The OverStich (Apollo) can close the defect in one layer with full-thickness bites endoscopically. This requires additional endoscopic attachments. The OverStich is attached to the end of the endoscope prior to insertion. Once at the area of perforation, the tissue is typically grasped with the helix device and brought into the path of the OverStitch swing arm. The swing arm has the needle with suture and can then take a full-thickness bite through the defect (**FIGURE 15**). Once the stitch is thrown, the bite is let go and then the process can be repeated until the entire defect has been addressed. Once suturing is complete, the needle is released. A suture cinch is then passed through the working channel of the endoscope. Once sufficient tension is pulled through the running bites, the suture cinch is then deployed. Any excess suture is cut via the suturing device and removed through the working channel. The device does allow for multiple sutures to be placed without removed the endoscope from the patient. Endoscopic suturing does require time familiarizing with the device and has a learning curve but does allow for primary closure without the need for an open procedure.

Endoluminal Vacuum Therapy

- Endoluminal vacuum therapy or E-Vac therapy uses the principles of negative pressure therapy used for wounds and applies it to esophageal perforations. Prior to placing the E-Vac, patient should have distal feeding access. A percutaneous endoscopic gastrostomy tube can be placed first. A 14 to 16 Fr NG tube should be used. First, the NG tube is placed through the nose then out the mouth. A piece of black polyurethane sponge should be sized to the defect. This should be secured with suture to the NG tube tip. A loop of suture should also be left at the tip (**FIGURE 16**). The NG tube is then inserted over the endoscope and advanced to the area of perforation. An endoscopic grasper is then placed through the port and used to grab the loop of suture on the NG tube and place the sponge into the defect. Commercially made device are available as well. Braun manufactures the Endo-Sponge or Eso-SPONGE, which has been utilized with good effect.[6] Suction is the applied prior to removing the scope. Suction should be applied with a wound vacuum system (**FIGURE 17**). Settings should be continuous suction at −125 to 100 mm Hg on the high setting. Some prescribe lowering the suction to −75 to 50 mm Hg once granulation tissue begins to appear. The tubing should be replaced every 3 to 5 days to promote wound healing.
- One advantage of this method is it avoids any need for a CT-guided mediastinal drain other modalities require. Similar to its use for cutaneous wounds, wound vacuum therapy promotes healing of the cavity via stimulating granulation tissue. This takes fibrous tissue in the abscess cavity and replaces it with granulation tissue that fills the defect while clearing contamination.
- Pines at al proposed an interesting alternative to this method. In patients who already have mediastinal or cervical drains but an indwelling traditional NG tube is not desired, the NG tube can be brought out through the drain site. A scope is first advanced to the area of perforation. A guidewire is then placed through the external drain and then grasped endoscopically and brought out through the mouth. An NG tube is then placed over the guidewire and

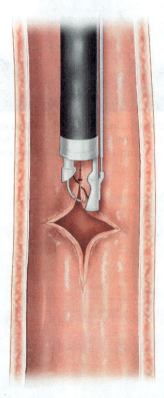

FIGURE 15 • This illustration shows how the OverStitch device is used to close an esophageal defect. (Reprinted by permission from Springer: Gurwara S, Clayton S. Esophageal perforations: an endoscopic approach to management. *Curr Gastroenterol Rep*. 2019;21(11):57.)

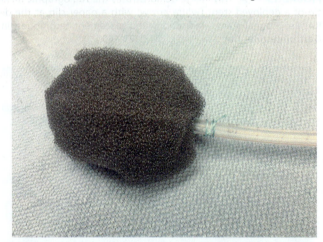

FIGURE 16 • A nasogastric (NG) tube ready for endoluminal vacuum therapy. Black wound vacuum sponge was sized to the defect and secured to the tip of an NG tube. A loop of suture can next be placed over the tip, so endoscopic graspers can grab it and place it into the cavity. (Reprinted with permission from Fischer JE. *Fischer's Mastery of Surgery*. 7th ed. Wolters Kluwer; 2019. Figure 79.5.)

Chapter 19 ENDOSCOPIC MANAGEMENT OF ESOPHAGEAL PERFORATION   153

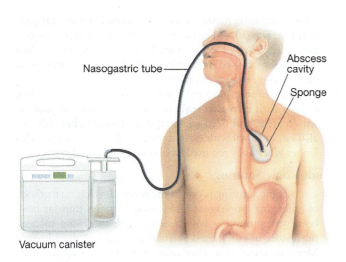

FIGURE 17 • The E-Vac system is connected to a vacuum-assisted closure system the same way an abdominal or incisional wound vacuum system would work. (Reprinted from Watkins JR, Farivar AS. Endoluminal therapies for esophageal perforations and leaks. *Thorac Surg Clin*. 2018; 28(4):541-554. Copyright © 2018 Elsevier. With permission.)

pulled out through the skin with the end that connects to suction brought out first. The smallest sized NG tube should be utilized to minimize the size of the fistula tract. The NG tube will have a black sponge affixed to the distal end. A loop of suture should be placed on the sponge to allow for retrieval later. The NG tube is the pulled out through the drain site incision until the sponge lies in proper place. This is confirmed and adjusted with endoscopy. The NG tube is then connected to suction. The tubing and sponge can later be retrieved in 3 to 5 days via endoscopy by grasping the loop of suture. Once the abscess cavity has been filled with granulation tissue, the fistula tract can be treated with fibrin glue once it is no longer utilized.[9]

- Another proposed combination treatment is the "stent-over-sponge" method. In this method, the endoluminal vacuum is placed as above. Once proper suction is achieved, a stent is then placed over it as described in the stent section. This method allows for infectious control and granulation of the abscess cavity using negative pressure and the stent provides the patient with the ability to have per oral intake of nutrition.[10]

CONSERVATIVE MANAGEMENT

- Cameron et al established the criteria for patients who may be managed nonoperatively. These include perforation contained within the mediastinum or between the mediastinum and the visceral lung pleural, drainage of contrast back into the esophagus, minimal symptoms, no perforation into the abdomen, and no signs of sepsis.[11]

- Nonoperative management should be abandoned and traditional surgical approaches used anytime a patient's status decompensations such as worsening pain, dyspnea, or worsening sepsis. If the patient develops an abscess or empyema, then surgical management is required.

PEARLS AND PITFALLS

Clips
- Clips are generally well tolerated. Occasionally clips can become dislodged or ulcerate the surrounding tissue. Occasionally, OTSCs may need to be removed and retrieval can be difficult. In many instances, removal of OTSC may require the use of an energy system and cutter (remOVE DC Cutter).

Stents
- Common complications of stents are nausea, dysphagia, retrosternal pain, and migration. Migration has been noted to occur in 20% to 60% of patients. There are some measures that can be done to combat this. One is to suture the stent proximally. Another is to place clips to hold it in place. Huh et al in their study had rates of only 3% migration when using a suture to secure the stent in place.[7] Occasionally, stents can prove difficult to remove. In this instance, argon beam coagulation can be tried to coagulate granulation tissue that has embedded the stent; however, this can time consuming.[12] Another option is "stent-in-stent" exchange when another stent of the same diameter and length is placed. This created a radial force that necroses the granulation tissue. This has been shown to have good success.[13]
- Freeman et al found four factors associated with stent migration and poor placement: cervical placement, coverage through gastroesophageal junction, esophageal injuries greater than 6 cm, and anastomotic leaks with more distal leak as well.[14]

Endoscopic Suturing
- The usage of endoscopic suturing for esophageal perforations is still developing. One of the largest drawbacks is access to the endoscopic suturing device and the learning curve. A strong foundation in interventional endoscopy may also be necessary prior to using the endoscopic suturing device.

Endoscopic Vacuum Therapy
- Most common complication of this method is failure to close the fistula tract and stenosis. A rare but devastating complication is hemorrhage from an esophageal-aortic fistula. Care should be taken to avoid placing negative pressure on an area of the esophagus overlying the aorta. This can be determined by both endoscopic identification as well as reviewing the CT.

POSTOPERATIVE CARE

- Patient should be admitted to a monitored floor. Level of care is determined by hemodynamics and comorbidities. Any change in clinical status should be treated as a leak until proven otherwise. Close attention should be paid to the amount and characteristics of the drainage, if applicable. Drain amylase can be used if a leak is suspected. Antibiotics, antifungals, and proton pump inhibitors should be continued for 7 to 10 days. If clinically stable, then an esophagogram should be done and then feeding started. Other drains can be pulled once output is minimal. If a stent is used, any concern for stent migration should be investigated with chest x-ray to check for placement.

OUTCOMES

Clips

- Overall, clips have been found to have a success rate from 50% to 100% in various studies.[4] Data show the average OTSCs have a success rate of 85% with containing upper GI perforations. OTSCs have only around a 1% complication rate.[15] A recent study by Morell found OTSC had a success rate of 60% for full-thickness perforation. The rates near 80% when comparing OTSC are utilized for acute perforations over chronic fistulas. Perhaps more importantly, complications rates near 0% in most published studies.[16] Lazar et al did a meta-analysis looking at success rate of both OTSC and TTSC in 127 patient applied both before and after the 24-hour window. They found in the early period both clips had success rates of about 90%, suggesting either is a viable option. Even with delayed presentation, success rate for TTSC and OTSC was still 100% and 88%, respectively. TTSCs were used for an average defect size of 10 mm. For larger defects, OTSCs were used. For large defects, a combination of clips can be used.[6]

Nasomediastinal Drainage

- There have been a few published case reports of successful treatment via this method. Two have been in the postintervention perforation and one was after a foreign body caused perforation.[12,16,17]

Stents

- When looking at stents overall, success rate for the treatment of esophageal perforations is reported to be 60% to 90% with migration rates of 8.8% to 40%.[4] A recent meta-analysis pooled 20 studies and complied over 600 patients looking at stent use for esophageal perforations, leaks, and fistulas. In all cases, self-expanding metal stents were used, with a majority being fully covered. The success rate was found to be 76%. However, when looking at perforations alone, the success rate was 86%. When comparing fully covered vs partially covered stents, success rates were roughly equal at 73% and 78%, respectively. Migrations rates were 16%. Migration rates were higher in fully covered stents, 21%, compared to partially covered stents, 11%. Mortality rate was found to be 0.5% mostly from bleeding due to erosion.[18] In another recent analysis by Dasari, both plastic and metallic stents were looked at for treatment of esophageal perforations and leaks. In this study, which looked at 340 patients, success rate was 81%. Success rates were similar when comparing plastic vs metallic stents. Their stent migration rate was 20%. Plastic stents had a much higher migration rate, 27% vs 11%. The study did mention that 2% had perforations caused by stenting as well as two patients who had bleeding from erosions.[19]
- Early use of stent, within the first 24 hours, has been shown to help with increased seal rates. Eighty percent of patients with a stent will need some type of drainage, but this can also be cut down with early stenting.[17] Success rates are also higher when they are used over smaller, <2 cm, defects.[20]

Endoscopic Suturing

- Endoscopic suturing is one of the newly developing methods of managing esophageal perforations. Studies thus far have been very promising with a recent series showing successful closure of esophageal perforations in 13 of the 13 cases. Many of these were after other methods had failed. They were able to close defects from 25 to 50 mm. Additionally, the study found that they were able to successfully close 40 fistulas of either the esophagus, stomach, or rectum with endoscopic suturing.[21] This is a challenge that other methods often struggle to produce good results with.
- A case series published by Granata looked at the use of endoscopic suturing in the closure of upper GI defects, mainly in the nonacute (>24 hours) setting. In endoscopic suturing alone, they had a success rate of 7/9 (77%). When defects were more complex, they treated with a combination of suturing and then stent placement. In this group, they achieved closure in 6/7 patients (87%). Endoscopic suturing has also shown in some instances to be successful in closing esophageal perforation that surgical suturing has failed.[22] Most of the data looking at endoscopic suturing in esophageal perforation are in conjure with stent placement.

Endoscopic Vacuum Therapy

- Studies looking at the success rate of healing perforations with this technique have been positive. Laukoetter et al have showed healing rate of 94% in esophageal and gastric perforations or anastomotic leaks treated with endoluminal suctioning. In the largest study thus far, they treated 52 patients with E-Vac therapy set to −125 mm Hg. The median initiation of therapy was 5.5 days with average length of 22 days. Sponges were exchanged every 3 to 5 days. Only two patients failed this therapy, one requiring OTSC and the other a stent. A few had strictures later that were managed with dilation. Two patients did die from massive hemorrhage from presumed erosion through to the aorta, emphasizing the need to avoid placing negative pressure near the aorta.[23] Similar results were seen in a German case series. Seven out of 10 patients were successfully managed with endoluminal vacuum therapy. They had success in both early, less than 24 hours, and late management. Patients who failed were due to filament sepsis, and one patient who had a complicated course with multiple previously failed interventions.[24]
- Stent-over-sponge method also has reported success rates of 75%. In Valli's study, 20 patients were treated with this method after mostly postsurgical leaks, although one was an iatrogenic perforation. In those who received it as first-line treatment, the success rate was 71%, but when it was used after failed previous interventions, the success rate was 80%. Median treatment course was 15 days with primary

treatment requiring a shorter time than secondary treatment. In patients who failed, two had cutaneous fistulas that failed to close and the other had a large thoracic leak. They too had two patients who developed strictures that were able to be treated with dilation. They had no mortality.[25]

- Dahyat et al looked at 52 patients with either anastomotic leak, perforation, or Boerhaave syndrome, treated with E-Vac therapy. Ninety-four percent of patients were successfully managed. They compared this to a control group treated with stenting or surgery. In follow-up that averaged about 20 months, none treated with E-Vac therapy had reoccurrence of their fistulas, although four patients required dilation. Twenty patients were lost to follow-up due to death from cardiovascular disease or progression of esophageal cancer.[26]

CONCLUSION

- Through the past few decades, esophageal perforation has been an area where endoscopic management has expanded greatly. What was once managed with thoracotomies and other open invasive procedures has shifted to endoscopic management. Along with this paradigm change, mortality and outcomes have improved. Esophageal perforations have become an example of the utility that endoscopy provides. While some of the techniques require more advance technique and equipment such as stenting and endoscopic suturing, much of this can still be managed in a surgeon's hands. Endoluminal vacuum therapy utilizes tools such as NG tubes and negative pressure therapy, equipment very familiar to the surgeon, placed with endoscopic guidance. TTSC can be placed by most clinicians with basic upper endoscopy skills. OTSCs require more equipment but do not add tremendously to the difficulty of the case. Stenting and suturing are more advanced skills, but through collaboration with gastroenterologists or through more training, these can be utilized.

- Endoscopic management certainly holds a strong place in the management of esophageal perforations and its use will likely increase in the future. Results thus far are very promising and already we are seeing endoscopy as the primary treatment modality of perforation with or without conventional surgical techniques. It then is upon surgeons, who are often called early in the management of these perforations, to be well informed on available modalities and, if possible, work them into their practice.

REFERENCES

1. Biancari F, D'Andrea V, Paone R, et al. Current treatment and outcome of esophageal perforations in adults: systematic review and meta-analysis of 75 studies. *World J Surg.* 2013;37(5):1051-1059.
2. Tellechea JI, Gonzalez JM, Miranda-García P, et al. Role of endoscopy in the management of Boerhaave syndrome. *Clin Endosc.* 2018;51(2):186-191.
3. Søreide JA, Viste A. Esophageal perforation: diagnostic work-up and clinical decision-making in the first 24 hours. *Scand J Trauma Resusc Emerg Med.* 2011;19:66.
4. Watkins JR, Farivar AS. Endoluminal therapies for esophageal perforations and leaks. *Thorac Surg Clin.* 2018;28(4):541-554.
5. Eroğlu A, Aydın Y, Yılmaz Ö. Minimally invasive management of esophageal perforation. *Turk Gogus Kalp Damar Cerrahisi Derg.* 2018;26(3):496-503.
6. Morrell DJ, Winder JS, Johri A, et al. Over-the-scope clip management of non-acute, full-thickness gastrointestinal defects. *Surg Endosc.* 2020;34(6):2690-2702.
7. Huh CW, Kim JS, Choi HH, et al. Treatment of benign perforations and leaks of the esophagus: factors associated with success after stent placement. *Surg Endosc.* 2018;32(8):3646-3651.
8. Docimo S, Pryor AD. Management of leaks with endoluminal stents. In: Chand B, ed. *Endoscopy in Obesity Management.* Springer; 2018.
9. Alakkari A, Sood R, Everett SM, et al. First UK experience of endoscopic vacuum therapy for the management of oesophageal perforations and postoperative leaks. *Frontline Gastroenterol.* 2019;10(2):200-203.
10. Lázár G, Paszt A, Mán E. Role of endoscopic clipping in the treatment of oesophageal perforations. *World J Gastrointest Endosc.* 2016;8(1):13-22.
11. Cameron JL, Kieffer RF, Hendrix TR, et al. Selective nonoperative management of contained intrathoracic esophageal disruptions. *Ann Thorac Surg.* 1979;27(5):404-408.
12. Shiratori Y, Nakamura K, Ikeya T, Fukuda K. Treatment of esophageal perforation with mediastinal abscess by nasomediastinal drainage placement. *Clin J Gastroenterol.* 2020;13(5):703-707.
13. Aiolfi A, Bona D, Ceriani C, et al. Stent-in-stent, a safe and effective technique to remove fully embedded esophageal metal stents: case series and literature review. *Endosc Int Open.* 2015;3(4):E296-E299.
14. Freeman RK, Ascioti AJ, Giannini T, Mahidhara RJ. Analysis of unsuccessful esophageal stent placements for esophageal perforation, fistula, or anastomotic leak. *Ann Thorac Surg.* 2012;94:959-964.
15. Kobara H, Mori H, Nishiyama N, et al. Over-the-scope clip system: a review of 1517 cases over 9 years. *J Gastroenterol Hepatol.* 2019;34(1):22-30.
16. Altintoprak F, Gundogdu K, Eminler AT, et al. An endoscopic nasomediastinal approach to a mediastinal abscess developing after Zenker's diverticulectomy. *Case Rep Gastrointest Med.* 2017;2017:8726706.
17. Abe N, Sugiyama M, Hashimoto Y, et al. Endoscopic nasomediastinal drainage followed by clip application for treatment of delayed esophageal perforation with mediastinitis. *Gastrointest Endosc.* 2001;54(5):646-648.
18. Van Halsema EE, Van JE, Emo H, et al. Clinical outcomes of self-expandable stent placement for benign esophageal diseases: a pooled analysis of the literature. *World J Gastrointest Endosc.* 2015;16:135-153.
19. Dasari BV, Neely D, Kennedy A, et al. The role of esophageal stents in the management of esophageal anastomotic leaks and benign esophageal perforations. *Ann Surg.* 2014;259:852-860.
20. Shim CN, Kim HI, Hyung WJ, et al. Self-expanding metal stents or nonstent endoscopic therapy: which is better for anastomotic leaks after total gastrectomy? *Surg Endosc.* 2014;28(3):833-840.
21. Sharaiha RZ, Kumta NA, DeFilippis EM, et al. A large multicenter experience with endoscopic suturing for management of gastrointestinal defects and stent anchorage in 122 patients: a retrospective review. *J Clin Gastroenterol.* 2016;50(5):388-392.
22. Granata A, Amata M, Ligresti D, et al. Endoscopic management of post-surgical GI wall defects with the overstitch endosuturing system: a single-center experience. *Surg Endosc.* 2020;34(9):3805-3817.
23. Valli PV, Mertens JC, Kröger A, et al. Stent-over-sponge (SOS): a novel technique complementing endosponge therapy for foregut leaks and perforations. *Endoscopy.* 2018;50(2):148-153.
24. Laukoetter MG, Mennigen R, Neumann PA, et al. Successful closure of defects in the upper gastrointestinal tract by endoscopic vacuum therapy (EVT): a prospective cohort study. *Surg Endosc.* 2017;31(6):2687-2696.
25. Pines G, Bar I, Elami A, et al. Modified endoscopic vacuum therapy for nonhealing esophageal anastomotic leak: technique description and review of literature. *J Laparoendosc Adv Surg Tech.* 2018;28(1):33-40.
26. Dhayat SA, Schacht R, Mennigen R, et al. Long-term quality of life assessment after successful endoscopic vacuum therapy of defects in the upper gastrointestinal tract quality of life after EVT. *J Gastrointest Surg.* 2019;23:280-287.

SECTION VII: Surgery of the Abdominal Wall

Chapter 20: Inguinal Hernia: Open Approaches

Kamal M.F. Itani and Samer Sbayi

DEFINITION

- Inguinal hernia is one of the most commonly encountered clinical problems for the general surgeon.
- An inguinal hernia is an opening in the myofascial plane of the oblique and transversalis muscles that can allow herniation of intra-abdominal or extraperitoneal organs.
- There are three potential spaces for an inguinal hernia: (1) an indirect hernia occurs lateral to the inferior epigastric vessels and through the opening that accommodates the cord structures in men and the round ligament in women, (2) a direct hernia occurs through Hesselbach triangle, and (3) a femoral hernia occurs through the femoral canal medial to the femoral vein.

DIFFERENTIAL DIAGNOSIS

- Patients present with complaints of either a bulge in the groin or groin pain.
- The differential diagnosis for a groin bulge includes inguinal lymphadenopathy, hydrocele, varicocele, a testicular mass, a cord lipoma, or an iliac or femoral aneurysm.
- The differential diagnosis for groin pain includes testicular pathology, ilioinguinal strain, or groin pain syndrome including athletic pubalgia.

PATIENT HISTORY AND PHYSICAL FINDINGS

- Patient can present with an incidental asymptomatic bulge in the groin, various amount of discomfort or pain, up to incarceration or strangulation of a hernia.
- The presence of an inguinal hernia can almost always be confirmed on physical examination. Both groins and testicles should be assessed for masses. A reducible mass is best felt with the patient standing and providing intermittent Valsalva such as a cough. A femoral hernia will be felt below the inguinal ligament, adjacent to the femoral vessels.

IMAGING AND OTHER DIAGNOSTIC STUDIES

- If the diagnosis cannot be definitely made with physical examination, ultrasound or computed tomography scan can be used to assess the integrity of the abdominal wall.
- The finding of fat on imaging in the inguinal canal in the absence of symptoms or clinical findings does not constitute a hernia.

SURGICAL MANAGEMENT

- The bulk of surgical treatment is discussed in the "Techniques" section. Here, consider indications and other more general concerns, such as the following:

Preoperative Planning

- The role of routine antibiotic prophylaxis for elective inguinal hernia remains controversial. There is a body of literature indicating no statistically significant advantage to the use of antibiotic prophylaxis in the performance of routine inguinal hernia repair with or without the use of mesh. Nevertheless, many surgeons argue that antibiotic prophylaxis with a first-generation cephalosporin to cover skin flora is both inexpensive and safe and that such practice should not be considered inappropriate. In the acute setting of a small bowel obstruction secondary to an incarcerated hernia, appropriate perioperative antibiotics should be given within 60 minutes of the initial skin incision.
- Patients should be asked to void preoperatively. In most elective cases, a Foley catheter is not necessary.
- Deep vein thrombosis prophylaxis with pneumatic compression devices starting prior to surgery and continuing in the recovery phase is now standard of care.
- Anesthesia options for inguinal herniorrhaphy include general, spinal, and local anesthesia with or without intravenous sedation. Emergent cases of small bowel obstruction secondary to an incarcerated inguinal or femoral hernia will require general anesthesia.

Positioning, Approach, and Exposure

- The patient is positioned supine with arms out on arm boards.

- The approach to the inguinal canal is the same for all anterior groin hernia repairs.
- Gentle palpation of the inguinal area allows the identification of the spermatic cord. An oblique incision or incision along a skin crease or hairline centered on the cord structures is then made (**FIGURE 1**).
- Using electrocautery, the soft tissue is dissected to the superficial epigastric vessels, which are ligated. The dissection is then carried down through Camper fascia and the more fibrous Scarpa fascia. The next layer is the transparent innominate fascia and the external oblique aponeurosis. Palpation along the external oblique aponeurosis moving laterally and inferiorly should exclude a femoral hernia.
- The external ring is identified and is covered with the external spermatic fascia, which is continuous with the innominate fascia. The external oblique aponeurosis is opened with a scissor, starting medial at the external ring and moving superior/lateral parallel to the inguinal ligament (**FIGURE 2**). Elevating the fascia and using a scissor protects the ilioinguinal nerve from sharp or thermal injury. The ilioinguinal nerve lies just below the aponeurosis of the external oblique and anterior to the cord. If injury to the nerve occurs, it is best divided and excised proximally, allowing the nerve to retract into the muscle or preperitoneal space.
- The medial and lateral external oblique flaps are then dissected free. Insertion of Weitlaner retractors below the flaps greatly facilitates exposure of the spermatic cord. The iliohypogastric nerve can be identified running between the internal and external oblique superior and medial to the spermatic cord. It exits the external oblique medial and superior to the external ring (**FIGURE 3**).
- The spermatic cord is mobilized and isolated in the inguinal canal at the pubic tubercle but not medial to it (**FIGURE 4**). This will reduce the chance of damaging the posterior inguinal canal and any collateral circulation to the testes. A Penrose drain is placed around the cord structures and can be used to provide traction during dissection of the cord.
- The spermatic cord is explored for evidence of an indirect hernia. The cremaster muscle fibers are not divided but are split parallel to the cord. The genital branch of the genitofemoral nerve lies posterior in the cord and is best preserved by splitting the cremasteric muscles. Inspection on the anterior medial aspect of the cord will identify an indirect hernia (**FIGURE 5**).

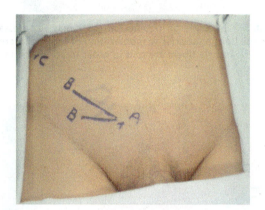

FIGURE 1 • Incision for repair of an inguinal hernia is centered over the palpable spermatic cord along a hairline crease (*AB*, lower line). Alternatively, incision is done parallel to the inguinal ligament (*AB*, upper line toward *C* representing the anterior superior iliac spine).

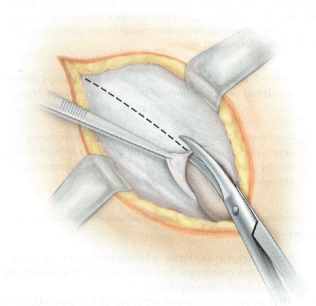

FIGURE 2 • The external oblique is opened from the superficial ring toward the deep ring while avoiding injury to the ilioinguinal nerve.

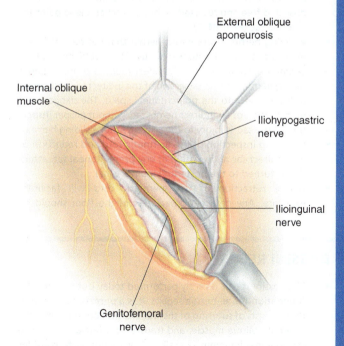

FIGURE 3 • Location of the ilioinguinal and genitofemoral iliohypogastric nerves.

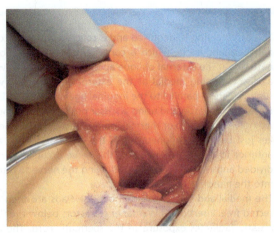

FIGURE 4 • The isolation of the spermatic cord is done above the pubic tubercle to prevent injury to the inguinal floor.

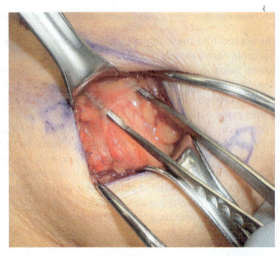

FIGURE 5 • In very large inguinal hernias, it may be necessary to isolate the hernia sac prior to mobilization of the cord. Here, the cremasteric muscle fibers are split in order to access the indirect sac.

- The indirect hernia sac is then dissected from the cord structures using sharp and blunt dissection. The sac is dissected down to the internal inguinal ring and freed from surrounding structures. Care must be taken to avoid damage to the vas deferens, which is closely associated with the sac proximally. The hernia sac is then reduced through the internal ring. The sac can also be transected and ligated. If ligated, the sac should be opened to assure that there is not a sliding component to the hernia.
- In female patients, the round ligament can be completely transected, allowing for closure of the internal ring during repair.
- A cord "lipoma" is not a lipoma (suggesting growth of adipose tissue) but is rather extra or preperitoneal fat. It is usually associated with an indirect hernia but could also be present without an associated sac. Cord lipomas should be dissected free and resected as they can act as a lead point for a hernia sac (**FIGURE 6**).
- A sliding hernia is an indirect hernia that has part of its sac made up of retroperitoneal viscus. This could be bladder, cecum, or sigmoid colon. The safest method of managing a sliding hernia is a safe dissection of the indirect sac and simple reduction back to the preperitoneal space. The danger with high ligation of an indirect hernia sac, without proper inspection of the sac, is injury to the bowel within a sliding hernia.
- Following inspection of the spermatic cord and reduction of any indirect sac and excision of any preperitoneal fat, attention is turned to the posterior inguinal canal.
- Gentle retraction of the spermatic cord will facilitate exposure. Any defects or weakness of the floor should be assessed. In large direct hernias, a purse-string suture around the defect or imbrications of the floor with figure-of-eight sutures will reduce the direct bulge, allowing one to work unencumbered by it.
- Awareness of nerve anatomy and identification during surgery is paramount in reducing the incidence of posthernior-rhaphy pain. A planned prophylactic iliohypogastric and/or ilioinguinal neurectomy is not recommended.[1]

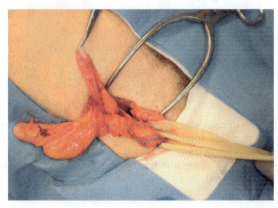

FIGURE 6 • Cord lipomas, which can act as leads to a sac, should be resected in order to reduce the incidence of recurrent inguinal hernias. The hernia sac lies anteromedial to the cord and is separated from a large cord lipoma.

BASSINI REPAIR

- The Bassini repair is rarely performed today but remains the foundation for all hernia repairs. It is a primary tissue repair that consists of suturing of the transversus abdominis muscle, internal oblique muscle, and transversalis fascia medially to the inguinal ligament laterally.[2,3] It is an option to consider in cases where contamination is likely and the use of mesh becomes contraindicated.

Steps

- Bassini's original description of the procedure included resection of the cremasteric fibers. Although still advocated by some, it is not routinely done.
- After elevation and lateral retraction of the spermatic cord, the inguinal canal is carefully inspected for defects and weaknesses.
- The muscular and aponeurotic arch formed by the lower fibers of the transversus abdominis muscle and the internal

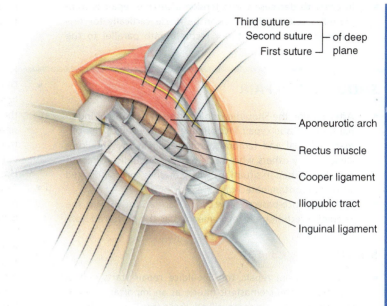

FIGURE 7 • If the transversalis fascia is opened in a Bassini repair, the iliopubic tract may be incorporated into the lateral stitch.

oblique muscle is used to identify the medial edge of the repair.[4] In his repair, Bassini opened the transversalis fascia,[2] but most surgeons today would often omit this step and place the sutures between the aponeurotic arch and the deeper transversalis fascia to the inguinal ligament. If the anatomic layers are not clear, as in recurrent hernia surgery, opening the floor and clearly defining the anatomy will ensure the incorporation of the three anatomic layers medially: the internal oblique muscle, the transversus abdominis muscle, and the transversalis fascia.

- If the decision is made to open the inguinal canal floor, it is done by incising the transversalis fascia from the pubic tubercle to the internal inguinal ring. Care should be taken not to injure the inferior epigastric vessels, which are directly posterior to the transversalis fascia. Once the transversalis fascia is opened and the undersurface of the fascial flaps is exposed, one can easily identify the three anatomic layers described earlier and more carefully inspect the femoral canal.
- Once the muscular aponeurotic arch and the inguinal ligament are properly exposed and a femoral hernia is ruled out, single interrupted permanent polypropylene sutures are used to perform the repair. The first stitch is the most medial and should include the lateral edge of the rectus sheath if possible. It is placed from the rectus sheath and aponeurotic arch to the fascia overlying the pubic tubercle and not the inguinal ligament. This is an important technical point in order to reduce recurrence at the pubic tubercle, a common site.
- Subsequent sutures should be placed from the muscular aponeurotic arch, incorporating all three layers, to the inguinal ligament. Medially, each suture is taken 2 cm from the edge of the arch. Laterally, the suture should incorporate few fibers of inguinal ligament, thus avoiding the underlying femoral vessels. Different fibers should be incorporated with each suture to avoid tearing the inguinal ligament. Upon reaching the internal inguinal ring, the ring is tightened,

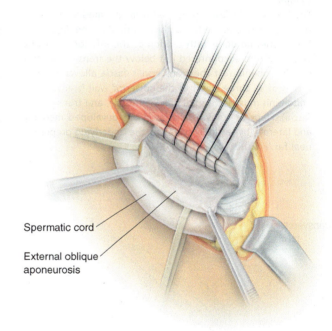

FIGURE 8 • The Bassini repair is carried lateral until the internal ring is re-created.

allowing the tip of a forceps to pass through the ring and avoiding strangulation of the cord structures.
- If the transversalis fascia has been opened, the iliopubic tract will be identified. The medial stitch should first incorporate the iliopubic tract and then the inguinal ligament (FIGURE 7).
- The spermatic cord is returned to its normal anatomic position, lying superior to the newly reconstructed inguinal floor, and closure of the superficial layers is performed in the standard fashion (FIGURE 8).

- In order to decrease tissue tension after the repair is completed, a relaxing incision can be made vertically for few centimeters on the anterior rectus sheath parallel to the repair line. This will allow relaxation of the aponeurotic arch toward the inguinal ligament.

SHOULDICE REPAIR

- After Bassini, the Shouldice repair is the most popular inguinal hernia tissue repair.[5] It continues to be used as the primary inguinal and femoral hernia repair in the Shouldice clinic and by others who trained at the Shouldice clinic.[6] It can also be used in situations where mesh is contraindicated such as in contaminated cases.
- In the evidence-based review by the Hernia Surge Group, the Shouldice technique is recommended as the preferred non-mesh repair.[1]

Steps (▶ Videos 1 and 2)

- Like the Bassini repair, the Shouldice repair starts with a resection of the cremasteric muscle as an important step of the repair. Although some still advocate this step, we do not think that this adds to the durability of repair and it potentially exposes the genital branch of the genitofemoral nerve to injury.
- The transversalis fascia is opened from the medial aspect of the internal ring to the fascial thickening of Cooper ligament. This should be done with caution as the inferior epigastric vessels will be encountered just below the transversalis fascia. The opening of the transversalis fascia allows identification of all three layers of the posterior wall (transversalis abdominis muscle, internal oblique muscle, and transversalis fascia). Flaps of transversalis fascia are developed medially and laterally by carefully sweeping the underlying preperitoneal fat (FIGURE 9).
- Dissection of the lateral flap should be carried to Cooper ligament to identify any femoral hernias and clearly expose the iliopubic tract. Although not done at our institution, incision of the superficial thigh fascia (cribriform fascia) to assess the femoral canal and to improve mobility of the external oblique has been reported and practiced at the Shouldice Hospital in Ontario.
- Originally performed with stainless steel wire, this repair is now performed with 2-0 Prolene sutures. A four-layer repair is performed using two continuous sutures. The first layer begins medially, anchoring the suture from the transversalis fascia to the fascia overlying the periosteum of the pubic tubercle. Leaving a portion of suture long enough to tie to, the stitch is run laterally, approximating the posterior rectus sheath to the iliopubic tract. When the rectus sheath can no longer be brought to the iliopubic tract without tension, the stitch is transitioned to the posterior transversalis fascia and is run superior and lateral until the internal ring is recreated (FIGURE 10).
- The suture is then reversed, and a second layer is started using the same Prolene suture. The second layer approximates the three layers, including the free edge of the medial transversalis fascia, the internal oblique, and the transversus abdominis to the inguinal ligament. The second suture line is brought over the anchoring stitch, reinforcing the medial aspect of the repair, and tied to the anchoring stitch of the first suture line. This effectively imbricates the first layer.
- The third and fourth layers are also run continuously. Starting at the internal ring, the first stitch is blindly placed in the internal oblique and transversus abdominis and approximated to the posterior external oblique aponeurosis, just above the inguinal ligament. This is run medially, creating a ridge just superior and parallel to the inguinal ligament (FIGURE 11).
- The fourth layer is run back to the internal ring, buttressing the third layer, again taking the transversus abdominis and internal oblique, and approximating them to undersurface of the external oblique. The suture is tied to its tail (FIGURE 12).

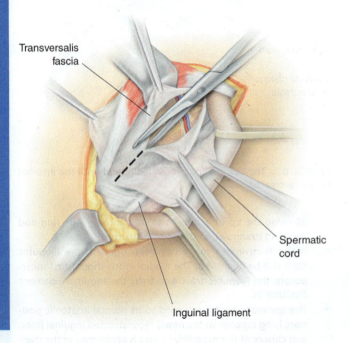

FIGURE 9 • In a Shouldice repair, the transversalis fascia is opened. It is necessary to protect the inferior epigastric vessels from injury.

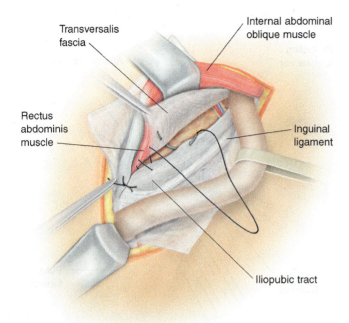

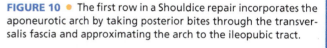

FIGURE 10 • The first row in a Shouldice repair incorporates the aponeurotic arch by taking posterior bites through the transversalis fascia and approximating the arch to the ileopubic tract.

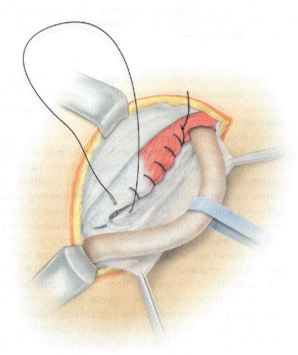

FIGURE 11 • Starting at the internal ring, the third suture layer of a Shouldice repair incorporates the internal oblique and the underlying transversus abdominis medially, which are approximated to the undersurface of external oblique just above and parallel to the inguinal ligament laterally.

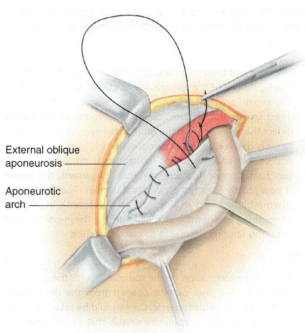

FIGURE 12 • In the Shouldice repair, the fourth layer reapproximates the internal oblique to the undersurface of the external oblique, thus effectively reinforcing the third layer.

THE MCVAY REPAIR OR COOPER LIGAMENT REPAIR

- The Cooper ligament repair is a primary tissue repair that was described and advocated by Dr. McVay in 1958. Following 300 cadaver dissections, he noted that the internal oblique and external oblique do not attach to the inguinal ligament. Rather, they attach to the pubic bone at the location of Cooper ligament attachment.[7] He concluded that repair of the inguinal defect would be anatomically correct if the three layers (internal oblique aponeurosis, transversus abdominis, and transversalis fascia) were sutured to Cooper

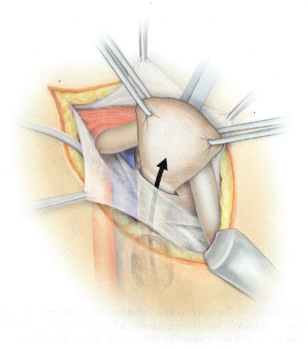

FIGURE 13 • When addressing a femoral hernia, the sac is opened and its contents inspected prior to reduction of the sac.

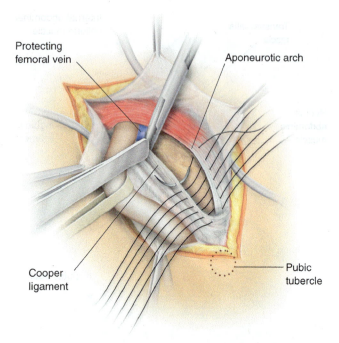

FIGURE 14 • In a McVay repair, the transversus abdominis, internal oblique aponeurosis, and transversalis fascia are approximated to Cooper ligament.

ligament and then transitioned to the inguinal ligament following closure of the femoral myopectineal defect.
- The repair provides closure of the femoral, indirect, and direct spaces and, as such, can be used to repair any hernia defect that may occur in the groin.[8] However, and due to the tension created by this repair, the risk of injury to the femoral vessels, and the risk of recurrence at the suture transition from Cooper ligament to inguinal ligament, this repair is now mostly reserved for femoral hernias. The postoperative morbidity and mortality increase significantly in patients undergoing emergent repair, highlighting the importance of repairing femoral hernias in an elective setting.

Steps (▶ Video 2)

- Following examination of the spermatic cord, the posterior wall of the inguinal canal is opened from the deep inguinal ring to the pubic tubercle. Care should be taken to avoid injury to the inferior epigastric vessels that lie just posterior to the transversalis fascia near the deep ring.[9]
- This provides exposure to the preperitoneal space (space of Bogros), femoral vein, and femoral canal. The femoral hernia sac is found medial to the femoral vein and is reduced.
- If an incarcerated or strangulated femoral hernia cannot be reduced with traction from the preperitoneal space and pressure from below the femoral ring on the anterior thigh, the medial lacunar ligament can be incised to enlarge the femoral ring. If still unable to reduce the hernia, the inguinal ligament can be divided and then repaired following reduction of the hernia (**FIGURE 13**).
- Incising the posterior wall of the inguinal canal exposes the three aponeurotic layers: the internal oblique muscle and aponeurosis, the transversus abdominis muscle and aponeurosis, and the transversalis fascia. Starting medially, simple interrupted sutures are used to approximate the internal oblique aponeurosis, transversus abdominis muscle and aponeurosis, and the transversalis fascia to Cooper ligament (**FIGURE 14**).
- A transition stitch is placed, incorporating the triple layer, Cooper ligament, the femoral sheath at its medial aspect, and the inguinal ligament. If the femoral sheath cannot be identified, it may be omitted. The femoral sheath is intimately associated with the femoral vein. If bleeding occurs following a stitch in the femoral sheath, it should be immediately removed and direct pressure applied. It should not be tied as this would result in tearing of the femoral vein. If the stitch is placed too lateral on Cooper ligament, the femoral vein can be compressed leading to thrombosis (**FIGURE 15**).
- The remainder of the inguinal floor is repaired by approximating the triple layer to the inguinal ligament and continuing, lateral, to the level of the internal ring (**FIGURE 16**).
- This repair creates tension. The distance to Cooper ligament from the aponeurotic arch of the transversus and internal oblique can be up to 8 cm. To release this tension, a relaxing incision is required. This involves first exposing the rectus sheath behind the external oblique aponeurosis. Sparing the external oblique component, the rectus sheath is then incised vertically from the tubercle extending cephalad for approximately 6 cm along its lateral edge. The relaxing incision should be performed before the sutures are tied (**FIGURE 17**).
- The external oblique and skin are closed as described previously.
- Alternatively, a mesh can be used to perform a McVay repair. This is outlined in the "Lichtenstein Repair" section. Laterally, the mesh is sutured to Cooper ligament up to the point where the femoral vein exits at which point the suture is transitioned to the inguinal ligament.

Chapter 20 INGUINAL HERNIA: OPEN APPROACHES   163

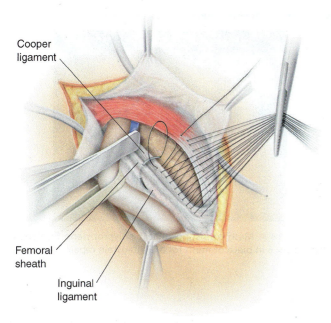

FIGURE 15 • The transition stitch of a McVay repair incorporates Cooper ligament, the medial femoral sheath, and the inguinal ligament. If bleeding occurs, the stitch is immediately removed and pressure should be held.

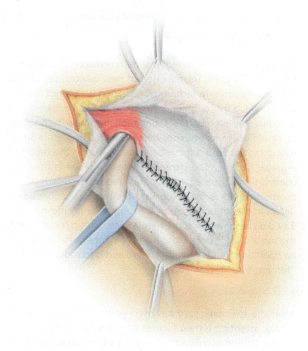

FIGURE 16 • The final step of a McVay repair is the approximation of the aponeurotic arch to the inguinal ligament beyond the transition stitch in order to re-create the internal ring.

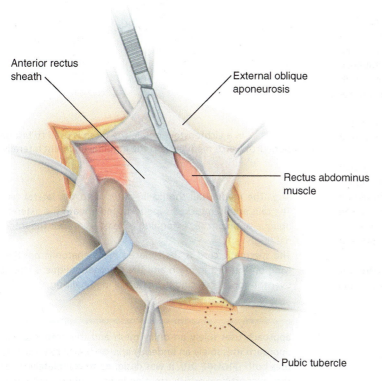

FIGURE 17 • A relaxing incision performed on the rectus fascia will relax the repair and should be performed prior to tying the sutures.

LICHTENSTEIN REPAIR

- The use of prosthesis in inguinal herniorrhaphy is a dynamic field with frequent introduction of new devices, prosthesis, and modifications in technique. Although we cannot include all of them, a thorough understanding of the mechanics and anatomy will provide the foundation that new technology can build on. In its evidence-based review, The Hernia Surge Group recommend a mesh-based technique in the repair of inguinal hernias.[1] The Lichtenstein hernia repair is the most commonly performed mesh-based repair. In this repair a prosthetic mesh is used to bridge the muscular aponeurotic defect in the inguinal region, creating an onlay mesh repair. Based on best evidence, the Hernia Surge Group recommends the use of a large pore monofilament synthetic flat mesh. It is an operation that is straightforward and is considered to be a "tension-free" repair.[10,11]

Steps (▶ Video 3)

- After the spermatic cord has been evaluated for an indirect hernia, attention is then focused on the inguinal floor.
- Any protrusion of a direct hernia can be imbricated to flatten the posterior wall.
- A sheet of at least 3 × 6 in mesh, preferably consisting of soft polypropylene, is fashioned so that the mesh overlaps the rectus by 1 to 2 cm and reaches the inguinal ligament. The mesh should extend underneath the external oblique past the deep inguinal ring. A slit is made on the proximal end of the mesh to accommodate the spermatic cord. This creates two tails of mesh. In females, if the round ligament is ligated, obviously, no slit is required (**FIGURE 18**).
- The mesh is first placed underneath the spermatic cord. With the medial aspect of the mesh overlying 2 to 3 cm on the pubic tubercle, a Prolene suture is used to anchor the mesh. The suture should include the fascia overlying the tubercle but not the periosteum. Overlapping the pubic tubercle with mesh is important as this is a frequent site of recurrence (**FIGURE 19**).
- The first stitch is run continuously from the patch to the inguinal ligament every 1 cm. This stitch is continued until it runs past the deep inguinal ring.
- The medial sutures are interrupted, attaching the patch to the rectus sheath, and eventually will include the internal oblique muscle or aponeurosis. These sutures should be spaced every 2 to 3 cm and are placed to prevent migration of the mesh. The mesh should wrinkle rather than lay flat in order to accommodate shrinking of the mesh and prevent tension.
- The tails are then sutured together around the spermatic cord and to the inguinal ligament, creating a new internal ring. The medial tail should lie anterior to the lateral tail. The tails are then tucked superiorly underneath the external oblique aponeurosis, extending at least 3 cm past the internal ring.
- The spermatic cord is then placed in its anatomic position lying on top of the mesh and the external oblique is closed over the cord recreating the external inguinal ring.

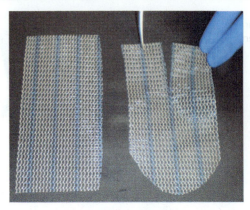

FIGURE 18 ● Mesh consisting of soft polypropylene fashioned from a 3 × 6 in piece of mesh for a Lichtenstein repair.

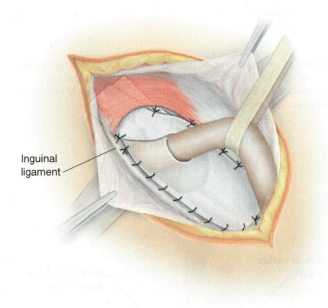

FIGURE 19 ● In a Lichtenstein repair, the mesh is used to bridge the aponeurotic arch medially and the inguinal ligament laterally.

PROLENE HERNIA SYSTEM AND PLUG SYSTEM

- First introduced in 1998, the Prolene Hernia System (PHS) is an evolution of both the Lichtenstein repair and the preperitoneal approach for inguinal hernia repair. The Lichtenstein approach uses solely an onlay mesh and the preperitoneal approach uses solely an underlay approach, whereas the PHS uses both (**FIGURE 20**). It was designed to completely cover the myopectineal orifice, treating indirect, direct, and femoral defects.[12,13] Direct and indirect hernias may be approached differently and are presented separately.

- Although the PHS and plug system are popular in open repairs among some surgeons, the Hernia Surge Group in their evidence-based review discourage the use of these implants over the flat mesh used by Lichtenstein due to excessive use of foreign material and the need to dissect the anterior and posterior planes and associated costs of the mesh.[1]

Steps

Indirect Hernia Approach

- After examination of the spermatic cord and complete reduction of the indirect sac, the floor of the inguinal canal is examined. If the posterior wall of the inguinal canal looks intact, the preperitoneal space is entered through the deep inguinal ring.
- The preperitoneal space is accessed through the internal ring. The preperitoneal fat and peritoneum are separated from the transversalis fascia. This is facilitated by introducing a Raytech sponge through the internal ring and doing this dissection bluntly with care not to injure the inferior epigastric vessels. The borders of dissection should be inferior to the pubic tubercle, below Cooper ligament, and lateral to past the deep inguinal ring. This creates a space where the posterior leaflet of the mesh will cover all defects within the myopectineal orifice.

Direct Hernia Approach

- If the direct hernia is easily reduced, the method described earlier for developing the preperitoneal plane can be used. Alternatively, the preperitoneal space can be accessed directly through transversalis fascia. The transversalis fascia is entered, and the epigastric vessels are identified. A Raytech sponge may be used to create a space that extends below the pubic tubercle and inferior to Cooper ligament. Because the dissection of the preperitoneal space was started more medially than the indirect method, it is important to ensure adequate dissection of the lateral defect. The space should be extended past the deep ring, ensuring adequate coverage of the lateral myopectineal orifice.

Insertion of Prolene Hernia System Mesh

- The PHS mesh consists of two leaflets connected in the middle (**FIGURE 20**). Proper preparation of the mesh is integral for proper deployment. The circular posterior leaflet is designed to sit in the preperitoneal space, and the oblong oriented leaflet is designed to lie on top of transversalis fascia with the short end toward the pubic tubercle. Insertion of the posterior leaflet starts with folding the oblong portion of the mesh and holding it with a ring forceps close to the connector. This will allow easier insertion of the posterior leaflet of the mesh through either the internal ring or the opening made into transversalis fascia by pushing the mesh with the ring forceps (**FIGURE 21**).
- The mesh is then fully inserted through the internal ring, or the direct defect, creating an umbrella shape of the circular mesh. When gently pulling the anterior leaflet mesh out of the defect, the posterior leaflet should expand above the preperitoneal fat and peritoneum. This could be assisted by gently pushing the edges of the posterior mesh with the back of a forceps. It is important to ensure that this mesh expands to below the pubic tubercle, below Cooper ligament, and lateral to cover the internal ring (**FIGURE 22**).

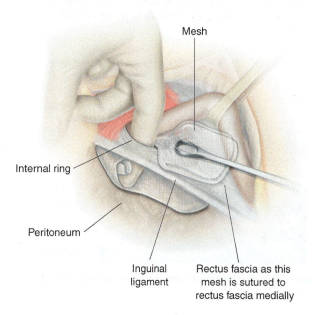

FIGURE 21 • In a PHS repair, the posterior leaflet of the mesh sits below the transversalis fascia above the peritoneum and reduced sac and covers the femoral defect. The anterior leaflet of the mesh lies above the transversalis fascia and is sutured to the inguinal ligament laterally and rectus fascia medially.

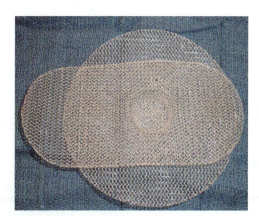

FIGURE 20 • PHS mesh comes in three different sizes: small, medium, and extended. The extended mesh is shown in this photograph.

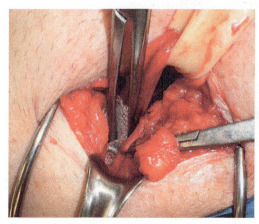

FIGURE 22 • Insertion of the posterior leaflet of the PHS mesh.

- The connector between the anterior and posterior leaflets is allowed to sit in the internal ring or within the opening made into transversalis fascia. This opening can be tightened around the connector with one or two interrupted 2-0 Prolene sutures (**FIGURE 23**).
- The anterior leaflet of the mesh is then treated as a Lichtenstein repair. A 2-cm overlap is allowed between the anterior leaflet of the mesh and the pubic tubercle. The anchoring suture to the fascia overlying the pubic tubercle is run between the lateral edge of the anterior leaflet and the inguinal ligament up to the level of the internal ring. The suture is then tied to itself. Medially, the mesh is anchored with few interrupted sutures to the rectus fascia.
- A slit is made in the lateral border of the anterior leaflet to accommodate the spermatic cord. The edges of the slit are then approximated to each other around the cord and to the inguinal ligament. The proximal portion of the anterior mesh is tucked flat underneath the external oblique aponeurosis proximally.
- The external oblique aponeurosis is closed in the standard fashion.

Closure

- The spermatic cord is placed in its normal anatomic position on the recreated floor of the inguinal canal.
- The external oblique aponeurosis is then closed with a continuous absorbable suture starting proximally and moving distally, thus recreating the external inguinal ring. The ilioinguinal and iliohypogastric nerves should be protected during this step to avoid injury and entrapment (**FIGURE 24**).
- Several interrupted absorbable sutures are placed to reapproximate Scarpa fascia and the subcutaneous tissue layers (**FIGURE 25**).
- The skin is closed with a running absorbable subcuticular suture, and an occlusive dressing is placed.
- Following the removal of the sterile drapes, the testicles at the site of repair should be examined. If retracted, gentle traction on the scrotum will reduce the testicle back to its anatomic position. If left in the inguinal canal, it may permanently scar in that location.

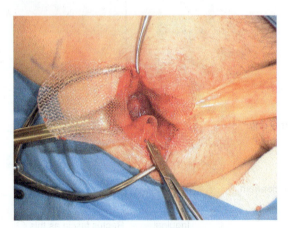

FIGURE 23 • The PHS mesh with the posterior leaflet in place.

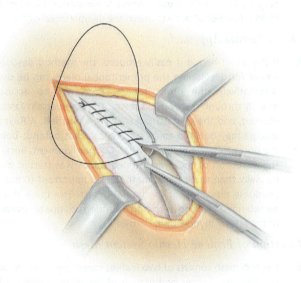

FIGURE 24 • The external oblique is reapproximated, avoiding the ilioinguinal or iliohypogastric nerve.

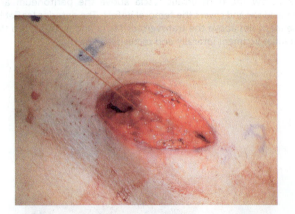

FIGURE 25 • Scarpa fascia is reapproximated.

PEARLS AND PITFALLS

Unable to locate the hernia defect	■ If unable to locate a direct or indirect hernia defect, then open the inguinal floor medial to the inferior epigastric vessels to examine the femoral canal.
Primary repair on tension	■ If the tissue quality is poor, use a mesh prosthesis to allow for a tension-free repair. ■ If mesh is contraindicated, a relaxing incision in the anterior rectus fascia should be performed. ■ Avoid use of mesh in contaminated operative fields.
Meticulous hemostasis	■ Patients undergoing hernia repair are often on antiplatelet or anticoagulants for cardiac disease. Meticulous hemostasis is important to prevent postoperative hematoma and wound complications.

POSTOPERATIVE CARE

- Most patients are discharged on the day of repair. Patients should void prior to leaving the recovery area.
- Patients are recommended to resume normal activities as soon as they feel comfortable.[1]

OUTCOMES

- Elective repair of inguinal hernia is associated with low recurrence rates. Tension-free mesh repairs have the lowest rates of recurrence in adult populations. The overall recurrence rate is 3% to 5% for mesh repairs and 10% to 15% for suture repairs.[14]

COMPLICATIONS

- The rate of complications after inguinal herniorrhaphy has been reported between 15% and 50%.[15] When evaluating patient-centered outcomes, the overall rate of complications is consistently above 30%. The knowledge of complications, experience with handling them, and anticipation of adverse events can reduce their occurrence and guide informed consent.
- The most frequent complication is the development of a seroma. This has been reported to be between 2.4% and 13.6%. The introduction of bacteria by aspiration of a seroma has been widely reported. In the presence of mesh, any attempt at aspiration should be reserved to patients with suspected infection for diagnostic purposes. A seroma should spontaneously resolve over 6 to 8 weeks. Careful ligation of vessels, limiting dissection of soft tissue, and closure of dead spaces can reduce seroma formation.
- The risk of hematoma is reported between 5.5% and 6.5%. Meticulous hemostasis and knowledge of the vascular anatomy of the groin can reduce occurrence. Small hematomas may be treated conservatively; however, large hematomas inducing significant pain or creating tension will usually require evacuation.
- The risk of hemorrhage requiring transfusion is very rare. Intraoperative injury to major vessels is most likely to occur when suturing to Cooper or the inguinal ligament. The femoral artery and vein are bordered by Cooper ligament posteriorly and the inguinal ligament anteriorly. Superficial bites under direct vision should reduce the chance of injury. If an injury does occur, immediate removal of the suture, without tying the suture, and holding direct pressure usually prevent excessive bleeding. If the injury is not recognized, or the suture is tied resulting in a tear of the femoral vein, the inguinal ligament should be divided and a vascular repair should be initiated.
- The reported rate of surgical site infection in clean, nonemergent, inguinal hernia repairs ranges from 0.5% to 3%. This rate of infection is higher for recurrent and emergent hernia operations. Guiding principles of surgical infection prevention are applicable. In case of infection, early opening of the wound and appropriate antibiotic therapy for cellulitis and systemic symptoms will treat the majority of superficial infections. Deep surgical site infections, which are likely associated with foreign material such as suture or mesh, require fastidious wound care and drainage. Although usually not required in the early stages of therapy with early recognition and proper wound care, the mesh may ultimately need to be removed or debrided.
- Urinary retention is reported to occur in 0.2% to 2.42% of the cases. Urinary retention is lowest in patients having regional anesthesia compared with general anesthesia. For those patients with retention, bladder catheterization is required. Bladder injury should be rare. In the case of an iatrogenic injury during a sliding hernia, a two-layer repair of the bladder with absorbable suture will suffice.
- Ischemic orchitis occurs in less than 1% of the cases. It may progress to testicular atrophy, but its clinical course is difficult to predict. Ischemic orchitis is most often caused by thrombosis of the testicular vein within the spermatic cord but can also be from arterial injury. A Doppler ultrasound can evaluate blood supply to the testicles. Reducing cord dissection, preventing overly tight internal ring reconstruction, and transecting large distal hernia sacs and leaving them in situ can reduce this risk.
- Injury to the vas deferens should be rare. When an injury is recognized, and surgical repair is indicated, microsurgical repair with an operating microscope gives superior outcomes. However, repair may also be performed over a 0 Prolene suture, which is brought through the vas at a point distal to the reanastomosis. The Prolene is then brought through the skin and removed on day 3. If unable to repair an injured vas, ligation with permanent suture, and preventing further dissection of the vas, may allow reconstruction in the future. When the vas is injured by rough handling or becomes entrapped by mesh, painful ejaculation or dysejaculation can develop from the resulting partially obstructed lumen.
- Chronic or severe pain following inguinal herniorrhaphy is reported in 10% to 14% of the cases. It remains a perplexing and challenging problem. It is associated with preoperative chronic pain and with recurrent inguinal hernia repair.[16] The identification and protection of the ilioinguinal, genitofemoral, and iliohypogastric nerves are important in preventing

nerve entrapment injuries. If a nerve is injured, it should be transected and ligated proximally, allowing it to retract into the muscle or preperitoneal space. Operative treatment with planned resection of the three nerves can improve or resolve the pain. However, a multidisciplinary pain team approach is imperative for optimal patient outcomes.

ACKNOWLEDGMENT

The authors would like to acknowledge the contributions of Michael D. Paul, MD, to this chapter.

REFERENCES

1. The HerniaSurge Group. International guideline for groin hernia management. *Hernia.* 2018;22:1-165.
2. Bassini E. Sulla cura radicale del ernia. *Arch Soc Ital Chir.* 1887;4:380.
3. Catterina A. *Bassini's Operation for the Radical Cure of Inguinal Hernia.* Lewis; 1934.
4. Fruchaud H. *Anatomie Chirurgicale Des Hernies Del'aine.* Bendavid R, Cunningham P, trans. Gaston Doin & Cie; 1956.
5. Shouldice EB. The Shouldice repair for groin hernias. *Surg Clin N Am.* 2003;83:1163-1187.
6. Glassow F. The Shouldice hospital technique. *Int Surg.* 1986;71(3):148-153.
7. McVay CB, Anson BJ. A fundamental error in current methods of inguinal herniorrhaphy. *Surg Gynecol Obstet.* 1942;74:746-750.
8. Barbier J, Carretier MD, Richer JP. Cooper ligament repair: an update. *World J Surg.* 1989;13:499-505.
9. Rutledge RH. The Cooper's ligament repair. In: Fitzgibbons RJ Jr, Greenburg AG, eds. *Nyhus and Condon's Hernia.* 5th ed. Lippincott Williams & Wilkins; 2002:139-148.
10. Lichtenstein IL, Shulman AG, Amid PK, et al. The tension-free hernioplasty. *Am J Surg.* 1989;157:188-193.
11. Shulman AG, Amid PK, Lichtenstein IL. The Lichtenstein open "tension-free" mesh repair of inguinal hernias. *Surg Today.* 1995;25:619-625.
12. Gilbert A, Graham M, Voigt W. A bilayer patch device for inguinal hernia repair. *Hernia.* 1999;3:161-166.
13. Awad SS, Yallampalli S, Srour AM, et al. Improved outcomes with the Prolene Hernia System mesh compared with the time-honored Lichtenstein onlay mesh repair for inguinal hernia repair. *Am J Surg.* 2007;193:697-701.
14. Bendavid R Complications of groin hernia surgery. In: Bendavid R, ed. *Abdominal Wall Hernias.* Springer-Verlag; 2001:693-700.
15. Matthews RD, Anthony T, Kim LT, et al. Factors associated with postoperative complications and hernia recurrence for patients undergoing inguinal hernia repair: a report from the VA Cooperative Hernia Study Group. *Am J Surg.* 2007;194:611-617.
16. Grant AM, EU Hernia Trialists Collaboration. Open mesh versus non-mesh repair of groin hernia: meta-analysis of randomized trials based on individual patient data [corrected]. *Hernia.* 2002;6:130-136.

Chapter 21 Inguinal Hernia: Laparoscopic Approaches

Courtney E. Collins and Benjamin Kuttikatt Poulose

DEFINITION

- Inguinal hernias can be divided into indirect, direct, and femoral based on location.
- Inguinal hernia repair is one of the most common procedures performed by general surgeons in the United States, with 750,000 to 800,000 cases annually.[1]
- Inguinal hernias affect nearly 27% of men and 3% of women over their lifetime.[2]
- The majority of femoral hernias occur in women (around 70%), but indirect inguinal hernias are still the most common type of hernia in women.[2]
- Indirect inguinal hernias result from a patent processus vaginalis and are responsible for most pediatric inguinal hernias.
- Direct inguinal hernias arise from protrusion of intra-abdominal contents through Hesselbach triangle.

ANATOMY

- The myopectineal orifice includes both the inguinal and femoral regions. The inguinal ligament divides the myopectineal orifice into the inguinal region superiorly and the femoral region inferiorly.
- The boundaries of the inguinal canal are as follows: anteriorly, the aponeurosis of the external oblique and the internal oblique muscle laterally; posteriorly, the transversalis fascia and the transversus abdominis muscle; superiorly, the arch formed by the internal oblique muscle; inferiorly, the inguinal ligament; and medially, the aponeurosis of the external oblique and its insertion on the pubic symphysis (**FIGURE 1**).
- An indirect hernia passes with the spermatic cord (or round ligament, in women) through the inguinal canal via the internal and external rings.
- Hesselbach triangle (the site of direct hernias) is bordered by the inferior epigastric vessels superolaterally, the inguinal ligament inferolaterally, and the edge of the rectus abdominis medially (**FIGURE 2**).
- The boundaries of the femoral canal consist of the lacunar ligament (medial), the femoral vein (lateral), the inguinal ligament (anterior), and the pectineal ligament (posterior).
- Femoral hernias pass through the femoral canal, medial to the femoral vessels, and inferior to the inguinal ligament.
- The nerves at risk for traction injury in most anterior inguinal hernia repairs include the ilioinguinal nerve, iliohypogastric nerve, and the genital branch of the genitofemoral nerve.

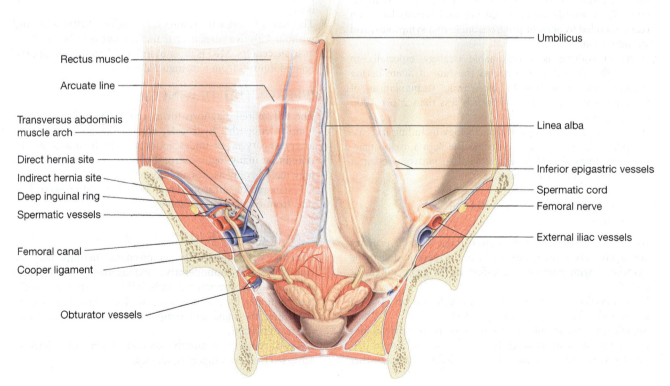

FIGURE 1 • Anatomy of the inguinal canal, intra-abdominal view.

169

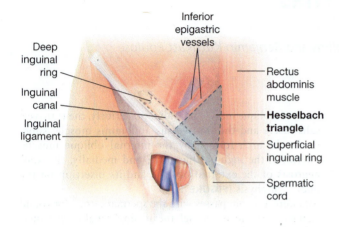

FIGURE 2 • Hesselbach triangle, the site of direct hernias, is bordered by the inferior epigastric vessels, the edge of the rectus abdominis, and the inguinal ligament.

PATHOGENESIS

- Indirect hernias occur as a result of a patent processus vaginalis and are congenital. The hernia involves a peritoneal sac passing through the inguinal canal alongside the spermatic cord or round ligament.
- Direct hernias tend to occur secondary to increased intra-abdominal pressure. Predisposing factors include chronic cough, constipation, straining and difficulty with urination, obesity, and ascites.

NATURAL HISTORY

- The natural history of untreated inguinal hernias is not fully known, although many believe that progression is inevitable. Traditionally, repair of all inguinal hernias has been recommended to prevent progression, hernia symptoms, and strangulation.
- Watchful waiting is a reasonable strategy especially in men with minimal symptoms, as the rate of acute hernia incarceration with bowel obstruction, strangulation of intra-abdominal contents, or both is less than 2 per 1000 patient-years.[3]
- Patients with escalating symptomatology including increasing pain/bulging, difficulty reducing the hernia, or obstructive symptoms should be encouraged to undergo repair if reasonable surgical candidates.

PATIENT HISTORY AND PHYSICAL FINDINGS

- Most patients present with a groin bulge as their primary complaint. Over time, this tends to increase and may be associated with pain or discomfort in the groin, thigh, or testicle.
- Some hernias are asymptomatic and detected on physical examination by a primary care physician.
- Significant pain at initial presentation, particularly if not accompanied by an obvious bulge, may not be due to hernia. Patients with pain and no bulge should undergo further diagnostic testing prior to surgery as these patients often have chronic pain even after groin exploration.
- Patients who develop progressive symptoms with increasing hernia size tend to have the best outcomes after surgical repair with significant improvement in pain.[4]
- Physical examination is the best way to diagnose inguinal hernias, and both sides should be evaluated for the presence of a hernia. The patient should be examined supine and upright, with a finger palpating the external ring while the patient performs a Valsalva maneuver. A bulge detected below the inguinal ligament in the medial thigh suggests a femoral hernia.

IMAGING AND OTHER DIAGNOSTIC STUDIES

- If history and physical examination are consistent with the diagnosis of inguinal hernia, routine imaging is not required.
- A recent systematic review found that overall ultrasound had the highest sensitivity and specificity for the diagnosis of inguinal hernias in addition to being the least expensive test.[5] However, it should be noted that ultrasound results are highly operator dependent and therefore results should always be interpreted in context. When performed, patients should be examined supine and standing, and Valsalva maneuvers should be employed.
- CT scan can also be useful for hernia diagnosis; however, specificity can be low and small hernias may be difficult to visualize in the supine position. Where possible, Valsalva maneuvers should be used during CT scans. A negative CT scan does not necessarily rule out a diagnosis of inguinal hernia.
- CT scan may also be considered in the event of large, complex, and/or recurrent hernias if clarification of the anatomy is needed.
- The role of magnetic resonance imaging (MRI) with and without Valsalva maneuver is unclear but may be available at some centers. MRI is most useful in differentiating sports-related injuries from true inguinal hernias.

DIFFERENTIAL DIAGNOSIS

- The differential diagnosis for a groin bulge includes hernia, lymphadenopathy, hydrocele, abscess, hematoma, femoral artery aneurysm, or undescended testicle. It should also be noted that many inguinoscrotal hernias in cirrhotic patients may include only ascites and not enteric contents.
- CT scan and/or ultrasound may be able to differentiate hernias from other groin pathology.

NONOPERATIVE MANAGEMENT

- Patients with minimally symptomatic hernias may be candidates for nonoperative management or watchful waiting.[3] This approach entails follow-up after 6 months and annually by a care provider, along with instructions regarding the signs and symptoms of acute incarceration or strangulation.
- Delay of repair for 6 months has been shown not to have an adverse effect on surgical outcomes.[6]

- Patients who experience significant pain with activity, those who have prostatism or constipation, and those with overall good health status are likely to benefit most from surgical repair.[4]
- After 2 years, about 25% of patients who are minimally symptomatic will develop worsening symptoms and request surgical repair.[3] This rate can be as high as 72% after 7 years.[7]

SURGICAL MANAGEMENT

- Techniques for the laparoscopic management of inguinal hernia include the transabdominal properitoneal (TAPP) approach and the totally extraperitoneal (TEP) technique. TEP and (more commonly) TAPP repairs can also be performed robotically.
- Laparoscopic repair is especially useful for bilateral inguinal hernias and recurrent hernias after a prior open repair.

Preoperative Planning

- General anesthesia is usually required for laparoscopic repairs, whereas open repairs can be performed with the use of local anesthesia.
- Immediately prior to surgery, the patient should be instructed to void, or a Foley catheter should be placed. Most patients can adequately void preoperatively, precluding the need for a urinary catheter, which may increase the risk of urinary retention as well as infection.
- For recurrent hernias, it is imperative that the surgeon review previous operative reports. In general, the approach used to repair a recurrence should use fresh surgical planes to facilitate the repair. For a previous open repair that has recurred, a laparoscopic approach is usually favored. If a mesh plug has been used, a TAPP approach may be significantly easier than TEP due to the high chance of peritoneal violation and need to debulk the plug.
- Large inguinoscrotal hernias, particularly those that do not reduce are difficult to repair from a TEP approach given the relative lack of operating space with this technique. For these patients, a TAPP or open approach should be considered.
- For a previous laparoscopic repair that has recurred, an open approach may be easier to perform. However, given the variety of laparoscopic inguinal hernia techniques used, repeat laparoscopic repair of a recurrence is possible in experienced hands.
- Caution should be taken in patients with previous prostatectomy or cesarean section with entrance into the space of Retzius, which can make laparoscopic repair much more challenging. In these cases, serious consideration should be given to an anterior approach. As with repairing laparoscopic inguinal hernia repair recurrences, a laparoscopic approach can be attempted, if deemed advantageous, by an experienced laparoscopic hernia surgeon. If a laparoscopic approach is used, care should be taken when dissecting near Cooper ligament to avoid a bladder injury.

Positioning

- The patient is positioned supine with arms tucked and legs secured in order to prevent slippage with changes in table position during the procedure.
- The surgeon stands on the contralateral side from the hernia being repaired.

LAPAROSCOPIC TRANSABDOMINAL PROPERITONEAL INGUINAL HERNIA REPAIR

Establishment of Pneumoperitoneum and Port Placement

- The first trocar is placed at the level of the umbilicus, typically beginning in the umbilicus, and extending the incision inferiorly. Pneumoperitoneum can be established either with a Veress needle or by placing a 12-mm Hasson port.
- Two 5-mm ports are then placed lateral to the rectus sheath approximately 1 to 2 cm above the level of the umbilicus (FIGURE 3). A 5-mm 30° laparoscopic camera is used and is placed in the port ipsilateral to the hernia. The surgeon uses the umbilical port and port contralateral to the hernia. If visualization is challenging in this configuration, the camera may also be moved to the middle port.
- The patient is placed in the Trendelenburg position with the hernia side of the patient up displacing the pelvic viscera cephalad and away from the defect.

Peritoneal Incision

- The inferior epigastric vessels are identified on the side of the hernia. Note that chronically incarcerated properitoneal fat may occupy the hernia defect precluding clear visualization of the defect itself. Therefore, during a TAPP approach, if there is a high suspicion for inguinal hernia by history and physical examination, dissection commences on the symptomatic side even if no obvious hernia is initially seen from the intraperitoneal view.
- The peritoneum is incised with laparoscopic scissors beginning lateral to the inferior epigastric vessels (FIGURE 4). This dissection can typically be done without the use of electrosurgery. The correct plane of dissection in the TAPP repair is the true properitoneal plane. It is extremely easy to inadvertently dissect the retrorectus plane with this approach (FIGURE 4). Should this occur, dissection can proceed (similar to the TEP approach) but dissection into the retrorectus space without the benefit of balloon tamponade can incur increased blood loss. Conversely, a retrorectus dissection may be preferred in patients with very thin peritoneum to avoid

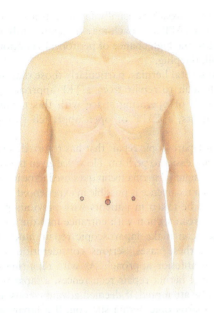

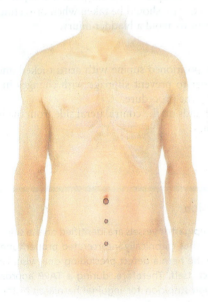

tears in the peritoneal flap. Some surgeons advocate intentional entrance into the retrorectus place medially due to the thin peritoneum medially.
- The peritoneal flap is mobilized high up on the lower abdominal wall, extending laterally to the anterior superior iliac spine and medially to the ipsilateral medial umbilical fold.
- Care should be taken to avoid injury to the inferior epigastric vessels, which lie posterior to the rectus muscles in the retrorectus plane. Maintaining a plane of dissection in the true properitoneal space minimizes the risk of injury to these vessels.

Dissection of the Properitoneal Plane

- Beginning laterally, retract the peritoneum medially, and dissect the properitoneal plane, leaving the fat against the abdominal wall to preserve small nerves and vessels.
- The inferior epigastric vessels are again identified and the properitoneal plane is developed medial to these vessels toward Cooper ligament. During the initial learning curve of this procedure, the overwhelming tendency is to dissect too far medially and posteriorly into the region of the bladder. Confirmation of the trajectory of dissection toward Cooper ligament can be obtained by a brief intraperitoneal view. Once Cooper ligament has been identified, it is exposed for about 2 cm anticipating fixation at its superior aspect (**FIGURE 5**). A direct sac may obscure Cooper ligament until the sac is reduced entirely into the true pelvis. It is important to expose the periosteum of Cooper ligament with care being taken not to injure the corona mortis venous plexus often in close proximity to Cooper ligament. Some patients may also have an aberrant obturator artery arising from the external iliac artery, which crosses Cooper ligament.
- After Cooper ligament has been identified, a dissection lateral to the inferior epigastric vessels is commenced attempting to dissect the properitoneal fatty tissue anteriorly while maintaining integrity of the peritoneum. This dissection is taken to the level of the iliopubic tract.

FIGURE 3 • Port placement. **A**, For transabdominal properitoneal approach, ports are placed at the umbilicus and lateral to the linea semilunaris at the level of the umbilicus. **B**, Totally extraperitoneal ports are placed in the midline at the umbilicus, 2 cm above the symphysis pubis, and the final in between the first two, at least 4 cm cranial to the second port.

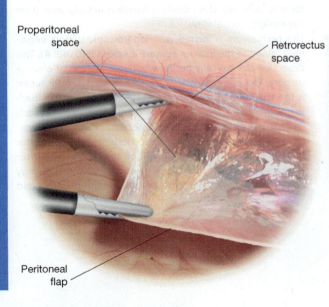

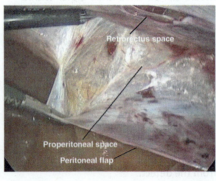

FIGURE 4 • Creation of the peritoneal flap during transabdominal properitoneal approach. Beginning lateral to the epigastric vessels, the peritoneum is incised and the properitoneal space dissected, creating a flap. The retrorectus space, seen at the top of this figure, may be inadvertently entered, resulting in increased bleeding.

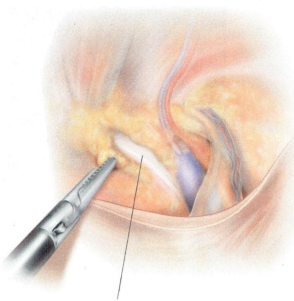
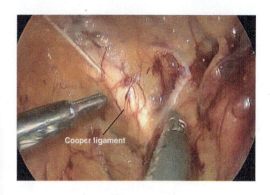

FIGURE 5 • Cooper ligament. Dissection proceeds medially toward Cooper ligament. Once identified, approximately 2 cm of the superior aspect of Cooper ligament is cleared for mesh fixation.

Reduction of the Hernia

Direct hernias often reduce easily as the peritoneal flap is taken down. If more dissection is needed, the peritoneum is gently grasped and retracted cephalad. The surgeon should look for the white edge of the pseudosac (attenuated transversalis fascia), which is then grasped with a dissector and peeled off the peritoneum.

- At this point, attention is turned to an indirect hernia sac if present, and it is dissected away from the cord structures. The peritoneum is now separated from the transversalis fascia overlying the inferior epigastric vessels. As the indirect hernia sac is approached, gentle but persistent cephalad traction is applied to reduce the hernia sac. Typically, if it can be done safely, the entire sac is reduced into the true pelvis. As the sac is reduced, the medial vas deferens and lateral testicular vessels are identified.
- In women, the round ligament is identified. The sac is dissected away from these structures. In women, the round ligament can often be separated from the peritoneum. Should this not be possible, efforts are made to divide the peritoneum along the axis of the round ligament, reapproximating the peritoneum after an adequate dissection has been performed. However, if transection is necessary to perform an adequate hernia repair, the round ligament can be divided.
- Once the hernia is reduced, the peritoneum is separated from the iliac vessels, vas, and testicular vessels posteriorly toward the umbilicus (**FIGURE 6**). This ensures a generous exposure of the entire myopectineal orifice. In addition, separation of the cord structures from the peritoneum ensures the ability to place a solid piece of mesh across the myopectineal orifice without the need for keyhole creation (**FIGURE 7**). Should a keyhole configuration be employed, the dissection proceeds caudally to the vas and testicular vessels, beginning at the level of the internal ring. Care should be taken to dissect well posteriorly to allow mesh overlap.

Mesh Placement and Fixation

- An appropriately sized (usually 14 cm [transverse axis] × 12 cm [craniocaudal axis]), macroporous mesh should be chosen, which will cover the hernia defect as well as the entire myopectineal orifice. Light or heavyweight mesh can be considered; however, a recent meta-analysis found that lightweight mesh increases the risk of recurrence particularly in large hernias or direct defects. Additionally, lightweight mesh was not found to provide a benefit in terms of pain or foreign body sensation.[8]
- The mesh is then grasped medially and inserted into the 12-mm port, aiming toward Cooper ligament. A Maryland dissector can be used to position the lateral and superior aspect of the mesh.
- Prior to fixation, precise placement of the mesh over the entire myopectineal orifice is ensured. Care is taken to ensure at least 3 cm of overlap over any hernia defect. All three hernia spaces (indirect, direct, and femoral) should be covered by the mesh.
- Minimal fixation is used to prevent migration of the mesh (**FIGURE 8**). For indirect hernias, two tacks are placed just above Cooper ligament: one high medially over the posterior aspect of the rectus sheath and one high laterally well above the iliopubic tract. For direct defects, some additional fixation is usually necessary to avoid early migration and recurrence. In general, no tacks should be placed below Cooper ligament or below the iliopubic tract. Counterpressure should be used to feel the tip of the tacking device on all tacks except those placed adjacent to Cooper ligament. There are little data to support any one

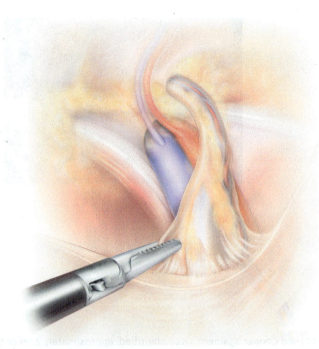
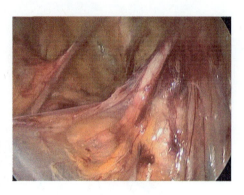

FIGURE 6 • Dissection of peritoneum off posterior structures. Once the hernia is reduced, the peritoneum is separated from the cord structures and iliac vessels to allow adequate exposure of the myopectineal orifice. This allows room for generous mesh overlap and is a key step in preventing hernia recurrence.

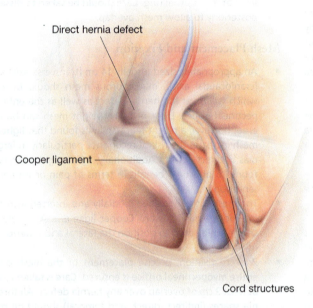
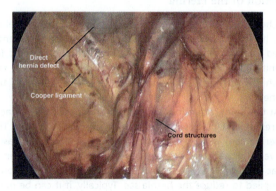

FIGURE 7 • Completed dissection. The hernia has been reduced and dissection completed prior to mesh placement. Note the direct hernia defect; Cooper ligament, which has been cleared superiorly; and the cord structures.

type of fixation (absorbable vs permanent). Initial results suggest that avoiding mechanical fixation with the use of sealants or glues may be feasible, especially with a TEP approach; however, more conclusive information is needed.[9,10]

Closing the Peritoneal Flap and Incisions

- The peritoneal flap can be closed with either tacks or absorbable suture fixation, taking care to avoid injury to the inferior epigastric vessels (FIGURE 9). All attempts are made to minimize exposure of dissected tissue and mesh to the peritoneal cavity. During flap closure, care is taken to ensure that the posterior aspect of the mesh does not buckle or twist, which can act as a lead point for recurrence.
- After desufflation, trocars are removed under direct visualization. Fascia at the 12-mm port site should be closed, and skin is approximated with 4-0 Monocryl sutures.

Chapter 21 INGUINAL HERNIA: LAPAROSCOPIC APPROACHES 175

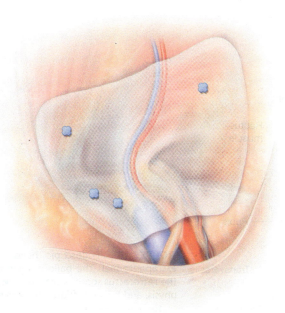
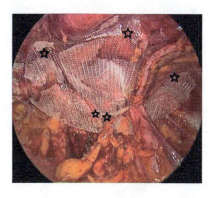

FIGURE 8 • Mesh fixation. The mesh can be either a solid piece or one with a keyhole and should be taut. Fixation tacks are used sparingly: two above Cooper ligaments, one in the posterior rectus sheath, and one laterally, well above the iliopubic tract.

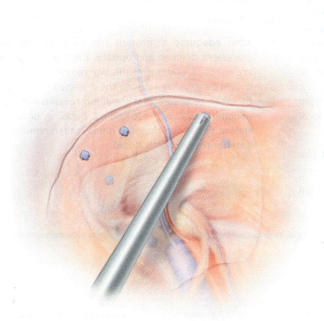
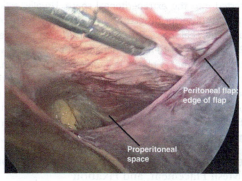

FIGURE 9 • Peritoneal flap closure for transabdominal properitoneal. The peritoneal flap is closed with sequential tacks.

TOTALLY EXTRAPERITONEAL INGUINAL HERNIA REPAIR

Establishment of the Operative (Properitoneal) Space and Port Placement

- A 1- to 2-cm longitudinal skin incision is made inferior to the umbilicus and the subcutaneous tissues are divided. The anterior rectus sheath is identified just lateral to linea alba on the ipsilateral side of the hernia. The anterior rectus sheath is then divided using electrosurgery. The rectus muscle is retracted laterally and the retrorectus space is entered. An endoscopic balloon dissector is advanced immediately beneath the rectus muscle and advanced to the pubic symphysis (**FIGURE 10**). A 10-mm 0° laparoscope is placed into the lumen of the balloon and it is fully inflated and held in position for 2 minutes

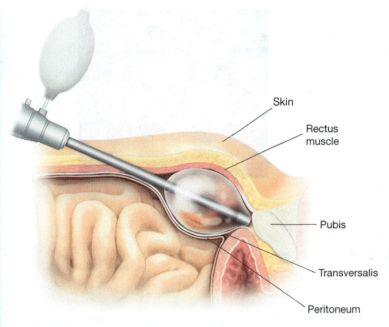

FIGURE 10 • Endoscopic balloon dissector, totally extraperitoneal. The balloon dissector is inserted into the retrorectus space, advanced toward the pubic symphysis, and fully insufflated for 2 minutes to allow adequate hemostasis.

to achieve hemostasis. The balloon is removed and either a Hasson cannula (with stay sutures) or a balloon-tipped cannula is inserted into the extraperitoneal space. Usually, action of the balloon dissector dissects both the retrorectus space and the properitoneal space. This space is insufflated to a pressure of 12 mm Hg and a 10-mm 30° laparoscope is used for visualization. The patient is placed in Trendelenburg position. Two 5-mm operating ports are inserted under direct visualization in the lower midline. The lowest is placed 2 cm above the pubic symphysis. The second port is placed at least 4 cm cranial from the first port (FIGURE 2). Use of a finder needle with local anesthetic can assist in placement of these ports.

Dissection of the Properitoneal Plane, Reduction of the Hernia, Mesh Placement, and Fixation

- These steps proceed similarly to that described for the TAPP approach discussed previously.

- Note that direct hernias often reduce with the inflation of the endoscopic balloons and may not be visible when the laparoscope is introduced.

Desufflation

- After adequate hemostasis has been assured and mesh placement deemed appropriate, the 5-mm operating ports are removed, and the insufflation removed. The peritoneum should be visualized closing the dissected space. Care should be taken to ensure that the mesh remains flat against the abdominal wall without folding, buckling, or twisting. The Hasson or balloon-tipped cannula is then removed, and the anterior rectus sheath closed.

PEARLS AND PITFALLS

TEP—entrance into properitoneal space	Entrance into the properitoneal space during TEP should be performed away from the umbilicus as the peritoneum and transversalis fascia are fused to the umbilical stalk, preventing easy mobilization. Entry can be made 5 mm below the umbilicus or slightly off midline can facilitate this step. Typically, the retrorectus space is first entered, with the balloon dissector expanding this plane. The dissector usually also expands the properitoneal plane. In some instances, the transversalis fascia may remain intact, requiring laparoscopic mobilization into the true properitoneal space.
TAPP—properitoneal dissection	Care is taken to enter the plane between the peritoneum and the transversalis fascia. If the transversalis fascia is inadvertently entered, attempts should be made to get back into the properitoneal plane. If this cannot be done, the dissection can proceed in the retrorectus space anterior to the transversalis fascia. This is usually a less hemostatic plane; care should be taken to avoid excessive bleeding and injury to the inferior epigastric vessels.

TEP—avoidance of pneumoperitoneum	▪ Maintaining integrity of the peritoneum and avoidance of pneumoperitoneum facilitates exposure with the TEP approach. Small tears in the peritoneum can often be left alone while larger ones should be repaired with either clips, absorbable loop ligatures, or sutures. A Veress needle can be placed into the peritoneal cavity in the upper abdomen to vent the pneumoperitoneum and reestablish visualization in the extraperitoneal space if needed. Inability to control the peritoneal gas leak may necessitate conversion to a TAPP approach.
TAPP/TEP—avoidance of injury to aberrant obturator vessels and corona mortis venous plexus	▪ Dissection of Cooper ligament often exposes aberrant obturator vessels and the corona mortis venous plexus. Great care should be taken to avoid injury to these structures as hemostasis can be challenging. Additionally, these structures should be taken into consideration when mesh fixation is used adjacent to Cooper ligament.
TAPP/TEP—large direct hernia sac	▪ With large direct sacs, identification of Cooper ligament can often be challenging. When a sizable direct hernia is encountered, the sac is reduced early in the dissection to identify Cooper ligament.
TAPP—large indirect hernia sac	▪ Reduction of a large indirect hernia sac is one of the most challenging maneuvers in laparoscopic inguinal hernia repair. Often, medial and lateral retraction of the sac can help facilitate dissection of the sac away from the cord structures and inferior epigastric vessels. Manual reduction (externally with fingers) can sometimes help dissect the entire sac back into the true pelvis. If complete reduction is unable to be achieved, transection of the sac can be performed. This should be seriously considered if there is concern for injury to spermatic cord structures (particularly devascularization) from difficult and/or prolonged dissection. In this case, the testicular vessels and vas are clearly identified and separated from the tenacious sac. Laparoscopic clips or absorbable sutures are used to clip the proximal aspect of the sac and the sac is divided, allowing the open distal aspect of the sac to "parachute" back into the inguinal canal. The sac can then be mobilized in the standard fashion to facilitate mesh placement.

POSTOPERATIVE CARE

- In addition to the typical postoperative monitoring for hydration and adequate analgesia, it is important that the patient be monitored for urinary retention in the immediate postoperative period and a Foley catheter inserted, if needed.
- Diet can be advanced quickly within 12 hours postoperatively. Ambulation can resume once appropriately recovered from anesthesia. Patients are typically ready for discharge on the day of surgery.
- Constipation and straining should be avoided postoperatively. Light activity can be resumed within 1 day of surgery. Patients should be advised to avoid strenuous activity, particularly heavy lifting and straining, for at least 3 to 4 weeks postoperatively.

OUTCOMES

- A recent meta-analysis demonstrated that both TAPP and TEP repairs were associated with significantly reduced early postoperative pain, faster return to work, less chronic pain, and fewer hematomas and wound complications compared to open repairs.[11]
- Hernia recurrence and hospital length of stay were no different between open vs minimally invasive approaches.[11]

COMPLICATIONS

- Complications after inguinal hernia repair (whether open or laparoscopic) include surgical site infection, seroma or hematoma, mesh infection (all <1%), hernia recurrence (2%-5% for primary inguinal hernia; around 10% for recurrent hernia), and chronic groin pain (around 0.5%).
- Men with bilateral hernias should be counseled regarding the slightly increased risk of decreased fertility associated with bilateral laparoscopic inguinal hernia repairs.[12]
- TAPP has been associated with an increased risk of intraabdominal and vascular injury, although this risk is low (<1%).
- Laparoscopic repair (TAPP and TEP) carries the risk of port site hernias (approximately 0.1%-2%).
- All male patients undergoing repair of very large inguinoscrotal hernias and/or complex recurrent hernias should be counseled on the risk of injury to the cord structures, particularly the vessels. Cord devascularization can result in orchitis or possibly (but rarely) the need for an orchiectomy either at the time of repair or postoperatively.

REFERENCES

1. Rutkow IM. Demographic and socioeconomic aspects of hernia repair in the United States in 2003. *Surg Clin North Am.* 2003;83(5):1045-1051, v-vi. doi:10.1016/S0039-6109(03)00132-4
2. Kingsnorth A, LeBlanc K. Hernias: inguinal and incisional. *Lancet.* 2003;362(9395):1561-1571. doi:10.1016/S0140-6736(03)14746-0
3. Fitzgibbons RJ Jr, Giobbie-Hurder A, Gibbs JO, et al. Watchful waiting vs repair of inguinal hernia in minimally symptomatic men: a randomized clinical trial. *J Am Med Assoc.* 2006;295(3):285-292. doi:10.1001/jama.295.3.285
4. Sarosi GA, Wei Y, Gibbs JO, et al. A clinician's guide to patient selection for watchful waiting management of inguinal hernia. *Ann Surg.* 2011;253(3):605-610. doi:10.1097/SLA.0b013e31820b04e9
5. Piga E, Zetner D, Andresen K, Rosenberg J. Imaging modalities for inguinal hernia diagnosis: a systematic review. *Hernia.* 2020;24(5):917-926. doi:10.1007/s10029-020-02189-4
6. Thompson JS, Gibbs JO, Reda DJ, et al. Does delaying repair of an asymptomatic hernia have a penalty? *Am J Surg.* 2008;195(1):89-93. doi:10.1016/j.amjsurg.2007.07.021
7. Mizrahi H, Parker MC. Management of asymptomatic inguinal hernia: a systematic review of the evidence. *Arch Surg.* 2012;147(3):277-281. doi:10.1001/archsurg.2011.914
8. Bakker WJ, Aufenacker TJ, Boschman JS, Burgmans JPJ. Heavyweight mesh is superior to lightweight mesh in laparo-endoscopic inguinal

hernia repair: a meta-analysis and trial sequential analysis of randomized controlled trials. *Ann Surg.* 2021;273(5):890-899. doi:10.1097/SLA.0000000000003831
9. Kaul A, Hutfless S, Le H, et al. Staple versus fibrin glue fixation in laparoscopic total extraperitoneal repair of inguinal hernia: a systematic review and meta-analysis. *Surg Endosc.* 2012;26(5):1269-1278. doi:10.1007/s00464-011-2025-2
10. Shah NS, Bandara AI, Sheen AJ. Clinical outcome and quality of life in 100 consecutive laparoscopic totally extra-peritoneal (TEP) groin hernia repairs using fibrin glue (Tisseel): a United Kingdom experience. *Hernia.* 2012;16(6):647-653. doi:10.1007/s10029-012-0936-z
11. Aiolfi A, Cavalli M, Del Ferraro S, et al. Treatment of inguinal hernia: systematic review and updated network meta-analysis of randomized controlled trials. *Ann Surg.* 2021;274(6):954-961. doi:10.1097/SLA.0000000000004735
12. Peeters E, Spiessens C, Oyen R, et al. Laparoscopic inguinal hernia repair in men with lightweight meshes may significantly impair sperm motility: a randomized controlled trial. *Ann Surg.* 2010;252(2):240-246. doi:10.1097/SLA.0b013e3181e8fac5

Chapter 22 Robotic Inguinal Hernia Repair

Andrew T. Bates and David M. Pechman

DEFINITION

- Inguinal hernias represent one of the most common problems faced by general surgeons, with greater than 20 million patients undergoing elective inguinal hernia repair worldwide annually.[1,2]
- An inguinal hernia is an opening in the myofascial plane which allows for intraperitoneal and preperitoneal contents to protrude through the inguinal canal. Inguinal hernias may be direct or indirect. Indirect inguinal hernias occur lateral to the inferior epigastric vessels and are due to a patent processus vaginalis; direct inguinal hernias occur medial to the inferior epigastric vessels and pass through a defect in the posterior wall of the inguinal canal.
- Herniation can occur at other potential spaces and include femoral hernias, obturator hernias, and suprapubic hernias.

DIFFERENTIAL DIAGNOSIS

- Differential diagnosis depends on chief complaint, which is most commonly groin bulge or groin pain.
- For patients complaining of groin bulge, differential diagnosis includes inguinal hernia, femoral hernia, inguinal lymphadenopathy, hydrocele, varicocele, undescended testicle, neoplasm, cord lipoma, and vascular aneurysm or pseudoaneurysm. In pregnant women, groin bulge may represent a round ligament varix.[3]
- For patients complaining of groin pain, the differential diagnosis consists of the above disorders and expands to include neurogenic pain, osteitis pubis, or muscle strain/tear (athletic pubalgia).
- Some male patients may present with chief complaint of testicular pain. In these cases, differential diagnosis includes testicular torsion and epididymitis. Testicular torsion is a urologic emergency and must be ruled out or reduced expeditiously.

PATIENT HISTORY AND PHYSICAL FINDINGS

- History and physical examination can confirm a diagnosis of inguinal hernia in the majority of cases. Common chief complaints for patients presenting with inguinal hernia are groin bulge and/or groin pain with or without radiation to the ipsilateral testicle (in men). Pain most commonly is "aching" in nature and may be made worse with activity or at the end of the day. Comprehensive patient history should include the presence or absence of similar symptoms on the contralateral side and surgical history. If the patient has a history of prior inguinal hernia repair, it is important to determine the type of repair that was performed.

Physical examination should include a careful assessment of bilateral groins and testicles (in men) to assess for palpable defects or masses. Reducible inguinal hernias may not be palpable when examination is performed in supine position. Leg lift may be helpful to palpate reducible hernias while patient is supine. Reducible hernias may be best appreciated with patient standing with Valsalva maneuver performed.

IMAGING AND OTHER DIAGNOSTIC STUDIES

- In the majority of cases, diagnosis and repair of inguinal hernias can occur without imaging. In some cases, computed tomography (CT) or ultrasound (US) imaging may be helpful to confirm or rule out the presence of inguinal hernia.
- US may be performed as a dynamic study, utilizing Valsalva maneuver to identify bulging hernia contents. As with any US study, sensitivity and specificity is variable and is operator-dependent. A 2013 meta-analysis determined that US sensitivity was 86% and specificity was 77% in the diagnosis of occult inguinal hernia.[4]
- CT imaging may be helpful in identifying hernias when physical examination is difficult due to body habitus or other factors. In the meta-analysis mentioned earlier, CT sensitivity was 80% and specificity was 65% in the diagnosis of occult inguinal hernia.
- Although US or CT may help identify small inguinal hernias not appreciated on physical examination, nonvisualization does not rule out the presence of hernia.

SURGICAL MANAGEMENT

Preoperative Planning

- As with all hernia repairs, patient selection is key to optimizing surgical outcomes. More recently, surgical prehabilitation has been a focus of many hernia centers to promote improved patients' functional status and nutrition.[5] Several authors have recommended preoperative weight loss for all patients with BMI above 35, as well as nutritional counseling for patients with albumin levels below 2.5. Patients should be able to achieve at least four METs of physical activity prior to hernia repair. Additionally, most centers will require smoking cessation (including all nicotine products) at least 30 days prior to all elective hernia surgeries.
- The size and morphology of the hernia also determines the most appropriate repair. Although robotic repairs benefit many patients, some massive inguinoscrotal hernias are likely better served with an open repair, especially if they are chronically incarcerated. Additionally, patients who have undergone previous posterior repair or preperitoneal urologic surgery represent a higher surgical complexity if robotic repair is attempted; robotic repair in these cases should be performed only by experienced robotic hernia surgeons.

SECTION VII SURGERY OF THE ABDOMINAL WALL

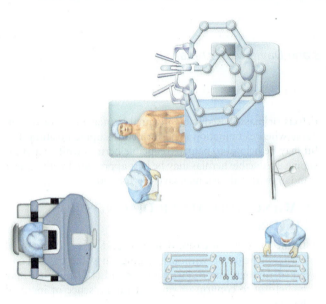

FIGURE 1 • Room setup for da Vinci Si platform.

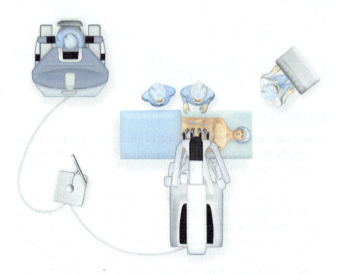

FIGURE 2 • Room setup for da Vinci Xi platform.

Positioning

- The patient will be placed supine on the operating table with both arms tucked to the side to avoid clashes with the robotic arms. The hinge of the bed should align with the angle between the patient's iliac crest and costal margin. The bed should be flexed to increase the abdominal space for port placement as well as to avoid injuries to the patient's face. Some method of facial protection should be used, such as foam padding or a low-profile metal tray. Routine use of urinary catheters is not required as long as the patient can void immediately prior to entering the operating room. However, in patients with a history of benign prostatic hyperplasia or incomplete voiding, catheterization may be useful to decompress the bladder.
- For those surgeons using a da Vinci Si robot, parallel docking or split-leg docking with the patient in lithotomy is preferred to have access to both sides of the groin (**FIGURE 1**). For surgeons using the Xi platform, the robotic cart can be positioned on any side of the patient, with the cart set for a pelvic docking (**FIGURE 2**).

TECHNIQUES

- The procedure is performed under general anesthesia. The abdomen is prepped from xiphoid to the scrotum and penis to prepare for the possibility of open conversion. A skin incision is made at the umbilicus. Entry and insufflation can be obtained via Hasson or Veress technique depending on the robotic platform being used. Right- and left-sided 8-mm ports are placed at least 10 cm lateral to the camera port at the level of the umbilicus.[6,7]
- On the side of the hernia, the peritoneum is incised just above the arcuate line, allowing for sufficient space for mesh coverage later in the procedure (**FIGURE 3**). This incision should extend from midline out laterally to the anterior superior iliac spine. The preperitoneal space is then dissection inferiorly using a combination of blunt dissection and electrocautery. During this dissection, the peritoneum should be pulled toward the camera to minimize tears. Medially, the pubic tubercle and Cooper ligament is exposed and the peritoneum is dissected to expose the obturator space. Laterally, the preperitoneal space (space of Bogros) is developed while taking care not to violate the

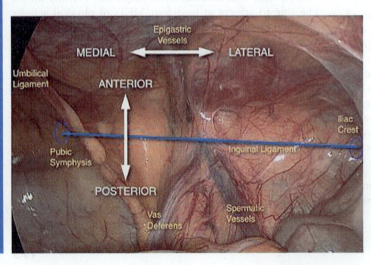

FIGURE 3 • Anatomy of the groin.

Chapter 22 ROBOTIC INGUINAL HERNIA REPAIR   181

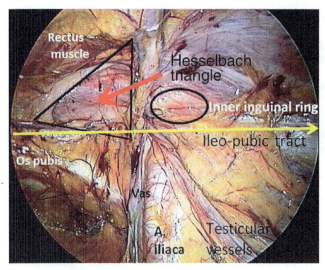

FIGURE 4 • The dissected myopectineal orifice.

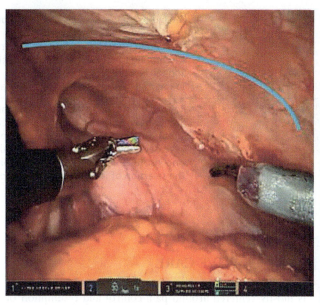

FIGURE 5 • Starting the peritoneal flap.

transversalis fascia and potentially injure the lateral femoral cutaneous nerve.[6,7]

- The femoral and direct inguinal spaces are inspected for the presence of any hernias and their contents are reduced. The hernia sac/peritoneum is dissected away from the spermatic cord with minimal/judicious use of electrocautery (FIGURE 4). The contents of the spermatic cord must be identified and protected. Once reduced, the peritoneum should be freed posteriorly to the base of the vas deferens. Hemostasis should be confirmed prior to insertion of the mesh.[6,7]
- A variety of inguinal hernia meshes can be used with equal efficacy, including anatomic and flat meshes. A lightweight, macroporous mesh is recommended. The medial border of the mesh should cross over the midline and extend under the pubic ramus to cover potential obturator and femoral defects. The inferior edge of the mesh should drape across the spermatic cord, ensuring the peritoneum is not anterior to the mesh. The superior edge of the mesh should lay posteriorly against the rectus abdominis muscle. Fixation of the mesh, although not required, is often undertaken with simple suture to help hold the mesh in place during closure of the peritoneal flap. The peritoneal flap is then closed with a running absorbable suture.[6,7]

PEARLS AND PITFALLS

Starting the peritoneal flap	■ The proper level for the incision of the peritoneal flap is important for visualization and later coverage of mesh. ■ Starting the flap at or just above the arcuate line is usually sufficient (FIGURE 5). ■ Using a robotic grasper, pinch a small amount of peritoneum and pull away from the posterior sheath. ■ Once the peritoneum is incised, either sharply or with cautery, the pneumoperitoneum should help dissect the correct plane. Although it is preferred to only enter the preperitoneal space, the surgeon may elect to incise the posterior sheath as well if they feel the peritoneum is very thin and will need greater thickness in order to close without tearing. If this technique is used, the surgeon must reenter the preperitoneal plane inferiorly.
Proper dissection technique	■ The preperitoneal space is relatively avascular and minimal cautery should be required. ■ Once the space is entered, the flap should be pulled toward the camera and the operative hand is used to push the areolar tissue away. ■ The grasper should be moved deeper inside the flap as needed to continue providing proper tension. ■ The wrist of the dissecting hand should be preferentially used to create more evenly distributed pressure and minimize the risk of injury to bladder or vessels.
Tearing the peritoneum	■ When grasping or manipulating the peritoneal flap, force should be applied as evenly as possible. ■ Secure grasp of the tissue with appropriate tension is key. ■ Once the dissection moves inferiorly toward the pubis and inguinal ring, gentle downward pressure with an open grasper is usually sufficient for dissection and helps to prevent tearing.

Sewing	▪ Sewing of the peritoneal flap should be performed in a "down-to-up" orientation, pronating the sewing hand toward the surgeon. ▪ This allows for the greatest mobility on the operative hand. ▪ Attempting to sew away from one's self often results in an error message due to inappropriate torque and tension on the instruments. ▪ To improve efficiency, multiple bites can be completed before pulling the suture taut.
Minimizing instrument usage	▪ Robotic hernia surgery is typically higher in cost than open or laparoscopic surgery, such that the surgeon should be conscientious of instrument and material usage. ▪ Robotic inguinal hernia repairs can typically be performed with three instruments, and some practitioners have developed two-instrument techniques. ▪ One instrument should be able to apply electrocautery, sew, incise the peritoneum, and grasp tissue. ▪ The selection of instruments that can perform multiple functions is key.

POSTOPERATIVE CARE

- Proper postoperative care after robotic inguinal hernia repair is mostly centered around pain control and resumption of normal activities. A multimodal pain control protocol is advised to help avoid the regular use of opioid pain control, which has the potential for dependency and side effects such as nausea and constipation. We utilize preoperative agents against neuropathic pain, such as gabapentin, as well as intraoperative nerve blocks using long-acting local anesthetics. Postoperatively, acetaminophen and anti-inflammatory medications are usually sufficient. Additionally, patients are advised to place cold compresses to the affected groin during the first postoperative day to help reduce swelling.
- Despite their widespread adoption, recommendations advising against physical activity after hernia repair are not supported by the literature. Furthermore, early ambulation has been shown to shorten the period of postoperative convalescence. We advise patients that they may return to normal activities as long as they are asymptomatic.
- Constipation is an extremely common occurrence after all abdominal surgeries. Hernia repair patients may be particularly affected due to discomfort with Valsalva maneuvers. Patients should be placed on a prophylactic bowel regimen and advised to maintain adequate fluid and fiber intake.

COMPLICATIONS

- The most common complications after robotic inguinal hernia repair are generally the same as laparoscopic transabdominal inguinal hernia repair.[8] The risk of bleeding and infection are quite low but can certainly occur. Prosthetic mesh infection after minimally invasive inguinal hernia repair is very rare. Hernia recurrence is highly dependent upon the proficiency of the surgeon with minimally invasive hernia repairs. However, once the surgeon is outside of their learning curve, the recurrence rate of open and minimally invasive repairs is equivalent.[9,10] Postoperative seroma can be frustrating to the patient but usually resolves spontaneously. The rate of seroma formation is highly dependent on the size of the original hernia and the volume of dead space created after reduction of the hernia sac. One disadvantage of the transabdominal approach is the formation of postoperative adhesions, with early bowel obstructions being described in the literature.[11,12]
- The risk of chronic groin pain after robotic inguinal hernia repair can approach 10% of cases and varies in severity.[13] The proper dissection of the preperitoneal plane with knowledge of the neuroanatomy of the groin is essential to avoid nerve injury. The most commonly injured nerves in the area are the genitofemoral nerve and the lateral femoral cutaneous nerve, both of which travel in the space lateral to the spermatic cord. The treatment of postsurgical neuropathic pain can involve a combination of medical therapy, regional nerve blocks, and possibly neurectomy in severe cases.

REFERENCES

1. The HerniaSurge Group. International guidelines for groin hernia management. *Hernia*. 2018;22(1):1-165.
2. Kingsnorth A, LeBlanc K. Hernias: inguinal and incisional. *Lancet*. 2003;362(9395):1561-1571.
3. Dent BM, Al Samaraee A, Coyne PE, Nice C, Katory M. Varices of the round ligament mimicking an inguinal hernia - an important differential diagnosis during pregnancy. *Ann R Coll Surg Engl*. 2010;92(7):W10-W11.
4. Robinson A, Light D, Kasim A, Nice C. A systematic review and meta-analysis of the role of radiology in the diagnosis of occult inguinal hernia. *Surg Endosc*. 2013;27(1):11.
5. Lyons NB, Bernardi K, Olavarria OA, et al. Prehabilitation among patients undergoing non-bariatric abdominal surgery: a systematic review. *J Am Coll Surg*. 2020;231(4):480-489.
6. Arcerito M, Changchien E, Bernal O, Konkoly-Thege A, Moon J. Robotic inguinal hernia repair: technique and early experience. *Am Surg*. 2016;82(10):1014-1017.
7. Davis SS, Dakin G, Bates A, eds. *The SAGES Manual of Hernia Surgery*. Springer; 2018.
8. Huerta S, Timmerman C, Argo M, et al. Open, laparoscopic, and robotic inguinal hernia repair: outcomes and predictors of complications. *J Surg Res*. 2019;241:119-127.
9. Neumayer L, Giobbie-Hurder A, Jonasson O, et al. Open mesh versus laparoscopic mesh repair of inguinal hernia. *N Engl J Med*. 2004;350(18):1819-1827.
10. Neumayer LA, Gawande AA, Wang J, et al. Proficiency of surgeons in inguinal hernia repair: effect of experience and age. *Ann Surg*. 2005;242(3):344.
11. Khan FA, Hashmi A, Edelman DA. Small bowel obstruction caused by self-anchoring suture used for peritoneal closure following robotic inguinal hernia repair. *J Surg Case Rep*. 2016;2016(6):rjw117.
12. Iraniha A, Peloquin J. Long-term quality of life and outcomes following robotic assisted TAPP inguinal hernia repair. *J Robot Surg*. 2018;12(2):261-269.
13. Bjurstrom MF, Nicol AL, Amid PK, Chen DC. Pain control following inguinal herniorrhaphy: current perspectives. *J Pain Res*. 2014;7:277.

Chapter 23 | Incisional Hernia: Open Approaches

Sean Michael O'Neill and Dana A. Telem

DEFINITION

- **An incisional hernia** is a fascial defect underlying the site of a previous surgical incision.
- These are distinct from **primary ventral hernias**, including **umbilical** and **epigastric** hernias, which may be congenital or acquired, but arise in the absence of a previous surgery. However, the repair options described here for incisional hernias can be applied to primary ventral hernias as well.
- The goals of incisional hernia repair are to durably close the fascial defect and recreate a functional abdominal wall.
- There is heterogeneity in the size, morphology, and infectious/recurrence risk of abdominal incisional hernias, and the repair approach should be tailored to best achieve the goals of the operation while minimizing complication risk.
- This chapter will describe in detail two approaches to ventral incisional hernias and one approach to flank hernias.
- The most commonly employed approach to ventral incisional hernia repair is the **retrorectus sublay**, also known as the **modified Rives-Stoppa-Wantz repair**.[1,2]
- A second option is the **anterior onlay**, also known as the **Voeller** or **modified Chevrel** repair.[3,4] This can be combined with an **anterior component separation** if necessary.[5,6]
- These approaches can typically be utilized for defects up to 8 to 10 cm in transverse dimension.
- Larger and more complex defects in most cases will require a **posterior components separation** approach with **transversus abdominis release (TAR)** in order to medialize the rectus abdominis and allow wide reinforcement of the visceral sac with mesh to achieve a functional outcome.[7,8] These techniques are described elsewhere in this book.
- Repair of flank hernias with an **open preperitoneal approach** is described.

DIFFERENTIAL DIAGNOSIS

- Diagnoses such as **diastasis recti** (thinning of the linea alba with a resultant bothersome midline bulge) and flank **pseudohernia** (denervation and resultant adynamic bulging of the flank musculature) without a discrete fascial defect do not constitute incisional hernia. Surgical interventions for these conditions are not described in this chapter.
- **Parastomal hernias** are also hernias at the site of previous operations (stoma creation), but these are a unique form of incisional hernia and are discussed elsewhere in this book.
- **Postoperative seroma** may occur immediately or weeks, months, or even years after the original operation and may mimic a hernia with a ballotable bulge and discomfort.
- Ultrasound or CT imaging is essential for distinguishing these entities from true fascial defects.

PATIENT HISTORY AND PHYSICAL FINDINGS

- By definition, the patient has a previous abdominal or flank surgical history. Frequently, patients present with a complex history of multiple operations. Obtain the indications for and details of each operation, including operative notes, paying particular attention to the closure technique and materials used (absorbable vs permanent suture, primary closure vs mesh placement). This is of paramount importance when the surgical history includes attempts at hernia repair.
- Asymptomatic incisional hernias are often diagnosed incidentally on routine physical examination or imaging obtained for other reasons.
- Symptoms are present in varying degrees, depending on the size and location of the hernia, the complexity of the previous operations, and the presence of mesh or contamination:
  - Bulging
  - Discomfort
  - Tenderness to palpation
  - Pain
  - Bowel sounds
  - Peristalsis
  - Erythema
  - Intestinal obstruction—acute or chronic
  - Skin attenuation
  - Skin ulceration
  - Enterocutaneous fistula
- Physical examination proceeds in a standard manner, with the following specific objectives:
  - Inspect for the presence and extent of previous incisions, paying particular attention to unusual or overlapping incisions.
  - Inspect the condition of the overlying skin, including erythema and attenuation, and being aware of the possibility of ulceration, necrosis, and fistula related to any existing wounds. Chronic wounds should receive focused regular wound care to achieve healing before an elective operation is considered.
  - Elicit a Valsalva maneuver while standing to demonstrate the degree of herniated contents.
  - Have the patient flex their rectus abdominis by lifting their head off the table while supine. This will demonstrate the presence of rectus diastasis.
  - Palpate around the edges of the bulge to establish whether a fascial defect is present, and, if so, the approximate dimensions.
  - Determine to what degree any herniated contents are reducible. This may be challenging in patients with a significant amount of subcutaneous adipose tissue.

IMAGING AND OTHER DIAGNOSTIC STUDIES

- For smaller hernias (<5 cm) that are well demarcated on physical examination without additional complicating factors such as incarceration, additional imaging is optional.
- For larger hernias, noncontrast computed tomography (CT) with and without Valsalva to assess the true dimensions and morphology of the defect is standard.
- For situations in which a clear diagnosis cannot be made with physical examination due to body habitus, additional imaging with either ultrasound or CT is essential. In particular, symptomatic areas without a palpable defect should raise suspicion for interstitial hernias, in which the anterior fascial layer is intact but a posterior defect has allowed herniation of contents between layers. This situation is akin to a primary Spigelian hernia. These are potentially high-risk hernias that are notoriously difficult to diagnose without dedicated imaging.
- MRI can be used when patients have contraindications to CT.
- In particular, CT imaging should be reviewed looking for the following specific elements:
  - Precise location of the fascial defect and layers affected.
  - Transverse (TV) and craniocaudal (CC) dimensions of the fascial defect. If multiple defects are visualized (particularly "Swiss cheese" defects that may only be seen on imaging), use a single measurement to include them all.
  - Presence of any previous implants or permanent materials such as metal tacks.
  - Integrity and condition of the lateral abdominal wall layers (external oblique, internal oblique, and transversus abdominis). For flank bulges, this is the key to ruling out pseudohernia, as these layers are often simply attenuated and adynamic without a discrete fascial defect.
  - Integrity and condition of the rectus abdominis. This can be attenuated or even absent at a previous stoma location.
  - Presence of loss of domain—does the volume of herniated contents exceed what could be reduced into the abdominal cavity? If this is the case, the techniques described in this chapter are unlikely to achieve a successful repair.

SURGICAL MANAGEMENT

Indications for Elective Surgical Intervention

- Symptomatic incisional ventral hernias can be considered for elective repair.
- Ventral incisional hernias less than 10 cm in transverse dimension are generally amenable to the techniques described in this chapter. For hernias larger than 10 to 15 cm, a posterior component separation with TAR is often necessary to achieve fascial closure.

Emergent Surgical Intervention—Indications and Technique

- In an emergent laparotomy mandated by bowel obstruction, strangulation, or perforation, a formal herniorrhaphy is most often ill-advised, particularly in the presence of a contaminated field.
- For these cases, primary closure of the fascia should be performed without permanent mesh reinforcement.
- This approach accepts a high (>50%) risk of recurrence, but by avoiding any intentional disruption of the myofasciocutaneous planes during the emergent operation, it allows for a formal mesh-based repair to be performed in the future in a clean field.
- If the fascia cannot be reapproximated primarily in the midline in these cases, a bridging absorbable mesh is employed.
- We favor use of an inexpensive mesh such as polyglycolic acid (Vicryl), which is typically 30 × 30 cm and can be folded on itself for additional reinforcement, as the goal is to prevent fascial dehiscence until the wound is fully closed.
- Biologic absorbable prosthetics are an acceptable alternative in these situations and yield similar rates of recurrence but at higher cost.

Timing of Operation

- A thorough discussion of the risks and benefits of the operation must be carried out with the patient, with appropriate setting of expectations.
- The most common indications for elective repair are pain and discomfort that limit a patient's ability to perform normal activities.
- Patients may also be experiencing chronic intermittent bowel obstruction.
- In most cases, the operation can be delayed over a period of months or longer to optimize the modifiable risk factors (obesity, diabetes, smoking, wound care) described in the next section.
- Postoperative restrictions include avoiding activities that significantly stress the abdominal core for 6 to 8 weeks. An easy guideline is to avoid lifting anything heavier than 10 lb and avoid any bending or twisting. Patients must be prepared to adhere to these guidelines during the recovery period, and the operation can typically be scheduled to allow this. Patients may already be on disability or on light duty at the time of initial surgical consultation.

Preoperative Preparation

- In our practice, we have developed a comprehensive preoperative optimization regimen.[9] Required elements include:
- Tobacco cessation. Patients must cease smoking and nicotine use at least 1 month prior to surgery.
- Weight loss. Patients with body mass index (BMI) >40 are at greatly increased risk of recurrence, and reduction to a BMI of 30 to 35 is strongly advised. For patients outside of this range, we offer weight loss counseling and referral to bariatric surgery when feasible. These are difficult conversations, but the presence of a symptomatic hernia can often serve as a strong motivator for patients to achieve weight loss through behavioral, medical, or surgical means.
- Diabetes. All patients must be screened for diabetes with HbA1c or fasting blood glucose. We ideally target a HbA1c of 6.5% or lower. For patients with HbA1c of 6.5% to 8.0%, referral to endocrinology or primary care for improved management is mandatory. For values higher than 8.0%, we delay surgery until diabetes is better controlled.
- Wound care. Dedicated wound care management should be instituted prior to an elective operation to minimize the possibility of creating a contaminated field.

Choice of Approach—Open Versus Minimally Invasive

- Techniques for minimally invasive ventral hernia repair, both laparoscopic and robotic assisted, continue to evolve and are covered elsewhere in this book. Outside of specialized centers, however, it is generally recommended to limit minimally invasive repairs to defects less than 6 cm in maximal transverse width.
- Multiple open techniques should be in the surgeon's armamentarium as a backup if a minimally invasive approach proves infeasible at the time of operation.

Choice of Open Technique

- Two techniques for ventral incisional hernia are described in this chapter and can be applied to defects up to 10 to 15 cm in transverse dimension. For most hernias greater than 10 to 15 cm, a TAR approach is necessary.
- The mainstay of open ventral incisional hernia repair, and our favored approach, is the **retrorectus sublay repair** (also known as the **modified Rives-Stoppa-Wantz**).
- This approach achieves closure of the posterior rectus sheath and allows prosthetic reinforcement in a well-vascularized plane separate from the bowel. In general, this approach results in fewer wound complications and recurrences compared with the anterior approach.
- The **anterior onlay repair** (also known as the **Voeller** or **modified Chevrel**), with or without an anterior component separation, may be a preferable option in certain cases and for specific reasons.
- Although there is a greater risk of wound complications due to raising extensive subcutaneous skin flaps, in patients with a frozen abdomen or with an increased risk of enterotomy (eg, Crohn disease, dilated small bowel from chronic obstruction), an anterior approach can often be accomplished with minimal lysis of adhesions and bowel manipulation.
- Furthermore, if a large hernia sac has already effectively created large subcutaneous skin flaps, the anterior sheath can be exposed with relatively minimal additional dissection.

Perioperative Management

- Pain Management. This begins with appropriate expectation setting with the patient preoperatively, as a multimodal, nonopioid analgesic regimen forms the basis of pain management for these patients.
- Acetaminophen, 1000 mg, is administered preoperatively.
- Transversus abdominis plane blocks with long-acting local anesthetics can be performed preoperatively under ultrasound guidance or intraoperatively under direct vision.
- Intraoperative administration of 30 mg of ketorolac intravenously is given routinely unless contraindicated.
- Postoperatively, 650 mg acetaminophen and 600 mg ibuprofen are administered every 6 hours on a scheduled basis for at least the first 72 hours.
- Additional nonopioid oral analgesic adjuncts include gabapentin 300 mg TID and methocarbamol 750 mg TID.
- Opioids, most commonly 5 mg oxycodone, are reserved for breakthrough pain only. Many patients are able to avoid the use of opioids entirely with a comprehensive multimodal approach.
- For larger defects requiring inpatient admission or postoperative nasogastric decompression and NPO status, the use of opiates with a patient-controlled analgesia device is often needed for breakthrough pain.
- Antibiotic prophylaxis. Two grams of cefazolin (3 g if patient weight is >120 kg) is given 30 to 60 minutes prior to incision, and redosed every 4 hours intraoperatively.
- Antiemetics. We seek to minimize postoperative nausea and vomiting (PONV) to protect the repair. Screen for risk factors (female, nonsmoker, history of motion sickness or PONV). Treatment adjuncts include ondansetron 4 mg given 15 minutes prior to case completion, a scopolamine patch placed at least 2 hours prior to induction, and 4 to 8 mg of dexamethasone given IV after induction. For large repairs requiring extensive bowel manipulation or lysis of adhesions, placement of a nasogastric tube that will remain postoperatively should be considered.
- Temperature Management. Normothermia (~36 °C) should be maintained with pre- and intraoperative forced-air warming blankets and management of ambient operating room temperature.
- Fluid Management. Tailor the administration of intraoperative fluids to prevent avoidable tissue edema. Foley catheters are avoided if possible, but if placed due to the length and complexity of the operation, removal in the operating room at the conclusion of the case should be considered.

Positioning

- Supine positioning is appropriate for most ventral incisional hernias.
- Flank hernias benefit from lateral decubitus position with the bed flexed.
- The abdomen is widely prepped and draped at least 10 to 15 cm beyond the extent of the previous incision.
- A sterile iodine-impregnated barrier drape such as Ioban (3M) is applied.

Mesh Principles

- Synthetic, macroporous, lightweight or mid-weight mesh is the preferred implant when the mesh can be placed in a position excluded from the bowel and in the absence of contamination.
- Macroporous mesh products have demonstrated greater salvageability in the event of mesh infection compared with microporous or nonporous synthetic meshes.
- If contact with viscera cannot be avoided, a barrier-coated synthetic mesh may be used in a fully intraperitoneal position. We would advise against placing a coated mesh in a protected space, as the coating will predispose to seroma and impair incorporation of the mesh. A biologic mesh can be considered in contaminated fields.

RETRORECTUS SUBLAY REPAIR: MODIFIED RIVES-STOPPA REPAIR

- This approach is the workhorse of open incisional ventral hernia repair. It can be applied to most defects less than 10 to 15 cm in transverse dimension without additional releases and isolates the mesh away from the bowel in the well-vascularized retromuscular field.

Incision

- The previous incision and scar with attenuated skin are excised as part of a midline laparotomy (**FIGURE 1A**).

Dissection of Hernia Sac and Lysis of Adhesions

- The dissection is carried down to the hernia sac, which is then freed circumferentially down to the edges of the fascial defect. Blunt, sharp and judicious cautery dissection are employed as needed.
- The hernia sac is opened sharply and extended to the length of the fascial defect.
- A lysis of adhesions is performed to allow greater mobilization of the lateral abdominal wall, and the hernia sac is excised (**FIGURE 1B**).

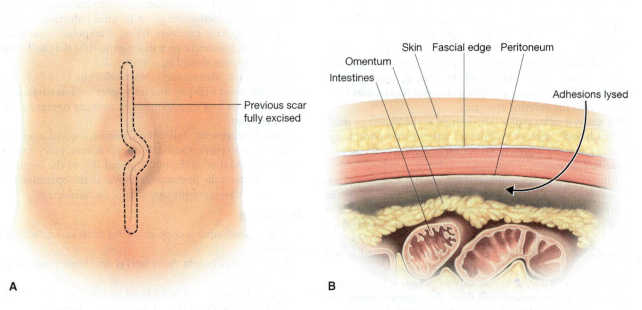

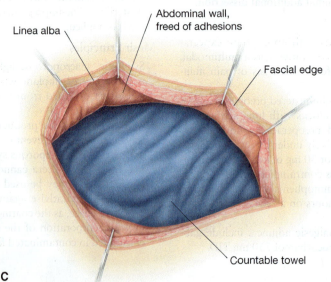

FIGURE 1 • Incision and lysis of adhesions. **A,** The existing scar is fully excised with a new laparotomy incision. Attaining healthy, well-vascularized skin and subcutaneous tissue is key for facilitating good wound healing postoperatively. **B,** A lysis of adhesions is performed to fully mobilize the anterior abdominal wall. Meticulous care is taken to avoid visceral injury. **C,** After the lysis of adhesions is completed, a large, radiopaque, countable towel is placed over the viscera for protection and visualization.

- After the intra-abdominal portion of the operation is completed, a radiopaque, countable towel is placed overlying the viscera for protection and visualization (**FIGURE 1C**).

Mobilization of Retrorectus Space

Entry

- The medial edge of the rectus sheath fascia is unambiguously identified and distinguished from the hernia sac.
- Kocher clamps are placed at the edge of the fascial defect and lifted upward to expose the posterior surface of the rectus sheath.
- The posterior rectus sheath is incised with cautery just lateral to the medial edge to enter the retrorectus space (**FIGURE 2A**).
- This must be confirmed by visualizing the fibers of the rectus abdominis muscle. If fatty tissue is encountered rather than muscle, it is most likely that the incision was made through the hernia sac or attenuated linea alba, which carries the dissection into the subcutaneous space. If this occurs, the incision should be made further lateral until the muscle is identified.

Extending the Incision

- This incision is then carried superiorly and inferiorly, at least 5 to 7 cm beyond the extent of the fascial defect. The line of incision in the posterior rectus sheath should be maintained as medially as possible, as the goal is to detach the posterior rectus sheath insertion from the linea alba.

Lateral Dissection

- Kocher clamps are placed on the posterior sheath and pulled medially, and the clamps on the anterior sheath are lifted upward to expose the interface of the posterior sheath and rectus abdominis. Dynamic retraction is essential for proper visualization of this space. An assistant should also

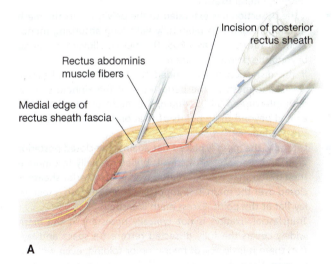

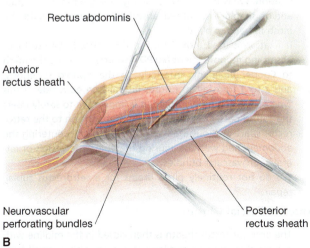

FIGURE 2 • Entering the retrorectus space. **A,** After clearly identifying the medial edge of the rectus sheath fascia, the posterior surface of the rectus sheath is incised just lateral to the medial edge to enter into the retrorectus space. The rectus muscle fibers should be clearly identified at this step before extending the incision. **B,** Lateral dissection of retrorectus space. The dissection of the rectus muscle from the posterior rectus sheath is carried laterally. Perforating neurovascular bundles will indicate the lateral extent of the retrorectus space. These bundles can be mobilized, but great care is taken to preserve them. Dynamic upward retraction on the fascial edge and medial retraction on the posterior rectus sheath are essential to adequately expose this space.

use Richardson retractors to lift up the muscle to maximize exposure.
- Using cautery, the muscle is freed from the posterior sheath. This proceeds laterally until the semilunar line is encountered. Typically this is first identified by the presence of perforating neurovascular bundles. These penetrate through the fascia overlying the transversus abdominis muscle (**FIGURE 2B**).
- Preservation of the neurovascular bundles is important for preservation of normal abdominal wall function.
- The posterior rectus sheath is mobilized off the muscle cephalad and caudad, beyond the extent of the fascial defect.
- The superior and inferior epigastric vessels and their branches will be encountered and care should be taken to avoid injury.

Cephalad Dissection

- As the dissection is carried cephalad and caudad, dynamic exposure is paramount. For work in both directions, Kocher clamps should be placed on the medial edges of the posterior rectus sheath and retracted toward the surgeon. The assistant should retract upward on the rectus muscle bellies with large Richardson retractors.
- Cephalad, the space is extended 5 to 7 cm above the furthest extent of the fascial defect. In many cases of upper abdominal hernias, this will require connecting the retrorectus spaces by dissecting deep to the xiphoid process.
- This is accomplished by carrying the incision in the posterior rectus sheath cephalad to its insertion on the xiphoid process. This insertion is then divided, which allows entry into the retroxiphoid "fatty triangle." After this is done on both sides, the retrorectus spaces can be connected across the midline. Care is taken to preserve the linea alba (the continuation of the anterior rectus sheath) anterior to this dissection (**FIGURE 3A-C**).

Caudal Dissection

- Caudad, a similar dissection 5 to 7 cm beyond the extent of the fascial defect is the goal.
- Care is taken as the dissection extends below the arcuate line, as the posterior rectus sheath disappears, and the thinner transversalis fascia and peritoneum must be preserved. Similarly to the cephalad dissection, the insertion of this posterior layer into the linea alba is divided and the anterior sheath is preserved.
- This can be carried down to Cooper ligaments and into the space of Retzius if needed, sweeping the bladder down off the pubis symphysis. As with an inguinal hernia dissection, care must be taken to preserve the iliac, gonadal, and epigastric vessels; the vas deferens in males; and the ilioinguinal, genitofemoral, and iliohypogastric nerves (**FIGURE 4**).

Posterior Fascial Closure

- Any off-midline defects in the posterior rectus sheath, such as those from a stoma site, are closed with 2-0 PDS. A transverse closure typically minimizes creation of additional tension on the midline. This is particularly true for larger defects (eg, former stoma sites).
- The countable towel is removed at this point.
- The posterior sheath is then pulled to the midline with Kocher clamps.
- If this can be accomplished without undue tension, this fascial layer is then closed with a long-absorbable suture in running fashion. Owing to the often thin tissue below the arcuate line, we recommend a 2-0 PDS with a small-bore needle (**FIGURE 5**).
- If this layer cannot be reapproximated in the midline without tension, a posterior component separation with transversus abdominis release can then be performed on one or both sides (Chapter 25).
- Partial closure of the posterior rectus sheath and use of a bridging mesh is not recommended. This creates the possibility of a recurrent interstitial hernia into the retrorectus space, deep to a closed anterior sheath. This is analogous to a Spigelian hernia and can be very difficult to diagnose until bowel incarceration develops.[10]

Mesh Placement and Fixation

- For large defects, our preference is to use a 30 × 30 cm piece of macroporous, mid-weight uncoated polypropylene mesh, which is then oriented in a diamond configuration and trimmed to fit the retrorectus space to obtain the widest overlap (**FIGURE 6**).
- For small defects with a more limited dissection, the use of self-gripping permanent mesh (with the adherent surface apposed to the muscle) is acceptable if adequate overlap of the defect can be obtained. This can obviate the need for transfascial fixation.
- Fixation is performed cephalad and caudad first before performing lateral fixation.
- If the dissection has extended to the pelvis, we fix the mesh to Cooper ligaments bilaterally with long-absorbing monofilament suture such as 0-PDS. The mesh is allowed to extend beyond the points of fixation.
- If the dissection has extended to the retroxiphoid space, we fix the mesh to the periosteum of the xiphoid process with interrupted 0-PDS. Again, the mesh can be allowed to extend beyond these points of fixation to achieve wider tissue overlap.
- Laterally, the mesh is placed flat against the closed posterior layer and the anterior sheath is pulled medially to simulate the tension that will be created when the anterior sheath is closed over the mesh. It is important that the mesh is seen to lay flat at this point. Excess mesh is excised.
- Transfascial fixation is not typically necessary. If the mesh widely covers the fully dissected retrorectus space and lays flat, there is little risk of migration or folding, even without fixation. We will typically use self-gripping mesh, fibrin glue, and/or simple interrupted absorbable sutures to hold the mesh flat and in place.
- If fixation is used (not shown in the figures), we use long-absorbing monofilament (#0 PDS) sutures to secure the mesh to Cooper ligaments inferiorly, to the xiphoid superiorly, and 2 to 3 transfascial sutures laterally on each side. If this type of fixation is performed, it is imperative to safely insert the suture passer directly from the stab incision to the retrorectus space without inadvertently and blindly entering the abdomen, and without injuring the epigastric vessels or lateral neurovascular bundles.
- We do not routinely place drains for a retrorectus sublay repair.

Anterior Fascial Closure

- The anterior rectus sheath is then closed in the midline with a long-absorbing monofilament suture with a small-bore

Chapter 23 INCISIONAL HERNIA: OPEN APPROACHES   189

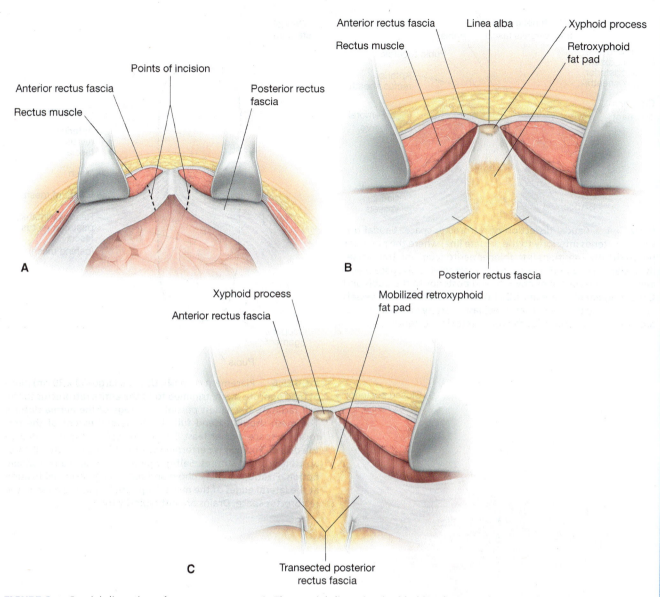

FIGURE 3 • Cranial dissection of retrorectus space. **A,** The cranial dissection is aided by placing a clamp on the midline fascia at the cranial-most extent of the hernia defect. Next, the medial insertion of the posterior rectus fascia into the anterior rectus fascia is transected, being careful not to disrupt the continuity of the anterior rectus fascia with linea alba cranially. **B,** When it is necessary to mobilize fully up to the xiphoid, the medial fascial insertions of the posterior rectus fasciae to the lateral xiphoid are transected and the triangular fat pad posterior to the xiphoid is mobilized posteriorly off the posterior surface of the xiphoid, allowing creation of a subdiaphragmatic space 3 to 5 cm behind the xiphoid/distal sternum. **C,** Fully mobilized retrosternal space, allowing the mesh to cross the midline behind the xiphoid.

needle (2-0 PDS on SH needle) in running fashion. With clear identification of the fascial edges, ideally this layer is closed with 5-mm suture bites every 5 mm, which achieves a 4:1 suture length to wound length ratio (**FIGURE 7**)
- Alternatively, #1 or #0 PDS with 1-cm bites is an acceptable approach.

If the anterior sheath cannot be completely closed medially, consideration should be given to a component separation procedure to achieve tension-free medialization. This is superior to only partially closing the anterior rectus sheath, which would essentially convert this into a bridged repair, requiring heavyweight mesh and extensive transfascial fixation.

Closure of the Wound

- The subcutaneous tissues are then closed in layers with a deep subcutaneous layer of 2-0 absorbable suture, a deep dermal layer of 3-0 absorbable suture, and a 4-0 running subcuticular layer. Sterile dressings are applied.

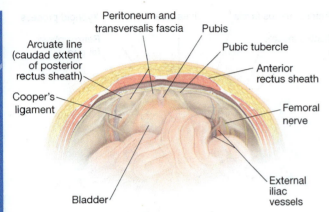

FIGURE 4 • Caudal dissection of retrorectus space. Caudal dissection extends inferiorly to the arcuate line, where the posterior rectus sheath transitions into thinner peritoneum and transversalis fascia. Staying in the retrorectus, pretransversalis space medially, dissection continues down to and posterior to the pubis and Cooper ligaments. Care must be taken to protect the iliac vessels and especially the deep inferior epigastric artery and vein, which are at the lateral aspect of the rectus muscles posteriorly.

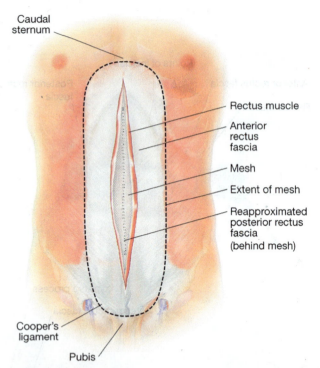

FIGURE 6 • Placement of mesh. Use of a large (30 × 30 cm) piece of macroporous mesh, trimmed to fit the entire retrorectus space, will facilitate the widest possible coverage of the hernia closure. The mesh should extend fully to the lateral extent of the retrorectus space and at least 5 to 6 cm cephalad and caudad to the defect. Fixation is performed with fibrin glue or with absorbable interrupted sutures. Self-gripping mesh is also a reasonable option. Fixation to the xiphoid and pubis, or transfascial fixation at the lateral edges of the mesh, is optional if placing mesh in the retrorectus space. Drains are not typically used.

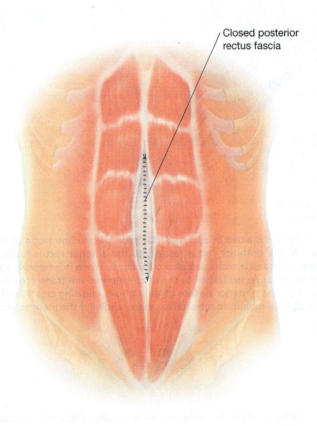

FIGURE 5 • Closure of the posterior rectus fascia. If the posterior sheaths can be brought to the midline without undue tension, this fascial layer is then closed with a long-absorbing suture on a small-bore needle in running fashion. We typically use 2-0 PDS on an SH needle. If this layer cannot be brought together without tension, a posterior component separation procedure may be necessary.

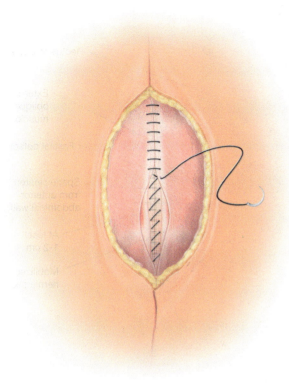

FIGURE 7 • Anterior fascial closure. The anterior rectus sheath is closed in the midline with a long-absorbing monofilament suture with a small-bore needle in running fashion. With clear identification of the fascial edges, ideally this layer is closed with 5 mm suture bites every 5 mm, which achieves a 4:1 suture length to wound length ratio.

ANTERIOR ONLAY AND ANTERIOR COMPONENT SEPARATION

- Circumstances that make this approach an advantageous option compared with a retrorectus repair include a hostile abdomen that confers an increased risk of bowel injury, as the operation can be accomplished in some cases without violating the peritoneum. In cases in which a wide hernia sac has effectively created a large subcutaneous pocket, the skin flaps are often able to be fashioned with minimal additional dissection.
- The major disadvantages of this approach arise due to the large skin flaps required for wide mesh placement, which can predispose to seroma formation, flap ischemia or vascular congestion, wound infection, and subsequent mesh infection. Therefore, meticulous hemostasis and the use of subcutaneous closed-suction drains are mandatory.
- Patients with multiple risk factors for wound infection (obesity, diabetes, history of wound infection) are not ideal candidates for this approach if the retrorectus technique is feasible.
- Patients with multiple overlapping scars such as a subcostal incision or stoma site in addition to a midline incision are at particularly increased risk of skin ischemia, and use of this technique must be employed thoughtfully.

Incision

- The previous incision and scar are excised as part of a midline laparotomy as with the sublay repair (see **FIGURE 1A**).

Dissection of Hernia Sac and Lysis of Adhesions

- The dissection is carried down to the hernia sac, which is then freed circumferentially down to the edges of the fascial defect. Blunt, sharp, and judicious cautery dissection are employed as needed.
- Care is taken to avoid thermal injury across the hernia sac.
- In certain cases with relatively smaller defects, the necessary dissection and fascial reapproximation can be accomplished extraperitoneally, without entry into the hernia sac (**FIGURE 8A**). After the edges of the fascial defect are identified, the dissection should be carried into the preperitoneal space approximately 1 to 2 cm from the defect in order to allow safe placement of fascial closing sutures (**FIGURE 8B**).
- In most cases, it is more advantageous to sharply enter the hernia sac and open it widely to safely reduce the bowel under direct vision and lyse intra-abdominal adhesions as necessary, in the same manner as with the retrorectus sublay operation. Lysis of adhesions to the anterior abdominal wall in particular allows greater fascial mobility for midline approximation (see **FIGURE 1B**).
- After the intra-abdominal portion of the operation is completed, a radiopaque, countable towel is placed overlying the viscera for protection (see **FIGURE 1C**).

Creation of Space for Prosthesis

- Raising subcutaneous skin flaps affords some additional mobility of the fascial defect, but additional releases may be needed and are described in the next section.

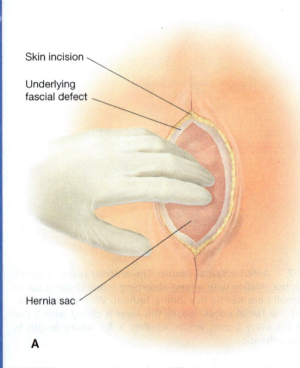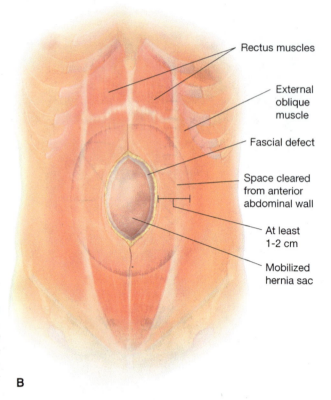

FIGURE 8 • Extraperitoneal mobilization. **A,** In certain cases with smaller defects, extraperitoneal mobilization of the hernia sac is possible. **B,** By preserving the hernia sac and identifying the fascial edges, the preperitoneal space can be entered and developed at least 1 to 2 cm past the fascial edges circumferentially. This allows a wider area for safe placement of fascial closing sutures.

- Kocher clamps are placed at the medial edge of the rectus fascia, and tension is pulled toward the surgeon.
- The assistant uses retractors to pull tension upward on the skin and subcutaneous tissues.
- The dissection plane is located just superficial to the anterior rectus sheath and is obtained with cautery dissection. There is a very thin (1-2 mm) layer of lymphatic channel-bearing tissue overlying the anterior rectus fascia that should be preserved, as this drainage plexus can help in reducing seroma formation risk (**FIGURE 9**).
- Take care to avoid entering the anterior rectus sheath during this dissection. Any defects are closed with 2-0 PDS.
- Significant cutaneous perforating vessels should be preserved to maintain tissue perfusion. It is acceptable to create a small split in the mesh to accommodate large perforating vessels.
- The extent of the dissection should be pursued as far as is necessary for wide mesh overlap, and ideally no further. In practice, this is at least to the semilunar line. In the event that an anterior component separation is required, the skin flaps must be taken at least 2 cm lateral to the semilunar line.
- This dissection is performed bilaterally.

Consideration of Component Separation Maneuvers

- At this point, the hernia defect is measured transversely and craniocaudally.
- Kocher clamps are used to reapproximate the fascia in the midline.
- If the fascial edges fully medialize at this point without undue tension, proceed with fascial closure and mesh placement.
- If the fascial edges do not fully medialize, one or two additional maneuvers will be needed to achieve reapproximation. We employ these techniques selectively to achieve the closure needed.
- These can each be performed unilaterally or bilaterally to achieve the needed distance.
- As described by Ramirez and Voeller, the minimal number of releases necessary should be performed to achieve a tension-free fascial reapproximation. Check the tension and closure after each step.
- A posterior rectus sheath release achieves 1 to 2 cm of additional distance per side.
- An external oblique release achieves a greater amount of distance, although this varies by location, with 3 to 5 cm in the epigastrium, 7 to 10 cm at the level of the umbilicus, and 1 to 3 cm in the suprapubic area.

Posterior Rectus Sheath Release

- Kocher clamps are used to elevate the fascial edges and expose the posterior rectus sheath.
- Cautery is used to enter the posterior rectus sheath 1 cm lateral to the medial border of the rectus, similar to the entry for the retrorectus dissection (**FIGURE 10**).
- The posterior sheath is then dissected free from the rectus muscle, which consequently allows the anterior sheath additional mobility.
- This is carried the length of the entire fascial defect.

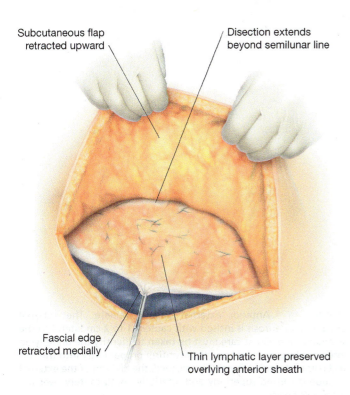

FIGURE 9 • Dissection of anterior subcutaneous space. Kocher clamps are placed at the medial edge of the rectus fascia, and tension is pulled toward the surgeon. The assistant uses retractors to pull tension upward on the skin and subcutaneous tissues. The dissection plane is located just superficial to the anterior rectus sheath and is obtained with cautery dissection. There is a very thin (1-2 mm) layer of lymphatic channel-bearing tissue overlying the anterior rectus fascia that should be preserved, as this drainage plexus can help in reducing seroma formation risk. Significant cutaneous perforating vessels should be preserved to maintain tissue perfusion. The extent of the dissection should be pursued as far as is necessary for wide mesh overlap, and ideally no further. In practice, this is at least to the semilunar line. In the event that an anterior component separation is required, the skin flaps must be taken at least 2 cm lateral to the semilunar line.

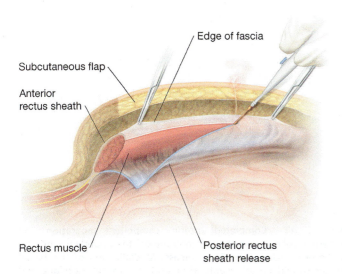

FIGURE 10 • Posterior rectus sheath release. Kocher clamps are used to elevate the fascial edges and expose the posterior rectus sheath. Cautery is used to enter the posterior rectus sheath 1 cm lateral to the medial border of the rectus, similar to the entry for the retrorectus dissection. The posterior sheath is then dissected free from the rectus muscle, which consequently allows the anterior sheath additional mobility. This is carried the length of the entire fascial defect and provides 1 to 2 cm of additional medialization.

External Oblique Release

- The semilunar line is identified by grasping the muscle bulk of the rectus abdominis and visualizing the change in fascial striations, which are craniocaudal over the anterior rectus sheath and diagonal over the external oblique ("hands in pockets").
- The external oblique aponeurosis is incised with cautery 1 to 2 cm lateral to the semilunar line. Great care must be taken to identify the underlying internal oblique muscle and thus confirm proper entry into the correct compartment.
- After this is achieved, the division of the external oblique is carried superiorly and inferiorly, using cautery over the surgeon's finger (FIGURE 11).
- Pulling medially on the fascial edges, the external oblique fascia is then further mobilized off the internal oblique to achieve maximal release (FIGURE 12).

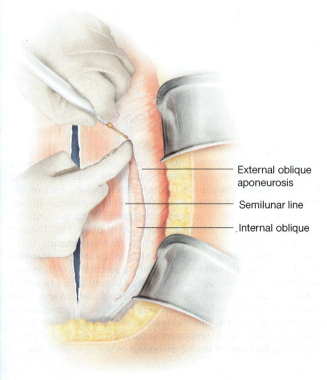

FIGURE 11 • Anterior external oblique release. The external oblique aponeurosis is incised with cautery 1 to 2 cm lateral to the semilunar line. Great care must be taken to identify the underlying internal oblique muscle and thus confirm proper entry into the correct compartment. After this is achieved, the division of the external oblique is carried superiorly and inferiorly, using cautery over the surgeon's finger.

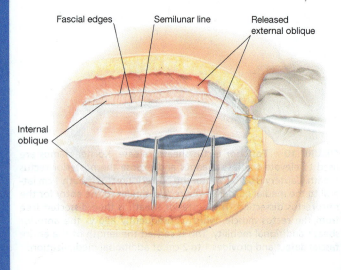

FIGURE 12 • Completed anterior component separation. The external oblique is mobilized laterally off the underlying internal oblique to achieve maximal release. Medialization of the fascial edges should be achievable after both the external oblique and posterior rectus sheath releases are completed.

Reapproximation of Fascial Edges

- The fascial edges are reapproximated in the midline without undue tension. If this is still not possible, a portion of the hernia sac should be preserved to act as a tissue barrier for a bridging mesh.
- The radiopaque towel is removed.
- The hernia sac is fully excised in almost all cases.
- Fascial closure is performed with long-absorbing monofilament suture with a small-diameter needle in running fashion. Suture sizes #1, 0, and 2-0 are reasonable options. Some surgeons prefer to use a barbed suture to minimize knot prominence underneath the mesh (FIGURE 13).

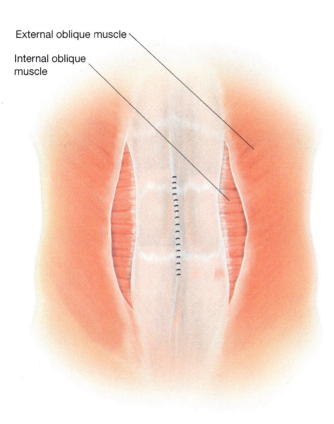

FIGURE 13 • Fascial closure. Fascial closure is performed with long-absorbing monofilament suture with a small-diameter needle in running fashion. Suture sizes #1, 0, and 2-0 are reasonable options. Some surgeons prefer to use a barbed suture to minimize knot prominence underneath the mesh.

Placement of Prosthetic Mesh

- The skin flaps should allow at least 5 to 8 cm of mesh overlap beyond the fascial edges.
- If an external oblique release was performed, the mesh should extend 1 to 2 cm beyond the lateral border of the external oblique to "cover" the release.
- A piece of mid-weight, macroporous, uncoated synthetic mesh is selected and trimmed to fit within the entire dissected space. We recommend beginning with a 30 × 30 cm piece and orienting it in a diamond orientation.
- As discussed earlier, making small slits in the mesh to accommodate large cutaneous perforating vessels is acceptable.

Fixation of Mesh

- Unlike the other techniques described in this chapter with transfascial fixation of prosthetics, an anterior onlay mesh can only be fixed to the anterior surface of the abdominal fascia. Therefore, both point fixation and fibrin glue are used.
- We prefer interrupted absorbable suture fixation at cardinal points around the periphery of the mesh as well as surrounding the fascial closure. Most importantly, the lateral fixation points must include the lateral external oblique aponeurosis.
- Both staples and tacks have been described for point fixation as well.
- Regardless of the technique, care must be taken to avoid placing fixation too deeply at thinner areas of the abdominal wall and risk inadvertent bowel injury.
- After this, a generous amount of fibrin glue is applied and massaged into the mesh to achieve flush contact with the anterior fascia. We use at least 20 to 30 mL, which typically requires multiple large applicators of the most common commercial products (FIGURE 14A).

Wound Closure

- Two closed-suction drains are laid along the lateral gutters of the dissection space (FIGURE 14B).
- We leave these in place until output is <30 mL/d for 2 consecutive days. Timing of removal is controversial, as it is believed that prolonged use allows a conduit for bacterial ingress. There is no evidence to support the use of postoperative prophylactic antibiotics in this situation.
- Closure of subcutaneous tissues and skin is performed in layers to minimize dead space, using absorbable suture.
- Excess skin, particularly that which is attenuated from scarring, is excised prior to final skin closure.
- Sterile dressings are applied.

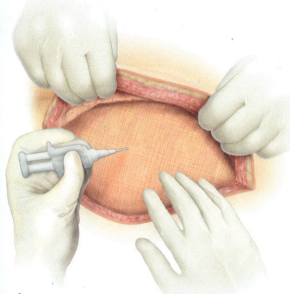

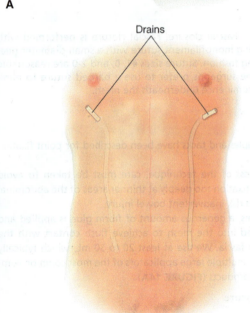

FIGURE 14 • Placement and fixation of mesh. **A,** A large piece of mid-weight, macroporous, uncoated synthetic mesh is selected and trimmed to fit within the entire dissected space. Fixation with interrupted absorbable suture at the edges of the mesh is optional. A generous amount of fibrin glue is applied and massaged into the mesh to achieve flush contact with the anterior fascia. We typically use at least 20 to 30 mL. **B,** Two closed-suction drains are laid along the lateral gutters of the dissection space.

FLANK HERNIAS

General Considerations

- Flank hernias arise most commonly from anterior/retroperitoneal spinal access and kidney/ureter operations, including transplants. Pseudohernias with painful bulging and lack of tone due to denervation can be mistaken for incisional hernias, making cross-sectional imaging essential for these patients.
- The technique described here is a preperitoneal dissection with sublay position of the mesh. Intramural sublay with placement of the mesh above the transversus abdominis and deep to the internal oblique has also been described. We believe that the preperitoneal position affords the widest possible mesh overlap.

Step 1: Patient Positioning

- For open flank hernias, full (**FIGURE 15**) or partial lateral decubitus position (secured with a moldable bean bag) and slight flexing of the bed to achieve greater exposure of the space between the lateral costal margin and anterior superior iliac spine is strongly recommended.
- The midline, umbilicus, costal margin, anterior superior iliac spine, pubic tubercle, inguinal ligament, and xiphoid process should be clearly marked.

Chapter 23 INCISIONAL HERNIA: OPEN APPROACHES   197

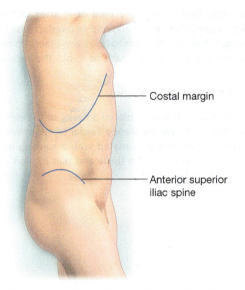

FIGURE 15 • Lateral Decubitus positioning for Flank Hernia Repair. For open flank hernias, full lateral decubitus position (secured with a moldable bean bag) and slight flexing of the bed to achieve greater exposure of the space between the lateral costal margin and anterior superior iliac spine is strongly recommended.

Step 2: Development of Preperitoneal Space

- The prior skin incision is excised and dissection carried through the subcutaneous tissues to identify the hernia sac. The sac is then followed down to the edges of the hernia defect.
- The preperitoneal plane is then developed with gentle blunt dissection. It is often easiest to identify the preperitoneal and retroperitoneal fat laterally and inferiorly (FIGURE 16).
- It is possible to remain extraperitoneal during this dissection. Any defects in the peritoneum are closed with absorbable suture prior to mesh placement.
- As with all hernia repairs, the goal of dissection is to create a space for wide prosthetic reinforcement of the fascial closure. We recommend obtaining at least 8 to 10 cm of distance from the defect.
- Division of the muscle layers along the extent of the previous incision may be necessary to obtain sufficient exposure for a safe preperitoneal dissection.
- Inferiorly and laterally, the preperitoneal dissection proceeds similarly to a preperitoneal inguinal hernia repair. The nerves (lateral femoral cutaneous, genitofemoral, ilioinguinal, and

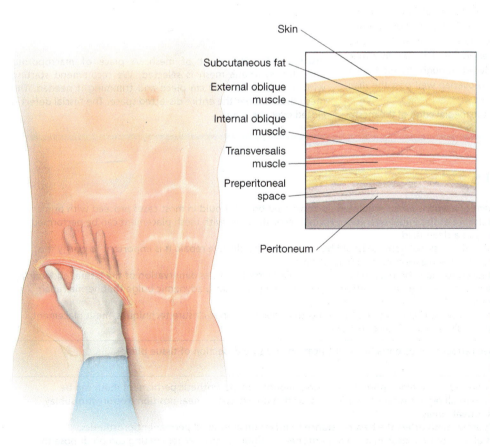

FIGURE 16 • Dissection of preperitoneal space. The prior skin incision is excised and dissection carried through the subcutaneous tissues to identify the hernia sac. The sac is then followed down to the edges of the hernia defect. The preperitoneal plane is then developed with gentle blunt dissection. It is often easiest to identify the preperitoneal and retroperitoneal fat laterally and inferiorly. It is possible to remain extraperitoneal during this dissection. Any defects in the peritoneum are closed with absorbable suture prior to mesh placement.

iliohypogastric); spermatic cord in males; and epigastric, gonadal, and iliac vessels are all identified and preserved as the space is developed down to Cooper ligament and the space of Retzius.
- Laterally, the dissection is extended to the border of the psoas, taking great care to avoid injury to the ureter and gonadal and iliac vessels.
- Medially, the preperitoneal space is extended to the lateral border of the rectus abdominis. Often, this will not allow sufficient mesh overlap of the defect. In that case, the posterior rectus sheath can be opened 1 to 2 cm medial to the semilunar line and the space extended to the linea alba. Great care must be taken to enter into the retrorectus space rather than directly through the semilunar line and into the subcutaneous space.
- The superior dissection is extended beyond the costal margin, carefully taking the peritoneum down off the diaphragm.

Step 3: Fixation of Prosthesis

- Once adequate margins have been obtained, and the peritoneum is closed to exclude the viscera, a piece of macroporous uncoated synthetic mesh is selected. We recommend starting with at least a 30 × 30 cm piece and trimming if needed (**FIGURE 17**).
- The mesh should cover the entire dissected space, inclusive of psoas, Cooper ligament, midline, and costal margin.
- Posterior transfascial fixation is performed with permanent suture, just lateral to the psoas, taking great care to avoid the ureter and iliac vessels.
- Inferiorly, the first option is to use the rim of fascia and soft tissue above the iliac wing for transfascial fixation sutures. If this tissue is too attenuated or absent, bone anchors with permanent suture can be placed in the iliac rim. In either case, the fixation sutures are placed through the mesh at a location that allows the mesh to overlap well past the iliac rim and down to Cooper ligament.
- Medial fixation is performed at the medial edge of the mesh.

- Superior fixation is performed only after unflexing the bed. Again, the mesh is allowed to overlap past the costal margin, but the fixation sutures are placed through the subcostal fascia, taking care to avoid the neurovascular bundle.

Step 4: Closure of the Wound

- A closed suction drain is placed anterior to the mesh.
- The muscle and/or weakened fascial layers anterior to the mesh are then reapproximated with a running absorbable suture; the subcutaneous tissue and skin incision are closed with absorbable suture.

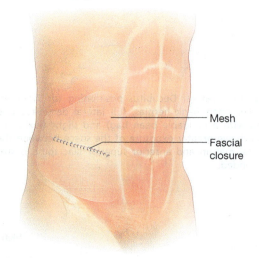

FIGURE 17 • Placement of mesh. A piece of macroporous uncoated synthetic mesh is selected. We recommend starting with at least a 30 × 30 cm piece and trimming if needed. The mesh should cover the entire dissected space. The fascial defect is closed over the mesh.

PEARLS AND PITFALLS

Indications	■ Emergent operations for strangulated or obstructed bowel should in most cases proceed with primary suture closure at the initial operation. Formal reconstruction with mesh placement can be performed electively in a clean field. ■ Symptomatic incisional hernias should be considered for elective repair. It is important to clarify the patient's goals and expectations ahead of time. ■ Expectations for flank hernia repairs are particularly important, as denervation of the lateral abdominal wall caused by the original operation may result in a permanent, adynamic bulge that hernia repair with mesh reinforcement will not fix. ■ Obtain and review previous operative notes to understand prior closure techniques, mesh placement, and previously violated dissection planes.
Intraoperative exposure	■ Effective retraction is essential for identification and safe dissection of tissue planes.
Choice of prosthetic	■ Mid- or light-weight, macroporous, uncoated, monofilament synthetic permanent mesh can be employed in all repairs where the mesh is placed in an extraperitoneal position (retrorectus sublay, preperitoneal, onlay). ■ Macroporous mesh offers the best resistance to infection among all permanent prosthetics. ■ Do not place a coated mesh in an extraperitoneal position, as the barrier coating can predispose to seroma formation and infection.

Exploration of hernia defect	■ Always look for a Swiss cheese defect along the prior fascial incision distant from the presumed "isolated" hernia defect. ■ When performing a Rives-Stoppa, retrorectus sublay repair in a patient who has had a prior enterostomal takedown (e.g., after takedown of a Hartmann procedure), be aware that a knuckle of bowel may protrude through a defect in the posterior rectus fascia. ■ If the patient has had a recent history of recurrent partial small bowel obstruction, consider an intraperitoneal adhesiolysis in addition to the hernia repair.
Early postoperative seroma	■ If asymptomatic, treat conservatively. ■ If there is evidence of infection, initiate antibiotics, percutaneous drainage, and reimaging. Consider local exploration and mesh excision if these measures are unsuccessful.

POSTOPERATIVE CARE

- For most patients undergoing repair of small (<5-6 cm) defects requiring limited dissection and adhesiolysis, these operations can be performed in the outpatient setting. Foley catheters are removed in the operating room.
- For larger defects or any operations requiring significant intra-abdominal lysis or component separation, inpatient admission is expected. Foley catheters should be removed no later than postoperative day 1.
- As discussed earlier, multimodal nonopioid analgesia is the basis of postoperative pain management. This has been shown to greatly reduce the use of opioids overall. Small doses of opioids should be made available on an as-needed basis for breakthrough pain.
- Epidural analgesic catheters are not used routinely and can prolong discharge from the hospital.
- Patients should wear an abdominal binder 24 hours a day to offload abdominal wall tension during the acute recovery period. We typically recommend 4 to 6 weeks, although there is little consensus or evidence surrounding this practice.
- Pharmacologic and mechanical deep venous thrombosis prophylaxis is employed, and early ambulation starting postoperative day 0 is encouraged.
- Most patients will not need a nasogastric tube, but in extended complex repairs, especially with an accompanying adhesiolysis, gastric decompression may be advisable.
- Drains are removed as expediently as possible. We recommend when output decreases to less than 30 mL/d for 2 consecutive days. There is no evidence for prophylactic antibiotic use due to drain placement.

OUTCOMES

- Recurrence. Retrorectus repairs generally have a lower rate of recurrence compared with anterior repairs in most published series, although meaningful comparisons are difficult to obtain due to heterogeneity in the size, morphology, and recurrence risk factors of different incisional hernias. Hernia recurrence in the best circumstances generally ranges from 5% to 10% and can be significantly higher for cases with multiple risk factors.
- The most recent systematic review and meta-analysis of 93 studies including 12,440 patients undergoing open retrorectus, open onlay, or laparoscopic intraperitoneal onlay mesh (IPOM) suggested a pooled recurrence rate of 3.2% at 12 months and 4.1% at 24 months. The authors noted a significant risk of bias in the included studies, so it is likely that recurrence rates in real-world practice are higher.[11] When comparing retrorectus vs onlay repair, retrorectus repair was associated with a lower likelihood of recurrence, surgical site infection, and seroma.
- Previously reported recurrence rates for open ventral hernia repair have ranged from 10% to 23% for low-risk cases less than 10 cm, to up to 46% or higher for hernias with multiple risk factors and/or width 10 to 20 cm or greater.[12-14]
- Wound infection (Late). Cross-sectional imaging can reveal potentially drainable fluid collections. With macroporous, monofilament mesh, it is rare to have to remove an entire prosthetic. These can often be managed with percutaneous drainage, limited exploration and mesh excision, and suppressive antibiotics.

COMPLICATIONS

- Unrecognized enterotomy or delayed perforation due to thermal bowel injury. As with all abdominal operations, a high degree of vigilance for this devastating complication must be maintained.
- Seroma/Hematoma. These are rare in the retrorectus space and much more common in the subcutaneous space created for an anterior onlay repair. In the absence of infection, these are treated conservatively.
- Wound infection (Early). Close monitoring of skin flaps and wound erythema is mandatory, particularly in onlay repairs. Expedient administration of antibiotics is recommended in these cases. If frank purulence is noted, the wound must be reopened and contamination controlled. With macroporous mesh, management with a negative-pressure wound therapy device in addition to suppressive antibiotics can facilitate mesh salvage and delayed wound closure.

REFERENCES

1. Stoppa R, Petit J, Abourachid H, et al. Procédé original de plastie des hernies de l'aine: l'interposition sans fixation d'une prothèse en tulle de dacron par voie médiane sous-péritonéale [Original procedure of groin hernia repair—interposition without fixation of Dacron tulle prosthesis by subperitoneal median approach]. Article in French. *Chirurgie*. 1973;99(2):119-123.
2. Rives J, Lardennois B, Pire JC, Hibon J. Les grandes éventrations. Importance du "volet abdominal" et des troubles respiratoires qui lui sont secondaires [Large incisional hernias. The importance of flail abdomen and of subsequent respiratory disorders]. Article in French. *Chirurgie*. 1973;99(8):547-563.
3. Shahan CP, Stoikes NF, Webb DL, Voeller GR. Sutureless onlay hernia repair: a review of 97 patients. *Surg Endosc*. 2016;30(8):3256-3261. doi:10.1007/s00464-015-4647-2

4. Alemanno G, Bruscino A, Martellucci J, et al. Chevrel technique for ventral incisional hernia. Is it still an effective procedure? *Minerva Chir*. 2020;75(5):286-291. doi:10.23736/S0026-4733.20.08463-1. PMID: 33210523
5. Ramirez OM, Ruas E, Dellon AL. "Components separation" method for closure of abdominal-wall defects: an anatomic and clinical study. *Plast Reconstr Surg*. 1990;86(3):519-526. doi:10.1097/00006534-199009000-00023
6. Read RC. Milestones in the history of hernia surgery: prosthetic repair. *Hernia*. 2004;8(1):8-14. doi:10.1007/s10029-003-0169-2
7. Novitsky YW, Elliott HL, Orenstein SB, Rosen MJ. Transversus abdominis muscle release: a novel approach to posterior component separation during complex abdominal wall reconstruction. *Am J Surg*. 2012;204(5):709-716.
8. Novitsky YW, Fayezizadeh M, Majumder A, Neupane R, Elliott HL, Orenstein SB. Outcomes of posterior component separation with transversus abdominis muscle release and synthetic mesh sublay reinforcement. *Ann Surg*. 2016;264(2):226-232.
9. Howard R, Delaney L, Kilbourne AM, et al. Development and implementation of preoperative optimization for high-risk patients with abdominal wall hernia. *JAMA Netw Open*. 2021;4(5):e216836.
10. Carbonell AM. Interparietal hernias after open retromuscular hernia repair. *Hernia*. 2008;12(6):663-666. doi:10.1007/s10029-008-0393-x
11. den Hartog FPJ, Sneiders D, Darwish EF, et al. Favourable outcomes after retro-rectus (Rives-Stoppa) mesh repair as treatment for non-complex ventral abdominal wall hernia, a systematic review and meta-analysis. *Ann Surg*. Published online February 18, 2022. doi:10.1097/SLA.0000000000005422
12. Ventral Hernia Working Group; Breuing K, Butler CE, et al. Incisional ventral hernias: review of the literature and recommendations regarding the grading and technique of repair. *Surgery*. 2010;148(3):544-558. doi:10.1016/j.surg.2010.01.008
13. Kanters AE, Krpata DM, Blatnik JA, Novitsky YM, Rosen MJ. Modified hernia grading scale to stratify surgical site occurrence after open ventral hernia repairs. *J Am Coll Surg*. 2012;215(6):787-793. doi:10.1016/j.jamcollsurg.2012.08.012
14. Petro CC, O'Rourke CP, Posielski NM, et al. Designing a ventral hernia staging system. *Hernia*. 2016;20(1):111-117. doi:10.1007/s10029-015-1418-x

Chapter 24: Incisional Hernia: Laparoscopic Approaches

Sullivan A. Ayuso, Sharbel A. Elhage, Paul D. Colavita, and B. Todd Heniford

DEFINITION

- An incisional hernia is defined as a fascial defect that arises at the site of a prior surgical incision. On long-term follow-up, nearly one quarter of patients who undergo laparotomy will develop an incisional hernia with certain patients having an even higher risk of hernia formation.[1] Factors that predispose patients to hernia development include obesity, surgical site infection, and a large-bite closure technique.[2,3]
- Each year in the United States more than 350,000 incisional hernia repairs are performed at an estimated cost of 3.2 billion dollars.[4] Although the majority of incisional hernia repairs are performed via an open technique, laparoscopic hernia repair accounts for 20% to 30% of total repairs.[5,6]
- Incisional hernias may be reliably repaired via an open, laparoscopic, or robotic technique, and the technique chosen for repair depends on hernia complexity, surgeon comfort, and patient preference. Laparoscopic incisional hernia repair was first described by Stoppa in 1989 and conventionally relies on intraperitoneal reinforcement with a mesh prosthesis.[7] A coated or composite synthetic mesh is typically used in order to provide a barrier between the mesh and the adjacent bowel, which can prevent dreaded complications such as mesh ingrowth and fistula formation.[8]
- Ensuring that a hernia repair is done correctly can minimize detrimental downstream effects for the patient and healthcare system. With each subsequent hernia repair, the risk of hernia recurrence increases and predisposes patients to further surgical intervention and potential for perioperative complications.[9]

DIFFERENTIAL DIAGNOSIS FOR INCISIONAL HERNIA

- Diastasis recti
- Rectus sheath hematoma
- Denervation of abdominal wall musculature
- Bulging of previously placed bridging mesh
- Hypertrophic scarring
- Seroma
- Abdominal wall abscess
- Lipoma
- Desmoid tumor
- Soft tissue sarcoma

PATIENT HISTORY AND PHYSICAL FINDINGS

- The workup of all patients with incisional hernias begins with a thorough but targeted history and physical examination.
- The patient history should focus on the location of the hernia, related symptoms (eg, pain, nausea), impact on quality of life, progression of the defect over time, and past medical and surgical histories. This should especially focus on previous abdominal surgery and previous hernia repairs. Reviewing previous hernia repair operative notes is often very helpful.
- Patients who have asymptomatic hernias should have their operative risk carefully evaluated. One of the main goals of any hernia operation is to improve patient quality of life. If the risks from anesthesia and postoperative complications outweigh the benefit of having the hernia repaired, then nonoperative management should be strongly considered.
- If patients have obstructive symptoms, such as nausea or vomiting, this could indicate that there is an incarcerated hernia, which could be chronic or acute. A marked change in pain and acute incarceration could be a sign of strangulation of the hernia contents. Such patients require appropriate imaging or urgent operative exploration to assess for bowel ischemia.
- A medical history must be elicited from patients and include information about pertinent comorbidities, including smoking, diabetes, immunosuppression, chronic obstructive pulmonary disease, coronary artery disease, vascular disease, or kidney disease, and assess medications the patient is currently taking, which should especially address those that would impact coagulation. It is also important to document patient allergies, particularly to antibiotics (eg, penicillin), and note any history of methicillin-resistant *Staphylococcus aureus* (MRSA) infection.[10]
- The preoperative use of opiates should be noted as should an existing relationship with a pain provider. Preoperative pain is the single most important predictor of postoperative pain, and patients must be appropriately counseled that their pain may not significantly improve following surgery.[11]
- If the history reveals symptoms of malignancy or perhaps recurrent disease, then an appropriate workup (ie, sigmoidoscopy or colonoscopy, tumor marker evaluation, CT scan) is warranted. Symptoms include bleeding, change in stool caliber, anemia, or unexplained weight loss.[12] For patients who are over the age of 45 to 50 years and due for colon cancer screen, colonoscopic evaluation might be considered prior to scheduled surgery.
- Knowing a patient's surgical history is one of the most important parts of the preoperative workup. Previous operative reports may not be readily available or accessible via the electronic medical record, so it is important to ask the patient directly about any operations they have had as well as their ability to obtain operative records. Patients who have had multiple prior abdominal operations or intra-abdominal sepsis are more likely to have intra-abdominal adhesions, which can increase the difficulty of dissection.
- Special attention should be paid to patients who have had a prior incisional hernia repair. Important details to consider for patients with recurrent hernias are prior mesh use (ie, biologic, synthetic, or absorbable synthetic, and if a synthetic mesh included a protective barrier), mesh location

(eg, intraperitoneal, retrorectus, preperitoneal, fascial onlay), method of fixation (eg, sutures or absorbable tacks), and operative complications (eg, surgical site infection, delayed wound healing, or reoperation).
- The potential degree of contamination needs to be assessed. For example, for patients who will have contaminated or dirty wounds at time of operation (eg, CDC wound class 2, 3, or 4—mesh infection, fistula, stoma, active wound infection), an open approach with a nonpermanent synthetic mesh may be favored with delayed primary closure.[13,14]
- Physical examination begins with inspection of the abdomen, which can help to identify prior surgical scars. Hernia specifics that should be noted and can influence the difficulty of a laparoscopic approach include the location (midline, lateral, subcostal, peri-iliac, suprapubic, etc), the size of the fascial defect, the amount of herniated abdominal contents (especially in regards to loss of abdominal domain), the quality and thickness of the overlying skin, compliance of the abdominal wall, and signs of infection (cellulitis, any draining sinuses, open wounds, etc).
- In addition, on physical examination, the presence of peritoneal signs, such as guarding, rigidity, rebound tenderness, or pain out of proportion on examination, indicate an acute intra-abdominal process and the need for emergent laparoscopy or laparotomy. Careful evaluation of patient vital signs may provide further evidence of the relative stability of the patient.
- A physical examination is not complete without concurrent evaluation for other hernias (eg, inguinal, femoral, parastomal, etc). If there are additional hernias noted on examination or imaging, consideration should be given to concurrent repair, which could spare the need for a subsequent operation.

IMAGING AND OTHER DIAGNOSTIC STUDIES

- Imaging serves as a diagnostic supplement to physical examination. Computed tomography (CT) of the abdomen and pelvis is the most common and useful imaging study for hernia evaluation. A CT scan can help to elucidate hernia defect size, including total area and width, hernia volume and organs contained, and proximity to other important structures, such as the iliac crest or costal margin.
- Knowing the size of the defect can help the surgeon anticipate what size mesh will be needed to obtain adequate mesh overlap (typically at least 5 cm in all directions) and if a minimally invasive approach will be feasible.[15] It can also aid in determining if the defect itself can be sutured closed. If the patient has a hernia that abuts a boney structure (eg, iliac crest or pubic symphysis), then consideration should be given to supplemental fixation devices, such as bone anchors, to ensure proper mesh fixation and overlap.[16]
- Not all hernia defects are easily palpable on physical examination. For patients who are obese, have had prior surgery significant scarring, it can be difficult to palpate fascial defects. A CT scan can help identify defects that are not picked up on physical examination or multiple "Swiss cheese" type defects.
- A CT scan can also be useful for planning the method and location of entry into the abdomen. The surgeon can assess whether or not entry at a specific point on the abdominal wall (eg, Veress technique at Palmer point) would be at higher risk for the patient or if a cut down procedure at a specific point might be most appropriate.

SURGICAL MANAGEMENT

Prehabilitation

- While the risk for postoperative wound complications is generally lower for patients undergoing laparoscopic operations in comparison with open surgery, patients should still be appropriately optimized if time permits in order to ensure the best possible outcomes and minimize complications.[17]
- There are three main tenets of preoperative prehabilitation: smoking cessation, glycemic control, and weight loss.
- Smoking cessation should take place at minimum 4 weeks prior to surgery to reduce the risk of wound and pulmonary complications.[18] Patients who are diabetic are also at increased risk for wound complications and have a hemoglobin A1c target of <7.2 g/dL.[19] In general, laparoscopic ventral hernia repair is a favored approach for obese patients due predominantly to decreased wound morbidity.[20] However, preoperative weight loss is encouraged through a combination of exercise and a ketogenic diet.
- Geriatricians may see patients over the age of 65 years to evaluate frailty and assess for risk of polypharmacy. Often perioperative medication adjustments can be made in conjunction with the geriatrics team preoperatively in clinic.
- Patients who are taking clopidogrel or acetylsalicylic acid have these medications held 5 to 7 days before surgery, respectively, in order to minimize the risk of bleeding.

Patient Positioning and Preoperative Planning

- For standard abdominal wall hernias, patients are taken to the operating room where they are placed in the supine position with their arms tucked at their sides (**FIGURE 1**). The patients have their arms placed in a supinated position to help avoid injury to the ulnar nerve.[21] Padding is used at pressure points, including the elbows, wrists, and heels, to prevent neurologic injury.

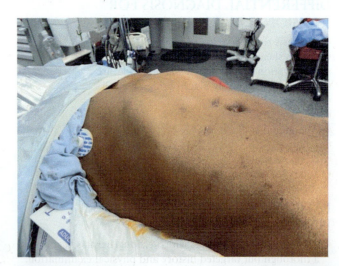

FIGURE 1 • The patient is placed in the supine position with both arms tucked. Both a padded chest strap and leg strap are used to secure the patient to the bed to allow for change in patient positioning intraoperatively.

- The lateral decubitus or semilateral position, with the hernia facing up, is utilized for patients who have lateral abdominal wall hernias.
- Regardless of patient positioning, patients are secured to the operating table with padded straps. These steps facilitate the ability of patients to be placed in Trendelenburg or reverse Trendelenburg positioning during the case.
- Laparoscopic monitors are positioned so that they are approximately at eye level and are typically placed on each side of the OR table allowing the surgeons, assistant, and scrub technologist to see the operative field.
- Preoperative hair removal is performed at the surgical site with electric clippers.
- The skin is prepped with chlorohexidine gluconate skin prep. Draping is then performed in sterile fashion making sure not to contaminate the field. Some surgeons prefer an iodine impregnated drape.
- Before the start of the case, all patients receive preoperative antibiotics, most commonly with a first-generation cephalosporin.[22] Patients are redosed with antibiotics if the case takes longer than 2 hours.
- Chemoprophylaxis with heparin is also administered before the start of the case, and sequential compression devices are applied to reduce the risk of venous thromboembolism.
- Gastric decompression with a nasogastric tube and urinary decompression with a Foley catheter are often performed.

INITIAL ACCESS AND PLACEMENT OF PORTS

- Once the patient has been appropriately placed under general anesthesia and prepping and draping is complete, attention is turned to entry into the abdomen.
- Abdominal access is obtained by one of two methods: open cutdown (**FIGURE 2**) or Veress technique. Direct cutdown may be performed at the site of the hernia or off of midline.
- There is typically a window of access present between the iliac crest and inferior costal margin. A common point of entry into the abdominal cavity occurs one fingerbreadth inferior to the costal margin on the left side of the abdomen at Palmer point.
- A balloon trocar can be used when a cutdown technique is performed to prevent the escape of air while establishing pneumoperitoneum. Pneumoperitoneum is set to 12 to 15 mm Hg using high-flow insufflation.
- A 5-mm port is placed at the access site, and the abdominal cavity is inspected using an angled 30° or 45° laparoscopic camera.
- For midline incisional hernias, two additional 5-mm ports are placed in the far lateral abdomen. The working ports must be placed far enough apart so that laparoscopic instruments move freely, and there are no collisions between the ports. There must also be enough distance between the ports and the hernia to make the dissection ergonomic and allow for visualization of mesh placement.
- If a cut down entry was performed and a 10- or 12-mm balloon port is placed there, that typically serves as the insertion site for the mesh. With this, all of the other ports can typically be 5 mm and a 5-mm 30° scope can therefore be moved from port to port to allow best visualization. As needed, additional 5-mm ports may be placed on the contralateral side of the hernia in order to aid with dissection or fixation of the mesh (**FIGURE 3**).
- For patients who have nonmidline hernias, the principles of port placement are the same. Two 5-mm trocars are placed as working ports.

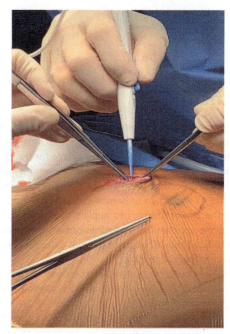

FIGURE 2 • Entry into the abdomen is gained via an infraumbilical cutdown. A 5-mm port is placed, without an obturator, in this position.

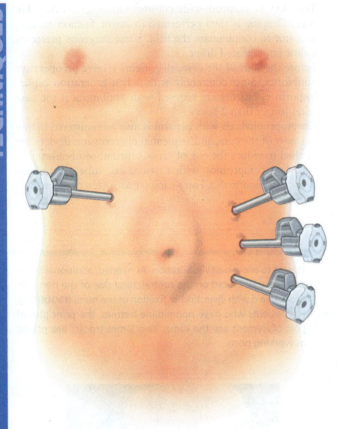

FIGURE 3 • There are three 5-mm ports placed ipsilaterally on the abdominal wall, and as needed, additional 5-mm ports are placed in order to facilitate reduction of the hernia sac and tacking of the mesh.

DISSECTION

- Two 5-mm bowel graspers, laparoscopic scissors (with or without monopolar electrocautery), and a laparoscopic clip applier are typically used and/or available for the dissection.
- Reduction of the hernia contents is carried out with blunt and sharp dissection using the bowel graspers and scissors (**FIGURE 4**). Reduction of hernia contents can be achieved by using the bowel graspers to apply steady, opposing retraction to the attachments and adhesions while the scissors are used to lyse them. The use of manual external pressure can aid in reduction of the sac.
- When electrocautery is used for the dissection, it is necessary to keep it away from the bowel to prevent immediate or delayed thermal injury.
- Care is taken to achieve hemostasis during the dissection as small, bleeding vessels have the tendency to retract and can result in delayed bleeding if not immediately clipped or cauterized.
- Laparoscopic adhesiolysis is continued until the entire hernia defect and the surrounding landing space for the mesh is completely visualized. If there are multiple defects, then each defect must be cleared.
- Any additional intestinal adhesions to the abdominal wall are taken down if they will interfere with mesh placement. Occasionally, the falciform ligament is taken down, so that

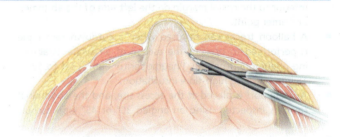

FIGURE 4 • Any adhesions to the anterior abdominal wall are lysed as needed in order to facilitate reduction of the hernia sac. There must be an appropriate amount of space to place the mesh.

the mesh can lay flat against the posterior fascia of the abdominal wall.
- The hernia sac itself is not taken and is left in situ.
- If, at any point, progress with dissection is halted or the dissection becomes too difficult to carry out laparoscopically, the operation should be converted to open. Similarly, if there is an enterotomy made during dissection, repair of that enterotomy becomes the priority. If it can be adequately repaired laparoscopically, that would be appropriate, but conversion to an open operation should be considered otherwise.

MESH PLACEMENT AND FIXATION

- Upon completion of the dissection, the hernia defect(s) is measured to allow for appropriate mesh sizing. For small and narrow hernias that have a width no more than 6 to 8 cm, it is recommended that fascial closure is achieved with 0 or 1-0 suture that can be placed using a transfascial suture passer or closed with laparoscopic suturing from inside the abdomen before mesh placement. When using a suture passer, typically interrupted or figure-of-eight stitches are utilized.
- Mesh is sized so that there is 5 cm or more of overlap circumferentially around the edge of the defect if possible. For small defects, especially if the defect is closed, a smaller overlap can be used.
- There are a number of ways to size the defect. We typically measure the length and width by placing spinal needles at the longest and widest sections of the hernia and using a ruler inside the abdomen (**FIGURE 5**), which is most often in the middle of the hernia head-to-foot and side-to-side. The use of the ruler gives precise hernia dimensions. Knowing the size of the defect accurately is very important. Having a too large or small mesh can lead to frustration and ultimately failure of the procedure. The mesh and the external abdominal wall at the midway points of the hernia are marked with a surgical marking pen in order to maintain orientation of the mesh (**FIGURE 6**). Four permanent, nonabsorbable 0 or #1 sutures are placed equidistant at each side of the tailored mesh before its insertion (**FIGURE 7**).
- Preferentially, a midweight, coated, wide-pore polypropylene or PTFE mesh is used. A coating is used to minimize adhesion formation between the mesh and the surrounding viscera.
- The mesh is rolled up (**FIGURE 8**) and then passed through the larger 11- or 12-mm trocar under direct visualization and unfurled using laparoscopic bowel graspers.
- The mesh is then reoriented based on the markings on the mesh and the external abdominal wall. Once orientation is achieved, each end of the preplaced sutures is brought through the abdominal wall with a suture passer (**FIGURE 8**). The suture that is closest to the structure of potential concern (eg, bone, stoma) should be passed first in order to maintain adequate visualization.
- The sutures are tied down extracorporeally. Sutures should not be tied down until the mesh is in the proper location and is lying flat against the abdominal wall (**FIGURE 8**).
- A 5-mm laparoscopic tacking device is used to further secure the mesh to the anterior abdominal wall. Laparoscopic hernia tacks are placed slightly less than 1 cm apart circumferentially

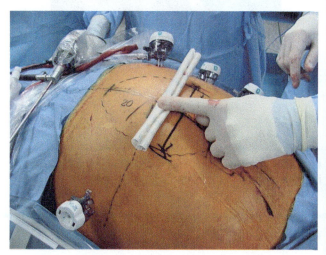

FIGURE 6 • The abdominal wall is marked based on the intracorporeally measurements.

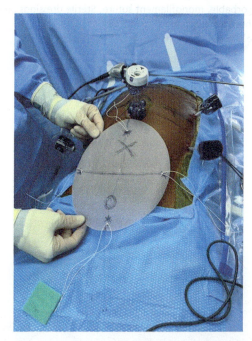

FIGURE 7 • The mesh is marked extracorporeally with a marking pen, which allows the surgeon to maintain orientation once the mesh is inserted in the body. Four sutures are preplaced in the four corners of the mesh, which are eventually externalized with a suture passer and tied down.

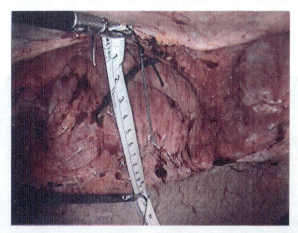

FIGURE 5 • Once the hernia sac is reduced and the anterior abdominal wall is completely freed, the hernia defect is measured intracorporeally with a ruler to allow for appropriate sizing of the mesh.

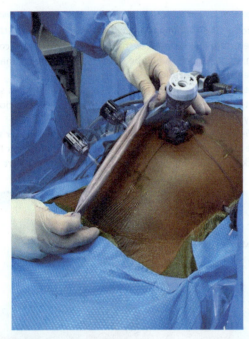

FIGURE 8 • The mesh is folded on itself longitudinally and then inserted through the 11-mm trocar.

along the edge of the mesh to make sure that there is no herniation of abdominal contents under the mesh. A second, inner row of tacks can be placed every 1 to 2 cm to secure the inner portion of the mesh if a double crown technique is to be used. If the fascial defect is closed, some surgeons will forgo the transfascial sutures and simply tack the mesh. Regardless, we prefer some form of permanent fixation to the peritoneum, either permanent sutures, permanent tacks, or both.

- For larger defects, buttressing transfascial sutures are placed every 6 cm or so at the edge of the mesh in addition to the spiral tacks. However, this is not done routinely as there is some evidence to suggest that transfascial sutures are associated with increased postoperative pain.[23]
- The abdomen is inspected once more to make sure everything is hemostatic and that there were no enterotomies made during dissection.
- A transversus abdominis plane (TAP) block using liposomal bupivacaine is performed from the anterior superior iliac spine to the costal margin. The TAP block is performed via extracorporeal injection, but it is visualized laparoscopically to ensure that the injection is being done in the proper plane (between the internal oblique and transversus abdominus muscle).
- The ports are removed under direct visualization.

CLOSURE

- Fascial closure is performed with an absorbable 0 or #1 suture using a suture passer for the 11-mm port site. Closing this port site helps to prevent the herniation of omentum or intestine.
- Each of the laparoscopic port sites are closed with a 4-0 absorbable, monofilament suture. Sterile dressings and skin adhesive are applied (FIGURE 9).
- See also FIGURES 10-12.

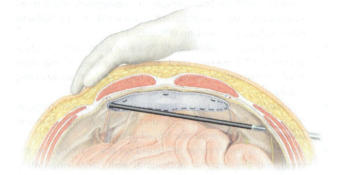

FIGURE 10 • A laparoscopic tacking device is used to place one or two rows of absorbable tacks circumferentially in for the mesh to lay flat on the abdominal wall.

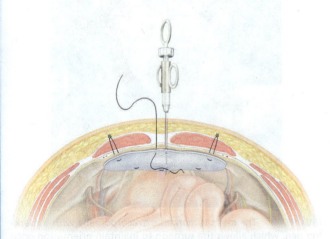

FIGURE 9 • Using a laparoscopic suture passer, the preplaced sutures are grabbed on both ends and pulled through the abdominal wall. They are tied down extracorporeally.

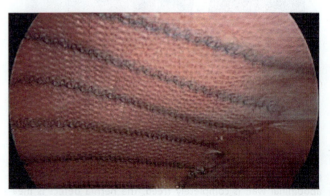

FIGURE 11 • Once the tacking is complete, the mesh should lay taut against the abdominal wall.

Chapter 24 INCISIONAL HERNIA: LAPAROSCOPIC APPROACHES 207

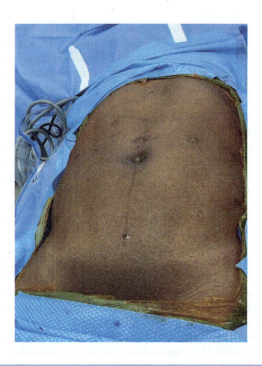

FIGURE 12 • This patient's skin incisions are closed with absorbable suture and then skin glue is placed over each of the incisions.

PEARLS AND PITFALLS

Incomplete preoperative workup	▪ An incomplete history and physical examination may lead to important missed details, such as the presence of other hernias. ▪ Failure to obtain a complete history regarding prior hernia repair may lead to unexpected intraoperative findings (eg, previous mesh placement). ▪ Similarly, failure to obtain preoperative imaging on a patient who does not have a reliable history and physical can lead to incorrect operative planning.
Inadequate prehabilitation	▪ Failure to adhere to stringent prehabilitation can result in unnecessary postoperative complications. ▪ Medications, such as anticoagulants, must be appropriately held to reduce the chance of postoperative bleeding. ▪ Multidisciplinary management of complex patients can lead to improved perioperative outcomes.
Port placement	▪ Safe entry into the abdomen can be one of the most difficult portions of the operation. ▪ When ports are located too close together or too close to the operative field, this can handcuff the surgeon and increase operative difficulty. ▪ More ports can always be added if needed if the surgeon is unhappy with initial port placement, especially on the opposite side of the abdomen.
Mesh fixation	▪ Mesh must be secured tautly to the abdominal wall, so there is little redundancy. ▪ Leaving the operating room before the mesh is properly secured can result in early postoperative recurrences or eventration of the mesh with a "mesh diastasis" or pseudorecurrence. ▪ Stretching the mesh out as additional tacks or sutures are placed can help to prevent the mesh from being too lax. ▪ Some form of permanent fixation to the peritoneum is preferred.
Failure to convert to an open procedure	▪ Conversion to an open procedure is not in and of itself a failure. ▪ Conversion to open should be considered when steady progress of the procedure has been halted. ▪ Ensuring the operation is done safely is most important.
Missed enterotomy	▪ A missed enterotomy can lead to significant postoperative complications, such as abscess, sepsis, or fistula formation. ▪ Primary laparoscopic repair can still be performed if the surgeon is appropriately skilled and comfortable with this. ▪ With contamination, avoidance of a permanent synthetic mesh should be considered.
Postoperative management and patient follow-up	▪ An early postoperative recurrence may occur if patients are quick to resume heavy lifting following their operation. ▪ Ideally, patients are seen in clinic within a few weeks of their operation to ensure that wound healing is adequate, pain is controlled, there is no sign of infection, and there is no acute recurrence. ▪ Seromas are common and will most often resolve with no intervention.

POSTOPERATIVE CARE

- Following surgery, patients are transferred to the postanesthesia care unit where they are monitored for a period of 2 to 3 hours before being discharged home or admitted for observation or otherwise to the hospital.
- Whether or not a patient is admitted to the hospital is multifactorial. Patient age, comorbidities, length and difficulty of the operation, and postoperative pain control should be considered when deciding whether to admit a patient.
- For patients admitted to the hospital, they are enrolled in an enhanced recovery after surgery (ERAS) pathway. As part of the ERAS pathway, patients receive multimodal pain control, are required to ambulate the day of the surgery, and are advanced to a regular diet once they have return of bowel function.[24]
- Early recognition and management of ileus is often required.
- Blood thinners are restarted on a case-by-case basis, but typically not sooner than 48 hours following surgery (other than subcutaneous heparin, etc).
- When patients are discharged, they are prescribed enough narcotics to supplement breakthrough pain for 2 to 5 days. Otherwise, first-line pain control is accomplished with anti-inflammatories and acetaminophen.
- Patients are instructed to avoid straining their abdomen for 6 weeks postoperatively. Heavy lifting or core exercises or other activities that place a significant strain on the abdomen can increase short-term recurrence.
- Patients typically follow up within 2 to 4 weeks after surgery.

COMPLICATIONS

- Enterotomy
- Other solid or hollow organ injury (eg, spleen, liver, bladder)
- Postoperative bleed
- Chronic pain
- Surgical site infection
- Seroma
- Deep venous thrombosis
- Symptomatic bulge
- Hernia recurrence
- Adhesive bowel obstruction
- Complications from anesthesia

OUTCOMES

- In one of the largest and earliest series published with 9 years of experience and 850 patients, overall complication rates were low (13.2%). The most frequent complications in this study were prolonged ileus (3%) and prolonged seroma (2.6%). Recurrence rates were comparable with open repair at 4.7%, and recurrence was associated with larger defects, obesity, recurrent hernias, and postoperative complications.[25] Morbidly obese patients had a more than 4-fold increase in recurrence rates compared with those of a normal body mass index.
- Multiple studies since then comparing laparoscopic vs open ventral hernia repair have shown that the techniques have comparable outcomes. A prospective evaluation of laparoscopic vs open repairs found that the two techniques had similar recurrence and overall complication rates, as well as similar long-term quality of life. Laparoscopic repairs did have fewer surgical site infections (0.3% laparoscopic vs 3.0% open) and decreased length of stay.[26]
- A randomized controlled trial with 10 years of follow-up comparing laparoscopic vs open repairs in 85 patients found that, when evaluating recurrence, reoperation, and death, there were no significant differences between the two groups. In addition, quality of life was assessed in the 47 patients without recurrence, reoperation, or death with a mean 13.8 years of follow-up and found to be similar between groups.[27]
- Many studies have been performed trying to identify the patients who would benefit most from laparoscopic repair over open ventral hernia repair. Laparoscopic repair can be safely performed and successful in obese and morbidly obese patients.[28] A study evaluating laparoscopic repair in 322 obese patients with 49 months follow-up found that class I, II, and III obesity did not individually affect long-term postoperative outcomes; however, patients with class III obesity did have increased length of stay. Multivariate analysis of these data found recurrent hernias and lateral hernia defects to be the only independent factors influencing recurrence.[29] However, this concept of recurrent hernias being at increased risk of recurrence after laparoscopic repair is countered by data comparing 786 laparoscopic repairs with 1120 open repairs, where it was found that laparoscopic repair affords patients with recurrent hernias and obese patients a decreased risk of postoperative infection.[17] Finally, evaluating 11,075 patients who underwent emergent ventral hernia repair showed that laparoscopic repair in the emergent setting is associated with decreased superficial surgical site infections and shorter hospital length of stay.[30]
- Recent adoption of robotic ventral hernia repair has led to studies comparing outcomes of the two minimally invasive techniques showing that robotic repair is safe and feasible when compared with laparoscopic repair.[31] However, in a randomized controlled trial of 75 patients, while laparoscopic and robotic repairs had similar outcomes, laparoscopic repair was cheaper and had shorter operative times. The authors concluded that robotic ventral hernia repair had increased cost and operative time without a measurable clinical benefit.[32]

REFERENCES

1. Fink C, Baumann P, Wente MN, et al. Incisional hernia rate 3 years after midline laparotomy. *Br J Surg*. 2014;101(2):51-54. doi:10.1002/bjs.9364
2. Walming S, Angenete E, Block M, Bock D, Gessler B, Haglind E. Retrospective review of risk factors for surgical wound dehiscence and incisional hernia. *BMC Surg*. 2017;17(1):1-6. doi:10.1186/s12893-017-0207-0
3. Deerenberg EB, Harlaar JJ, Steyerberg EW, et al. Small bites versus large bites for closure of abdominal midline incisions (STITCH): a double-blind, multicentre, randomised controlled trial. *Lancet*. 2015;386(10000):1254-1260. doi:10.1016/S0140-6736(15)60459-7
4. Poulose BK, Shelton J, Phillips S, et al. Epidemiology and cost of ventral hernia repair: making the case for hernia research. *Hernia*. 2012;16(2):179-183. doi:10.1007/s10029-011-0879-9
5. Funk LM, Perry KA, Narula VK, Mikami DJ, Melvin WS. Current national practice patterns for inpatient management of ventral abdominal wall hernia in the United States. *Surg Endosc*. 2013;27(11):4104-4112. doi:10.1007/s00464-013-3075-4
6. MacDonald S, Johnson PM. Wide variation in surgical techniques to repair incisional hernias: a survey of practice patterns among general surgeons. *BMC Surg*. 2021;21(1):259. doi:10.1186/s12893-021-01261-9

7. Stoppa RE. The treatment of complicated groin and incisional hernias. *World J Surg.* 1989;13(5):545-554. doi:10.1007/BF01658869
8. Cevasco M, Itani KMF. *Ventral hernia repair with synthetic, composite, and biologic mesh: characteristics, indications, and infection profile.* In: *Surgical Infections.* Vol. 13. Mary Ann Liebert, Inc; 2012:209-215. doi:10.1089/sur.2012.123
9. Holihan JL, Alawadi Z, Martindale RG, et al. Adverse events after ventral hernia repair: the vicious cycle of complications. Abstract presented at the Abdominal Wall Reconstruction Conference, Washington, DC, June 2014. Elsevier Inc. *J Am Coll Surg.* 2015;221(2):478-485. doi:10.1016/j.jamcollsurg.2015.04.026
10. Ousley J, Baucom RB, Stewart MK, et al. Previous methicillin-resistant *Staphylococcus aureus* infection independent of body site increases odds of surgical site infection after ventral hernia repair. Presented at the American College of Surgeons 100th Annual Clinical Congress, Surgical Forum, San Francisco, CA, October 2014. *J Am Coll Surg.* 2015;221(2):470-477. doi:10.1016/j.jamcollsurg.2015.04.023
11. Yang MMH, Hartley RL, Leung AA, et al. Preoperative predictors of poor acute postoperative pain control: a systematic review and meta-analysis. *BMJ Open.* 2019;9(4):e025091. doi:10.1136/bmjopen-2018-025091
12. Mayor S. One in five with bowel cancer diagnosed as emergency had previous "red flag" symptoms. *BMJ.* 2016;354:i5277. doi:10.1136/bmj.i5277
13. CDC, Oid, Ncezid, DHQP. *9 Surgical Site Infection (SSI) Event.* 2020. Accessed July 21, 2020. https://www.cdc.gov/nhsn/pdfs/ps-analysis-
14. Ayuso SA, Elhage SA, Aladegbami BG, et al. Delayed primary closure (DPC) of the skin and subcutaneous tissues following complex, contaminated abdominal wall reconstruction (AWR): a propensity-matched study. *Surg Endosc.* 2022;36(3):2169-2177. doi:10.1007/s00464-021-08485-z
15. SAGES. *Guidelines for Laparoscopic Ventral Hernia Repair.* A SAGES Publication. Accessed June 7, 2021. https://www.sages.org/publications/guidelines/guidelines-for-laparoscopic-ventral-hernia-repair/
16. Yee JA, Harold KL, Cobb WS, Carbonell AM. Bone anchor mesh fixation for complex laparoscopic ventral hernia repair. *Surg Innov.* 2008;15(4):292-296. doi:10.1177/1553350608325231
17. Schlosser KA, Arnold MR, Otero J, et al. Deciding on optimal approach for ventral hernia repair: laparoscopic or open. *J Am Coll Surg.* 2019;228(1):54-65. doi:10.1016/j.jamcollsurg.2018.09.004
18. Sørensen LT. Wound healing and infection in surgery: the clinical impact of smoking and smoking cessation. A systematic review and meta-analysis. *Arch Surg.* 2012;147(4):373-383. doi:10.1001/archsurg.2012.5
19. Heniford BT, Ross SW, Wormer BA, et al. Preperitoneal ventral hernia repair: a decade long prospective observational study with analysis of 1023 patient outcomes. *Ann Surg.* 2020;271(2):364-374. doi:10.1097/SLA.0000000000002966
20. Novitsky YW, Cobb WS, Kercher KW, Matthews BD, Sing RF, Heniford BT. Laparoscopic ventral hernia repair in obese patients: a new standard of care. *Arch Surg.* 2006;141(1):57-61. doi:10.1001/archsurg.141.1.57
21. Parekh PS, Gupta V. *Anatomy, Hand Positioning.* StatPearls Publishing; 2021. Accessed June 9, 2021. http://www.ncbi.nlm.nih.gov/pubmed/32491633
22. Hendren S, Fritze D, Banerjee M, et al. Antibiotic choice is independently associated with risk of surgical site infection after colectomy: a population-based cohort study. *Ann Surg.* 2013;257(3):469-475. doi:10.1097/SLA.0b013e31826c4009
23. Beldi G, Wagner M, Bruegger LE, Kurmann A, Candinas D. Mesh shrinkage and pain in laparoscopic ventral hernia repair: a randomized clinical trial comparing suture versus tack mesh fixation. *Surg Endosc.* 2011;25(3):749-755. doi:10.1007/s00464-010-1246-0
24. Shao JM, Deerenberg EB, Prasad T, et al. Adoption of enhanced recovery after surgery and intraoperative transverse abdominis plane block decreases opioid use and length of stay in very large open ventral hernia repairs. *Am J Surg.* 2021;222(4):806-812. doi:10.1016/j.amjsurg.2021.02.025
25. Heniford BT, Park A, Ramshaw BJ, Voeller G, Hunter JG, Fitzgibbons RJ. Laparoscopic repair of ventral hernias: nine years' experience with 850 Consecutive hernias. *Ann Surg.* 2003;238(3):391-400. doi:10.1097/01.sla.0000086662.49499.ab
26. Colavita PD, Tsirline VB, Belyansky I, et al. Prospective, long-term comparison of quality of life in laparoscopic versus open ventral hernia repair. *Ann Surg.* 2012;256(5):714-722. doi:10.1097/sla.0b013e3182734130
27. Asencio F, Carbó J, Ferri R, et al. Laparoscopic versus open incisional hernia repair: long-term follow-up results of a randomized clinical trial. *World J Surg.* 2021;45(9):2734-2741. doi:10.1007/s00268-021-06164-7
28. Tsereteli Z, Pryor BA, Heniford BT, Park A, Voeller G, Ramshaw BJ. Laparoscopic ventral hernia repair (LVHR) in morbidly obese patients. *Hernia.* 2008;12(3):233-238. doi:10.1007/s10029-007-0310-8
29. Maspero M, Bertoglio CL, Morini L, et al. Laparoscopic ventral hernia repair in patients with obesity: should we be scared of body mass index? *Surg Endosc.* 2022;36(3):2032-2041. doi:10.1007/s00464-021-08489-9
30. Kao AM, Huntington CR, Otero J, et al. Emergent laparoscopic ventral hernia repairs. *J Surg Res.* 2018;232:497-502. doi:10.1016/j.jss.2018.07.034
31. Dhanani NH, Olavarria OA, Holihan JL, et al. Robotic versus laparoscopic ventral hernia repair. *Ann Surg.* 2021;273(6):1076-1080. doi:10.1097/sla.0000000000004795
32. Petro CC, Zolin S, Krpata D, et al. Patient-reported outcomes of robotic vs laparoscopic ventral hernia repair with intraperitoneal mesh: the PROVE-IT randomized clinical trial. *JAMA Surg.* 2021;156(1):22-29. doi:10.1001/jamasurg.2020.4569

Disclaimer: *Dr. Colavita has an investigated sponsored agreement with Medtronic. Dr. Heniford receives surgical research/education grants as well as honoraria for speaking from Allergan and W.L. Gore.*

Chapter 25 Incisional Hernia Repair: Abdominal Wall Reconstruction Options

Lucas R. Beffa and Michael J. Rosen

DEFINITION

- The field of abdominal wall reconstruction has seen significant surgical advances in the past decade, yet the basic principles for abdominal reconstruction remain unchanged. A renewed interest in recreating a functional dynamic abdominal wall through reconstructing the linea alba and restoring normal anatomy of the abdominal wall unit has fostered several innovative techniques to achieve these goals. The foundation for much of our understanding of abdominal wall reconstruction can be linked to pioneering surgeons such as Oscar Ramirez, Renee Stoppa, and Jean Rives. These reconstructive surgeons brought forth the concepts of performing fascial releases of the abdominal wall compartments to provide advancement of the midline fascia. The principles laid forth by these surgeons are the basis for component separation techniques and remain unchanged since the original techniques were first described. Although newer techniques that will be described in this chapter may differ in the exact mechanism in which fascial advancement is obtained, the underlying concept of achieving fascial advancement to reconstruct the midline is a constant.
- When considering which approach is indicated for reconstructing the abdominal defect that the surgeon is faced with, it is helpful to provide general categories of the various abdominal wall reconstructive techniques. In the authors' opinion, the most clinically relevant classification scheme is based on preservation of the anterior abdominal wall neurovascular blood supply and the need to raise large lipocutaneous flaps to gain access to the lateral abdominal wall. In general, minimally invasive approaches preserve the abdominal wall blood supply and avoid large skin flaps. Examples of such techniques include endoscopic component separation, robotic posterior component separation, and periumbilical perforator sparing approaches, whereas the standard open approach does not typically preserve the anterior abdominal wall blood supply.
- This chapter will focus on some of the more advanced reconstructive techniques to repair large abdominal wall defects. Prior to discussing each of these approaches, it is imperative to understand that not all ventral hernia repairs will require these approaches. In fact, most abdominal wall defects less than 10 to 15 cm in maximal width can be repaired using a standard Rives-Stoppa-Wantz approach. This technique will be described in detail in another chapter in this textbook. In the authors' opinion, this approach should always be initially considered prior to moving on to more advanced techniques.

DIFFERENTIAL DIAGNOSIS

- When planning an abdominal wall reconstruction, the most important first step is to clarify patient's expectations for a successful outcome as well as the surgeon's. Not all defects, particularly in the setting of contamination or infection, can or should be repaired in a single setting. Often, the initial attempt at clearing the infectious source or reconstructing the gastrointestinal (GI) tract takes precedence and formal reconstruction should be delayed. In these cases, the patient should understand that they will likely have a ventral hernia at the end of the procedure that eventually will need to be repaired.

PATIENT HISTORY AND PHYSICAL FINDINGS

- Basic cardiac and pulmonary risk stratification is essential.
- Skin preparation is critical, and an experienced wound care nurse is invaluable. Treating any subcutaneous cellulitis or breakdown can significantly improve soft-tissue coverage at the time of formal reconstruction.
- Optimization of nutritional status is also important. This can include supplemental, enteral, or parenteral feeding when necessary. It is also important to point out that patients with an ongoing infectious nidus, particularly infected synthetic mesh, can be very difficult to obtain a positive nitrogen balance.
- Many patients with large ventral hernias also suffer from morbid obesity. The ideal approach to managing obesity in the setting of a complex ventral hernia is challenging. It is clear that there is increased risk of hernia recurrence with higher body mass index and weight loss prior to surgical intervention is optimal. There are several options for weight loss including medically supervised weight loss and weight loss surgery. This can be particularly challenging in symptomatic incarcerated hernias in which there is little time to achieve or obtain clearance for weight loss surgery.
- Preoperative smoking cessation is advisable prior to elective hernia repair. Clearly there is increased risk for surgical site occurrences with active smokers; however, infectious complications and hernia recurrences appear to be unaffected. We recommend examining individual outcomes at your own practice or institution regarding mandatory smoking cessation. (Does active smoking really matter before ventral hernia repair? An Americas Hernia Society Quality Collaborative analysis.)
- Obtaining and reviewing all old operative records is vital. Understanding what type of mesh and in what layer in the abdominal wall it was placed can help guide your approach. In addition, it is important to clarify if one of the lateral abdominal wall muscles were already released because it can lead to lateral abdominal wall laxity if it is rereleased. Likewise, the surgeon might choose another muscle to release to access an undissected plane.

Chapter 25 INCISIONAL HERNIA REPAIR: ABDOMINAL WALL RECONSTRUCTION OPTIONS

IMAGING AND OTHER DIAGNOSTIC STUDIES

- Routine radiologic imaging with an abdominal-pelvic computed axial tomography scan is particularly useful in complex ventral hernia repairs. These scans can provide valuable information as to the size of the defect and presence of loss of domain, the absence or destruction of important components of the abdominal wall, and the presence of remnant prosthetic materials.
- More advanced radiologic imaging such as magnetic resonance imaging or angiogram to look for periumbilical perforator vessels is not routinely performed in our practice.
- Preoperative antibiotic and deep venous thrombosis prophylaxis is routinely given. Typically, a first-generation cephalosporin will suffice, but in cases of prior or active methicillin-resistant *Staphylococcus aureus* infection, vancomycin is added.
- Foley catheters are routinely inserted; however, postoperative nasogastric decompression is rarely needed.
- Perioperative anesthesia management is critical to success in large abdominal wall reconstructions. It is important that the patient remains completely relaxed during the procedure as this greatly improves exposure of the abdominal wall. In addition, in larger abdominal wall reconstruction, there is often some level of compartment syndrome at the conclusion of the procedure. It is important to monitor plateau airway pressures changes both at the initiation of the case and once the abdomen is closed. High plateau airway pressures indicate compromised pulmonary compliance due to increased abdominal pressures, which place the patient at increased risk of postoperative respiratory failure. We typically keep patients intubated postoperatively if the plateau pressures change by more than 6 mm Hg until preoperative pulmonary compliance is achieved. This can take 24 to 72 hours depending on the magnitude of the case.

SURGICAL MANAGEMENT

- As with any hernia repair, it is critically important that the surgeon has a firm understanding of the anatomy of the abdominal wall prior to manipulation. The abdominal wall is basically composed of the two rectus muscles running longitudinally and the three lateral muscles on each side of the abdominal wall. Each performs a valuable function for the abdominal wall, and any disruption can cause impairment in core physiology. Understanding the neurovascular anatomy of the anterior abdominal wall is particularly important for optimizing the results of each of these approaches. The rectus muscle receives its innervation from the T7-T11 intercostal nerve routes. These nerves run between the transversus abdominis and internal oblique muscles in the lateral abdominal wall. They penetrate the linea semilunaris and segmentally innervate the rectus muscle. It is very important to preserve these nerves in any reconstruction; otherwise, the rectus muscle will atrophy and prevent any hope for a functional abdominal wall (**FIGURE 1**). One important consideration for a posterior

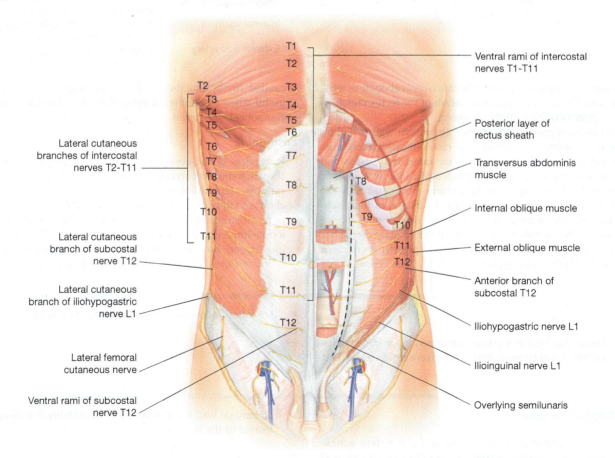

FIGURE 1 • Innervation of the anterior abdominal wall. Note the intercostal nerves run in the lateral abdominal wall in between the internal oblique and transversus abdominis muscle.

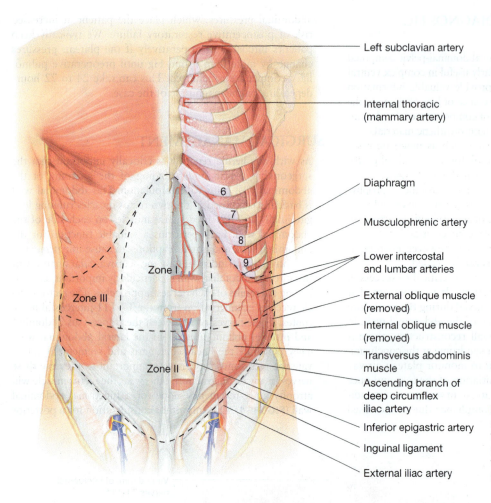

FIGURE 2 • Blood supply to the anterior abdominal wall. Note the location of the medial row of perforators off the inferior epigastric providing blood supply to the medial aspect of the skin.

component separation is that the transversus abdominis muscle actually forms the posterior sheath of the rectus muscle in the upper two-thirds of the abdomen.
- The blood supply of the anterior abdominal wall is slightly more complex (FIGURE 2). The rectus muscle receives its blood supply both laterally from the intercostal vessels and from a superior and inferior branch of the inferior epigastric vessel. The blood supply to the skin and subcutaneous tissues of the midline is also important to understand to limit ischemic problems during reconstruction. The skin does receive some limited supply from the lateral intercostal vessels, but the majority comes from deep inferior epigastric perforator vessels. These vessels typically lie within 5 cm cephalad and caudad to the umbilicus. This relationship is particularly useful when performing a periumbilical perforator sparing component separation.

Positioning

- Regardless of the abdominal wall reconstructive technique chosen, some basic technical aspects remain constant. A wide surgical preparation including the entire abdomen, lower chest, and upper legs is performed with a chlorhexidine solution. All stoma sites are oversewn to minimize spillage. An iodine-impregnated dressing is utilized at the discretion of the surgeon; however, it does not have any proven benefit to decrease wound complications or mesh infections.
- For robotic approaches, please refer to Chapter 26.

TECHNIQUES

INCISION

- The surgical incision is typically performed in a midline fashion and all other old scars or skin ulcerations are completely excised.

ADHESIOLYSIS

- The abdominal cavity is entered and a complete adhesiolysis is performed to free up the entire abdominal wall all the way to the colic gutters. This step is critical, as the abdominal wall will be limited in its mobility if it remains fixated to the viscera.

CONCOMITANT PROCEDURES AND REMOVAL OF ALL FOREIGN MATERIAL

- Any concomitant GI surgery is completed and all prior synthetic material is removed from the abdominal wall. In our opinion, removing prior synthetic material allows the new prosthetic to better incorporate into the abdominal wall and reduces seromas and mesh infections. After the intraperitoneal portion of the procedure is completed, a countable towel is placed over the abdominal viscera to prevent inadvertent injury during dissection of the abdominal wall.

POSTERIOR COMPONENT SEPARATION TECHNIQUE

- A posterior component separation is basically an extension of the standard Rives-Stoppa-Wantz repair.
- The initial procedure begins in a similar fashion. The linea alba is identified and grasped with Kocher clamps. To avoid confusion and misidentification of appropriate planes, the clamps must be placed on the medial edge of the rectus muscle and not on the hernia sac. If the clamps are on the hernia sac, the dissection will proceed in a subcutaneous plane. Next, an incision of the posterior sheath is made approximately 1 cm off the linea alba. It is important to identify the rectus muscle, which will avoid creating a subcutaneous or preperitoneal plane of dissection (**FIGURE 3**). The use of cautery to observe rectus musculature contraction is a useful aid in identifying the border of the rectus muscle, which can sometimes be challenging.
- The posterior rectus sheath is then separated off the rectus muscle using electrocautery, carefully preserving the inferior epigastric vessel. This dissection plane is facilitated by placing upward traction on the rectus muscle and medial traction on the posterior sheath with Kocher clamps. Typically, small posterior branches off the epigastric vessels can be coagulated.
- The lateral extent of this dissection continues until the perforating neurovascular bundles are identified. The nerves associated with the perforators are critical to maintain a functional innervated rectus muscle. They also are the landmark of the linea semilunaris, that is, the lateral extent of the rectus muscle. In a standard Rives-Stoppa-Wantz repair, the dissection is completed at this point (**FIGURE 4**).
- If more advancement is needed to provide mobilization for the posterior sheath for a safe tension-free closure, or anterior sheath, or provide a larger compartment for an adequate-sized piece of mesh, then a posterior component separation is performed.
- This dissection is usually started in the upper third of the abdomen. The initial release of a posterior component separation involves transecting the posterior lamella of the internal oblique. This fascia is the only posterior muscle/fascia that likely provides some advancement of the anterior components. Thus, if the surgeon only requires some additional release to achieve midline closure, this will suffice. After transecting the posterior lamella of the internal oblique, the transversus abdominis is exposed. In the upper third of the abdomen, the transversus abdominis muscle belly actually forms the posterior sheath and does extend medial to the linea semilunaris. The release of the transversus abdominis is begun approximately 0.5 cm medial to the intercostal nerves. When performing this release, it is always important to confirm that it is not disrupting the intercostal nerves.
- The transversus abdominis muscle release is facilitated by the use of a right-angle clamp in the upper third of the abdomen under the muscle (**FIGURE 5**). Below this muscle is the peritoneum and transversalis fascia and can be quite thin on the medial side.

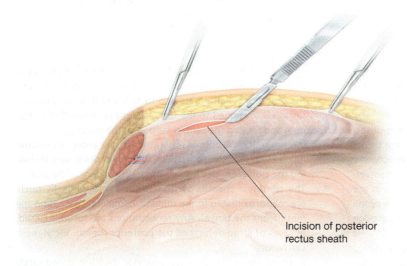

FIGURE 3 • The posterior rectus sheath is incised 1 cm lateral to the linea alba to gain access to the retrorectus space.

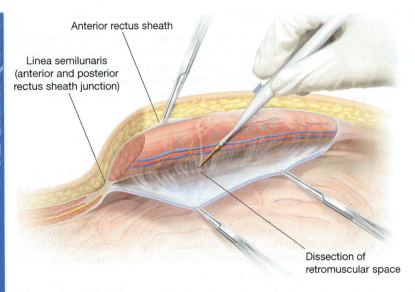

FIGURE 4 • The posterior rectus sheath is separated off the rectus muscle until the lateral edge of the rectus is identified by the presence of the perforating intercostal nerves.

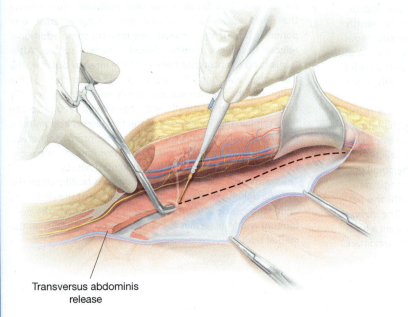

FIGURE 5 • The transversus abdominis muscle is incised to expose the peritoneum below. Note the intercostal nerves are preserved as this release occurs medially.

- As the dissection continues caudally, the muscle belly of the transversus abdominis is replaced with a fascial layer. This layer is also incised, leaving the transversalis fascia and peritoneum in the lower third of the abdomen (**FIGURE 6**).
- Once the entire transversus abdominis is released, the dissection is continued laterally. Again, this dissection plane is below the transversus abdominis muscle and above the peritoneum/retroperitoneum. It can either be achieved in the pretransversalis plane, which tends to be slightly more vascular, or in the preperitoneum, which can be slightly thinner and more prone to holes. The lateral extent of this dissection is the lateral edge of the psoas muscle. This plane can be extended cephalad to the costal margin, sweeping the peritoneum off the diaphragm.
- The posterior sheath is incised at its insertion into the linea alba to connect each side of the abdomen. This is continued at least 5 cm above the incision and typically can be performed to the xiphoid process. In upper abdominal hernias, the insertion of the posterior sheath is released from the xiphoid, and the dissection is continued to the fatty triangle underneath the sternum and toward the central tendon of the diaphragm.
- Inferiorly, the bladder is separated off the anterior abdominal wall. In suprapubic hernias, the pelvis is exposed, including the pubis, Cooper ligaments, and the space of Retzius.
- The posterior sheath, peritoneum, and transversalis fascia are reapproximated in the midline, completely excluding the mesh from the bowel. Any fenestrations are sutured closed. In cases of large defects of the posterior sheath, Vicryl mesh can be used.
- It is very important that the posterior sheath is closed safely because bowel can herniate through the posterior closure

Chapter 25 **INCISIONAL HERNIA REPAIR: ABDOMINAL WALL RECONSTRUCTION OPTIONS** 215

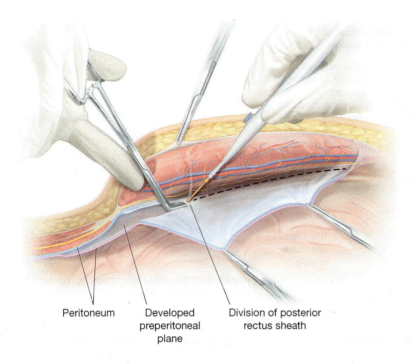

FIGURE 6 • In the lower third of the abdomen, the transversus abdominis is mainly fascia and is released to expose the peritoneum.

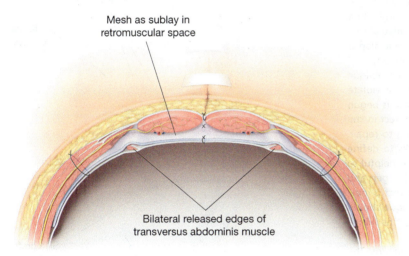

FIGURE 7 • Mesh is placed as a sublay with lateral transfascial sutures and the midline closed without buckling of the mesh.

and become incarcerated below the mesh resulting in an intraparietal hernia.
- A large sheet of unprotected medium-weight or heavy-weight polypropylene mesh is typically placed in the retrorectus space.
- If transfascial fixation is deemed necessary by the surgeon, several transfascial sutures are placed at the lateral edge of the mesh. The sutures are placed under tension so as to allow the midline closure to be off weighted. These sutures also set the tension on the mesh that prevents buckling when the midline is closed over the mesh (**FIGURE 7**).
- Drains are placed over the mesh and below the rectus muscle and removed when less than 30 mL/d of output.
- The midline fascia is reapproximated with running or interrupted slowly absorbable monofilament sutures. The skin is closed in layers.

ANTERIOR COMPONENT SEPARATION TECHNIQUE

- Anterior component separation is typically performed if the skin will require undermining to gain advancement for closure. In addition, if the retrorectus space or the preperitoneal or retroperitoneal space cannot be accessed, an anterior component separation can be performed with intraperitoneal mesh placement.
- Placing Kocher clamps on the linea alba provides medial retraction, whereas rake retractors are placed on the dermis and retracted superiorly. Using electrocautery, the

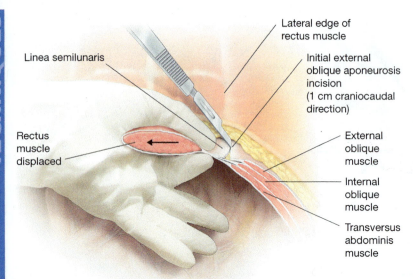

FIGURE 8 • Bimanual palpation to confirm the linea semilunaris location.

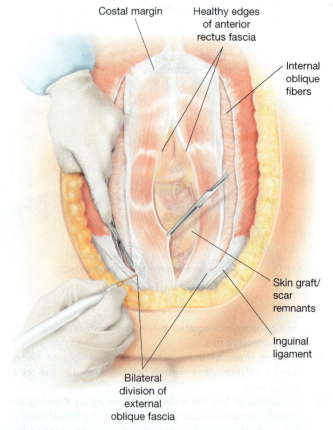

FIGURE 9 • Bilateral open component separation procedure completed.

- subcutaneous tissues are undermined to the lateral abdominal wall.
- These lipocutaneous flaps are created to the inguinal ligament and several centimeters above the costal margin. In a standard open component separation, all of the medial row perforator vessels are sacrificed. Therefore, the skin flap is supplied by the intercostal vessels approaching laterally.
- The release is performed by incising the external oblique muscle. It is imperative that this incision does not violate the linea semilunaris. This can occur if the release is begun too medially and will result in a full-thickness defect in the lateral abdominal wall, which is very challenging to repair. There are no clear anterior anatomic landmarks to define the linea semilunaris or the external oblique. It is helpful to grip the rectus muscle in between the thumb and fingers and feel the indentation at the lateral extent of the rectus muscle (FIGURE 8). The incision in the external oblique should be placed approximately 2 cm lateral to the identified linea semilunaris.
- A 1-cm incision is made parallel to the linea semilunaris. The orientation of the muscle fibers below should be confirmed. If the fibers are oriented in a vertical direction, it is likely that the anterior rectus sheath has been incised. To confirm, a right-angle clamp can be placed below the external oblique muscle and passed medially. If in the correct plane, the tip of the instrument will not be able to traverse the linea semilunaris. If the incision was erroneously placed on the anterior rectus sheath, the clamp will not meet resistance, and the incision should be closed and the dissection continued laterally.
- The external oblique is then released from the inguinal ligament to 3 to 4 cm above the costal margin. This can typically be performed with electrocautery (FIGURE 9). It is important to avoid injuring the internal oblique fascia or muscle complex below to avoid bulging and herniation.
- A component separation is more than a fasciotomy of the external oblique muscle. After the muscle is released, the external oblique muscle is dissected in the avascular plane in between the external and internal oblique to the posterior axillary line. This dissection allows the rectus complex to slide medially.
- A component separation should typically be performed bilaterally to allow for equal redistribution of forces on the eventual repair. In certain circumstances, such the presence of a stoma or a prior transverse incision, unilateral releases can be performed.

Chapter 25 INCISIONAL HERNIA REPAIR: ABDOMINAL WALL RECONSTRUCTION OPTIONS

- If further advancement is necessary, the posterior rectus sheath can be separated off the rectus muscle. This incision is made approximately 1 cm lateral to the linea alba on the posterior rectus sheath. The posterior rectus sheath can be separated off the rectus muscle to the linea semilunaris if necessary.
- An appropriately sized mesh is placed as a sublay or in the onlay position. In a sublay mesh, this is placed in the intraperitoneal position. Depending on the indications of the case, a synthetic or biologic mesh might be appropriate. If choosing to place an onlay mesh, then this would be placed between the closed fascia of the midline and lipocutaneous flaps raised during the external oblique release. This would allow placement of extraperitoneal mesh and the use of non–barrier-coated mesh implant.
- One of the major drawbacks of the anterior component separation is skin flap ischemia and wound breakdown. There are several techniques to minimize this risk. First, the skin flap should only be created as far lateral as needed to access the external oblique release and not all the way to the posterior axillary line. Second, redundant skin should be readily excised. This will limit the dead space and remove the most ischemic area. In certain cases, this can require a formal panniculectomy. However, most cases can just be performed using a vertically oriented elliptical incision. Some authors have advocated quilting sutures, securing the flaps to the anterior abdominal wall.

PEARLS AND PITFALLS

Operative planning	■ One of the most common pitfalls associated with abdominal wall reconstruction is underestimating the limitations of what each of these procedures can accomplish. In patients with massively large defects more than 30 cm in width and damaged, fibrotic, fixed abdominal walls, there is little hope for a definitive repair. It is critically important that both the patient and the surgeon have reasonable expectations as to what abdominal wall reconstruction procedures can actually achieve. ■ Preoperative optimization of the patient is one of the most important steps in predicting a successful outcome. Weight loss is encouraged; optimization of diabetes control essential to reducing postoperative complications.
Difficult anatomy	■ The xiphoid and suprapubic region can be difficult to achieve maximal advancement and should be avoided early in one's experience. ■ In many cases of complex abdominal wall reconstruction, the umbilicus must be resected. Patients must be aware of this issue preoperatively.
Avoid denervation	■ Understanding the anatomy of the anterior abdominal wall is very important to ensure a successful outcome. Special consideration should always be given to the innervation and blood supply to the abdominal wall musculature and skin during manipulation.
Inability to reapproximate the midline	■ Although it is always optimal to bring the midline together and reconstruct the linea alba, it is not always safe or feasible. If excessive tension results and the patient manifests hemodynamic instability or respiratory embarrassment, the closure should be aborted and a bridged repair is appropriate. ■ These advanced reconstructive procedures are not simply fasciotomies. Much of the advancement achieved is a result of separating the muscle layers from each other to provide advancement.

POSTOPERATIVE CARE

- Abdominal wall reconstruction is a major surgical procedure that results in a significant physiologic impairment to the patient. Because many patients undergoing abdominal wall reconstruction have multiple comorbidities, careful perioperative management is important to maximize outcomes.
- Reestablishing the midline in a large defect can have early consequences to respiratory mechanics. If the plateau pressures rise by greater than 6 mm Hg after fascial closure, patients remain intubated overnight. Airway pressures are reassessed in the morning to plan for extubation.
- Our group has largely abandoned epidural catheters and prefers surgeon-directed transversus abdominis plane (TAP) blocks. A TAP block can be effective in combination with a multimodal analgesic regimen for postoperative pain control.
- Enhanced recovery after surgery protocols have been helpful in decreasing patient discomfort after large surgeries as well as decreasing length of stay. We encourage a multimodal analgesic approach preoperatively as well as postoperatively, in conjunction with blocks. This does include preoperative carbohydrate loading, liberalization of per oral intake prior to surgery, and early enteral nutrition when possible.
- Most patients undergoing complex abdominal wall reconstruction are hospitalized for 5 to 7 days. Depending on the complexity of the procedures, some patients remain in the intensive care unit for several days.
- Patients are encouraged to ambulate early.
- Because these procedures create significant dead space, drains are placed. Drains should be removed when the output is less than 30 mL/d. In patients with subcutaneous drains, these may remain for several weeks.

- Perioperative antibiotics are continued for up to 24 hours, unless otherwise indicated.
- Most patients are allowed to return to activity within 6 weeks of surgery and unrestricted activity at 3 to 6 months, depending on the case. Abdominal binders are continued for the first 6 weeks and then as needed for comfort.

OUTCOMES

- There are very little comparative studies evaluating the outcomes of each of these approaches head-to-head. In fact, it is likely that these studies will never be completed, as the heterogeneous nature of the patients who develop incisional hernias precludes any one approach ever being ideal. Most series are from single centers with high-volume abdominal wall reconstructive practices. In the selected references, each article provides reasonable outcomes as to the expectations for each procedure.

COMPLICATIONS

- Wound morbidity is common after complex abdominal wall reconstruction.
- Wound cellulitis should initially be treated with broad-spectrum antibiotics. In most cases, the skin does not need to be opened. If the erythema does not improve within 24 to 48 hours, the incision should be opened, cultured, and drained. In cases with clinical signs of sepsis, the surgeon should have a low threshold to perform an abdominal pelvic computed tomography scan.
- Skin necrosis should be treated with early debridement and wound care. In certain cases, delayed primary closure can be performed.
- Seromas are very common after abdominal wall reconstruction and most do not require any intervention. If they are symptomatic, they can be drained under sterile conditions.

SUGGESTED READINGS

1. Blatnik JA, Krpata DM, Pesa NL, et al. Predicting severe postoperative respiratory complications following abdominal wall reconstruction. *Plast Reconstr Surg.* 2012;130(4):836-841.
2. Carbonell AM, Warren JA, Prabhu AS, et al. Reducing length of stay using a robotic-assised approach for retromuscular ventral hernia repair. *Ann Surg.* 2018;27(2):210-217.
3. Krpata DM, Blatnik JA, Novitsky YW, et al. Posterior and open anterior components separations: a comparative analysis. *Am J Surg.* 2012;203(3):318-322; discussion 322.
4. Novitsky YW, Elliott HL, Orenstein SB, et al. Transversus abdominis muscle release: a novel approach to posterior component separation during complex abdominal wall reconstruction. *Am J Surg.* 2012;204(5):709-716.
5. Rosen MJ, Fatima J, Sarr MG. Repair of abdominal wall hernias with restoration of abdominal wall function. *J Gastrointest Surg.* 2010;14(1):175-185.

Chapter 26

Robotic Ventral Hernia Repair: Transversus Abdominis Release

Charlotte M. Horne and Ajita S. Prabhu

DEFINITION

- Minimally invasive approaches allow a surgeon to perform a complex hernia surgery while minimizing recovery time and decreasing the rate of wound complications in appropriate candidates.[1]
- For larger more complex defects a standard laparoscopic sublay repair with tissue-separating mesh may be inadequate.
- First described in 2012, the transversus abdominus release (TAR) component separation facilitates wide mesh overlap by creating a large preperitoneal pocket and, in most cases, allows for fascial reapproximation.[2]
- The transversus abdominus muscle is the deepest of the oblique muscles that comprise the lateral abdominal wall and is identified by the horizontal orientation of the muscle fibers. Incising this allows the surgeon to connect the retrorectus plane to the preperitoneal plane creating a space to accommodate a large prosthetic.
- While a laparoscopic approach to a transversus abdominus release has been described,[3] its widespread utilization is limited due to the technical challenge associated with closure of the anterior fascia.
- Advantages of the robotic platform is the increased degrees of freedom and wristed instruments that facilitate a suture closure of the fascial defect.
- The robotic approach to TAR has demonstrated that it is safe and feasible compared with a laparoscopic approach[4] and allows for the surgeon to complete the same technical aspects of the open operation but in a minimally invasive fashion.
- A robotic approach has been shown to significantly decease length of stay, with similar rates of wound morbidity and decreased rate of systemic complications when compared with an open approach.[5,6]

PATIENT HISTORY AND PHYSICAL FINDINGS

- Ideal candidates are patients with centrally located defects that are between 7 and 15 cm in length and ideally without previously placed mesh.
- The patient should be examined to determine if there is a need for significant soft tissue resection and scar revision as these patients should be offered and open approach. Another key physical examination finding is whether or not the hernia can be reduced as this may predict the complexity of the adhesiolysis.
- Patients who present with obstructive symptoms that are unrelated to the hernia defect should also be offered an open approach and complete adhesiolysis.
- All previous operative reports, specifically previous hernia repairs, should be reviewed to determine the presence, type, and location of previously placed mesh.
- Patients who are not candidates for a robotic approach include those with loss of domain hernias or those with defects greater than 15 cm as these defects can be technically challenging to close robotically. Palpation of the edges of the fascia can help determine the size of the defect, but this should always be confirmed with cross-sectional imaging.
- Patient optimization prior to operative intervention is essential for successful outcomes. Patients with a history of diabetes should have an HbA1c < 8%, smoking cessation should occur preoperatively, and patients who have a body mass index > 40 kg/m^2 should either be referred for a surgical weight loss evaluation or be encouraged to lose weight prior to operative intervention.

IMAGING AND OTHER DIAGNOSTIC STUDIES

- It is our routine practice to perform cross-sectional imaging on all patients prior to consideration for a minimally invasive hernia repair.
- Cross-sectional imaging allows the surgeon to determine defect size, complexity of adhesiolysis, locations for safe entry into the abdominal cavity, and the presence of previously placed prosthesis.
- Additional key findings on imaging include the width of the rectus muscle as well as the location of the hernia as these will guide operative decision making. It is our standard to have at least 5 cm of mesh overlap in every aspect of the hernia defect.
- Imaging is utilized to predict the need to perform a transversus abdominis release. If the patient is found to have a narrow retrorectus space in relation to the defect size on cross-sectional imaging, the space is likely to be unable to accommodate the required size of mesh, necessitating a transversus abdominis release (**FIGURE 1**).
- Love et al demonstrated this principle by retrospectively analyzing preoperative cross-sectional imaging in patients undergoing open ventral hernia to determine the ability to predict whether an additional component separation was necessary after the retromuscular dissection was completed.[7]
- Love et al identified that, when the rectus to defect ratio was <2, a myofascial release was required in >90% of the cases to obtain fascial closure. In these situations, a TAR may be required in defects that are <10 cm.

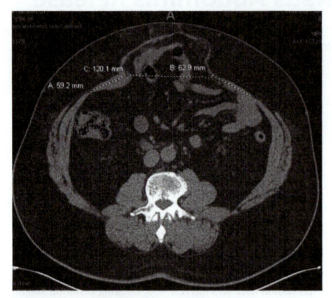

FIGURE 1 • Determining the need for transversus abdominis release: The retrorectus space is measured and compared with the defect width to determine the need for transversus abdominis release to ensure adequate mesh overlap is achieved.

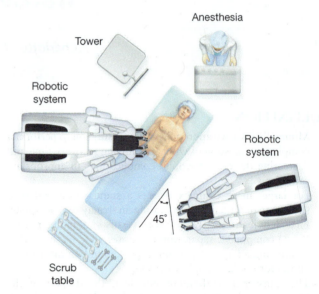

FIGURE 2 OR setup: The robot can be docked from either the right or left side. We angle the robot 45° to the patient's hip. We also flex the bed to increase working space between the costal margin and iliac crest.

- Defects that are <10 cm but off midline or in close proximity to the linea semilunaris may require a TAR to achieve appropriate mesh overlap.
- Determining the need for the transversus abdominus release preoperatively is imperative as doing a bilateral component separation will require additional port placement and redocking the robot, and so preparing for these logistical challenges preoperatively is essential.

SURGICAL MANAGEMENT

Positioning

- The patient is placed supine on the operating room table with either one or both arms tucked to allow for robot docking and to minimize collision with the extremity. This provides room for the bedside assistant to access the robotic arms and facilitates docking.
- The robot can be docked at either side of the patient, and the operative table can be angled slightly to facilitate docking. In addition, we position the base at a 45° angle to the hip to allow for enough room for the boom to swing and to maximize the range of motion between the robotic arms (**FIGURE 2**).
- The patient's umbilicus is aligned with the break point of the bed, and the bed can then be flexed slightly to allow for increased working room between the ribs and iliac crest.

ABDOMINAL ACCESS/PORT PLACEMENT

- Access into the abdomen is obtained using a 5-mm optical trocar in the left upper quadrant. We choose this site of access as it provides a safe place for entry into the abdomen. It also facilitates port placement to optimize adhesiolysis.
- Careful review of prior operative reports prior to gaining abdominal access is imperative, and one should ensure that their planned point of entry is in a location free of intra-abdominal adhesions.
- Other options for access include a standard cutdown or a Veress needle. If unable to gain access with an optical trocar, it is our preference to perform a cutdown for access over a Veress needle. Once pneumoperitoneum is established, additional ports can be placed to facilitate adhesiolysis.
- We place our initial ports to facilitate adhesiolysis. While this can be performed robotically or laparoscopically, one advantage of performing the adhesiolysis laparoscopically is the ability to create adequate working space prior to docking the robot. To minimize the risk of inadvertent thermal injury to the bowel, the adhesiolysis should be performed sharply.
- Three 8-mm robotic ports are utilized with the Xi platform. These are positioned 3 to 4 cm from the ipsilateral edge of the fascial defect as visualized through the entry port. On the contralateral side, the ports are placed slightly more laterally to accommodate closure of the anterior fascia. An assistant port can also be placed to allow for easy passage of sutures through the duration of the case.
- Ports placed too medially can result in the difficulty or inability to visualize the "near" side of the fascial defect, which can make it challenging to close this defect.
- A bariatric trocar can be utilized in the inferiormost port placement position to provide more degrees of freedom and decrease the restriction encountered with the anterior superior iliac spine.
- Robotic ports should be placed approximately 8 cm apart to minimize arm collisions. If the Si platform is being utilized, this distance should be increased to at least 10 cm where possible.

RETROMUSCULAR DISSECTION

- The retromuscular dissection is initiated by identifying the rectus muscle as close to the contralateral aspect of the defect as possible. The posterior sheath is then incised (**FIGURE 3**, ▶ **Video 1**). It is imperative that the muscle is identified before the dissection is continued. Failure to identify the rectus muscle initially can result in dissection in the wrong plane.
- Once the retromuscular plane is identified, the posterior sheath is incised both cephalad and caudally. We utilize a grasping instrument (Prograsp, Force Bipolar, or Caudiere grasper) and a scissor with monopolar cautery to perform this dissection.
- Unlike our typical approach to open TAR, we tend to develop the plane from medially to laterally as we make the initial posterior rectus sheath incision. This minimizes unnecessary repositioning of the camera and grasper and therefore provides a better economy of motion. Downward tension on the posterior rectus sheath allows the pneumoperitoneum to assist in exploiting the retromuscular plane, allowing for an efficient retromuscular dissection.
- When maturing the retromuscular plane, dissection should occur in the avascular plane between the rectus muscle and the posterior rectus sheath to maximize hemostasis (**FIGURE 4**).
- The retromuscular plane is matured until the perforating neurovascular bundles (T7-T11) are identified laterally and preserved (**FIGURE 5**, ▶ **Video 2**). This marks the extent of the retromuscular plane as the neurovascular bundles insert just medial to the linea semilunaris. The superior epigastric vessels are identified running along the costal margin, and the deep inferior epigastric vessels are identified lateral to the arcuate line in the caudal aspect and reflected away with the rectus abdominus muscle.

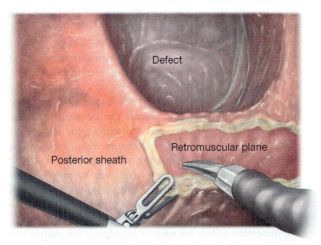

FIGURE 3 • Initial Retromuscular Dissection: The posterior sheath is incised just below the defect taking care to expose the rectus muscle to facilitate dissection in the appropriate plane.

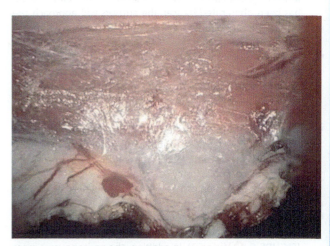

FIGURE 4 • Retromuscular plane: The posterior sheath is retracted downward and into the port. Dissection should proceed along the loose areolar tissue to maximize hemostasis.

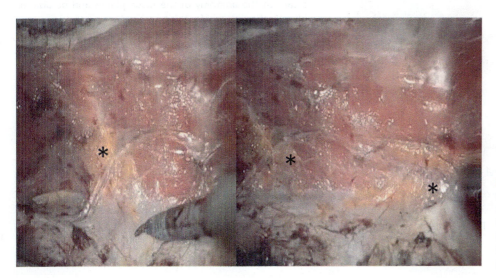

FIGURE 5 • Completed retromuscular dissection: Dissection of the retromuscular plane is performed until the neurovascular bundles (*) are identified, indicating the lateral extent of the retromuscular plane.

TRANSVERSUS ABDOMINIS RELEASE

- Once the lateral extent of the dissection has been achieved, the posterior rectus sheath and the posterior lamella of the internal oblique muscle are incised to reveal the underlying transversus abdominus muscle and its associated connective tissue.
- The abdominal wall can be divided into three sections based on the appearance and makeup of the transversus abdominis muscle. Superiorly, the transversus abdominus is identified by its wide muscular belly. Inferiorly, the transversus abdominus consists solely of thin investing fascia. In the middle, the muscle body of the transversus abdominus thins to an aponeurosis that inserts into the posterior sheath.
- The division of the transversus abdominus can begin either superiorly, where there is a thick muscle belly or inferiorly at the arcuate line where the transversus consists of fascia but can be easily identified.
- Decision of where to start is dictated by not only surgeon preference but also the level of scarring. If the caudal aspect has been obliterated by scar, the authors will approach the transversus abdominus release from the cephalad aspect preferentially.
- It is the preference of the authors to initiate this dissection at the caudal-most aspect at the juncture of the arcuate line and the deep inferior epigastric muscles, which have been reflected away with the body of the rectus abdominus muscle as previously described.
- The "TAR-UP" is our preferred approach to initiating the release of the transversus abdominis where the division is started at the arcuate line. Anatomically, the transversus abdominis consists of only a fascial layer here as it is easily identified. Dissection progresses from a caudal to a cephalad direction.
- Division at this point facilitates entrance into the preperitoneal plane and allows for further lateral dissection (FIGURE 6, ▶ Video 3). In addition, the peritoneum is more robust inferiorly, which minimizes the risk of injures to the posterior sheath.
- Entry into the preperitoneal plane followed by lateral maturation of the plane facilitates further division of the transversus abdominus cephalad.
- Dissection laterally allows the surgeon to work from a lateral to medial approach superiorly, which facilitates easier identification and division of the transversus abdominis fibers.
- As the dissection continues superiorly, the thin fascial layer of the transversus abdominus becomes more defined in the middle third of the abdominal wall and then at the superior aspect develops into the thick muscular layer.
- Superiorly, the fascia and then the muscle is divided to expose the peritoneum. The muscle fibers can then be pushed laterally to mature the preperitoneal plane.
- Maturing the plane as lateral as possible first allows for dissection of the posterior components off the inferior muscle, which facilitates further safe division of the transversus abdominis muscle (FIGURE 7). The lateral extent of the dissection is marked by identification of the retroperitoneal fat as well as the psoas muscle.
- When starting superiorly (top-down technique), the TAR begins just below the costal margin. First, the posterior rectus sheath and the posterior lamella of the internal oblique muscle is incised just medially to the neurovascular bundles to expose the transversus abdominis muscle (FIGURE 8, ▶ Video 4).
- Regardless of the orientation of the dissection (bottom to top or top to bottom), the grasper can be used to further create a "tunnel" underneath the transversus abdominis tissue, wherein the pneumoperitoneum will dissect a plane between the peritoneum and the overlying tissue.
- Exposure in this fashion can be achieved by gently applying downward pressure with the grasper to the peritoneum and upward pressure with the scissor toward the transversus abdominis muscle and its associated fascial layers. The resulting dissection allows for ease of visualizing the muscle and fascia, which must be divided, while minimizing rents in the peritoneum.
- If the peritoneum is prohibitively thin, the surgeon may opt to keep the transversalis fascia intact and with the peritoneum rather than divide it in its entirety. Surgeons must be aware of the anatomy of the tissue planes and be able to identify them clearly for this to occur.
- The TAR is completed when the posterior sheath lies on top of the viscera without tension. At this time the contralateral ports are placed, and the robot is redocked to perform the TAR on the contralateral side.
- We recommend closing any rents in the posterior sheath using 3-0 long-absorbing monofilament barbed sutures or braided absorbable nonbarbed sutures.
- The inferior dissection in the space of Retzius should cross midline to allow for easy identification of the retromuscular plane on the ipsilateral side. Dissection here should also include reduction of any inguinal or femoral hernia that can be repaired simultaneously.
- Inferior dissection in the space of Retzius facilitates the creation of the retromuscular plane on the ipsilateral side once the ports are inserted on the contralateral side.

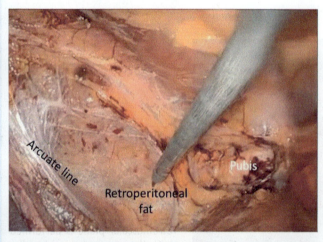

FIGURE 6 • TAR-Up dissection: The TAR is initiated at the arcuate line and carried upward.

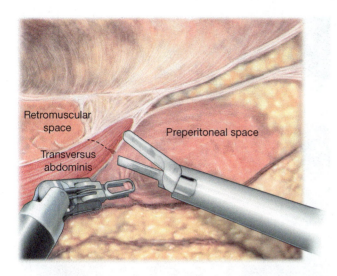

FIGURE 7 • TAR Dissection: Dissection is facilitated by dissection laterally in the preperitoneal space and posterior to the transversus abdominis muscle. This facilitates further division of the transversus abdominis muscle and minimizes holes made in the peritoneum.

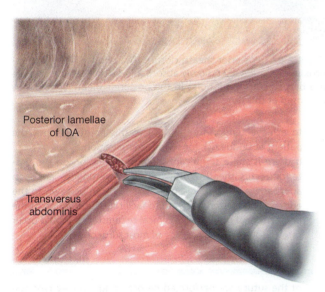

FIGURE 8 • Top-Down TAR: Just medial to the neurovascular bundles below the costal margin, the posterior lamella of the internal oblique aponeurosis is incised to expose the thick muscle belly of the transversus abdominis muscle, which is subsequently divided.

CONTRALATERAL TAR

- Ports on the contralateral side are placed more laterally to maximize the distance to the ipsilateral edge of the hernia defect, to improve visualization for defect closure.
- An important distinction is that the ports on this side are placed into the retromuscular plane as opposed to the intraabdominal plane. As noted previously, this is performed with three additional 8-mm ports, and the caudal-most port may be exchanged for a bariatric port to avoid limitations related to the anterior superior iliac spine.
- If utilizing the Xi platform, the boom is rotated until it is reversed in orientation without moving the base of the patient cart. When utilizing the Si platform, options for red-ocking include reversing the orientation of the bed, which may be accomplished efficiently by extending anesthesia tubing or alternatively repositioning the patient cart if there is sufficient space in the operating room.
- The initiation of the retromuscular dissection on the contralateral side is often already initiated by the pelvic dissection on the opposite (initial) side, and as such it is the practice of the authors to take advantage of this exposure to begin developing the retromuscular plane.
- The retromuscular dissection should take advantage of the pneumoperitoneum to facilitate exposure and division of the avascular areolar tissue. Dissection proceeds from a medial to lateral direction and continues until the costal margin is identified.
- The deep inferior epigastric vessels are reflected away with the rectus abdominus muscle in a hemostatic fashion, and the perforating neurovascular bundles are also identified and preserved. As noted, these structures signify that the dissection has reached its lateral extent. Dissection should not be pursued lateral to this point.
- The development of the retromuscular plane on the second side is notable for the presence of the previously placed intraperitoneal ports, one 5-mm port and three 8-mm ports. These must be liberated from the posterior rectus sheath during the dissection, and the bedside assistant can facilitate this by gently pulling back on the ports and allowing them to

- remain in the retromuscular plane, which exposes four holes from the ports in the peritoneum, which must be closed prior to the conclusion of the operation.
- Again, the posterior rectus sheath and the posterior lamella of the internal oblique are incised to reveal the transversus abdominus muscle and its associated aponeurotic and fascial portions, respectively. The transversus abdominis is incised either superiorly or inferiorly. Dissection occurs in the same manner as the previous side with incision of the transversus abdominus, lateral maturation of the plane, and then further division of the transversus abdominus. The authors prefer caudal to cephalad dissection for efficiency and economy of motion.
- Violations in the posterior sheath should be closed to prevent intraparietal hernias that may result in bowel herniating through these defects, causing an early postoperative bowel obstruction. It is our practice to close these with absorbable multifilament suture; however, closure can also be achieved with a barbed, knotless suture. Of note, failure to progress from a gastrointestinal function standpoint associated with vomiting after surgery should raise suspicion for posterior rectus sheath closure breakdown until proven otherwise by computed tomography imaging.
- The TAR dissection is deemed to be complete when the posterior sheath can be reapproximated at midline without tension. This layer is reapproximated with a 2-0 slowly absorbable barbed suture (FIGURE 9, ▶ Video 5).
- It is imperative that this layer is closed without tension, and dehiscence of this layer can result in an intraparietal hernia. If there is a significant amount of tension, the hernia sac or omentum may be utilized to facilitate closure and minimize tension.
- Difficulty resolving tension in this layer robotically should signal an indication to convert to an open operation, as failure

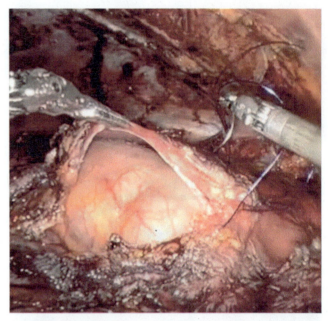

FIGURE 9 • Posterior sheath closure: The two leaflets are reapproximated using a 2.0 slowly absorbable suture. Our preference is a barbed suture. All holes in the posterior sheath should also be closed at this time.

to achieve tension-free closure at this point may put the patient at undue risk for serious complication.
- If there is still a significant amount of tension on the posterior rectus sheath closure after converting to an open approach, an absorbable piece of mesh can be sewn to the edges of the posterior sheath to facilitate the creation of the preperitoneal pocket. This clinical circumstance should occur rarely in the routine practice of most surgeons.

FASCIAL DEFECT CLOSURE

- Upon completion of the TAR and closure of the posterior sheath, the defect is subsequently measured intracorporeally to ensure appropriate mesh overlap. The defect is then subsequently closed in a running manner utilizing slowly absorbable barbed suture.
- We utilize a 1-0 slowly absorbing barbed suture for the fascial defect closure due to its tensile strength. Three or four throws of the suture are performed before using a pulley-type system to sequentially approximate the defect (▶ Video 6). The hernia sac may be included with this closure; however, caution must be taken to ensure that the dermis does not become tethered and puckered as a result. The bedside assistant may be engaged to perform surveillance of this step to prevent skin injury.
- In wider defects, to assist with fascial closure, the intra-abdominal pressure can be decreased to 10-12 mm Hg.

MESH IMPLANTATION

- We routinely choose bare polypropylene mesh when repairing the defect. It is our practice to reinforce the defect ensuring 5 cm of mesh overlap is obtained. It is not our routine practice to fixate the mesh, while sutures and fibrin sealants can be utilized for mesh fixation.[8]
- To ensure adequate overlap and prevent mesh migration and folding, we also measure the preperitoneal pocket to size the mesh to fit into the pocket. The edges of the mesh are rolled in the midline to create a side-to-side oriented scroll.
- The mesh is placed in the retroperitoneal pocket upon the completion of both sides of the TAR. A 12-mm port may be required for introducing the mesh into the retromuscular plane. The authors typically upsize the middle 8-mm port from the first side for this purpose.
- We typically undock the robot prior to introducing the mesh and perform the penultimate portion of the operation laparoscopically. The mesh is introduced using a locking laparoscopic grasper and then unrolled using a side-to-side motion laparoscopically. We then utilize one of our ports to place a drain retromuscular plane. Drain placement is at the discretion of the operating surgeon.

ALTERNATIVE APPROACHES

Hybrid TAR

- Patients may be deemed inappropriate candidates for a robotic abdominal wall reconstruction if they have multiple or large pieces of mesh that need to be removed, fascial defects that can be challenging to close with the robot, or voluminous hernia sacs or disfiguring scars that will require extensive soft tissue resection.
- Halka et al have described a hybrid approach where the lysis of adhesions, retromuscular dissection, and transversus abdominus release are done utilizing the robotic platform.[9]
- Upon completion and closure of the preperitoneal pocket, a midline laparotomy is made. The midline laparotomy incision is typically notably shorter in length than if the case were to be approached from an open incision at the outset.
- The midline laparotomy facilitates removal of any mesh, implantation of large pieces of mesh for reinforcement, fascial closure, as well as hernia sac debridement.
- The hybrid approach may still confer a decreased length of stay and decreased postoperative narcotic. When compared with the purely robotic approach a hybrid approach was also associated with a lower rate of surgical site occurrences.

Extended Totally Extraperitoneal TAR

- When performing a robotic TAR, one must close the two leaflets of the posterior sheath as well as close peritoneal defects made by placing trocars through the abdominal wall to perform the dissection. One method to mitigate this is to utilize an extended view totally extraperitoneal approach.
- This technique extrapolates the anatomic planes utilized during a totally extraperitoneal inguinal hernia repair to complex midline defects. This approach, described by Belyansky et al, utilizes port placement into the retromuscular plane. Dissection of the ipsilateral retromuscular plane is performed using a laparoscope and a combination of blunt dissection and cautery.
- The surgeon then uses a "crossover" technique to arrive at the contralateral retromuscular plane by incising just deep to the linea alba and dissecting in the preperitoneal space to the contralateral rectus muscle where the posterior sheath of the contralateral rectus muscle is incised to connect both retromuscular spaces.[10]
- It is of utmost importance to preserve the linea alba without disruption, as inadvertent injuries to the linea alba in this portion of the dissection will result in further hernia creation.
- Once the retromuscular dissection has been completed, the surgeon can then continue with the transversus abdominis release as described above. This approach eliminates holes made in the peritoneum from the trocars and can potentially eliminate the closure of the two posterior sheath leaflets if no holes are made during the dissection.

PEARLS AND PITFALLS

- The retromuscular dissection is complete when the neurovascular bundles and inferior epigastric vessel have been identified.
- Working lateral to medial allows for the pneumoperitoneum to provide retraction and facilitate dissection.
- The surgeon must be consciously aware of the location of the neurovascular bundles and ensure all division of the transversus abdominis occurs medial to this to prevent injuries to the linea semilunaris.
- Contralateral port placement should allow for at least 10 cm from the defect edge to the port to optimize visualization for defect closure.
- Crossing over midline in the space of Retzius facilitates the contralateral posterior sheath dissection and transversus abdominis release.
- The posterior sheath should be able to be closed without tension. If this is not possible, insufflation pressure should be decreased and the surgeon should perform more dissection laterally; however, if there is still tension, the surgeon should consider converting to an open procedure.

POSTOPERATIVE CARE

- Patients are instructed to wear a binder postoperatively, which may help minimize postoperative pain and provide some sense of protection to the hernia repair.
- We routinely start clears on postoperative day 0, and their diet is advanced as the patient is able to tolerate.
- We aim to minimize postoperative narcotics. As part of our enhanced recovery after surgery protocol, patients are given scheduled Tylenol as well as Gabapentin for postoperative pain. In addition, transversus abdominus plane blocks are administered to help minimize narcotic usage.
- Patient-controlled analgesia pumps are avoided where possible, in favor of oral narcotic pain medication when needed. Patients are discharged home when they are tolerating a diet and their pain is controlled on an oral pain regimen. The drain is removed when the output is less than 50 mL/d.

COMPLICATIONS

- Adhesiolysis should be performed without cautery, and the surgeon must ensure that is done with the utmost caution. Missed bowel injuries present with postoperative leukocytosis, severe abdominal pain, tachycardia, and fevers. Surgeons

should have a low threshold to obtain imaging or return to the operating room (OR) to evaluate patients with these symptoms.
- If there is an enterotomy identified upon return to the OR, the mesh should be explanted and primary defect closure should be performed.
- The large retromuscular space does create the potential for large hematomas to develop. These may originate from periumbilical perforators, branches of the inferior epigastric vessels, or the epigastric vessels themselves. If a retromuscular drain is placed, its output can help identify ongoing bleeding, which may necessitate operative intervention.
- Management of postoperative hematomas is dependent on the size and stability of the patient. Unstable patients or those with significant ongoing blood loss should return to the OR. Smaller hematomas in stable patients may be managed expectantly if the patient remains stable and asymptomatic.
- If a hematoma necessitates return to the OR, a laparoscopic approach may be feasible and the clot can be evacuated, and the retroperitoneal space drained.
- Dehiscence of the posterior sheath closure can result in an intraparietal hernia (**FIGURE 10**). This can be challenging to diagnose as the anterior sheath and mesh are closed so the patient may not have a significant bulge on examination. In the early postoperative period these may present with an early postoperative bowel obstruction and patients should be evaluated with cross-sectional imaging to exclude this potential complication.
- Division of the transversus abdominis lateral to the neurovascular bundles results in an injury to the linea semilunaris (**FIGURE 11**). This often presents as a lateral complication as the patient may note lateral bulges to their abdominal wall. These injuries are characterized by cross-sectional imaging.

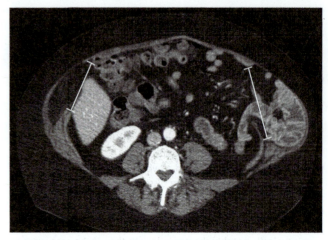

FIGURE 11 • Linea Semilunaris Injury: Division of the transversus abdominis muscle lateral to the neurovascular bundles can result in an injury to the linea semilunaris (marked with bars). This detaches the oblique muscles from the rectus muscle creating a lateral hernia.

Repairing these injuries is technically challenging as patients will require a redo component separation and reattachment of the oblique muscles to the rectus muscles. This injury can be prevented by ensuring the neurovascular bundles are identified and the transversus abdominis is divided medial to these.

OUTCOMES

- Robotic transversus abdominis release may be associated with improved postoperative pain and decreased length of stay when compared with an open approach.[5,6]
- The ideal candidates for this approach are patients who have defects between 7 and 15 cm width or patients with an inadequate retromuscular space to accommodate appropriate mesh overlap. Patients with defects wider than 15 cm or those that require extensive soft tissue revision should be evaluated for their candidacy for a hybrid TAR as these patients may still benefit from the robot despite the additional midline incision.[9]
- Surgeons on the learning curve for these operations should prepare by gaining familiarity with surgical anatomy and operative steps and should have a reasonable threshold for converting to an open approach if there is concern for the integrity of the closure.

REFERENCES

1. Beldi G, Ipaktchi R, Wagner M, Gloor B, Candinas D. Laparoscopic ventral hernia repair is safe and cost effective. *Surg Endosc*. 2006;20(1):92-95. Epub 2005 Dec 7. PMID: 16333538. doi: 10.1007/s00464-005-0442-9
2. Novitsky YW, Elliott HL, Orenstein SB, Rosen MJ. Transversus abdominis muscle release: a novel approach to posterior component separation during complex abdominal wall reconstruction. *Am J Surg*. 2012;204(5):709-716. Epub 2012 May 16. PMID: 22607741. doi: 10.1016/j.amjsurg.2012.02.008
3. Belyansky I, Zahiri HR, Park A. Laparoscopic transversus abdominis release, a novel minimally invasive approach to complex abdominal wall reconstruction. *Surg Innov*. 2016;23(2):134-141. Epub 2015 Nov 24. PMID: 26603694. doi: 10.1177/1553350615618290

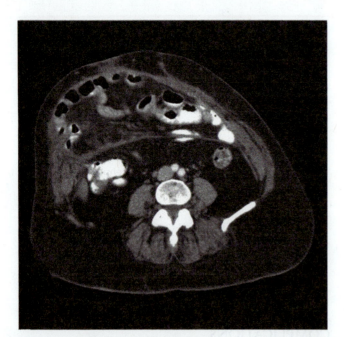

FIGURE 10 • Intraparietal Hernia: Tension on the closure of the posterior sheath can result in dehiscence of this layer creating an intraparietal hernia. These are technically challenging to repair as there is uncoated mesh adherent to bowel as well as the patient already has had a posterior component separation.

4. Warren JA, Cobb WS, Ewing JA, Carbonell AM. Standard laparoscopic versus robotic retromuscular ventral hernia repair. *Surg Endosc*. 2017;31(1):324-332. Epub 2016 Jun 10. PMID: 27287903. doi: 10.1007/s00464-016-4975-x

5. Bittner IVth JG, Alrefai S, Vy M, Mabe M, Del Prado PAR, Clingempeel NL. Comparative analysis of open and robotic transversus abdominis release for ventral hernia repair. *Surg Endosc*. 2018;32(2):727-734. Epub 2017 Jul 20. PMID: 28730275. doi: 10.1007/s00464-017-5729-0

6. Martin-Del-Campo LA, Weltz AS, Belyansky I, Novitsky YW. Comparative analysis of perioperative outcomes of robotic versus open transversus abdominis release. *Surg Endosc*. 2018;32(2):840-845. Epub 2017 Jul 21. PMID: 28733746. doi: 10.1007/s00464-017-5752-1

7. Love MW, Warren JA, Davis S, et al. Computed tomography imaging in ventral hernia repair: can we predict the need for myofascial release? *Hernia*. 2021;25(2):471-477. Epub 2020 Apr 10. PMID: 32277369. doi: 10.1007/s10029-020-02181-y

8. Weltz AS, Sibia US, Zahiri HR, Schoeneborn A, Park A, Belyansky I. Operative outcomes after open abdominal wall reconstruction with retromuscular mesh fixation using fibrin glue *versus* transfascial sutures. *Am Surg*. 2017;83(9):937-942. PMID: 28958271.

9. Halka JT, Vasyluk A, Demare A, Iacco A, Janczyk R. Hybrid robotic-assisted transversus abdominis release versus open transversus abdominis release: a comparison of short-term outcomes. *Hernia*. 2019;23(1):37-42. Epub 2018 Nov 19. PMID: 30456551. doi: 10.1007/s10029-018-1858-1

10. Belyansky I, Daes J, Radu VG, et al. A novel approach using the enhanced-view totally extraperitoneal (eTEP) technique for laparoscopic retromuscular hernia repair. *Surg Endosc*. 2018;32(3):1525-1532. Epub 2017 Sep 15. PMID: 28916960. doi: 10.1007/s00464-017-5840-2

Chapter 27 Parastomal Hernia

Melissa M. Alvarez-Downing and Susan M. Cera

DEFINITION
- Parastomal hernia is defined as an incisional hernia which occurs at the site of or immediately adjacent to an existing ostomy.

DIFFERENTIAL DIAGNOSIS
- Abdominal wall mass (tumor, hematoma, abscess)
- Eventration of the abdominal wall

PATIENT HISTORY AND PHYSICAL FINDINGS
- A thorough history should be obtained to determine the timeframe of onset, severity of symptoms, and degree of size change. Patients should also be questioned about their satisfaction with stoma site location because relocation is an option for repair of parastomal hernia.
- The most common symptoms associated with an uncomplicated parastomal hernia include bulging near the stoma that worsens with activity and difficulty of adherence of the stoma wafer due to irregularities and bulging of the skin surface. The results are frequent leakages and skin excoriation. In addition, patients complain of the associated expense of increased appliance/wafer usage. Occasionally, wafer leakage may be the presenting complaint and parastomal hernia should be included in the differential diagnosis.
- Other symptoms associated with a complication of the parastomal hernia (obstruction, incarceration, and strangulation) include abdominal pain, decreased ostomy output, cramping, nausea, or vomiting.
- Characteristic findings on physical examination will render the diagnosis of parastomal hernia in most patients. Examination should be performed with the stoma wafer off with the patient in both the supine and standing positions. The patient should be asked to perform a Valsalva maneuver. A characteristic bulge adjacent to the stoma site will be present and confirmed with digital palpation (**FIGURE 1**). A search for concomitant hernias should be undertaken, especially at previous laparotomy scars, because these can occur in up to 41% of patients.[1]
- Abdominal tenderness or skin discoloration associated with a nonreducible hernia is indicative of incarceration and/or strangulation and requires urgent/emergent intervention.

IMAGING AND OTHER DIAGNOSTIC STUDIES
- Computed tomography (CT) scan of the abdomen and pelvis performed with intravenous (IV) and oral contrast can confirm the presence of a hernia and help guide operative intervention (**FIGURE 2A** and **B**). Having the patient perform Valsalva during the CT may unmask a hernia and/or reveal the true extent of the hernia. The use of oral contrast will assist in identification of partial or complete obstruction associated with the hernia. The CT scan will also aid in the identification of other associated hernias, that is, at the site of previous laparotomy scars. The size of the neck of the hernia is important and is especially useful in determining the size of the mesh needed in cases where it will be used in the repair. Knowing the contents of the hernia sac (omentum, small bowel, large bowel) preoperatively aids in minimizing bowel injury during surgery because the peritoneum of the hernia sac and bowel serosa can appear similar during dissection. In addition, the planes between the hernia sac and intestine are often distorted by adhesions.

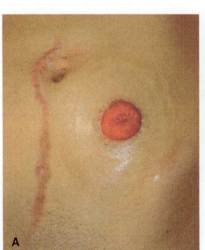
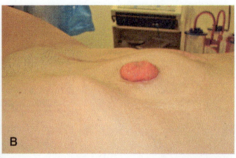

FIGURE 1 • **A** and **B**, Characteristic parastomal bulge seen on physical examination in a patient with a parastomal hernia.

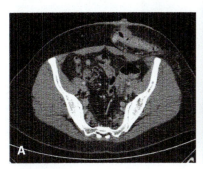
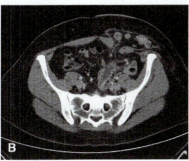

FIGURE 2 • **A** and **B**, Computed tomography images demonstrating a parastomal hernia with bowel present in the hernia sac at and below the level of the colostomy.

- If the stoma was created for inflammatory bowel disease, thorough evaluation of the entire gastrointestinal tract to evaluate for active disease that may necessitate surgical intervention at the time of the hernia repair is warranted. In addition to endoscopic examinations (see below), radiologic testing may include barium small bowel follow-through and capsule endoscopy.

SURGICAL MANAGEMENT
Preoperative Planning
- Patients should be counseled that parastomal hernia is the most frequent complication following the construction of a stoma and can occur in up to 50% of patients because the stoma itself creates a weakened area in the abdominal wall.[2]
- Patients should also be counseled on the various techniques/options available for treatment. Nonsurgical options are appropriate for asymptomatic patients and include use of a hernia belt (secured to the stoma wafer) or an abdominal binder. Surgical intervention is reserved for an enlarging hernia or those associated with symptoms or decreased quality of life because of inadequate stoma pouching. If surgical intervention is considered, the choice of procedure should be tailored to the individuals' life expectancy, operative risk/benefit analysis, degree of physiologic function (which often corresponds to the degree of weakness of the abdominal wall and ability to successfully sustain repair), and risk of recurrence.
- Type of surgical technique chosen is based on patient factors, surgeon experience, and safety of laparoscopic approach.
- Risk of initial occurrence and recurrence after repair is associated with obesity and/or weight gain, smoking, emergent intervention, poor nutritional status, immunosuppression, infection, and persistent underlying malignancy or inflammatory bowel disease.
- Informed consent should include a possibility of conversion to open in laparoscopic procedures and possible placement of a mesh, particularly in large hernia repairs.
- If stoma relocation is planned, preoperative stoma marking for a new stoma site is an important step. Consultation with a stoma nurse is advised. Stoma relocation may include placing the stoma in either of the upper quadrants as opposed to the lower quadrants because less tangential pressure is generated in the upper abdominal wall. This type of placement is also beneficial in morbidly obese patients with a large abdominal wall pannus. Additionally, it is important to explain to patients that the new ostomy site is associated with the same risk of hernia formation.[3]
- In morbidly obese patients, preoperative weight loss can assist with durability of parastomal hernia repair.
- Colonoscopy/ileoscopy should be performed to ensure no concomitant lesions are present, which would require simultaneous surgical resection. This can be performed the day prior to planned hernia repair so that the patient can undergo a single bowel preparation.
- After obtaining appropriate preoperative medical clearance, a standard bowel preparation with an isoosmotic lavage (polyethylene glycol solution) and oral antibiotics is used for parastomal hernias associated with colostomy. Bowel preparation is not needed for paraileostomy hernias. These patients are instructed to take a liquid diet the day prior to surgery. As with all abdominal surgery, perioperative IV antibiotics should be administered within 1 hour prior to incision and routine venous thromboprophylaxis should be instituted.

Positioning
- The patient is placed in a modified lithotomy position (**FIGURE 3**) for all cases whether open or laparoscopic because of the possibility of encountering extensive adhesions, which may require surgeon repositioning between the patient's legs. The arm on the working side (opposite the stoma and hernia) should be abducted. Securing the patient to the operative table with use of a bean bag and safety strap or silk tape across the chest is recommended to allow for rotational adjustment during the procedure if laparoscopic approach is planned.
- After induction of general anesthesia, a nasogastric and sterile indwelling bladder catheter are placed. A nasogastric tube (NGT) and inpatient hospitalization is advocated for larger hernia repairs to prevent postoperative vomiting that may result in immediate postoperative disruption of the repair.

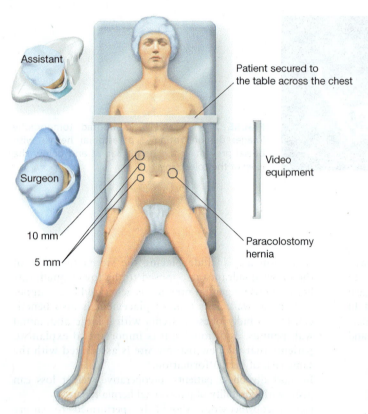

FIGURE 3 • Lithotomy position and positioning of surgeon and assistant.

STOMA RELOCATION

Existing Ostomy

- The new planned stoma site is marked prior to the procedure either during consultation with a stoma nurse or with a pen in the preoperative holding area and an 18-gauge needle after induction of anesthesia.
- A circumferential parastomal incision is made to isolate the stoma from the skin and subcutaneous tissue.
- Dissection is then carried down to the fascia identifying the hernia, reducing its contents, and excising the hernia sac. The bowel is placed into the abdomen using a marking stitch to easily retrieve it when necessary.

Division of Adhesions

- Lysis of adhesions is performed through the stoma site circumferentially and under direct vision. Placement of a wound protector and use of a headlight will facilitate visualization and adhesiolysis.

Relocation of the Ostomy

- Two fingers are now placed into the wound and underneath the abdominal wall to the new stoma site. A disk of skin is removed at the new stoma site. The anterior fascia and rectus muscle is divided vertically, directly over the fingers underneath the abdominal wall. The ostomy site is dilated two fingerbreadths. Using a Babcock clamp, the previously mobilized stoma is passed via the abdominal cavity and brought up through the new fascial opening. Care should be taken to ensure there is no twisting, rotation, or undue tension of the bowel mesentery.
- If extensive adhesions are found or the bowel does not reach the new stoma site, exploratory laparotomy may be necessary.
- A Babcock clamp should be left on the bowel at the new stoma site to prevent it from slipping back into the abdominal cavity until stoma maturation (final step).

Hernia Repair

- The hernia at the old stoma site is repaired by approximating the fascial edges with interrupted nonabsorbable sutures (0 Ethibond). Use of a prosthetic or biologic mesh should be done to ensure adequate closure, especially for fascial defects greater than 4 cm due to the high failure rate with primary repair.[3]

Closure

- If a midline laparotomy was made, it is closed with running 0-polydioxanone (PDS) sutures.
- The skin edges are reapproximated with running 4-0 Monocryl sutures or skin staples.
- The new stoma is matured with interrupted 3-0 chromic sutures and a stoma appliance is placed.

OPEN UNDERLAY TECHNIQUE (MODIFIED SUGARBAKER TECHNIQUE)

Exploratory Laparotomy and Lysis of Adhesions

- The abdomen is prepped, and a sterile 4 × 4 gauze is placed over the existing stoma. Ioban is included in the draping to keep the stoma covered but in the operative field.
- A midline incision is made and lysis of adhesions is performed. Caution should be used when dissecting in the vicinity of the stoma (which is why it is visually kept in the operative field).
- The stoma itself is not typically mobilized for this procedure unless the patient is unsatisfied with the extent of the brooking. In this case, the stoma can be mobilized and rebrooked, and the hernia repair should be performed with a biologic mesh to reduce mesh infection.

Hernia Repair

- Once the proximal bowel of the stoma is freed from surrounding adhesions, the hernia sac is resected and the hernia contents are reduced.
- A dual-sided expanded polytetrafluoroethylene (ePTFE, Gore-Tex DualMesh Biomaterial, WL Grove Associates, Newark, DE, USA) or biologic mesh is selected based on the size of the fascial defect, ensuring there is at least 4 cm additional reach on all sides.
- A precise keyhole incision is made in the mesh, making certain the central opening is small enough to only allow passage of the bowel to the stoma. The mesh is placed around the stoma on the undersurface of the abdominal wall and the ends are secured to itself (**FIGURE 4**). Placement of mesh above the fascia (onlay technique) or into the abdominal wall defect (inlay technique) has been abandoned because of high failure rates.[4]
- The mesh is sutured to the anterior abdominal wall using interrupted 0-Vicryl sutures. Additional sutures made of 2-0 Prolene may be passed through the entire abdominal wall ensuring no migration of the mesh, although this is not necessary because the stoma itself anchors it in place.

Closure

- The midline fascia is closed using running 0-PDS suture.
- The skin edges are reapproximated with running 4-0 Monocryl sutures or skin staples.

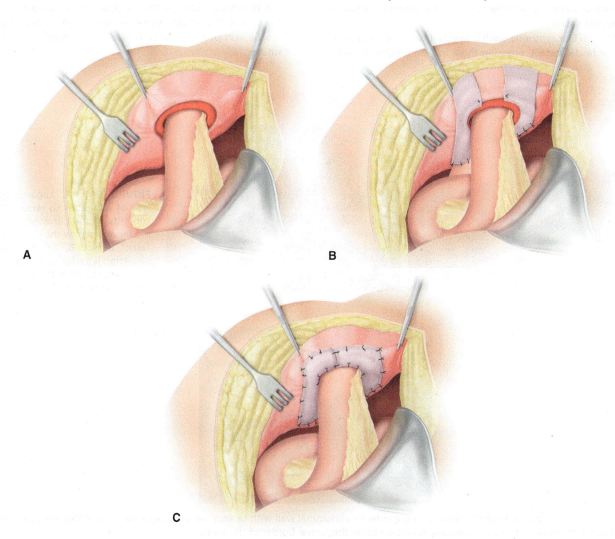

FIGURE 4 • **A-C,** Example of mesh placement in the open underlay technique. A precise keyhole incision is made in the mesh to ensure the central opening is small enough to only allow passage of the bowel of the stoma. The mesh is placed around the stoma on the undersurface of the abdominal wall and secured to the anterior abdominal wall and the ends to itself.

LAPAROSCOPIC MESH UNDERLAY TECHNIQUE

Entering the Abdominal Cavity

- A 10-mm subcostal incision is made on the side opposite of the stoma. Direct access is gained and a port is placed into the abdominal cavity. Pneumoperitoneum is achieved, and inspection of the abdominal cavity is performed to assess if a laparoscopic approach is both feasible and safe.
- Two additional 5-mm ports are placed under direct visualization laterally according to **FIGURE 3**.

Lysis of Adhesions

- Laparoscopic lysis of adhesions and reduction of the hernia sac and contents is performed (**FIGURE 5**). Careful dissection should be performed sharply with gentle countertraction to ensure no injury occurs to the bowel.

Hernia Repair

- The fascial defect is measured using a spinal needle passed intra-abdominally and by marking the external abdomen appropriately.
- An ePTFE or synthetic mesh is selected based on the size of the fascial defect, ensuring there is 4-cm additional reach on all sides. Permanent 0-0 sutures are placed on all four sides and the mesh is rolled up and introduced into the abdomen via the 10-mm port. A 5-mm camera should be used in an ipsilateral port to insert the mesh under direct visualization.
- The mesh is unrolled in the abdominal cavity ensuring correct orientation. The previously placed sutures are brought through the abdominal wall using stab incisions and a suture passer.
- A mechanical fixation device, for example, ProTack (Covidien, Mansfield, MA, USA), is used to place tacks around the circumference of the mesh to ensure no bowel can herniate between the mesh and the abdominal wall (**FIGURE 6**). Additional Prolene sutures are placed 2 cm apart through the abdominal wall around the mesh, except for the side of the mesh through which the bowel to the stoma passes.

Closure

- Once the mesh has been secured in place, the ports are removed under direct visualization and pneumoperitoneum is released. A 0-Vicryl suture is used to close the fascia of the 10-mm port site. 4-0 Monocryl sutures are used to close the skin at all port sites. Adhesive tape or glue can be used on the skin of the small stab incisions created to pass the sutures.

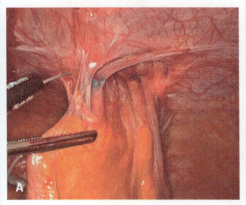
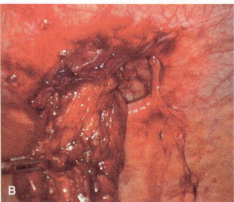

FIGURE 5 • **A,** Laparoscopic lysis of adhesions to reduce the contents of the parastomal hernia sac and define the size of the fascial defect. **B,** Careful sharp dissection is performed with gentle countertraction to ensure no injury occurs to the bowel wall.

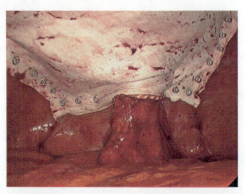

FIGURE 6 • Underlay mesh (ePTFE) secured to the anterior abdominal wall with tackers placed using a mechanical fixation device in a laparoscopic approach. The existing ostomy is visible exiting the lateral border of the mesh.

PEARLS AND PITFALLS

Indications	▪ Parastomal hernia repair should be undertaken only in patients who are symptomatic and/or with quality-of-life issues. Relocation is reserved for those who wish more desirable stoma location.
Preoperative planning	▪ Preoperative imaging is important to assess the extent of the parastomal hernia as well as address any confounding factors. ▪ When considering relocating a stoma, preoperative stoma marking is essential.
Type of hernia repair	▪ Open vs laparoscopic approach without stoma relocation is based on surgeon experience and comfort with laparotomy. Minimally invasive approach offers faster recovery and less pain.
Lysis of adhesions	▪ When performing lysis of adhesions, it is important to take extra caution around the stoma.
Hernia repair	▪ Primary closure of the hernia site should only be undertaken in hernias <4 cm in size. In patients with larger hernias, use of a mesh for repair will improve success rates. ▪ It is important to ensure the keyhole incision made in the mesh is exact to only allow passage of the stoma, therefore preventing future herniation at this site.

POSTOPERATIVE CARE

- Perioperative antibiotics can be administered during the first 24 hours after surgery.
- For small hernia repairs, diet can be resumed and the patient can be discharged after the recovery room. In most cases, however, the extent of the lysis of adhesions dictates at minimal inpatient observation and possibly an NGT until the ileus resolves.
- Patients should be encouraged to avoid heavy lifting and strenuous activity for 4 weeks following surgery.

OUTCOMES

- Long-term durability of parastomal hernia repair is variable, with recurrence rates reported in up to 50% of patients.[5] Although some studies have suggested that stoma relocation is superior to fascial repair, both approaches carry a high recurrence rate (33% vs 75%) because neither addresses the underlying pathophysiology driving hernia formation.[3] To address this, use of a mesh to aid in repair has been employed and dramatically reduces hernia recurrence rate to 16%, with no difference between synthetic and biologic mesh.[6,7] Additionally, mesh infection rates are similar, therefore making the less expensive synthetic mesh a more favorable option.[7]
- Mesh repair performed in a laparoscopic approach offers the best results, with a low recurrence rate of 6.6% and an ability to identify additional hernias not evident clinically.[1,6,8]
- Addressing patient risk factors such as obesity, nutritional status, immunosuppression, and comorbid conditions can aid in overall repair success.

COMPLICATIONS

- Postoperative wound infection
- Ileus
- Enterotomy
- Obstruction
- Recurrent hernia

REFERENCES

1. Hansson BM, Morales-Conde S, Mussack T, et al. The laparoscopic modified Sugarbaker technique is safe and has a low recurrence rate: a multicenter cohort study. *Surg Endosc.* 2013;27:494-500.
2. Carne PW, Robertson GM, Frizelle FA. Parastomal hernia. *Br J Surg.* 2003;90(7):784-793.
3. Rubin MS, Schoetz DJ, Matthews JB. Parastomal hernia: is stoma relocation superior to fascial repair? *Arch Surg.* 1994;129:413-419.
4. Hawn MT, Snyder CW, Graham LA, et al. Long-term follow-up of technical outcomes for incisional hernia repair. *J Am Coll Surg.* 2010;210(5):648-657.
5. Hotouras A, Murphy J, Thaha M, et al. The persistent challenge of parastomal herniation: a review of the literature and future developments. *Colorectal Dis.* 2013;15(5):202-214.
6. Hansson BM, Slater NJ, van der Velden AS, et al. Surgical techniques for parastomal hernia repair: a systematic review of the literature. *Ann Surg.* 2012;255(4):685-695.
7. Slater NJ, Hansson BM, Buyne OR, et al. Repair of parastomal hernias with biologic grafts: a systematic review. *J Gastrointest Surg.* 2011;15:1252-1258.
8. Berger D, Bientzle M. Laparoscopic repair of parastomal hernias: a single surgeon's experience in 66 patients. *Dis Colon Rectum.* 2007;50:1668-1673.

Chapter 28 Umbilical, Epigastric, Spigelian, and Lumbar Hernias

Andrew T. Strong and Jin Soo Yoo

DEFINITION

- A primary ventral hernia is an abnormal protrusion of the contents of the abdominal cavity or of preperitoneal fat through a defect in the abdominal wall, whether the defect is congenital, spontaneous (acquired), or the result of prior surgical incision.[1]
- An umbilical hernia is a primary ventral hernia with its center at the umbilicus.
- An epigastric hernia is a primary ventral hernia in the midline between the umbilicus and the xiphoid.
- A spigelian hernia is a primary ventral hernia in the area of the fascia spigelian aponeurosis.
- A lumbar hernia is a primary ventral hernia in the lumbar region.
- In contrast to umbilical and epigastric hernias, the hernia sac of a spigelian hernia or lumbar hernia is covered with an intact layer of abdominal wall muscle. For spigelian hernias, this is the external oblique muscle, and for lumbar hernias, the latissimus dorsi muscle (**FIGURE 1**).
- Primary ventral hernias are classified according to the location and diameter of the hernia defect as shown in **FIGURE 2**.[2]
- Groin hernias may be classified according to a similar schema,[3] shown in **FIGURE 3**.

DIFFERENTIAL DIAGNOSIS

- Subcutaneous lesions at the site where primary ventral hernias occur, such as lipomas, sebaceous cysts, lymph nodes, metastatic lesions, and trocar site metastasis.
  - Caveat: Epigastric lipoma: In a patient with a clinical subcutaneous lipoma near the midline above the umbilicus, an epigastric hernia should always be suspected.
- Abdominal wall tumors: desmoid tumors (or fibromatosis), soft tissue sarcoma, metastatic lesions.
  - Caveat: A "Sister Mary Joseph's nodule" is an umbilical swelling that might be mistaken for an umbilical hernia but is the manifestation of intraperitoneal carcinomatosis.
- Secondary ventral hernias: incisional hernia, trocar site hernia, and recurrent ventral hernias after previous repair.
- Parastomal hernias and ventral hernias resulting from enlargement of the aperture made in the abdominal wall during creation of a colostomy, ileostomy, ileal conduit, or other stoma.

PATIENT HISTORY AND PHYSICAL FINDINGS

- Symptoms can range from an asymptomatic presentation to acute incarceration with bowel obstruction and/or strangulation.
- Many small umbilical or epigastric hernias are asymptomatic, and often, the patient is not even aware of having a small abdominal wall defect.
- A bulge or swelling is often the first sign of a hernia. This swelling is often present for a long period and gradually increases in size (**FIGURE 4**).
- The presence of a reducible swelling, enlarging when straining (Valsalva maneuver), is pathognomonic for an abdominal wall hernia, but not all hernias are reducible and can hinder the clinical diagnosis in those hernias.
- The swelling of an epigastric hernia is often mistaken for a subcutaneous lipoma.
- Hernia defect size and pain intensity are not well correlated. Small hernias can cause a sharp pain, whereas umbilical hernias can be quite large without significant pain. The pain is caused by herniation of abdominal contents or of preperitoneal fat through the defect.
- For some hernias that are not palpable, such as spigelian hernias, abdominal wall pain can be the first presenting symptom and diagnosis might only be possible by imaging.
- Acute pain due to incarceration of intestines or omentum is intense and sharp. Incarceration can be intermittent and resolve by lying down and manual compression of

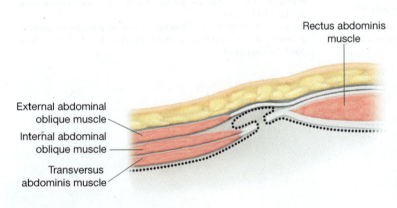

FIGURE 1 • Spigelian hernias are defects of the insertion of the transversus abdominis muscle and/or internal oblique muscle to the lateral border of the rectus muscle sheath (the spigelian aponeurosis). The external oblique muscle covers the hernia sac superficially.

Chapter 28 UMBILICAL, EPIGASTRIC, SPIGELIAN, AND LUMBAR HERNIAS

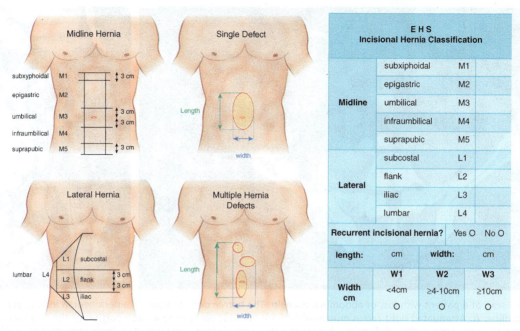

FIGURE 2 • Classification schema for ventral and incisional hernias, using a description for either midline or lateral hernias, position relative to the umbilicus and maximal width and length. For multiple or "Swiss cheese" defects the total length is from the top of the uppermost defect to the bottom of the lowermost defect, and width is measured to the further lateral extent of any defect. (Image and table modified by permission from the Springer: Muysoms FE, Miserez M, Berrevoet F, et al. Classification of primary and incisional abdominal wall hernias. *Hernia.* 2009;13(4):407-414.)

P = primary hernia
R = recurrent hernia

0 = no hernia detectable
1 = < 1.5 cm (one finger width)
2 = < 3 cm (two finger width)
3 = > 3 cm (more than two finger width)
x = not investigated

L = lateral / indirect hernia
M = medial / direct hernia
F = Femoral hernia

FIGURE 3 • Classification scheme for inguinal hernias. (Modified by permission from Springer: Miserez M, Alexandre JH, Campanelli G, et al. The European Hernia Society groin hernia classification: simple and easy to remember. *Hernia.* 2007;11(2):113-116.)

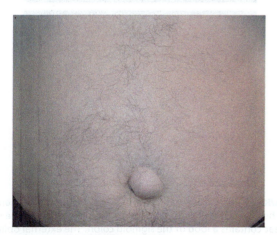

FIGURE 4 • Typical clinical presentation of an umbilical hernia with an umbilical swelling increasing in standing position and while straining (Valsalva maneuver).

the hernia sac and contents. Reduction of an incarcerated hernia allows the patient to be operated on electively after appropriate preoperative workup. If manual reduction is not possible, an emergency operation to reduce the hernia is indicated.

- Intestinal obstruction and associated vomiting due to incarcerated small bowel sometimes is the primary presentation in patients who have a subclinical hernia. In obese patients and for spigelian or lumbar hernias, the incarcerated hernia is sometimes not clinically visible or palpable.
- Late presentation of an incarcerated hernia includes sepsis from bowel ischemia and intestinal perforation. This can evolve into peritonitis or enterocutaneous fistula.
- Large hernias may be chronically incarcerated and lead to a "loss of domain" wherein the majority (>50%) of abdominal contents exist outside the normal contours of the abdominal cavity (**FIGURE 5**).

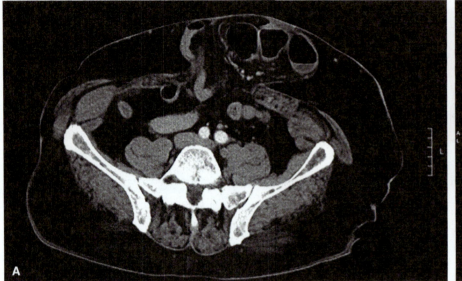
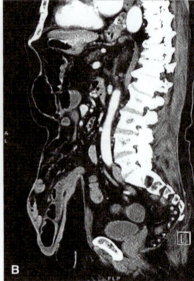

FIGURE 5 • CT scan of a patient with loss of abdominal domain. The hernia defect began as a paramedian incisional hernia but now includes the midline. **A**, Attenuated right rectus muscle with the hernia sac containing a large portion of the small bowel. **B**, Sagittal section demonstrating multiple midline defects and hernia sacs that contain large portions of multiple segments of small bowel.

IMAGING AND OTHER DIAGNOSTIC STUDIES

- For diagnosis of an umbilical or epigastric hernia, clinical examination is sufficient for the majority of patients. Imaging is not needed for most patients.
- Imaging with ultrasound or computed tomography (CT) scan can be helpful to measure the hernia defect size in irreducible hernias or obese patients. Sometimes the size of the hernia defect will influence the therapeutic approach, for example, open or laparoscopic technique.
- For spigelian and lumbar hernias, imaging with ultrasound or CT scan is often needed to make the diagnosis: spigelian hernia (**FIGURE 6**), lumbar hernia (**FIGURE 7**).
- CT scan imaging of the abdominal wall allows sizing the defect to see the hernia sac contents and to detect signs of intestinal obstruction.

SURGICAL MANAGEMENT

- Small primary umbilical, epigastric, or lumbar hernias do not require an operation, unless they are painful or increase in size or repair is desired for cosmesis. For spigelian hernias, a surgical repair is indicated even for asymptomatic patients because they hold an increased risk of incarceration compared with the other primary ventral hernias.
- Current guidelines recommend mesh for repair of primary ventral umbilical hernias. However, given little evidence for repair of hernias with defects smaller than 1 cm, suture-only repair is an acceptable alternative to mesh.[4] For inguinal hernias and incisional hernias, the current recommendation is to use mesh in all patients because of the proven decrease in recurrences. Recurrent umbilical or epigastric hernias should be repaired using a mesh prosthesis, as they are considered to be incisional hernias.
- The mesh used to repair abdominal wall hernias can be placed at different positions in relation to the abdominal wall layers. Five positions can be defined: onlay, inlay, retromuscular, preperitoneal, and intraperitoneal (**FIGURE 8**).
- Laparoscopic repair of ventral hernias, when feasible, is associated with a lower rate of perioperative wound complications, with similar operative times and recurrence rates.[5]

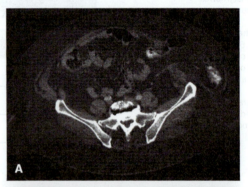
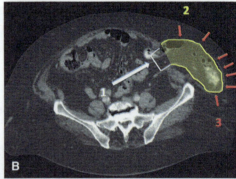

FIGURE 6 • **A**, CT of a patient with a left-sided spigelian hernia. The hernia defect is located lateral to the rectus sheath. The hernia sac contains a loop of the sigmoid colon. The external oblique muscle covers the hernia sac. **B**, 1 (white) The hernia defect in the abdominal wall muscles just lateral to the recuts sheath. 2 (yellow) The hernia sac with a sigmoid colon loop. 3 (red) The intact external oblique muscle covers the hernia sac.

Chapter 28 UMBILICAL, EPIGASTRIC, SPIGELIAN, AND LUMBAR HERNIAS 237

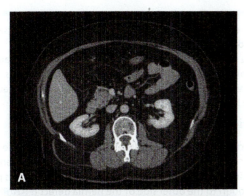

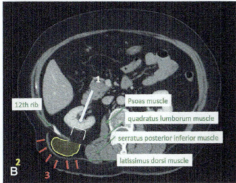

FIGURE 7 • A, CT of a patient with a right-sided lumbar hernia. The hernia defect is located lateral to the quadratus lumborum muscle. The hernia contains some retroperitoneal fat. The latissimus dorsi muscle covers the hernia sac. B, 1 (white) The hernia defect in the abdominal wall muscles just lateral to the quadratus lumborum muscle. 2 (yellow) The hernia sac with retroperitoneal fatty tissue. 3 (red) The intact latissimus dorsi muscle covers the hernia sac. *Green arrows*: the names of the different muscles involved.

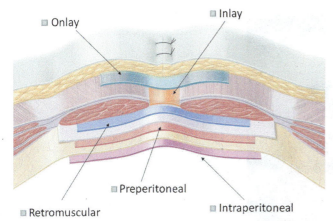

FIGURE 8 • Different positions of the mesh in relation to the abdominal wall layers to repair a ventral hernia by mesh reinforcement. (Reprinted by permission from Springer: Winkler MS, Gerharz E, Dietz UA. Narbenhernienchirurgie. Übersicht und aktuelle Trends. *Urologe*. 2008;47:740-774.)

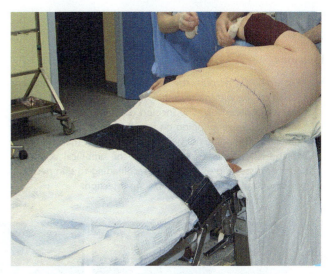

FIGURE 9 • Intraoperative positioning of a patient with a 45° lateral decubitus for open approach of a left-sided lumbar hernia.

Preoperative Planning

- Based on the size and the localization of the hernia, a decision will be made about the preferred approach in the individual patient: mesh or primary repair/open or laparoscopic technique.
- Although some centers perform the repair of small umbilical or epigastric hernias under local anesthesia as a routine, most centers prefer a general anesthesia for the comfort of the patient and the surgeon. Regional anesthesia through a sensory blocking of the anterior abdominal wall, by a transversus abdominis plane block (TAP block), is another less practiced option for postoperative pain control.
- For incarcerated hernias with bowel obstruction, adequate preoperative measures with nasogastric tube suction and rapid sequence intubation should be considered to minimize aspiration risk at the time of induction.
- Preoperative cleaning and disinfection of the umbilicus is helpful in decreasing the bacterial load during the operation.
- Antimicrobial prophylaxis for hernia repairs remains controversial, as hernia repairs are clean operations, with a <2% chance of surgical site infection. Given the low incidence of infection, most randomized controlled trials fail to show a benefit of antimicrobial prophylaxis, but are generally underpowered. As a result, reviews and meta-analyses are similarly inconclusive.[6] Thus, there is weak evidence to suggest a benefit of antimicrobial prophylaxis for clean hernia repairs; however, many surgeons do administer prophylaxis as a matter of routine.

Positioning

- Patients treated for primary ventral hernias are usually positioned in a supine position. Lumbar hernias are positioned in a 90° or 45° lateral decubitus to expose the lumbar region (**FIGURE 9**).
- For laparoscopic approach of ventral hernias, the position of the surgeon and the video equipment is determined by the localization of the hernia. It is important to have a wide lateral accessibility of the abdominal wall, because the trocars are placed very laterally to obtain access to hernias on the midline.

SUTURE REPAIR

Incisions

- For umbilical hernias, the incision of the skin for primary repair can be within the umbilical rim, in order to reduce the scar postoperatively. The incision can be placed either cranial or caudal, depending on the site of the hernia sac. The umbilical rim should not be incised for greater than 180°, due to the risk of devascularization of the umbilical skin after further dissection of the hernia sac, leading to skin necrosis, poor wound healing, and/or wound infection.
- For epigastric, spigelian, or lumbar hernias, the incision will be directly above the hernia.
- The skin is retracted with small retractors (eg, Volkmann, skin hooks, S-retractors), and the subcutaneous layer is incised down to the fascia, exposing one side, cranial or caudal of the hernia defect (**FIGURE 10A**).

Dissection of the Hernia Sac

- Starting at the lateral side of the hernia defect, the hernia sac, usually containing preperitoneal fat and/or omentum, is encircled using a curved hemostat clamp. The clamp is pushed through to the other side of the hernia defect (**FIGURE 10B**).

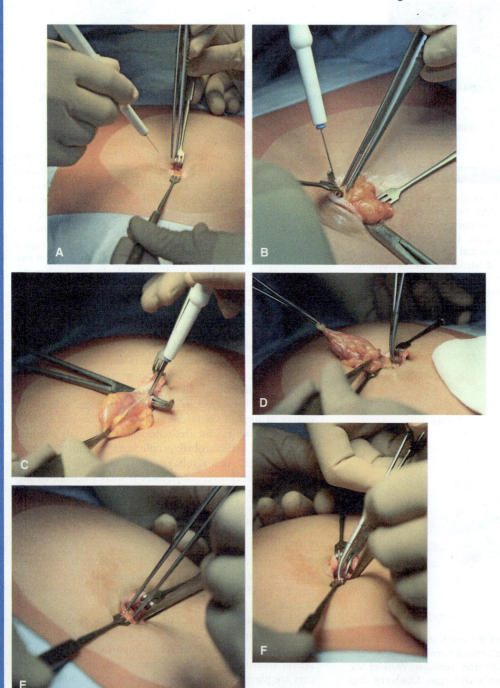

FIGURE 10 • A–F, Intraoperative pictures of an umbilical hernia repair by open approach.

Chapter 28 UMBILICAL, EPIGASTRIC, SPIGELIAN, AND LUMBAR HERNIAS

- The top of the hernia sac is dissected of the umbilical skin, taking care not to injure the skin (**FIGURE 10C**). This will expose the opposite side of the hernia defect (**FIGURE 10D**).

Reduction of the Hernia Sac

- The hernia sac and its contents are reduced through the hernia defect behind the abdominal wall muscles (**FIGURE 10E**). Careful control of hemostasis of the preperitoneal region is performed.
- Sometimes, the contents of the hernia sac are too voluminous to be reduced through the hernia defect. This is often the case in umbilical hernias with herniation of the preperitoneal fat pad, the falciform ligament and/or omentum, and epigastric hernias with preperitoneal fat. In these cases, the herniated fatty tissue may either be ligated and resected or the hernia defect can be enlarged to facilitate reduction of the herniated contents.
- In patients with acutely incarcerated hernias, the hernia sac should be opened and the herniated bowel inspected for viability. If concerns of ischemia, a bowel resection should be considered.

Closure of the Hernia Defect by Primary Closure

- The fascial edges of the defect are identified and isolated from the subcutaneous tissue and from the preperitoneal tissue for 5 to 10 mm (**FIGURE 10F**).
- We close the umbilical and epigastric hernias in a horizontal line. Several options for suturing technique (separate sutures, running suture, or "vest-over-pants" plication sutures) (**FIGURE 11A-C**) and materials (monofilament vs braided sutures; nonabsorbable, slowly absorbable, rapid absorbable) are available.
- Our preference is a braided permanent suture in a closely spaced, interrupted technique. Extrapolating data for the closure of midline laparotomy incisions, a 5-mm distance from the fascial edge and 5-mm distance between sutures is reasonable.

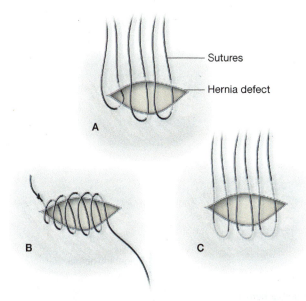

FIGURE 11 • Several techniques are available for closure of the hernia defect. **A**, Closure with separate sutures. **B**, Closure with running sutures. **C**, Closure with a vest-over-pants plication, commonly known as the Mayo Clinic technique.

Closure of the Skin

- The skin is sutured either subcutaneously or with separate superficial sutures.
- A commercially available skin adhesive is typically used to create a watertight barrier.

OPEN MESH REPAIR WITH A FLAT MESH

Incision

- This depends on the localization of the hernia. For umbilical hernias, placing a flat mesh will require an incision that is larger than the incision needed for primary closure or for placement of an umbilical ventral patch. Often, a horizontal omega or inverted omega incision (Ω) is chosen. For epigastric, spigelian, or lumbar hernias, the incision is directly over the hernia sac (**FIGURE 12**).

Dissection of the Hernia Sac and the Hernia Defect

- For umbilical and epigastric hernias, this is similar as for primary hernia repair (**FIGURE 10B-E**).
- For spigelian and lumbar hernias, an intact muscle layer covers the hernia sac. This is why these hernias can become quite large before they become clinically evident. For a spigelian hernia, the overlying external oblique muscle has to be opened to access the hernia sac. The muscle fascia is split in the direction of its fibers, which is from lateral downward in a ±45° angle toward the midline. The hernia sac is thus exposed and contains preperitoneal fat. The sac is reduced underneath the other abdominal wall muscles, and the defect is measured.

Closure of the Hernia Defect and Mesh Augmentation

- Usually in open surgery, the mesh is used to augment the primary fascial closure of the hernia defect. There are several options for positioning the mesh in relation to the abdominal wall as shown in **FIGURE 8**.
- Onlay position: The mesh is positioned on top of the fascia underneath the subcutaneous tissue. After closure of the hernia defect, a dissection of the subcutaneous plane is performed for several centimeters around the defect to allow enough overlap of the mesh beyond the margins of the defect.
- Inlay position: The mesh is placed inside the hernia defect, which is not closed, and the mesh is sutured to the margin of the defect. There is consensus among surgeons that this is not a preferred way to perform a mesh repair because of the lack of overlap between the mesh and the defect. The amount of overlap is considered to be critical to diminish the risk for recurrence. We rarely utilize this technique, except in the presence of a contaminated wound and utilized bioresorbable mesh as a temporizing measure to prevent evisceration and plan a formal repair using a permanent mesh in a staged fashion.

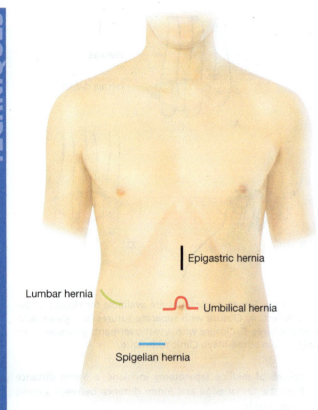

FIGURE 12 • Incisions to perform an open primary ventral hernia repair will depend on the localization of the hernia.

- Retromuscular position for midline hernias: For umbilical and epigastric hernias, the mesh will be placed behind the rectus abdominis muscle and in front of the posterior rectus fascia. To get enough overlap, a dissection in this plane is needed in all directions for several centimeters. In the cranial and caudal direction, this dissection involves incision of the posterior rectus fascia to allow placement of the mesh behind an intact linea alba. The posterior layer of the rectus fascia is closed. The flat mesh is placed in the dissected retromuscular plane. The anterior rectus fascia is closed in front of the mesh.
- Retromuscular position for lateral hernias: For spigelian and lumbar hernias, the mesh is placed behind the intact superficial muscle layer, the external oblique muscle, or the latissimus dorsi muscle, respectively. The mesh is placed on top of the closed hernia defect, on the internal oblique muscle, or on the quadratus lumborum muscle, respectively.
- Preperitoneal position: Another option is to place the mesh behind the posterior rectus fascia, or for lateral hernias, behind the transversus abdominis muscle. The preperitoneal space has to be created by dissecting the peritoneum of the fascia of the deepest abdominal muscle. It is not always easy to develop this plane without creating holes or tears in the peritoneum. These have to be closed if a regular mesh without a protective antiadhesive layer is used.
- Intraperitoneal position: There is a consensus that, if a mesh is placed in the intraperitoneal position, and thus in contact with the intestines, then a composite mesh that includes a protective antiadhesive layer should be used. Unprotected polypropylene or polyester meshes hold an increased risk of causing adhesions and complications such as bowel obstructions, bowel erosions, and fistulae.

Fixation of the Mesh

- Several options for fixation of the mesh are available, depending on the mesh positioning.
- For meshes in an intraperitoneal or preperitoneal position, transabdominal sutures and partial thickness tacks can be used. These sutures will fixate the mesh underneath the abdominal wall muscles.
- Suturing or tacking the mesh to the posterior fascia or muscular layer can hold the meshes in a retromuscular position. Avoiding transabdominal sutures will avoid the pain related to these sutures.
- For a mesh in the onlay position, sutures or tacks can be placed from the mesh to the anterior fascia.
- Fixation with glue, such as a fibrin glue, applied to the surface of the mesh is a first alternative to the use of sutures.
- Another alternative to the sutures is self-fixating meshes. These meshes have a mechanical fixation either with small gripping hooks or by glue impregnated in the mesh, which becomes active in contact with the moisture of the tissues.
- The size of the mesh and the overlap of the mesh beyond the hernia defect are of critical importance to avoid recurrences.

Closure of the Hernia Defect

- It is recommended that the fascia defect be closed, if possible, which is usually the case in primary ventral hernias. A mesh augmentation rather than a bridging of the hernia defect by the mesh is preferred.
- The anterior fascia is closed over the mesh in all repairs except an onlay mesh. In the onlay position, the hernia defect is closed before placing the mesh.

Closure of the Skin

- The skin is sutured either subcutaneously or with separate superficial sutures.
- A commercially available skin adhesive is typically used to create a watertight barrier.

OPEN MESH REPAIR WITH A VENTRAL PATCH

Incision

- The incision needed for repair with a ventral patch is smaller than the incision to place a flat mesh. It is similar to the incision for suture repair. It is recommended not to incise the umbilical rim for more than 180° because of the increased risk of devascularization of the umbilical skin after further dissection of the hernia sac, leading to skin necrosis and wound infection.
- The skin is retracted with small Volkmann retractors and the subcutaneous layer incised down to the fascia, exposing one side, cranial or caudal of the hernia defect (FIGURE 10A).
- The dissection of the hernia sac and reduction of contents is the same as the open primary repair technique.

Dissection of the Plane to Position the Mesh Device

- The mesh devices have an antiadhesive layer similar to the meshes used in an intraperitoneal position. Thus, the intraperitoneal placement is considered to be safe. If this is done, we consider it of utmost importance that the preperitoneal fat around the hernia is dissected from the abdominal wall around the hernia defect to allow contact between the mesh and the muscular fascia. This is most important cranial to the umbilical hernia, where the round ligament of the liver and its fatty tissue will hinder a correct flat placement of the mesh.
- Alternatively, it is possible in most patients to develop the plane behind the posterior rectus fascia without major damage to the peritoneum. The development of the preperitoneal plane is done through the hernia defect. This allows placement of the mesh device in a preperitoneal position and may allow for better contact between mesh and fascia, resulting in better ingrowth while avoiding the possible disadvantages of an intraperitoneal mesh. When using a mesh device, I (personal opinion of the author [JY]) always try the preperitoneal placement. In cases of failure to develop the preperitoneal plane, an intraperitoneal position is chosen.
- The hernia defect can be measured using Hegar dilators to correctly evaluate the size of the defect and classify the hernia accordingly. Because the diameter of the mesh devices does not allow a large overlap beyond the hernia defect, we recommend limiting the repair of ventral hernias with mesh devices to small hernias not larger than 2 cm (**FIGURE 13A**).
- Isolate the fascia margin from its underlying peritoneum, grasping the fascia edge with the small Volkmann retractors.
- Develop the preperitoneal plane by blunt dissection with the finger if the hernia defect is large enough to allow this (**FIGURE 13B**). Sometimes, slightly enlarging the hernia defect is needed to allow introducing a digit.
- The dissection of the preperitoneal plane is helped by introducing a gauze in the space created.
- The preperitoneal dissection should be extended far enough to allow easy and flat application of the mesh (**FIGURE 13C** and **D**).
- It is important to perform a good hemostatic control of the dissection plane to avoid postoperative hematoma around the mesh.

Introduction of the Mesh Device

- The mesh device is removed from the package after changing surgical gloves.
- Our preferred mesh device is 6.4 cm in diameter and has two central strips allowing the mesh to be pulled against the abdominal wall and fixed to the hernia defect (**FIGURE 13E**).

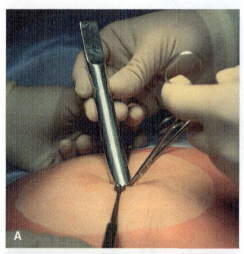
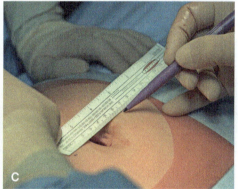
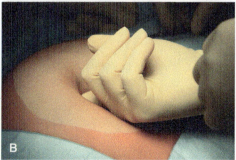

FIGURE 13 • A-K, An umbilical hernia is repaired using a round mesh device (Proceed Ventral Patch, Ethicon, Johnson & Johnson) of 6.4 cm diameter. We preferably place the mesh in a preperitoneal position if possible. The mesh is fixed with sutures to the hernia defect, using two central fixation strips, and we usually close the hernia defect on top of the mesh. Note: **FIGURE 13C** and **D**—In this patient, a mesh of 6.4 cm diameter will be placed. To illustrate the size of dissection needed underneath the posterior rectus fascia, we have measured and drawn a circle of 6.4 cm diameter.

242 SECTION VII **SURGERY OF THE ABDOMINAL WALL**

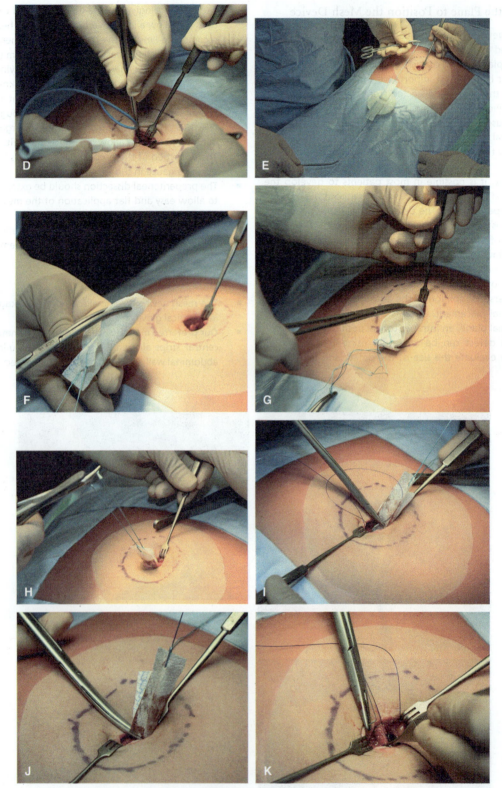

FIGURE 13 • Cont'd

- The mesh is folded in a manner not to break the internal memory ring at the margin of the mesh and grasped with a clamp (**FIGURE 13F**).
- While lifting the cranial fascia edge with the retractor, the mesh is pushed in the preperitoneal plane through the hernia defect (**FIGURE 13G**).
- With two nontraumatic forceps, the mesh is unfolded and checked for a correct flat position.
- The mesh is pulled against the abdominal wall by the central strips, controlling for a correct flat positioning of the mesh (**FIGURE 13H**).

Fixation of the Mesh Device

- Most round mesh devices for the treatment of small ventral hernias have two central fixation strips to fix the device to the margins of the hernia defect. The caudal strip is fixed to the lower margin of the hernia defect with a U-shaped suture of a slowly absorbable monofilament suture (**FIGURE 13I**).
- The strip is cut directly above the suture, leaving no mesh material above the fascia (**FIGURE 13J**).
- The same is done with the cranial strip that is sutured to the upper margin of the hernia defect.

Closure of the Hernia Defect

- Closure of the hernia defect is recommended. It separates the mesh device in the intraperitoneal or preperitoneal position from possible postoperative wound infections (**FIGURE 13K**).
- As for the primary hernia repair, several options for suturing technique and materials are available: separate sutures, running suture, or vest-over-pants plication sutures (**FIGURE 11A-C**).

Closure of the Skin

- The skin is sutured either subcutaneously or with separate superficial sutures.
- A commercially available skin adhesive is typically used to create a watertight barrier.

LAPAROSCOPIC MESH REPAIR

Creation of the Pneumoperitoneum and Trocar Placement

- The surgical field should be prepped and draped widely, with good exposure of the lateral parts of the abdomen. The trocars are placed very laterally to allow for a good view of the anterior abdominal wall and optimal angles when placing the tacks to fixate the mesh (**FIGURE 14**). For a midline hernia or for a right spigelian hernia, the trocars will be placed on the left side. For a left-sided spigelian hernia, the trocars are placed on the right side.
- The pneumoperitoneum is created with the use of a Veress needle placed in a subcostal position.
- Three trocars are placed in the flank on the anterior axillary line (**FIGURE 14**). When a large mesh is used, fixation on the surgeon's side will need an extra contralateral trocar to allow the tacks to be applied. For most primary ventral hernias, three trocars on one side are sufficient.

Adhesiolysis, Hernia Reduction, and Preconditioning of the Abdominal Wall

- Adhesiolysis, which is sometimes very difficult and time consuming in laparoscopic incisional hernia repair, is usually not a major issue in primary ventral hernias. If any adhesions are present, they are most often between the omentum and the hernia sac. Adhesiolysis has to be performed carefully, avoiding the use of cautery or other energy sources to minimize the risk of an inadvertent bowel injury.
- The mesh must lay flat on the abdominal wall; however, there is often fatty tissue that prevents this from easily occurring. The clearance of such fatty tissue has been termed "preparing the landing zone."[7] Out approach to this is to begin by incising the peritoneum at the lateral junction of the preperitoneal fat pad (**FIGURE 15**), and using monopolar energy to develop a plane between the preperitoneal fat pad and the posterior rectus fascia. This is performed cephalad and caudal

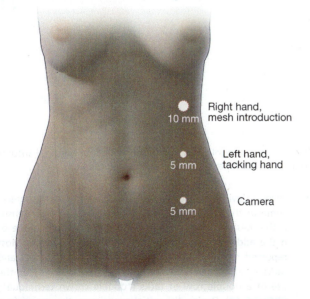

FIGURE 14 • Drawing of the intraoperative setting and trocar positions for a laparoscopic ventral hernia repair.

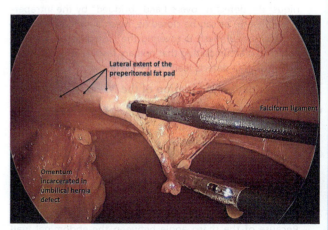

FIGURE 15 • Intraoperative image from laparoscopic umbilical hernia repair demonstrating mobilization of the preperitoneal fat pad and development of a subfascial plane.

SECTION VII SURGERY OF THE ABDOMINAL WALL

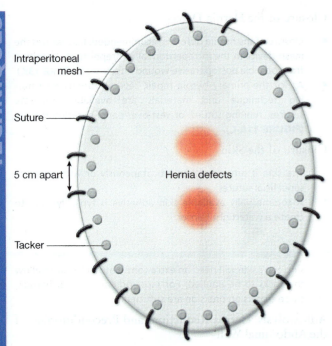

FIGURE 16 • Fixation with sutures and tacks during laparoscopic ventral hernia repair.

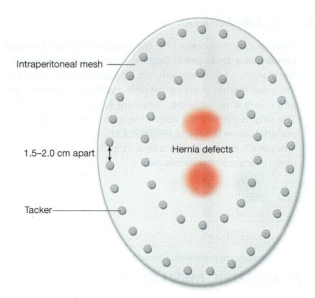

FIGURE 17 • "Double crown" fixation during laparoscopic ventral hernia repair.

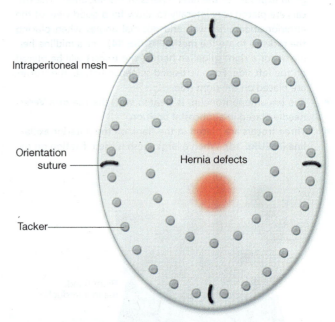

FIGURE 18 • Double crown fixation with four cardinal sutures orientation for laparoscopic ventral hernia repair.

to the hernia defect, leaving the hernia contents unreduced. This dissection thus also removes the plica umbilicalis mediana and the falciform ligament of the liver. Care should be taken to avoid thermal injury to the posterior rectus fascia, as this creates a new fascial defect (see ▶ Video 1).

- The fibrous attachments to the herniated contents are then lysed, and the herniated contents reduced. The subfascial plane is then developed to the contralateral junction of the preperitoneal fat pad with the posterior rectus fascia. Care is taken not to injure the overlying skin while dissecting the sac. The skin above an umbilical hernia may be very thin (see ▶ Video 1).

- The defect of the hernia can be left open (ie, bridging technique: the defect is covered and "bridged" by the intraperitoneal mesh) or can be closed (ie, mesh augmentation: the intraperitoneal mesh is covering the closed hernia defect). Evidence is accumulating that primary fascial closure of small ventral hernia defects leads to less recurrence.[8,9]

Mesh Placement and Fixation of the Mesh

- The mesh used during laparoscopic ventral hernia repair needs an antiadhesive side that will be in contact with the viscera. Many different meshes are available for this purpose.[7]
- It is mandatory to have a good overlap of the mesh beyond the hernia defect. An overlap of at least 5 cm in all directions is considered a minimum. This is necessary because all meshes shrink over time. Moreover, it is important to position the mesh symmetrically around the hernia defect. Because of the sharp angle between the abdominal wall and the tacker device, there is a tendency to push the mesh away from the surgeon's side, resulting in an asymmetric mesh placement.

- Several devices are available for the fixation of the mesh.[7] Some of the tackers are absorbable. There is no consensus if the mesh can be adequately fixed with tackers alone or if the addition of transabdominal sutures is needed. Most reported techniques involve a combination of sutures and tacks ("suture and tacks technique") (**FIGURE 16**) or the use of a double row of tacks ("double crown technique") (**FIGURE 17**). During the initial experience, the use of four cardinal sutures to orient and position the mesh is very helpful (**FIGURE 18**) (see ▶ Video 1).

PEARLS AND PITFALLS

Indications	- Small asymptomatic umbilical, epigastric, or lumbar hernias do not need repair, and a "watchful waiting" policy can be proposed. - Spigelian hernias need surgical treatment because they hold an increased risk of incarceration. - Strangulated hernias should be operated in emergency.
Medical imaging	- For most umbilical and epigastric hernias, medical imaging is not necessary for diagnosis and treatment planning. - Spigelian and lumbar hernias can often only be diagnosed with medical imaging, if they are clinically not palpable.

Mesh repair	- Suture repair is only applicable in small ventral hernias.
	  - A mesh repair will decrease the risk for recurrent ventral hernia.
	  - Several mesh positions and surgical approaches are possible.
	  - A good overlap of the mesh beyond the hernia defect margin is important to compensate for mesh shrinkage.

Laparoscopic repair	- A mesh with antiadhesive properties has to be used for intraperitoneal placement. - Flat and symmetric positioning of the mesh around the hernia defect is the goal. - The abdominal wall around the hernia in contact with the mesh should be adequately prepared and fatty tissue removed. - Several mesh fixation alternatives exist, without a clear consensus on the optimal approach. - Closure of the hernia defect is optional during laparoscopic ventral hernia repair.

POSTOPERATIVE CARE

- Repair of primary ventral hernias can most often be performed in an ambulatory setting. Restriction of lifting heavy weight and intense sporting activities for 2 weeks is advocated. An abdominal binder to support the hernia repair can have a positive impact on early ambulation and pain control.

OUTCOMES

- Nationwide Danish follow-up data 41 months after surgery show a reoperation rate for recurrence of 4% and a total clinical recurrence rate of 15%.[10]
- From the same Danish database, we know that umbilical and epigastric hernia repair has a low morbidity and mortality but a high readmission rate mostly because of wound problems, seroma formation, or pain.[11] Moreover, many patients complained about pain and discomfort 3 years after elective repair of a small umbilical or epigastric hernia.[12]

COMPLICATIONS

- Seroma
- Hematoma
- Surgical site infection
- Mesh infection
- Recurrence
- Chronic pain

REFERENCES

1. Muysoms F, Campanelli G, Champault GG, et al. Eurahs: the development of an international online platform for registration and outcome measurement of ventral abdominal wall hernia repair. *Hernia.* 2012;16(3):239-250. doi:10.1007/s10029-012-0912-7
2. Muysoms FE, Miserez M, Berrevoet F, et al. Classification of primary and incisional abdominal wall hernias. *Hernia.* 2009;13(4):407-414. doi:10.1007/s10029-009-0518-x
3. Miserez M, Alexandre JH, Campanelli G, et al. The European hernia society groin hernia classification: simple and easy to remember. *Hernia.* 2007;11(2):113-116. doi:10.1007/s10029-007-0198-3
4. Henriksen NA, Montgomery A, Kaufmann R, et al. Guidelines for treatment of umbilical and epigastric hernias from the European Hernia Society and Americas Hernia Society. *Br J Surg.* 2020;107(3):171-190. doi:10.1002/bjs.11489
5. Al Chalabi H, Larkin J, Mehigan B, mccormick P. A systematic review of laparoscopic versus open abdominal incisional hernia repair, with meta-analysis of randomized controlled trials. *Int J Surg.* 2015;20:65-74. doi:10.1016/j.ijsu.2015.05.050
6. Orelio CC, van Hessen C, Sanchez-Manuel FJ, et al. Antibiotic prophylaxis for prevention of postoperative wound infection in adults undergoing open elective inguinal or femoral hernia repair. Cochrane Colorectal Group, ed. *Cochrane Database Syst Rev.* 2020;4(4):CD003769. doi:10.1002/14651858.CD003769.pub5
7. Muysoms FE, Novik B, Kyle-Leinhase I, Berrevoet F. Mesh fixation alternatives in laparoscopic ventral hernia repair. *Surg Technol Int.* 2012;22:125-132.
8. Bernardi K, Olavarria OA, Holihan JL, et al. Primary fascial closure during laparoscopic ventral hernia repair improves patient quality of life: a multicenter, blinded randomized controlled trial. *Ann Surg.* 2020;271(3):434-439. doi:10.1097/SLA.0000000000003505
9. Christoffersen MW, Westen M, Rosenberg J, et al. Closure of the fascial defect during laparoscopic umbilical hernia repair: a randomized clinical trial. *Br J Surg.* 2020;107(3):200-208. doi:10.1002/bjs.11490
10. Helgstrand F, Rosenberg J, Kehlet H, et al. Reoperation versus clinical recurrence rate after ventral hernia repair. *Ann Surg.* 2012;256(6):955-958. doi:10.1097/SLA.0b013e318254f5b9
11. Bisgaard T, Kehlet H, Bay-Nielsen M, et al. A nationwide study on readmission, morbidity, and mortality after umbilical and epigastric hernia repair. *Hernia.* 2011;15(5):541-546. doi:10.1007/s10029-011-0823-z
12. Erritzøe-Jervild L, Christoffersen MW, Helgstrand F, Bisgaard T. Long-term complaints after elective repair for small umbilical or epigastric hernias. *Hernia.* 2013;17(2):211-215. doi:10.1007/s10029-012-0960-z

SECTION VIII: Surgery of the Stomach and Duodenum

Chapter 29 | Vagotomy: Truncal and Highly Selective

George A. Sarosi Jr. and Mary T. Hawn

DEFINITION

- Truncal vagotomy is defined as the division of the anterior and posterior vagus nerves, which innervate the stomach and remainder of the gastrointestinal (GI) tract, at the level of the distal esophagus. Vagotomy eliminates cholinergic stimulation to gastric parietal cells and decreases parietal cell response to gastrin and histamine, thereby reducing gastric acid secretion. By transecting at the entrance point into the abdomen, all innervation to the liver, gallbladder, pancreas, and small intestine is also divided. Truncal vagotomy requires a drainage procedure due to the disruption of antral and pyloric muscular innervation.
  - For many years, vagotomy was one of the cornerstones of surgical treatment of ulcers. However, with further understanding of the role of *Helicobacter pylori* in ulcer pathogenesis and advancement in pharmacologic management including proton pump inhibitors (PPIs) and histamine blockers, the role of surgery has changed. Of the classic indications for ulcer, surgery, bleeding, perforation, obstruction, and intractability, vagotomy is only commonly used in those patients who require surgical control of ulcer bleeding and with intractability/obstruction.
  - Level one evidence suggests that vagotomy is not necessary in the treatment of duodenal perforation in patients who are *H. pylori*–positive,[1] and the number of patients requiring operation for gastric outlet obstruction and intractability has declined dramatically with the advent of improved pharmacologic and endoscopic therapy of peptic ulcer disease (PUD). The incidence of definitive acid reduction surgery decreased by more than 50% from 1993 to 2006 and continues to decrease.[2,3]
- Highly selective vagotomy (HSV) is defined as the division of the gastric branches of the nerves of Latarjet. The nerves of Latarjet, celiac division of posterior vagus, and hepatic division of anterior vagus are preserved. Therefore, cholinergic stimulation is selectively eliminated to reduce acid secretion by parietal cells in the body and fundus, and the innervation of the antrum and pylorus, biliary tract, and small and large intestines are untouched. A drainage procedure is not required with HSV. This is also known as "parietal cell vagotomy" or "proximal gastric vagotomy."
  - The operation was developed to avoid the need for a gastric drainage procedure, which is required with truncal vagotomy, as up to one-third of patients will develop delayed gastric emptying following this procedure. Despite the elegance of parietal cell vagotomy, it is a technically demanding operation with a higher ulcer recurrence rate in inexperienced hands and a much longer learning curve than truncal vagotomy. This is a legacy operation with only a few indications in the current era. In an era when few vagotomies are performed, it has largely fallen out of favor.[4]
- Of historical note, a selective vagotomy sections the anterior vagus just distal to the point where the branch to the gallbladder and liver and the posterior vagus just distal to the branch to the pancreas and small intestines. Although in theory this might reduce the side effects of vagotomy, it is unclear in practice that this had any effect on outcomes.

DIFFERENTIAL DIAGNOSIS

- In a patient with acute severe upper GI bleeding, the differential diagnosis includes a bleeding peptic ulcer, bleeding esophageal or gastric varices secondary to portal hypertension, esophageal mucosal diseases such as severe esophagitis and Mallory-Weiss tears, gastric arteriovenous malformations and Dieulafoy lesion, and rarely, ulcerated tumors or hemobilia.
- In a patient with acute abdominal pain and free air, the differential diagnosis should include a perforated peptic ulcer, perforated diverticulitis, perforated appendicitis, and small bowel perforation.
- In a patient with gastric outlet obstruction, the differential diagnosis includes PUD, gastric cancer, duodenal web, functional delay in gastric emptying, and chronic ulcer disease related to nonsteroidal anti-inflammatory drug (NSAID) or aspirin use.

PATIENT HISTORY AND PHYSICAL FINDINGS

- The majority of operations for PUD performed now are urgent or emergent operations for complicated ulcer disease.
- A thorough history and physical examination should be obtained with key focus on the duration of symptoms, previous ulcer therapy, NSAID or aspirin use, and smoking history. Consider investigation into hypersecretory and malignant etiologies in patients with refractory ulcer disease.
- Patients should be specifically questioned regarding *H. pylori* status and prior *H. pylori* treatment including a history of eradication. In patients unable to stop anti-inflammatory

drug use, those with *H. pylori*-negative ulcer disease, or those unable to tolerate PPI therapy, it may be reasonable to consider performing an acid-reducing procedure at the time of perforated ulcer repair.
- Bleeding can occur in 15% to 20% of patients with PUD and is the most common ulcer-related complication.[3] The majority will resolve with conservative or endoscopic treatment. In patients undergoing operation for a bleeding duodenal ulcer, the best available evidence suggests that vagotomy should be combined with oversewing of a duodenal ulcer.[5] As such, the patient's *H. pylori* status, history of prior NSAID use, or prior ulcer disease will not affect the use of vagotomy in the management of their bleeding duodenal ulcer.
- Obstruction is the least common complication of ulcer disease at 5% to 8% and occurs as a result of scarring of the pylorus.[3] Endoscopy often delineates location and degree of the obstruction and also allows for therapeutic balloon dilation of the pylorus. Surgery is reserved for failure of less invasive treatments and may include vagotomy.[6]
- Intractable disease encompasses failure of medical management to heal the ulcer, relapse of disease while on current therapy, or multiple courses of medical therapy. Medical management includes acid suppression, *H. pylori* eradication, and NSAID cessation. Symptoms should be substantiated with endoscopic visualization of a persistent or recurring ulcer.

IMAGING AND OTHER DIAGNOSTIC STUDIES

- In a patient with sudden onset of acute abdominal pain and physical exam findings of peritonitis, an upright chest radiograph confirming the finding of free intraperitoneal air is a sufficient workup prior to proceeding to the operating room (OR) for a presumed perforated ulcer.
- In patients with a history and physical examination consistent with a perforated ulcer, but without free air on radiograph, a computed tomography (CT) scan or upper GI contrast study using water-soluble contrast can help to make the diagnosis.
- Testing for *H. pylori* is used to confirm presence of or gauge the eradication of disease. Antibody testing assesses overall exposure but is not specific for active disease. Urease breath test and stool antigen test can be used to confirm eradication. Full treatment of *H. pylori* should be attempted before definitive acid reduction surgery is considered.
  - Stool antigen testing for *H. pylori* should be performed prior to operation for PUD, as knowledge of *H. pylori* status may help determine the need for vagotomy. As mentioned earlier, it may not be necessary to perform vagotomy for *H. pylori*–positive disease, but may be considered in treatment of *H. pylori*–negative ulcer disease.
- Serum gastrin levels should be tested to rule out hypergastrinemic syndromes.
- Endoscopy is part of standard investigation of ulcer disease when symptoms persist despite medical therapy. Endoscopy is also used to assess ulcer healing and perform biopsies to evaluate malignancy, gastritis, and *H. pylori* infection.
- In patients with a bleeding peptic ulcer, the surgeon should be present at the time of upper endoscopy to gain an accurate anatomic understanding of the location of the ulcer. Patients with gastric ulcers not caused by acid, such as ulcers along the lesser curvature proximal to the incisura or near the gastroesophageal (GE) junction, will not require a vagotomy. Patients with duodenal or prepyloric ulcer should undergo vagotomy at the time of their operation for bleeding control.

SURGICAL MANAGEMENT

Preoperative Planning

- Patients undergoing emergency surgery for peptic ulcer bleeding will have a stomach full of blood and are at significant risk of aspiration. A nasogastric tube should be placed prior to induction for all vagotomy procedures, and rapid sequence induction should be used if possible.
- When performing an emergency operation for bleeding, the surgeon should ensure that blood is cross-matched and available.
- For laparoscopic procedures, having the ability to perform intraoperative esophagogastroduodenoscopy (EGD) can facilitate the identification of the ulcer in difficult cases.
- With truncal vagotomy, the gastric antrum and pylorus are denervated and concomitant drainage procedure must be performed.
  - Options include pyloroplasty, gastrojejunostomy, or gastric resection with reconstruction (see Chapter 30).
- HSV preserves antral muscular function and the pylorus mechanism. It is not necessary to perform a drainage procedure.
- Transthoracic vagotomy requires double lumen intubation tube and separate lung ventilation; for sufficient exposure to distal esophagus, the left lung must be collapsed.
- Perioperative antibiotics should be administered; cefazolin is standard, clindamycin plus a fluoroquinolone or aminoglycoside for penicillin allergy.

Positioning—Open

- Open approach: Patient is supine with the arms tucked or extended.
  - Space is left on the patient's left side to attach a Bookwalter or Omni retractor to the bed rail.
- Reverse Trendelenburg position of the table will help with exposure of the hiatus.

Positioning—Laparoscopic

- Laparoscopic approach: Patient is supine with right arm tucked. Surgeon stands on patient's right and assistant stands on patient's left.
- Reverse Trendelenburg position of the table will help with exposure of the hiatus.

Positioning—Transthoracic

- Patient is placed in right lateral decubitus position.

TRUNCAL VAGOTOMY—OPEN

Skin Incision and Retractor Positioning

- Use a standard upper midline incision, from just below xiphoid process to level of the umbilicus.
- A body wall retractor blade is placed on either side of the upper half of the incision to facilitate exposure.
- Depending on the size of the left lateral segment of the liver, it may be necessary to divide the avascular portion of the left triangular ligament to allow the left lateral segment to be retracted in order to facilitate visualization of the abdominal esophagus (**FIGURE 1**).

Exposure of the Esophagus

- The pars flaccida and the phrenoesophageal ligament are divided to expose the right crus and anterior esophageal wall. Take caution to recognize and preserve an accessory left hepatic artery when dividing the pars flaccida. The position of the esophagus can be verified by palpation of the nasogastric tube within the lumen of the esophagus.
- Identify the right crus of the diaphragm; gently dissect to expose the anterior surface of the esophagus. This peritoneal incision should be carried across the anterior surface of the esophagus and onto the left crus of the diaphragm to expose the anterior surface of the esophagus (**FIGURE 2A**). By applying downward and rightward traction on the stomach, the surgeon can place the esophagus on tension to enhance exposure (**FIGURE 2B**).
- Continue to develop a plane between right crus and the esophagus; extend posteriorly to create a retroesophageal window.

- The esophagus is then dissected circumferentially and this, again, can be facilitated by palpating the nasogastric tube in the lumen of the esophagus.
- A Penrose drain is placed around the GE junction to assist with downward traction on the GE junction.

Identification and Division of the Anterior (Left) Vagus Nerve

- The vagus nerves rotate counterclockwise at the level of the esophageal hiatus with the right vagus nerve coursing more posterior and the left vagus nerve anterior with respect to the esophagus.
- The left (anterior) vagus nerve is typically anterior and just right of midline at the 1- to 2-o'clock position. It is often almost within the longitudinal muscle layer (**FIGURE 3**).
  - Downward traction of the GE junction via the Penrose drain can help tense the nerve like a guitar string to help with palpation.
  - Dissect the nerve off the anterior surface of esophagus using a right angle with sharp dissection, minimal cautery.
  - Any additional anterior vagus nerve should be dissected free of esophagus if present. In about 10% of cases, two or rarely more anterior vagal branches may be found.[7]
- A medium clip is then placed on the nerve(s) at the level of the diaphragm and a second clip is placed on the nerve 3 to 4 cm distal to the first. The segment of nerve(s) between the clips is excised and sent for pathology to verify nervous tissue was excised (**FIGURE 4**).

Identification and Division of the Posterior (Right) Vagus Nerve

- The right (posterior) vagus is found at the 7-o'clock position and is often up to a centimeter away from the esophageal wall between the esophagus and the right crus (**FIGURE 5**).
  - In about 15% of cases, it may be located to the left of midline.[7]
- To identify the posterior vagus trunk(s), the surgeon should again apply downward traction on the Penrose drain while sweeping the index finger of the right hand posterior to the esophagus from the left crus to the right.
  - The surgeon's finger should be right on the esophageal wall and any tense bands identified should be hooked with a right angle and dissected free from the esophageal wall (**FIGURE 6**).
- A clip should be placed at the level of the diaphragm and a second clip is placed on the nerve 3 to 4 cm distal. The segment of nerve(s) between the clips is excised and sent for pathology to verify nervous tissue.
- Continue with gastric drainage procedure as indicated: pyloroplasty, gastrojejunostomy, or gastric resection with reconstruction (see Chapter 30).

Assessment of Hemostasis and Closure

- After verifying that no additional vagal trunks can be identified, the surgeon should inspect the diaphragmatic hiatus. During blunt mobilization of the GE junction, a hiatal hernia is sometimes created.

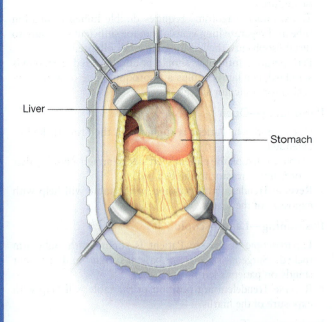

FIGURE 1 • A Bookwalter-style self-retaining retractor provides excellent exposure of the stomach and duodenum for drainage procedures. Placement of four abdominal wall blades, two on either side of the upper and lower aspect of the wound will provide the optimum exposure. A Harrington or malleable retractor on the left lobe of the liver can facilitate exposure.

Chapter 29 VAGOTOMY: TRUNCAL AND HIGHLY SELECTIVE 249

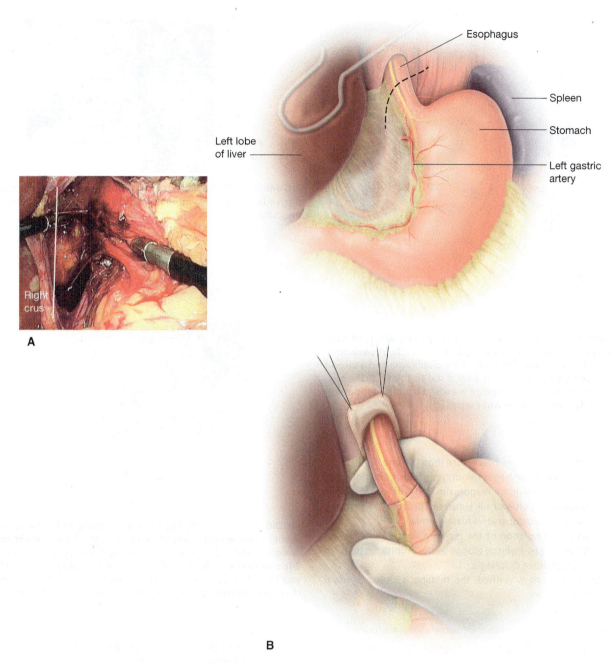

FIGURE 2 • A, Photo (left) and illustrations showing incision of the peritoneum of the pars flaccida to expose the right crus of the diaphragm and the esophagus. This peritoneal incision should be carried across the anterior surface of the esophagus and onto the left crus of the diaphragm to expose the anterior surface of the esophagus. B, Beginning on the left of the esophagus, blunt dissection with a finger or a Kittner dissector will allow the surgeon to separate the esophagus from the left crus. With gentle blunt dissection, it is possible to encircle the esophagus with the right index finger.

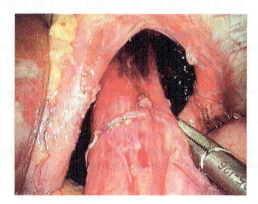

FIGURE 3 • As seen in this intraoperative photo, the anterior vagus trunk is a large band intimately associated with the muscular wall of the esophagus and often located on the right anterior surface of the esophagus.

SECTION VIII SURGERY OF THE STOMACH AND DUODENUM

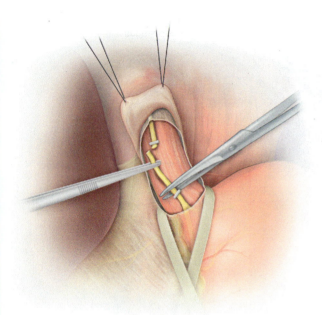

FIGURE 4 • The anterior vagus trunk is carefully dissected from the anterior surface of the esophagus, and a medium clip is then placed on the nerve(s) at the level of the diaphragm and a second clip is placed on the nerve 3 to 4 cm distal to the first. The segment of nerve(s) between the clips is excised and sent for pathology to verify nervous tissue was excised.

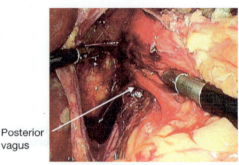

FIGURE 5 • As shown in this intraoperative photo, the posterior vagal trunk is less intimately associated with the esophageal musculature.

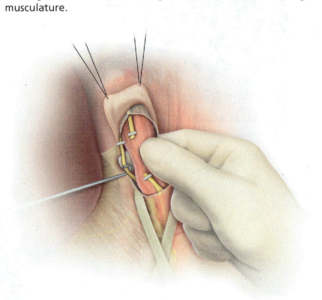

FIGURE 6 • To identify the posterior vagus trunk(s), the surgeon should again apply downward traction on the Penrose drain while sweeping the index finger posterior to the esophagus from the left crus to the right. The surgeon's finger should be right on the esophageal wall and any tense bands identified should be hooked, dissected free from the esophageal wall, and divided between clips.

- If the surgeon can insert more than the one finger adjacent to the esophagus through the hiatus, the right and left crura should be reapproximated with one or two 0 braided polyester or silk sutures to prevent the development of a postoperative hiatal hernia.
- At the completion of the repair, a single finger should be able to be inserted alongside the esophagus to avoid postoperative dysphagia.
- After hemostasis is verified, the midline is closed in usual standard fashion.

LAPAROSCOPIC TRUNCAL VAGOTOMY

Port Placement and Liver Retraction

- Port placement (**FIGURE 7**)
  - 5-mm periumbilical camera port 2 cm to the left of midline
  - 5-mm subxyphoid trocar for liver retraction
  - 5-mm right midclavicular line, two fingerbreadths below costal margin: left hand working port
  - 5-mm trocar between the right midclavicular line and camera trocar
  - 5-mm left anterior axillary line, below costal margin: stomach retraction
- A Nathanson liver retractor is placed to elevate the left lobe of the liver.
  - The patient is positioned supine with the right arm tucked.
  - The surgeons stands to the patient's right and the assistant to the patient's left.

Exposure of the Esophagus

- The peritoneum of the pars flaccida and the phrenoesophageal ligament is incised with a Harmonic scalpel or bipolar cautery device to expose the right crus of the diaphragm onto the anterior surface of the esophagus and across to the left crus to expose the entire surface of the esophagus.
- The position of the esophagus can be verified by palpation of the nasogastric tube within the lumen of the esophagus or by performing an intraoperative EGD.
- The peritoneum overlying the medial edge of the right crus of the diaphragm is identified and incised, and then, blunt dissection is used to elevate the esophagus off of the right and left crus to make a retroesophageal window.
- A grasper is then passed through the window and a Penrose drain is used to encircle the esophagus.

Chapter 29 VAGOTOMY: TRUNCAL AND HIGHLY SELECTIVE   251

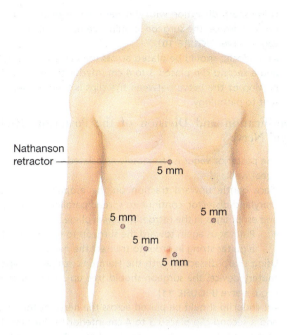

FIGURE 7 • Shows the standard port placement used for a laparoscopic vagotomy.

Identification and Division of the Anterior (Left) Vagus Nerve

- With the magnification inherent in laparoscopy, the anterior vagus can often be visualized directly on the anterior surface of the esophagus (FIGURE 3).
    - If the nerve cannot be easily visualized, downward traction on the GE junction obtained by having the assistant pull down on the Penrose drain will make the nerve tense like a guitar string and will allow for either visual or tactile identification of the anterior vagus.
- Using a Maryland dissector, the surgeon should carefully dissect the anterior vagus away from the esophageal muscle and elevate the nerve.
- Using sharp dissection with the Harmonic scalpel or bipolar cautery device, the surgeon should free up the vagus to the diaphragmatic hiatus.

- An endoclip should be placed across the nerve at the hiatus and a second clip placed 3 to 4 cm inferior to the first. The portion of the nerve between the clips is then excised and sent to pathology.
- A search for additional anterior trunks should be conducted as discussed previously.

Identification and Division of the Posterior (Right) Vagus Nerve

- The posterior vagus is less closely associated with the esophageal wall.
- To identify the posterior vagus trunk(s), the assistant should apply caudal and leftward traction on the Penrose drain with a grasper inserted through the left upper quadrant port.
    - The posterior vagus should become visible at this point as a tight band traversing between the posterior wall of the esophagus and the right crus of the diaphragm (FIGURE 5).
    - Many times, the posterior vagal trunk will be encircled within the Penrose drain, and the Penrose drain will need to be repositioned to allow the dissection of the nerve trunk away from the esophagus.
- Using sharp dissection with the Harmonic scalpel or bipolar cautery device, the surgeon should free up the vagus to the level of the diaphragmatic hiatus
- An endoclip should be placed at the level of the diaphragm and a second clip is placed on the nerve 3 to 4 cm distal. The segment of nerve(s) between the clips is excised and sent for pathology to verify nervous tissue was excised.

Assessment of Hemostasis and Closure

- Again, verify no additional vagal trunks.
- Inspect the diaphragmatic hiatus, if a more than 2-cm space (the size of an open 5-mm grasper) is noted next to the esophagus consider reapproximating the diaphragmatic crura.
- Remove laparoscopic ports under direct vision to ensure hemostasis.
- Close skin in the usual standard fashion, with fascial closure for port sites greater than 5 mm.

TRANSTHORACIC VAGOTOMY

Port Placement

- We use standard laparoscopic ports for this procedure.
- 5-mm camera port in 7th or 8th intercostal space, posterior axillary line.
- 10-mm instrument trocar along anterior axillary line at 6th and 10th intercostal space, forming a semicircle with the camera port.
- 5 mm can be placed in 10th or 11th intercostal space along posterior axillary line if needed (FIGURE 8).
- An additional 5-mm port can be placed for the surgeon's left hand inferior to the 10-mm port.

Exposure of the Esophagus

- The left lung will need to be collapsed to visualize the distal esophagus.
- Transect the pulmonary ligament with scissors or electrocautery and retract the collapsed lung superiorly (FIGURE 9).
- Incise the mediastinal pleura to expose the esophagus.

Identification and Division of the Anterior (Left) Vagus Nerve

- With the magnification in laparoscopy, the anterior vagus can often be visualized directly on the anterior surface of the esophagus.

- Using a Maryland dissector, the surgeon should carefully dissect the anterior vagus away from the esophageal muscle and elevate the nerve, placing tension by pulling toward the surgeon.

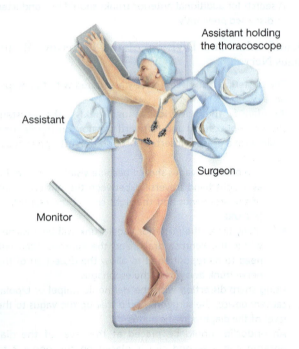

FIGURE 8 • Positioning and port placement for the transthoracic vagotomy. Patient is in the right lateral decubitus. Note: hand ports are as far away as possible from each other but forming semicircle with video port.

- Using sharp dissection with the Harmonic scalpel or bipolar cautery device, the surgeon should free up 3 to 4 cm of the vagus nerve (**FIGURE 10**).
- An endoclip should be placed across the nerve at the hiatus and a second clip placed 3 to 4 cm inferior to the first. The portion of the nerve between the clips is then excised and sent to pathology.

Identification and Division of the Posterior (Right) Vagus Nerve

- The posterior vagus is less closely associated with the esophageal wall.
- Place gentle upward traction on the esophagus. Using a Maryland dissector, continue to spread parallel to the nerve and esophagus in the retroesophageal plane.
    - Pull vagus again toward the surgeon to tense nerve like a guitar string in order to transect the nerve.
- Using sharp dissection with the Harmonic scalpel or bipolar cautery device, the surgeon should free up 3 to 4 cm of the vagus nerve (**FIGURE 11**).
- An endoclip should be placed across the nerve at the hiatus and a second clip placed 3 to 4 cm inferior to the first. The portion of the nerve between the clips is then excised and sent to pathology.

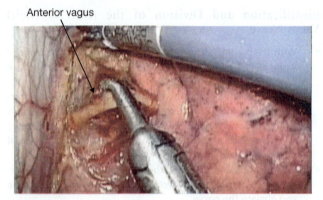

FIGURE 10 • Anterior vagus is identified on top of the esophagus. It is carefully dissected by spreading parallel to esophagus and then placed on tension by pulling toward the surgeon. A segment is then clipped for removal and sent to pathology.

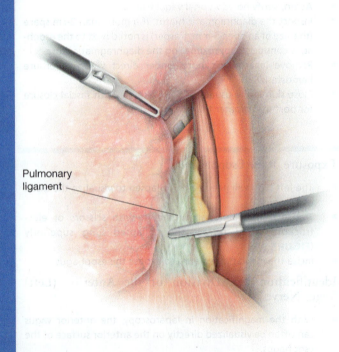

FIGURE 9 • To expose the distal esophagus, transect the pulmonary ligament and retract the collapsed left lung superiorly.

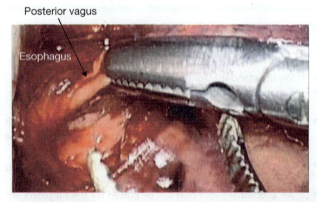

FIGURE 11 • Gentle traction placed on esophagus to pull anterior in the chest. The posterior vagus nerve is dissected from the tissue below the esophagus. This is again pulled toward surgeon to aid in excision.

Chapter 29 VAGOTOMY: TRUNCAL AND HIGHLY SELECTIVE   253

Assessment of Hemostasis and Closure

- After hemostasis is ensured, the lung should be re-expanded under direct vision. If concerns for an air leak exist, a soft 20-Fr chest tube can be inserted through on the camera ports and fed proximally over the lung tissue to evacuate any retained air.
- The camera port is then withdrawn.
- Closure of laparoscopic port sites in usual standard fashion.

HIGHLY SELECTIVE VAGOTOMY

Exposure of Esophagus

- The phrenoesophageal ligament overlying the esophagus is incised and the esophagus is encircled with a Penrose drain.

Exposure of Vagus Nerves, Nerve of Latarjet

- The anterior and posterior vagus nerves are identified and each encircled with a vessel loop. Dissection is carried far enough into the posterior mediastinum to identify main vagal trunks.
- Examine the lesser curvature of the stomach to identify the nerve of Latarjet (**FIGURE 12**).
- Dissect 6 to 7 cm proximal to the pylorus along the lesser curvature of the stomach at the incisura angularis. It is key to leave the terminal branches of the nerve, referred to as "crow's foot," to maintain innervation to the antrum and pylorus (**FIGURE 13**).
- Divide the lesser omentum from the lesser curve from the incisura angularis and continue to divide the vagal branches to 6 cm proximal to the GE junction. Stay inside the main vagal braches.
    - Clamp and divide neurovascular branches along the lesser curve as close to the stomach as possible to avoid injury to the nerve of Latarjet (**FIGURE 14**).
    - There is an anterior and posterior bundle and they should be divided separately.
- Invert the lesser curvature of the stomach with interrupted Lembert sutures.

Hemostasis and Closure

- Midline is closed in usual standard fashion.
- Laparoscopic ports close in usual standard fashion, with fascial closure for port sites greater than 5 mm.

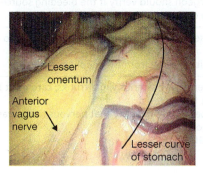

FIGURE 12 ● Identify the lesser curve of the stomach; see the anterior vagus nerve coursing in on the lesser omentum.

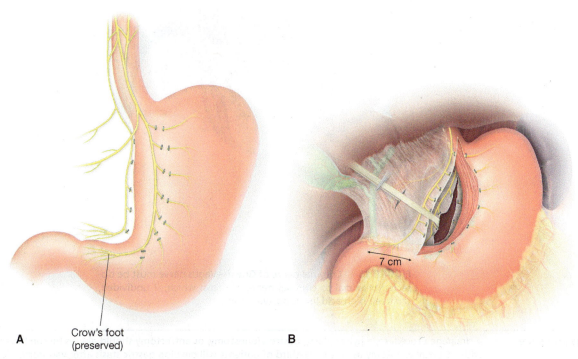

FIGURE 13 ● **A** and **B**, Dissection occurs along the lesser curvature of the stomach from proximal to the GE junction to the incisura angularis, 6 to 7 cm proximal to the pylorus. Leave the terminal branches of the nerve, referred to as "crow's foot," to maintain innervation to the antrum and pylorus.

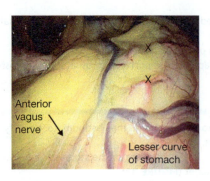

FIGURE 14 • Clamp and divide neurovascular branches along the lesser curve as close to the stomach as possible to avoid injury to the nerve of Latarjet. Marked by the X. There is an anterior and posterior bundle and they should be divided separately.

PEARLS AND PITFALLS

Indications	■ In patients with evidence of active *H. pylori* infection, treatment of the ulcer complication and antihelicobacter therapy may be sufficient. ■ When the operative indication is GI bleeding, the surgeon should verify if the bleeding source is in a location associated with a high acid state such as the duodenum or prepyloric stomach.
Exposure	■ Take caution when encircling the esophagus and dissecting the vagus off of the esophagus to prevent injury. ■ Avoid the use of cautery when dissecting the vagal fibers away from the esophageal surface.
Vagotomy	■ Ten percent of patients will have more than one anterior or posterior vagal trunks; care must be taken to look for additional fibers after division of the first trunk. ■ Always send a section of the excised vagal trunk to pathology to verify that nervous tissue was excised. ■ Most ulcer reoccurrences result from incomplete vagotomy. ■ Care to resect above the criminal nerve of Grassi (FIGURE 15). ■ Injury to thoracic duct in transthoracic approach.

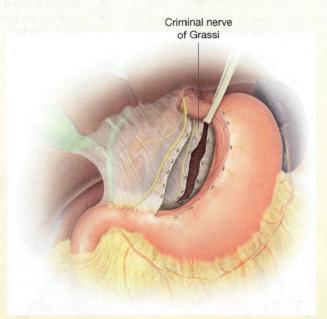

FIGURE 15 • Criminal nerve of Grassi—Vagus nerve must be dissected proximal to criminal nerve of Grassi which, if undivided, can keep high acid levels postvagotomy.

Drainage procedure	■ A drainage procedure, a pyloroplasty, gastrojejunostomy, or antrectomy should always be combined with a truncal vagotomy as up to one-third of patients will develop gastric stasis after vagotomy alone.
Paraesophageal herniation	■ Inspect the esophageal hiatus at the conclusion of the procedure to verify that an iatrogenic paraesophageal hernia has not been created.

POSTOPERATIVE CARE

- Nasogastric suction may be used in the early postoperative period. In patient who has undergone gastric drainage procedure or perforation repair, postoperative ileus may last as long as 7 to 10 days.
- Consistent with other foregut surgery, diet advancement is as tolerated.
- Intolerance to diet should prompt investigation for delayed gastric emptying.
- In patients operated on for perforated ulcers, broad-spectrum antibiotic therapy including antifungal agents should be administered postoperatively.
- Patients who are found to be *H. pylori*–positive should receive 10 to 14 days of antibiotic therapy directed at *H. pylori* eradication. Eradication should be confirmed by repeat testing.
- Patients operated on for bleeding should be carefully monitored for rebleeding for up to 96 hours.
- Patients chronically using NSAIDs or aspirin products should be counseled to avoid further use of these medications. Patients who are medically unable to discontinue these drugs should be started on a PPI.
- Transthoracic patients should be monitored with daily chest radiographs until the chest tube is removed appropriately.

OUTCOMES

- **Vagotomy**
  - Truncal vagotomy has demonstrated 80% reduction in basal acid secretion.[8]
  - Truncal vagotomy has the lowest reoccurrence rates (1%-10%) but have the highest morbidity (20%-25%) and mortality (0.5%-2%).[9,10] Ulcer recurrence rates also vary based on drainage procedure, with best results from total vagotomy with antrectomy.
  - Common postoperative morbidity includes diarrhea (10%-25%), dumping syndrome (10%-20%), and bile reflux gastritis (2%).[9,10]
  - Vagal-mediated receptive relaxation of the stomach is abolished; there may be more rapid emptying of liquids and solids.
- **HSV**
  - Lower mortality and morbidity including diarrhea and dumping syndrome (1%-5%).[4]
  - Higher ulcer recurrence rates, greater than 10% at 5 years.[4]
  - Vagal-mediated receptive relaxation of the stomach is abolished, and therefore, there is more rapid emptying of liquids. However, with preservation of antrum innervation, emptying of solids is unaffected.

COMPLICATIONS

- Esophageal perforation
- Bleeding
- Incomplete vagotomy—failure to identify accessory vagus nerves. Vagus must be taken proximal to the criminal nerve of Grassi, the first gastric branch of the posterior vagus.
- Delayed gastric emptying
- Dumping syndrome
- Pleural effusion

Disclaimer: The authors would like to acknowledge the substantial contributions made by Ashley Augspurger Davis to the prior edition of this chapter.

REFERENCES

1. Ng EK, Lam YH, Sung JJ, et al. Eradication of *Helicobacter pylori* prevents recurrence of ulcer after simple closure of duodenal ulcer perforation: randomized controlled trial. *Ann Surg.* 2000;231(2):153-158. doi:10.1097/00000658-200002000-00001
2. Wang YR, Richter JE, Dempsey DT. Trends and outcomes of hospitalizations for peptic ulcer disease in the United States, 1993 to 2006. *Ann Surg.* 2010;251(1):51-58. doi:10.1097/SLA.0b013e3181b975b8
3. Olufajo OA, Wilson A, Yehayes B, Zeineddin A, Cornwell EE, Williams M. Trends in the surgical management and outcomes of complicated peptic ulcer disease. *Am Surg.* 2020;86(7):856-864. doi:10.1177/0003134820939929
4. Lagoo J, Pappas TN, Perez A. A relic or still relevant: the narrowing role for vagotomy in the treatment of peptic ulcer disease. *Am J Surg.* 2014;207(1):120-126. doi:10.1016/j.amjsurg.2013.02.012
5. Schroder VT, Pappas TN, Vaslef SN, De La Fuente SG, Scarborough JE. Vagotomy/drainage is superior to local oversew in patients who require emergency surgery for bleeding peptic ulcers. *Ann Surg.* 2014;259(6):1111-1118. doi:10.1097/SLA.0000000000000386
6. Wang A, Yerxa J, Agarwal S, et al. Surgical management of peptic ulcer disease. *Curr Probl Surg.* 2020;57(2):100728. doi:10.1016/j.cpsurg.2019.100728
7. Skandalakis JE, Rowe JS Jr, Gray SW, Androulakis JA. Identification of vagal structures at the esophageal hiatus. *Surgery.* 1974;75(2):233-237.
8. Ashley S, Evoy D, Daly J. Stomach. In: Schwartz S, ed. *Principles of Surgery.* 7 ed. McGraw-Hill; 1999:1191.
9. Lee CJ, Simeone DM. Gastric ulcer. In: Bland KI, Büchler MW, Csendes A, Sarr MG, Garden OJ, Wong J, eds. *General Surgery.* Springer London; 2009:539-548.
10. Postier RG, Havron WS. Chapter 57—vagotomy and drainage. In: Yeo CJ, ed. *Shackelford's Surgery of the Alimentary Tract.* 7th ed. W.B. Saunders; 2013:720-730.

Chapter 30 | Drainage Procedures: Pyloromyotomy, Pyloroplasty, Gastrojejunostomy

George A. Sarosi Jr

DEFINITION

- Drainage procedures, or more properly gastric drainage procedures, are a variety of surgical approaches used to either render incompetent or bypass the pylorus. Drainage procedures are often performed in conjunction with procedures that interrupt vagal innervation of the pylorus, and the purpose is to facilitate gastric drainage. Originally performed in conjunction with a truncal vagotomy for the treatment of peptic ulcer disease, drainage procedures are also performed to facilitate gastric emptying when the stomach is used as an esophageal replacement and occasionally to address poor gastric emptying in patients who have undergone fundoplication or paraesophageal hernia repair. Gastrojejunostomy is also frequently used to treat duodenal or gastric outlet obstruction.

DIFFERENTIAL DIAGNOSIS

- In patients who have undergone prior gastroesophageal junction surgery, the differential diagnosis for abdominal bloating includes visceral hypersensitivity (irritable bowel syndrome), gastroparesis, postsurgical delayed gastric emptying secondary to vagal injury, paraesophageal herniation of the fundoplication or portions of the stomach, and overeating or excess consumption of inappropriate foods such as carbonated beverages.
- In patients who have undergone esophageal replacement with a gastric conduit, the differential diagnosis of dysphagia, early satiety, or regurgitation of undigested foods includes anastomotic structure, an inadequate-sized hiatal opening, torsion of the conduit, paraesophageal hernia, and competent pylorus.

PATIENT HISTORY AND PHYSICAL FINDINGS

- Depending on the indication for a drainage procedure, certain historical elements and physical findings should be sought.
  - For patients with peptic ulcer disease, the duration of symptoms and any prior treatment of peptic ulcer disease should be sought. In addition, knowledge of the patients' *Helicobacter pylori* status and prior *H. pylori* treatment is important. Finally, a history of use of nonsteroidal anti-inflammatory drugs (NSAIDs) or aspirin products should be sought.
    - In patients with a prior history of peptic ulcer disease who are undergoing surgical treatment of a bleeding ulcer, a history of prior ulcer disease should alert the surgeon to the possibility of encountering a scarred and possibly fibrotic duodenum.
    - Patients known to be *H. pylori* positive who have not had treatment for their *H. pylori* may not require an acid-reducing procedure at the time of surgical bleeding control. Simple ligation of the bleeding site may be sufficient.
    - Patients with a significant history of NSAID or aspirin product use are at a significant risk of recurrent ulcers and must be counseled to avoid all these products in the future.
  - For patients undergoing drainage procedures after esophageal replacement with a gastric conduit, patients should be questioned carefully about their symptoms. Patients with poor gastric drainage will describe early satiety, bloating, regurgitation, or emesis of undigested food. Patients with anastomotic strictures typically will describe dysphagia.
  - For patients undergoing or who have undergone a fundoplication, a history of postprandial abdominal pain, bloating, or early satiety should be sought, as this can be a symptom of poor gastric emptying, which can be confirmed with a gastric emptying study.

IMAGING AND OTHER DIAGNOSTIC STUDIES

- In patients undergoing emergency operations for upper gastrointestinal hemorrhage, all patients should undergo esophagogastroduodenoscopy (EGD) prior to operation with an attempt at endoscopic hemostasis. The operating surgeon should make every effort to be present during the endoscopy, as accurate anatomic information regarding the location of the ulcer will facilitate the operation.
- In patients suspected of having poor emptying of their gastric conduit after esophageal replacement, gastric emptying studies are of limited use due to the altered anatomy and the lack of reference values for emptying. The author has used EGD and botulinum toxin injection as a diagnostic test for patients with poor emptying of the conduit.[1] Those who have an improvement in symptoms have been offered surgical drainage procedures.
- In patients with prior fundoplication or paraesophageal hernia repair suspected of having delayed gastric emptying, nuclear medicine gastric emptying studies are helpful in identifying patients who could benefit from a drainage procedure. Hamrick et al,[2] in a large series of revisional paraesophageal hernia patients, used a T1/2 emptying time of 90 minutes as an indication for the addition of a gastric drainage procedure with good results. Alternatively, EGD and botulinum toxin injection of the pylorus can also be used as a diagnostic study.[3]

SURGICAL MANAGEMENT

Preoperative Planning

- Patients undergoing drainage procedures will have poor gastric emptying and will be at risk for aspiration during induction of anesthesia. For elective procedures, patients should be placed on a clear liquid diet 24 hours prior to surgery and made NPO the night before the procedure. Patients undergoing emergency surgery for peptic ulcer bleeding will have a stomach full of blood and are at significant risk of aspiration. Whenever feasible, rapid sequence induction should be used. Antibiotic prophylaxis with 1 to 2 g of cefazolin is the standard approach; clindamycin plus a fluoroquinolone or aminoglycoside is the appropriate choice for those patients with allergies to cefazolin. When performing an emergency operation for bleeding, the surgeon should ensure that blood is crossmatched and available. For laparoscopic procedures, having the ability to perform intraoperative EGD can facilitate the identification of the pylorus and bleeding source in difficult cases.

Positioning

- For open drainage procedures, the patient is positioned in the supine position with both arms extended. Space is left on the patient's left side to attach a Buchwalter or Omni retractor to the bed rail. During the surgical procedure, the patient will often be placed in reverse Trendelenburg to facilitate exposure of the upper abdominal organs. In a laparoscopic approach, the same position is used, but a footboard and safety strap should also be added to prevent the patient from sliding when steep reverse Trendelenburg position is used.

OPEN PYLOROPLASTY

Skin Incision and Retractor Positioning

- An upper midline incision is used for all open drainage procedures. This should begin at the level of the umbilicus and extend to just below the xiphoid process. Body wall retractor blades are placed on either side of the upper half of the incision to facilitate exposure. If necessary, a malleable or Harrington retractor blade can be placed on the left lobe of the liver to expose the pylorus (**FIGURE 1**).

Kocher Maneuver

- A Kocher maneuver is performed to facilitate exposure of the duodenum and pylorus and to eliminate tension on the suture line. A forceps is used to grasp the peritoneum lateral to the duodenum, which is then incised with scissors or the electrosurgical device. The surgeon then can insert an index finger behind the duodenum and head of the pancreas and sweep the finger to the right, elevating the lateral duodenal ligament and avascular retroperitoneal tissues, which can then be divided with the electrosurgical device (**FIGURE 2**). The plane of dissection should remain close to the duodenal wall to avoid injury to the gonadal vein on the anterior surface of the inferior vena cava. The duodenum and head of the pancreas should be mobilized from the junction of the duodenal bulb and second portion of the duodenum to just before the lateral aspect of the superior mesenteric vein. If the procedure is being performed for a bleeding duodenal ulcer, the Kocher maneuver step can be deferred until after control of the bleeding vessel has been achieved.

Pyloric Incision

- The pylorus is identified either visually or by palpation of the muscular ring with a finger inserted from the gastric side. Beginning roughly 2 cm proximal to the pylorus on the gastric antrum, incise the gastric wall, enter the lumen, and extend the incision distally parallel to the long axis of the bowel across the pylorus onto the duodenum to a distance of roughly 5 cm using the electrosurgical device (**FIGURE 3**). This incision will provide reasonable exposure of the duodenal bulb. If the operation is being performed for ulcer bleeding, the incision can be extended further along the duodenum to expose the bleeding site. The pyloroplasty incision can be facilitated by placing a seromuscular stay stitch on the superior and inferior edge of the pylorus.

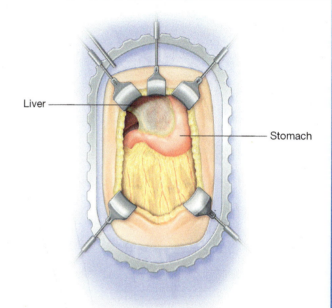

FIGURE 1 • A Bookwalter style self-retaining retractor provides excellent exposure of the stomach and duodenum for drainage procedures. Placement of four abdominal wall blades, two on either side of the upper and lower aspect of the wound, will provide the optimum exposure. A Harrington or malleable retractor on the left lobe of the liver can facilitate exposure.

Bleeding Control

- If the operation is being performed for a bleeding duodenal ulcer, the ulcer is identified on the posterior aspect of the duodenal bulb. Temporary hemostasis is achieved by digital pressure, and then definitive hemostasis is achieved by placing three 2-0 silk suture ligatures. The first suture is placed at the cranial margin of the ulcer, encircling the proximal gastroduodenal artery (GDA). The second suture is placed at the caudal edge of the duodenal ulcer encircling the distal GDA. The final suture is a U suture placed underneath the

SECTION VIII SURGERY OF THE STOMACH AND DUODENUM

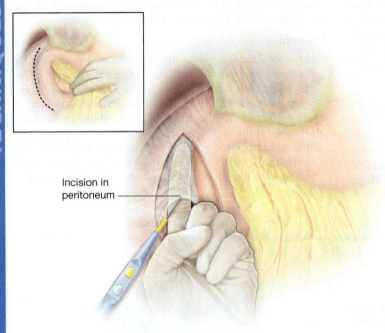

FIGURE 2 • Application of leftward traction on the stomach and duodenum will allow the surgeon to score the peritoneum lateral to the duodenum with the electrosurgical device as shown in the *inset*. The surgeon's index finger can then bluntly elevate the avascular tissues between the duodenum, pancreas, and vena cava, making division of these tissues with the electrosurgical device easy.

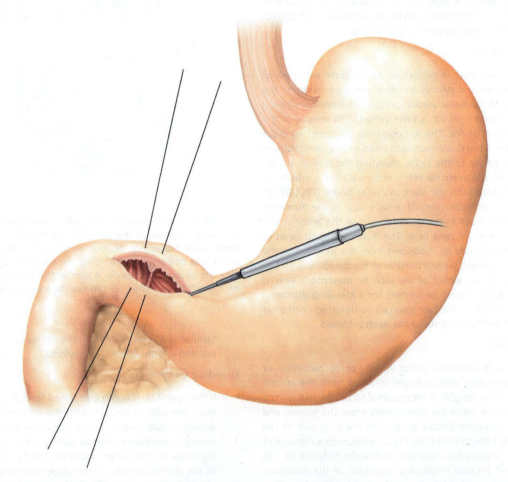

FIGURE 3 • Placing silk stay sutures superior and inferior to the proposed pyloroplasty incision will make the entry into the duodenum easier. (Reprinted with permission from Nussbaum MS. *Master Techniques in Surgery: Gastric Surgery*. Wolters Kluwer Health/Lippincott Williams & Wilkins; 2013.)

Chapter 30 DRAINAGE PROCEDURES: PYLOROMYOTOMY, PYLOROPLASTY, GASTROJEJUNOSTOMY

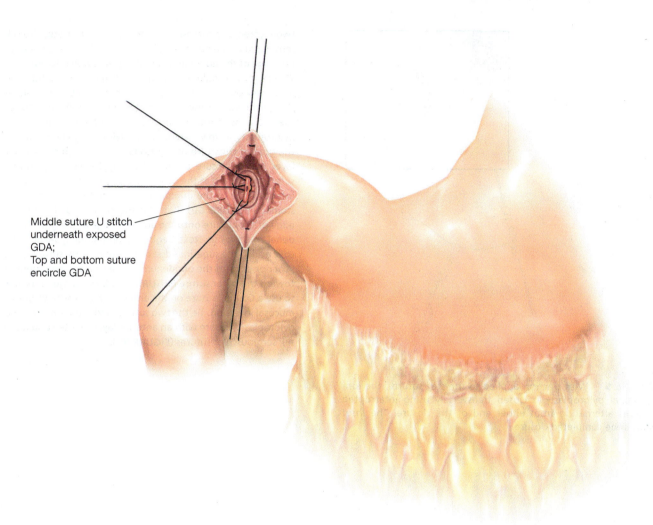

FIGURE 4 • When operating to ulcer bleeding, placing the pyloroplasty incision directly over the ulcer crater will optimize exposure. Control of bleeding from the GDA is achieved with three sutures. A simple or figure-of-eight suture is placed at the cranial and caudal edge of the ulcer to ligate the trunk of the GDA. A third horizontal U stitch is placed under the ulcer crater to control the transverse pancreatic branches. GDA, gastroduodenal artery. (Reprinted with permission from Nussbaum MS. *Master Techniques in Surgery: Gastric Surgery.* Wolters Kluwer Health/Lippincott Williams & Wilkins; 2013.)

ulcer crater to control the posterior entry of the transverse pancreatic artery into the back wall of the GDA (**FIGURE 4**).

Closure of Pyloroplasty—Heineke-Mikulicz

- The most common closure of the pyloroplasty is the Heineke-Mikulicz approach, closing the longitudinal pyloroplasty with a single layer of sutures in a transverse fashion. This closure is appropriate when the duodenum is not distorted or scarred and the pyloroplasty incision is shorter than 6 to 7 cm. The closure is performed by applying superior and inferior traction on the stay sutures, converting the longitudinal gastroduodenal incision into a transverse incision. The incision is then closed with interrupted 3-0 silk sutures or 3-0 polyglycolic acid sutures with either a full-thickness simple stitch or a Gambee stitch. The closure is best performed by starting at the top corner of the incision and alternating from the top to the bottom proceeding toward the middle. The sutures may be tied as they are placed until the last three sutures, which should be left untied until all of the sutures are placed to ensure that the mucosal layer is included in all of the bites (**FIGURE 5**). A vascularized pedicle of omentum is then placed over the closure and the stay sutures tied over the omental pedicle to hold it in place in the fashion of a Graham patch.

Closure of Pyloroplasty—Finney

- If the duodenum is significantly inflamed or scarred from chronic peptic ulceration or if a longer duodenotomy is required to obtain hemostasis on a bleeding source beyond the duodenal bulb, a Finney closure of the pylorus is appropriate to prevent tension on the closure and gastric outlet obstruction. The Finney closure is in essence a side-to-side gastroduodenostomy with the pylorus at the cranial apex of the anastomosis. The duodenum will need to be completely mobilized to allow this closure to be tension free. Remove the inferior stay suture and apply cranial tension on the superior stay suture to convert the longitudinal incision into an inverted U shape. The Finney closure is a standard

260 SECTION VIII SURGERY OF THE STOMACH AND DUODENUM

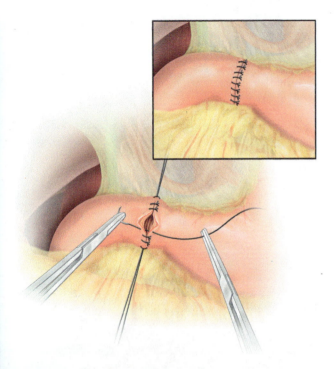

FIGURE 5 • With traction applied to the stay sutures, the longitudinal pyloroplasty is closed transversely using interrupted sutures alternating from either end of the closure. The *inset* shows the completed closure.

two-layered anastomosis. A back row of interrupted 3-0 silk seromuscular (Lembert) sutures is placed between the inferior edge of the duodenum and the gastric wall (**FIGURE 6A**). These sutures should be placed 5 to 10 mm from the cut edge of the mucosa. It is often necessary to extend the incision on the gastric side of the pylorus to ensure that the lengths of the two arms of the incision are equal. When extending the pyloroplasty in this fashion, it is advisable to cheat toward the greater curvature of the stomach. Next, begin the inner layer of the closure using a 3-0 polyglycolic acid running suture beginning at the divided pylorus muscle, suturing the inferior edge of the duodenum to the inferior edge of the stomach (**FIGURE 6B**). Run this suture around the inferior edge of the closure onto the anterior edge of the gastroduodenal anastomosis. Next, begin a second running 3-0 polyglycolic acid at the superior edge of the cut pylorus, suturing the superior edge of the duodenum to the stomach and running toward the other suture (**FIGURE 7A**). Many surgeons prefer to use a Connell suture on the anterior wall to achieve better mucosal inversion. Tie the two sutures and then complete the pyloroplasty closure with an anterior layer of interrupted 3-0 silk seromuscular sutures (**FIGURE 7B**).

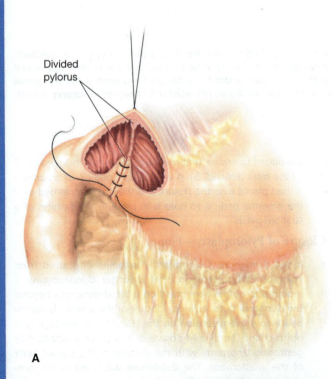
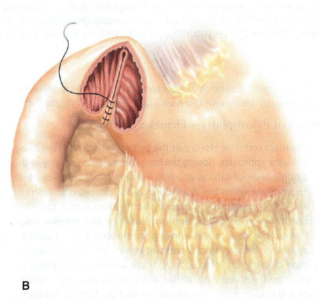

A   **B**

FIGURE 6 • **A,** With superior traction on the superior stay suture, the back row of the Finney pyloroplasty is created by approximating the duodenum to the greater curvature of the stomach with seromuscular sutures. **B,** The back portion of the inner row is begun using a running suture approximating the duodenal mucosa to the gastric mucosa beginning at the inferior edge of the transected pylorus. This suture is then run up to the anterior surface of the pyloroplasty.

Chapter 30 DRAINAGE PROCEDURES: PYLOROMYOTOMY, PYLOROPLASTY, GASTROJEJUNOSTOMY **261**

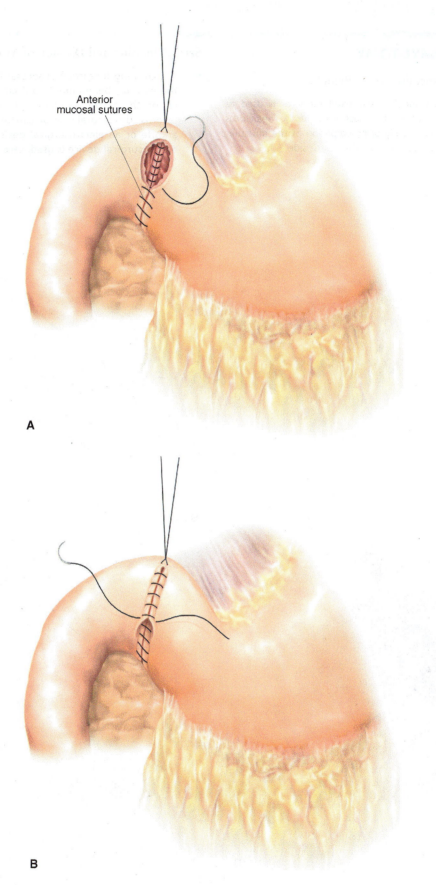

FIGURE 7 • In panel **(A)**, after the inner mucosal suture is run to the middle of the anterior surface of the closure, a second inner running suture is begun at the superior cut edge of the pylorus, approximating the duodenal and gastric mucosa. This suture is run to the posterior suture and they are tied together, completing the inner row of sutures. In panel **(B)**, the pyloroplasty is completed with a second layer of seromuscular sutures. (Reprinted with permission from Nussbaum MS. *Master Techniques in Surgery: Gastric Surgery*. Wolters Kluwer Health/Lippincott Williams & Wilkins; 2013.)

OPEN PYLOROMYOTOMY

Incision and Identification of the Pylorus

- An upper midline incision and fixed retractor is used as described previously for pyloroplasty (FIGURE 1). The pylorus is identified either visually or by palpation of the muscular ring with a finger inserted from the gastric side.

Serosal Incision and Division of Muscular Fibers

- A 3-cm long longitudinal serosal incision is made across the pylorus, beginning 1 to 2 cm proximal to the pylorus on the gastric side and extending 1 cm distal to the pylorus. This serosal incision can be performed either with a knife or an electrosurgical device (FIGURE 8A). If the electrosurgical device is used, care should be exercised to

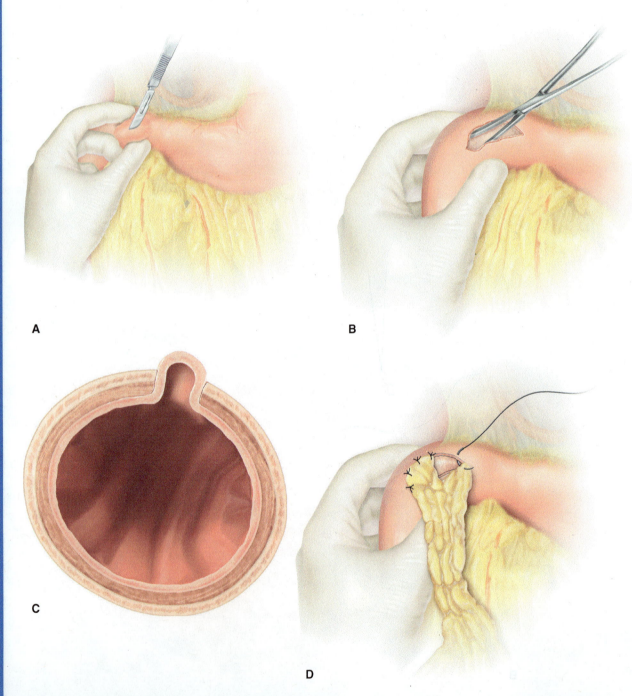

FIGURE 8 • In panel (A), the surgeon scores the serosa with a scalpel blade exposing the muscular layer. In panel (B), a hemostat is used to spread the longitudinal muscle fibers and dissect the circular fibers away from the mucosa for division with a scalpel. When the myotomy is completed, the mucosa will bulge as shown in panel (C). An omental patch is then sewn to the serosal edges of the myotomy to cover the mucosa as shown in panel (D).

Chapter 30 DRAINAGE PROCEDURES: PYLOROMYOTOMY, PYLOROPLASTY, GASTROJEJUNOSTOMY   263

avoid deep penetration into the muscularis and thermal injury to the mucosa. Beginning on the gastric side of the incision, use a fine tipped hemostat to dissect the muscular fibers off of the submucosa and divide the circular muscular fibers with a knife (FIGURE 8B). Muscular bleeders can usually be controlled with pressure, and there is a very limited role for cautery at this point of the operation. Great care should be taken to avoid mucosal injury especially on the duodenal side, as the submucosa is thinner and more fragile. When properly performed, the mucosa and submucosa will bulge out of the incision (FIGURE 8C).

Omental Patch

- A vascularized pedicle of omentum is placed over the pyloromyotomy and sutured with three 3-0 silk sutures. The first is placed through the superior edge of the divided pyloric ring and the superior edge of the omental pedicle to prevent the two cut edges of the pylorus from coming into contact. The next two are placed between each lateral edge of the serosal incision and the lateral edges of the omental patch to ensure that the patch covers the entire pyloromyotomy. Additional sutures are then placed between the superior edge of the serosal defect and the omentum to completely cover the pyloroplasty (FIGURE 8D).

OPEN GASTROJEJUNOSTOMY

Skin Incision and Retractor Positioning

- An upper midline incision is used for all open drainage procedures. This should begin at the level of the umbilicus and extend to just below the xiphoid process. Body wall retractor blades are placed on either side of the upper half of the incision to facilitate exposure (FIGURE 1). If necessary, a malleable or Harrington retractor blade can be placed on the left lobe of the liver to expose the stomach and pyloric region.

Preparation of the Stomach and Identification of Proximal Jejunum

- There is insufficient evidence to recommend a posterior gastrojejunostomy over an anterior gastrojejunostomy, and an antecolic, anterior gastric wall gastrojejunostomy is the easiest to create. Identify the pylorus, and then identify a point, 5 cm proximal to the pylorus, as the gastric site of the anastomosis. Next, identify the ligament of Treitz, and select a section of the jejunum 15 to 30 cm distal to the ligament of Treitz, which will easily reach the distal stomach without tension.

Construction of the Anastomosis

- A standard double-layered side-to-side anastomosis is constructed by aligning the small bowel with the stomach in an isoperistaltic fashion, with the distal portion of the small bowel located closest to the pylorus. The back row of the anastomosis is first created by suturing the jejunum to the greater curvature of the stomach using seromuscular 3-0 silk interrupted sutures. The tails of the sutures at either corner are left long to allow them to be used as stay sutures (FIGURE 9A). Using the electrosurgical device, a full-thickness jejunotomy is made in the small bowel, and a gastrotomy is made in the stomach roughly 5 to 10 mm from the outer layer of the anastomosis (FIGURE 9B). Beginning in the middle of the posterior portion of the anastomosis, the inner layer of the anastomosis is constructed by running two 3-0 polyglycolic acid sutures from the middle of the back row in opposite directions (FIGURE 10A). Many surgeons prefer to use Connell sutures on the anterior row to achieve better eversion, but this step is not necessary (FIGURE 10B). The anastomosis is completed with an outer anterior layer of seromuscular 3-0 silk interrupted sutures.

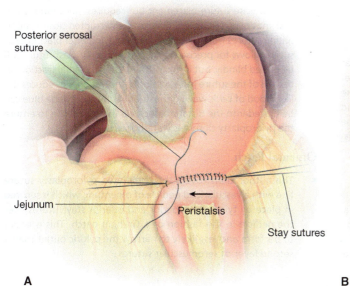
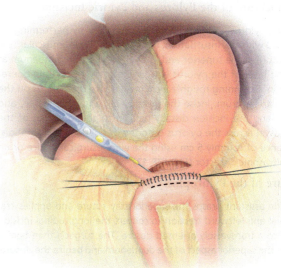

FIGURE 9 • An antecolic, isoperistaltic gastrojejunostomy is begun by placing a back row of seromuscular sutures between the greater curvature of the stomach and the antimesenteric edge of the jejunum over a distance of 8 cm as shown in panel (A). The stomach and the jejunum are then opened with the electrosurgical device in panel (B).

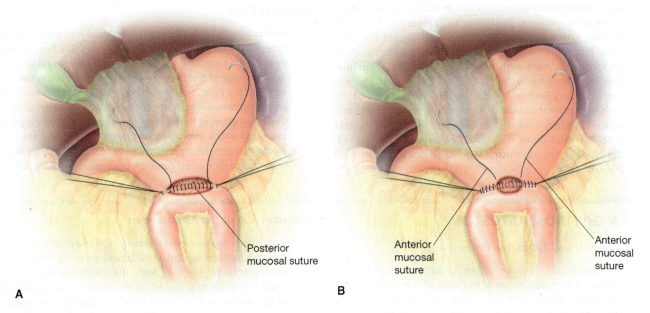

FIGURE 10 • A double-armed suture is placed in the center of the back row of the anastomosis and run to the corners of each side as shown in panel (A). This same suture is then run to the middle of the anterior row as shown in panel (B). The anterior row can either be Connell sutures or simple sutures based on surgeon preference.

LAPAROSCOPIC PYLOROPLASTY

Port Placement and Liver Retraction

- We use a standard four-trocar approach for gastric procedures, with a 5-mm port in the left upper quadrant, a second 5-mm trocar just to the left of the umbilicus, a 12-mm trocar at the level of the umbilicus in the midclavicular line, and a 5-mm trocar in the right upper quadrant. A Nathanson liver retractor is placed to elevate the left lobe of the liver (FIGURE 11).

Identification of the Pylorus and Pyloric Incision

- The pylorus is identified either visually or by performing an EGD with CO_2 insufflation. Placing a 3-0 silk seromuscular stay suture at the superior and inferior edge of the duodenum at the level of the pylorus will facilitate the rest of the operation. Beginning roughly 2 cm proximal to the pylorus on the gastric antrum, incise the gastric wall, enter the lumen, and extend the incision distally parallel to the long axis of the bowel across the pylorus onto the duodenum to a total distance of roughly 5 cm using the electrosurgical device or an ultrasonic dissector (FIGURE 12).

Closure of the Pyloroplasty

- The assistant grasps the superior stay suture and applies cranial and leftward traction to convert the longitudinal incision into a transversely oriented closure. The surgeon then begins at the superior aspect of the duodenum and begins the closure. The easiest method is a running closure with 3-0 or 2-0 silk or polyglycolic suture. The surgeon should run this suture toward the inferior aspect of the duodenum stopping about two-thirds of the way down. A laparoscopic clip is placed on the suture to maintain tension while the surgeon focuses on the lower aspect of the closure. A second suture is then run from the inferior edge of the pyloroplasty to the middle and tied to the upper suture after first removing the clip from the suture. The assistant can facilitate the suturing angles by retracting the inferior stay suture caudal and rightward. An alternative approach is to perform an interrupted closure. This allows for more precise suture placement but requires more intracorporeal knot tying (FIGURE 13). With an interrupted closure, alternating sutures from the either end and tying after placing each suture allows for precise suture placement. The last suture will be placed blindly, but if the assistant applies cranial traction on the tail of the suture just superior to the last one, it reduces the likelihood of back-walling the duodenum. Methylene blue can be placed into the distal stomach via the EGD scope to ensure the pyloroplasty closure is watertight.

Omental Patch

- The author then covers the completed pyloroplasty suture line with a vascularized pedicle of omentum, which is secured in place by tying the superior and inferior stay sutures over the pedicle in the fashion of a Graham patch. This is easier to perform and less likely to narrow the pyloric outlet than a second layer of seromuscular sutures.

Chapter 30 DRAINAGE PROCEDURES: PYLOROMYOTOMY, PYLOROPLASTY, GASTROJEJUNOSTOMY 265

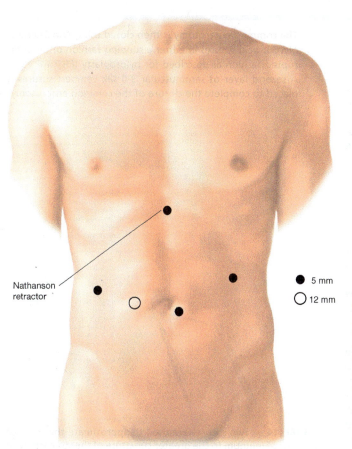

FIGURE 11 • Shown is the standard port placement used for all laparoscopic drainage procedures. The surgeon stands on the patient's right. The first port placed is the left upper quadrant 5-mm port, which will be the assistant's instrument. The left periumbilical port is for the camera, and right 12-mm port is for the surgeon's dominant hand instrument. The lateral right port is for the surgeon's nondominant hand. A Nathanson liver retractor is placed in the subxiphoid position to retract the left lobe of the liver. (Reprinted with permission from Nussbaum MS. *Master Techniques in Surgery: Gastric Surgery*. Wolters Kluwer Health/Lippincott Williams & Wilkins; 2013.)

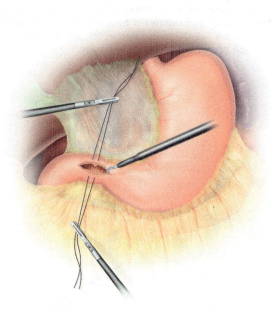

FIGURE 12 • Two stay sutures are placed above and below the proposed pyloroplasty incision. The surgeon retracts the superior suture with their nondominant hand, and the assistant retracts the inferior suture from the far left port. A hooked cautery is then used to incise the pylorus beginning from the gastric side.

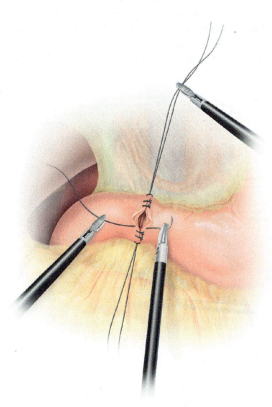

FIGURE 13 • Although the assistant provides cranial traction on the superior stay suture to convert the longitudinal pyloroplasty incision into a transversely oriented incision, the surgeon closes the pyloroplasty with either interrupted or running sutures.

LAPAROSCOPIC GASTROJEJUNOSTOMY

Port Placement

- We use a standard four-trocar approach for most gastric procedures, with a 5-mm port in the left upper quadrant, a second 5-mm trocar just to the left of the umbilicus, a 12-mm trocar at the level of the umbilicus in the midclavicular line, and a 12-mm trocar in the right upper quadrant. A Nathanson liver retractor is sometimes placed to elevate the left lobe of the liver and facilitate exposure of the anterior and inferior gastric wall (FIGURE 11).

Preparation of the Stomach and Identification of Proximal Jejunum

- First, identify the pylorus by either palpation with a grasper or by performing an intraoperative EGD. Identify a point 5 cm proximal to the pylorus, and then select a section of the jejunum 15 to 30 cm distal to the ligament of Treitz, which will easily reach the distal stomach without tension in an antecolic fashion.

Construction of the Anastomosis

- A stapled side-to-side gastrojejunostomy is then constructed in an isoperistaltic fashion by aligning the distal portion of the small bowel with the pyloric side of the stomach. Placement of two interrupted 2-0 silk seromuscular sutures between the greater curvature of the stomach and the small bowel 6 cm apart serves to align the bowel for the stapled anastomosis. Using the electrosurgical device, an enterotomy is made in the stomach and small bowel (FIGURE 14). A 60-mm Endo GIA stapler is inserted via the most lateral right side port and fired to construct the anastomosis (FIGURE 15A). A blue or green load of the stapler device should be used depending on the thickness of the stomach.

The common enterotomy is then closed using two 3-0 polyglycolic acid sutures in either a running fashion or an interrupted fashion as described for pyloroplasty (FIGURE 15B). A second layer of seromuscular 3-0 silk Lembert sutures is placed to complete the closure of the common enterotomy.

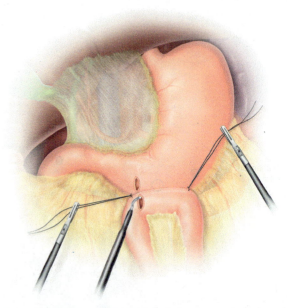

FIGURE 14 • Two sutures are used to approximate the selected segment of jejunum to the greater curvature of the stomach in an antecolic, isoperistaltic fashion. With the assistant providing cranial traction from the left on the proximal suture and the surgeon providing caudal and rightward traction, the hooked cautery is used to make a full-thickness open in the stomach and jejunum for insertion of a linear endocutting stapler.

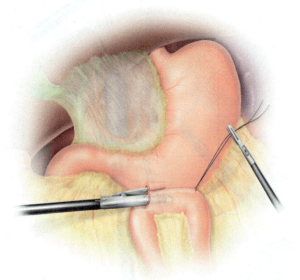

A

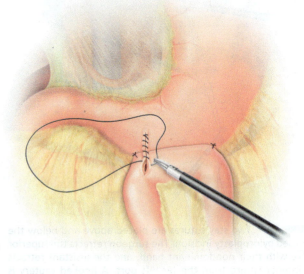

B

FIGURE 15 • In panel (**A**), a blue or green load 60-mm endostapler is fired to construct the anastomosis. In panel (**B**), the common enterotomy defect is then closed in two layers with sutures. The assistant can facilitate the suturing with cranial traction on the distal stay suture.

PEARLS AND PITFALLS

Indications	▪ When performing a drainage procedure for delayed gastric emptying with a fundoplication, documentation of poor emptying with a gastric emptying study is strongly recommended prior to surgery. ▪ When operating for gastrointestinal bleeding, being present at the initial endoscopy to see the precise bleeding location will help avoid having to make an excessively large pyloroplasty incision.
Pyloroplasty incision	▪ Incisions longer than 7 or 8 cm are difficult to close in a Heineke-Mikulicz fashion without narrowing the pyloric lumen and may require a Finney closure.
Kocher manuever	▪ Is not always necessary with a short pyloroplasty and a Heineke-Mikulicz closure but is always required with a Finney closure.
Pyloromyotomy	▪ Is very hard to perform without mucosal perforation in the setting of any duodenal inflammation. If a significant mucosa perforation occurs during pyloromyotomy, the safest approach is to convert to pyloroplasty.
Gastrojejunostomy	▪ Predisposes to marginal ulceration if a vagotomy is not performed. Patients undergoing gastrojejunostomy drainage without vagotomy will require lifetime proton pump inhibitor therapy. ▪ In the setting of a prior gastric outlet obstruction, a prolonged period of delayed gastric emptying may be encountered despite an adequate anastomotic lumen.

POSTOPERATIVE CARE

- Most patients will require nasogastric decompression for 24 to 48 hours after a drainage procedure.

OUTCOMES

- When performed in conjunction with fundoplication in patients with delayed gastric emptying, 80% of patients report an improvement in bloating symptoms.[4]
- The incidence of diarrhea reported when pyloroplasty is performed in conjunction with fundoplication in the setting of delayed gastric emptying is reported to be as high as 25%.[5]
- The incidence of clinically significant dumping syndrome after drainage procedures is less than 10%.[6]

COMPLICATIONS

- Leak from suture or staple line
- Delayed gastric emptying
- Surgical site infection
- Dumping syndrome
- Diarrhea
- Duodenogastric reflux is quite rare after pyloroplasty.
- Bile reflux gastritis following gastrojejunostomy

REFERENCES

1. Nevins EJ, Rao R, Nicholson J, et al. Endoscopic botulinum toxin as a treatment for delayed gastric emptying following oesophagogastrectomy. *Ann R Coll Surg Engl.* 2020;102(9):693-696. doi:10.1308/rcsann.2020.0136
2. Hamrick MC, Davis SS, Chiruvella A, et al. Incidence of delayed gastric emptying associated with revisional laparoscopic paraesophageal hernia repair. *J Gastrointest Surg.* 2013;17(2):213-217. doi:10.1007/s11605-012-1989-0
3. Gilsdorf D, Volckmann E, Brickley A, Taylor LJ, Glasgow RE, Fang J. Pyloroplasty offers relief of postfundoplication gastroparesis in patients who improved after botulinum toxin injection. *J Laparoendosc Adv Surg Tech A.* 2017;27(11):1180-1184. doi:10.1089/lap.2017.0099
4. Masqusi S, Velanovich V. Pyloroplasty with fundoplication in the treatment of combined gastroesophageal reflux disease and bloating. *World J Surg.* 2007;31(2):332-336. doi:10.1007/s00268-006-0723-z
5. Khajanchee YS, Dunst CM, Swanstrom LL. Outcomes of Nissen fundoplication in patients with gastroesophageal reflux disease and delayed gastric emptying. *Arch Surg.* 2009;144(9):823-828. doi:10.1001/archsurg.2009.160
6. Tack J, Arts J, Caenepeel P, De Wulf D, Bisschops R. Pathophysiology, diagnosis and management of postoperative dumping syndrome. *Nat Rev Gastroenterol Hepatol.* 2009;6(10):583-590. doi:10.1038/nrgastro.2009.148

Chapter 31

Endoscopic Management of Gastroparesis and Gastric Outlet Obstruction

Juan S. Barajas-Gamboa and John H. Rodriguez

DEFINITION

- Gastroparesis and gastric outlet obstruction are conditions characterized by a delay or complete absence of gastric emptying. The cause is highly variable and includes a number of conditions that result in either functional or mechanical etiology. Gastroparesis specifically implies the absence of an obstructive component and is the term used to define an underlying functional syndrome. The etiology commonly falls under three categories: idiopathic, diabetic, or postsurgical.[1]
- Gastric outlet obstruction encompasses a wide variety of etiologies that result in either internal or external compression that affect the gastric-duodenal drainage basin. Gastric or duodenal pathology such as neoplastic or inflammatory processes can result in the typical symptoms, which include epigastric abdominal pain, bloating, nausea, and postprandial vomiting. External compression can result from a wide variety of intra-abdominal and retroperitoneal neoplastic processes and tend to manifest later in the course of the underlying disease.

DIFFERENTIAL DIAGNOSIS

- Patients presenting with typical symptoms will have to be classified in one of two broad categories: functional vs mechanical etiology. This differentiation will be the main determinant and predictor of outcomes when considering treatment options. Current endoscopic interventions will either be palliative or therapeutic based on the differential diagnosis.
- Evaluation of patients presenting with nausea and vomiting will include a combination of imaging and functional studies that will help further understand the differential diagnosis. These include a variety of processes that can result in gastric outlet obstruction. Among others, they can be peptic ulcer disease, duodenal or gastric malignancy, pyloric stenosis, and external compression from malignancy.
- In cases where a mechanical component cannot be identified, functional studies will help understand underlying gastrointestinal (MI) motility. Studies have shown that a significant number of patients with gastroparesis may suffer from additional motility alterations in the GI tract including colonic inertia and small bowel dysmotility.[2] In this population, it is very important to rule out other conditions that may mimic motility disorders. Many psychiatric illnesses and eating disorders, such as anorexia nervosa and bulimia, may mimic gastroparesis and should be ruled out. Other conditions, such as cyclical vomiting syndrome, irritable bowel syndrome, and celiac sprue, may present with overlapping symptoms and need to be differentiated as well.

PATIENT HISTORY AND PHYSICAL FINDINGS

- History taking is extremely important as it may help to clarify the etiology and develop an adequate treatment plan. Time from onset of symptoms can help determine chronicity as well as a potential association with a trigger, such as prior surgery or viral illness. Many patients suffering from motility disorders may have associated conditions.
  - To name a few, they can be diabetes, postural tachycardia syndrome, chronic abdominal pain, and fibromyalgia. Patients presenting with gastric outlet obstruction may have a history of peptic ulcer disease, *Helicobacter pylori* infection, use of nonsteroidal anti-inflammatory drugs, smoking, etc.
  - They may also present with signs of symptoms that may point to an underlying malignancy, such as weight loss, jaundice, type B symptoms, and melena, among others.[3]
- Prior surgical history is extremely important. Patients with a history of foregut surgery may develop postsurgical gastroparesis as a result of vagal nerve injury. Those with a history of fundoplication or hiatal hernia repair can develop symptoms related to the surgery that may mimic gastroparesis or a gastric outlet obstruction. Patients with history of esophagectomy can present with a poorly draining conduit or anastomotic stricture.
- Patients with a history of peptic ulcer disease who have undergone prior surgical intervention may have severe scarring involving the pyloric and duodenum. This may affect candidacy for future endoscopic interventions. The patient's nutritional status can be determined by obvious physical findings. Many patients will present with severe nutritional deficiencies due to poor oral tolerance.[2]

IMAGING AND OTHER DIAGNOSTIC STUDIES

- Esophagogastroduodenoscopy (EGD) is likely the most valuable diagnostic test that can determine the differential diagnosis between a functional or mechanical disorder. Special consideration should be taken when planning EGD in patients presenting with nausea and vomiting. Airway management should be considered as many of these patients are at high risk of aspiration during sedation. Large amount of food bezoars are a common finding and may obscure proper visualization. Patient preparation with an extended course of clear liquid diet for 48 to 72 hours prior may help improve visualization.
- Upper GI barium series is the most valuable imaging study. It can delineate anatomy in the entire upper GI tract and identify a mechanical etiology. Patients with long-standing gastric outlet obstruction or gastroparesis may present with a very large and distended stomach. This may warrant further

Chapter 31 ENDOSCOPIC MANAGEMENT OF GASTROPARESIS AND GASTRIC OUTLET OBSTRUCTION

consideration at the time of endoscopic intervention, as a longer scope may be required. This is a very useful study in patients with prior foregut surgery to evaluate a fundoplication and rule out the presence of a recurrent hiatal hernia with a significant mechanical component.
- Computed tomography of the abdomen and pelvis can be very useful in evaluating patients with a gastric outlet obstruction in which an external source is suspected. It is usually not a routine study required in patients with a motility disorder.[3] Gastric emptying scintigraphy has become the gold standard for evaluating gastric motility. This study is widely available and involves ingestion of a meal tagged with a radionuclide that can be traced at different time intervals. Protocols are not standardized and there can be wide variability between meals and measurement intervals. Most experts agree that a 4-hour study with ingestion of a solid meal yields the most accurate results. Discontinuation of promotility agents is recommended to avoid any potential interaction with test results.

SURGICAL MANAGEMENT

Preoperative Planning

- Patients undergoing endoscopic intervention for management of gastroparesis or gastric outlet obstruction will need to be treated as high-risk patients due to the frequent aspiration risk. Each facility will have special and individual setups that may require these procedures be performed in an operating room or endoscopy suite accordingly. Equipment and anesthesia availability can also vary and should be the main factor to consider in selecting the best environment.

Patient Positioning

- Patients should be positioned either in a supine or left lateral position based on the proceduralist's preference. In cases where fluoroscopy is planned, a supine position is preferred. This situation will also require using a fluoroscopy compatible surgical bed with no interruptions in the upper portion.

Equipment

- Selecting the proper endoscopic equipment ahead of time is crucial. Endoscopes have wide variability in terms of length, diameter, size, and number of working channels. A standard upper endoscope with a single 2.8-mm working channel will accommodate most instruments required for intramural surgery: through-the-scope (TTS) dilatation, medication delivery, and guidewire deployment. If stent deployment is planned, an endoscope with a 3.7-mm working channel will be required.
- Patients with marked gastric distention may require a longer endoscope to reach the pylorus and beyond. Most standard gastroscopes are in the range of 1000 mm, while colonoscopes can vary between 1300 and 1600 mm. Diameter is also variable and should be accounted for when trying to traverse stenosis areas or for tunneling during intramural intervention.
- Fluoroscopy is an excellent aid during endoscopic intervention. It is necessary for safe advancement of wires, stent deployment, and navigating through difficult anatomy. When the potential for using x-rays exist, patient positioning as well as surgical bed selection should be accounted for.

TECHNIQUES

ENDOSCOPIC DILATATION AND STRICTUROPLASTY

- Endoscopic dilatation of the pylorus for management of benign gastric outlet obstruction was described nearly 4 decades ago. The use of TTS balloon dilators has made this technique easy to perform and highly replicable. Effectiveness has been reported in up to 80% of patients. The procedure carries a low risk of complications, with perforation being the most feared. The risk of perforation tends to increase with balloon diameter, and the highest risk is when the balloons are over 15 mm.[4,5]

Equipment and Technique

- A standard upper endoscope with a 2.8-mm working channel is required. Use of fluoroscopy can be necessary in cases of severe stenosis to navigate a guidewire through the stricture. Endoscopic TTS balloons are classified by their ability to be advanced over a wire or not. Some commercially available balloons have a built-in guidewire that can be advanced or retracted with a locking mechanism. Balloons are further classified by diameter with sizes ranging from 5 to 20 mm (**FIGURE 1**). Balloon expansion is controlled with a pressure pump and balloon guides typically describe a pressure to diameter relationship.
- The endoscope is advanced to the stricture and the diameter inspected. Knowledge of the scope diameter is usually the easiest way to determine the size of the narrowing. If the scope can be advanced past the stricture, the starting diameter of the balloon should be around 12 to 15 mm. In this case, the balloon is extracted past the stricture under direct endoscopic vision at the same time the scope is withdrawn. If the stricture does not allow passage of the scope, the balloon can be advanced gently or over a guidewire with or without fluoroscopy as deemed necessary. It is important to remember that the guidewire will add stiffness to the system and can increase the risk of perforation when the balloon is advanced with the wire close to the tip.[4]
- The working length of the balloon is then positioned across the narrowed area and the balloon inflated to the corresponding diameter while the endoscopist ensures that the balloon remains stable during the inflation process. Once the balloon is inflated, the scope can be approximated to the balloon to allow direct visualization of the tissue during balloon expansion.

Intralesional Steroid Injection

- Steroid delivery at the time of dilatation can further enhance the effectiveness of this intervention by preventing stricture reformation.[6] The technique requires the use of an endoscopic injection needle (23-25 G) for medication delivery in a radial pattern. A four-quadrant injection pattern is applied in a circumferential fashion.

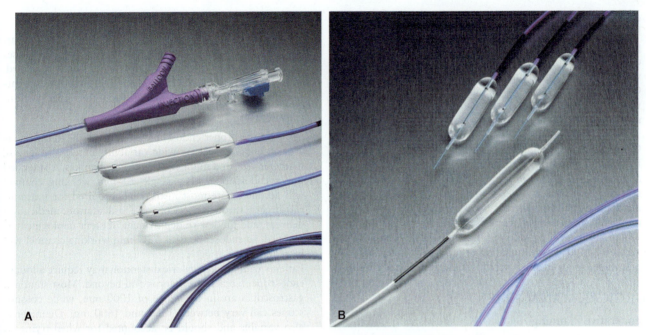

FIGURE 1 • Balloon dilatation catheters: **(A)** and **(B)**. Endoscopic CRE(TM) balloon dilation catheters.

ENDOSCOPIC STRICTUROPLASTY

- Use of electrosurgical endoscopic knives has been described for the management of strictures along the GI tract, mostly for the management of complications from inflammatory bowel disease.[7] Limited data exist supporting its role. Clinical experience has shown benefit in cases where a short stricture with a fibrotic component exists. The theory is that controlled cutting of the fibrotic ring can prevent uncontrolled tearing and perforation.

Equipment and Technique

- The technique involves radial cutting with an endoscopic electrosurgical knife along the circumference of a fibrotic ring. This can be done at multiple sites varying typically between 3 and 6 radial cuts. The cuts should be limited to the fibrotic component and avoid full-thickness incision. Insulated tip knives can be helpful to avoid inadvertent injury to tissues beyond the stricture that are not being visualized during the procedure.

ENDOSCOPIC STENTING

- Self-expanding metal stents (SEMS) have been used for the management of gastric outlet obstruction since it was first reported in the early 1990s. Stents are commercially available in a wide variety of sizes, materials, and delivery systems. Application has been described mostly for malignant obstruction. Metal stents designed for this application are uncovered and therefore not designed for retrieval. This must be taken into consideration in cases where the potential for later removal exists (**FIGURE 2**).[8]

Equipment and Technique

- Advancement and deployment of stents through the scope requires a 3.7-mm working channel. The delivery system can be advanced across the stenosis with or without the use of a guidewire. Size and stiffness are factors to be considered when selecting an adequate wire to allow proper navigation of the delivery system. Wire diameter should not exceed 0.035 in. Stiffer wires with a soft tip are preferred to help guide the delivery system through sharp turns typically encountered in the duodenum. Fluoroscopy is always recommended.
- Stent selection is based on the desired intent. In cases with a malignant obstruction where retrieval is unlikely, an uncovered stent is preferred. In patients where surgical intervention or later retrieval is desired, a partially covered stent is preferred. Stents designed for duodenal application have a diameter around 22 mm with a wider proximal flange to reduce the risk of migration. Length can vary between 60 and 120 mm.
- The endoscope is advanced to the level of the stenosis. Therapeutic endoscopes have a wider diameter that in many cases may preclude passage through the stricture. In this situation, the guidewire can be advanced under fluoroscopy for a significant extent past the stricture to avoid losing the wire during manipulation. The stent is then advanced over the wire and under fluoroscopy, to ensure safe navigation around turns. In challenging cases, placing tension on the wire while pushing the delivery system will help advancement around a tight corner. Once the stent is located across the stricture, the deployment process begins.

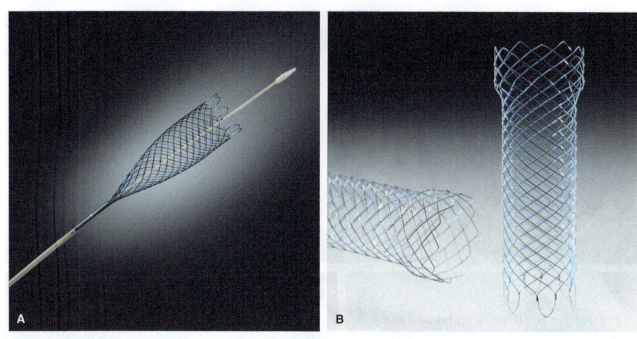

FIGURE 2 • Duodenal stents: **(A)** and **(B)**. Endoscopic through the scope uncovered duodenal stent.

- Most delivery systems will have radiologic markers that help identify the proximal and distal extent of the stent. There is a tendency toward shortening throughout the deployment process, which will need to be taken into account to avoid missing the desired target. Deployment typically requires pulling back a sheath that will uncover the SEMS. There is typically a "point of no return" at which the stent can no longer be resheathed. The proceduralist needs to be certain about the right position before passing this point in the deployment process.
- After deployment, SEMS will continue a slow expansion process to reach maximum diameter over 24 hours. Many endoscopists will recommend against passing the scope through a recently deployed stent to minimize the risk of distal migration.

ENDOSCOPIC PYLOROMYOTOMY

- Endoscopic per-oral pyloromyotomy (POP) has revolutionized management of gastroparesis.[9] Surgical treatment options have been limited to gastric electrical stimulation, gastric emptying, and, in advanced cases, gastric diversion or removal. Prior to the introduction of POP, endoscopic management of gastroparesis was limited to injection of botulinum toxin and transpyloric stenting. Neither of these options have gained traction due to inconsistent results or high complication rates.

Equipment and Technique

- A standard upper endoscope with a 2.8-mm working channel allows passage of all necessary instruments for this procedure. The endoscope should be fitted with a soft beveled cap to improve visualization and aid with dissection and tissue retraction. A 23-G endoscopic needle is needed for injection. A triangle-tip endoscopic electrosurgical knife is preferred, but many alternatives exist and can be modified based on the individual preference. A dyed solution is utilized to create a mucosal blob and improve visualization during the procedure. Diluted methylene blue at a ratio of 10 to 100 mL of normal saline is prepared prior to the procedure. This ratio can be adjusted to allow for a darker or lighter colored solution based on individual preference. Commercially available solutions with higher viscosity can also be utilized and have the advantage of slower dissipation through the tissues. An electrosurgical unit is also required (▶ Video 1).
- Two different techniques for endoscopic pyloromyotomy have been described. The first involves creation of a long tunnel along the greater curvature of the stomach. This technique has been modified to a lesser curvature approach, in which the tunnel is shortened and positioned along the lesser curvature of the stomach starting at a point, distal to the incisura angularis. Potential advantages to this technique include shorter operating time, easier identification of the pyloric ring, and higher technical feasibility.[10] This technique can be simplified into four steps (**FIGURE 3**):

Step 1—Mucosal Incision

- The procedure starts with a diagnostic EGD. The lesser curvature is carefully examined to identify any potential contraindication to the procedure such as ulcers or large food bezoars that preclude visualization. The pylorus is traversed and the duodenum inspected. In cases where pylorospasm is encountered, we avoid passing the scope through the pylorus to avoid any mucosal trauma.
- A site is selected 3 to 6 cm proximal to the pylorus along the lesser curvature. The preferred location is highly dependent on

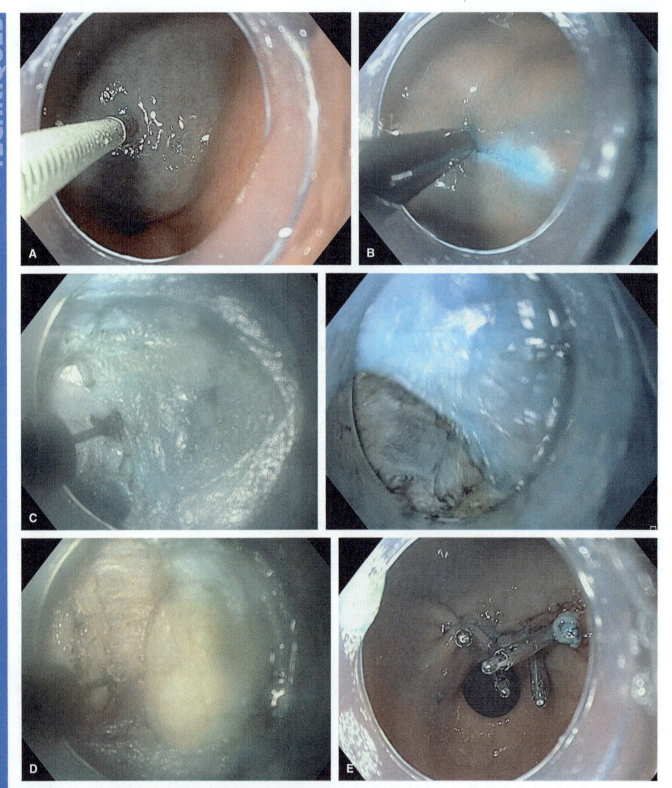

FIGURE 3 • Per-oral pyloromyotomy: **(A)** injection of methylene blue, **(B)** mucosotomy using triangle-tip knife, **(C)** submucosal tunneling, **(D)** myotomy, and **(E)** mucosotomy closure.

anatomy. It is recommended to start at least 2 cm distal to the incisors angularis, but no less than 3 cm proximal to the pylorus. The injection needle is then inserted and the blue dyed solution injected to create a mucosal bleb. In many cases, the

initial position of the needle can be too deep, so this maneuver involves slow and gentle withdrawal while injecting until the submucosal plane is reached. This can be confirmed by mucosal lifting. Once the needle is in the proper position, 5 to 10 mL of

solution is injected to create separation between the mucosa and muscle layers. The blue dye will stain the submucosal space, but the mucosa and muscle fibers will show very little uptake of the dye, preserving a whiter hue.
- Following mucosal lift, a transverse incision is made using an endosurgical knife. The submucosal injection helps avoid any muscle injury. The incision is carried for 1.5 to 2 cm in order to accommodate the endoscope while avoiding tearing of the incision. Cut current modes are preferred for this step to avoid charring of the mucosa.

Step 2—Tunneling

- After the incision is completed, the bevel of the cap is used to create gentle tension in the mucosa. This allows visualization of the submucosal plane. Using the endosurgical knife in spray coagulation mode, the space is further developed toward the muscle layer. The muscle can be clearly identified by a more pale color when compared to the submucosal plane. Once the muscle fibers are visualized, dissection continues in a distal fashion using gentle spray coagulation along the muscle, avoiding any potential thermal injury to the mucosa. The antrum of the stomach is cone shaped with the apex representing the pylorus.
- As the dissection continues distally, the position of the endoscope and cap will provide gentle tension to the mucosa. The pylorus can be clearly visualized by the configuration and orientation of the muscle fibers when compared to the surrounding tissue. It is important to recognize that the mucosa of the duodenum tends to be in a perpendicular position at the level of the bulb. Distal extension of the tunnel past the pylorus is unnecessary and increases the risk of mucosal injury and potential perforation.
- Bridging mucosal vessels may be encountered during this portion of the procedure. Preservation is preferred when feasible to avoid mucosal ischemia. However, they may need to be divided. This can be done with the endosurgical knife in coagulation mode for vessels between 1 and 2 mm in diameter. Larger vessels may need to be controlled using a coagulation grasper.

Step 3—Myotomy

- Once the distal extent of the tunnel allows proper visualization of the pylorus, the myotomy is performed. Hybrid cut energy modes are preferred to avoid excess charring, which may preclude proper visualization of the muscular planes. The preferred technique involves positioning of the shaft of the endosurgical knife across the pylorus. Energy is applied at the same time that upper deflection of the endoscope is performed. Careful visualization after each application can help determine the depth of the incision until all the pyloric fibers are divided. There tends to be a clear change in the pattern of the muscle fibers that can be visualized once pyloric division is completed. In many cases the blue dye will dissect between the muscle layers, adding an additional landmark for complete division.

Step 4—Mucosal Closure

- Once the myotomy is completed, a hemostasis is ensured to prevent postoperative bleedings. After this, the endoscope is removed from the tunnel and the pylorus is visualized from the lumen of the stomach. The mucosotomy is closed stepwise with multiple endoscopic clips to reapproximate the mucosal edges. Finally, the gastroscope is withdrawn and the patient is extubated.

PEARLS AND PITFALLS

- During endoscopic dilatation, perforation can occur during balloon insufflation. It is important to constantly communicate with the operator of the insufflation device to get feedback on resistance. Slow balloon expansion can also help avoid this complication.
- During stenting, miscalculation of the area for deployment can occur. However, the use of fluoroscopy and slow deployment can help prevent this mistake. Most commercially available stents have a deployment stage where the stent can no longer be resheathed. It is advised to always verify proper positioning before pulling the deployment mechanism past this point.
- Patients undergoing POP who have very distended and "J"-shaped stomach can present additional challenges. The retroflexed position of the endoscope during initial mucosotomy and tunneling can inadvertently misguide the proceduralist into creating a proximal tunnel along the lesser curvature of the stomach. Forced downward deflection of the endoscope, as well as reduction into a "short scope" position, can help avoid this mistake.

POSTOPERATIVE CARE

- Endoscopic management can be performed safely as an outpatient procedure. After the procedure, the patients are transferred to the postanesthesia care unit for monitoring. Patients are discharged the same day and begin a clear liquid diet. Patients continue with clear liquid diet for 7 to 10 days, and posteriorly, the diet is advanced to full liquid diet for 1 month. Generally, patients are prescribed with proton pump inhibitor and sucralfate therapy for 6 weeks to prevent ulcers and bleedings.

COMPLICATIONS

- Nausea
- Epigastric discomfort
- Bleeding
- Perforation
- Capnoperitoneum/pneumoperitoneum
- Pulmonary embolism
- Infections

REFERENCES

1. Soykan I, Sivri B, Sarosiek I, Kiernan B, McCallum RW. Demography, clinical characteristics, psychological and abuse profiles, treatment, and long-term follow-up of patients with gastroparesis. *Dig Dis Sci.* 1998;43(11):2398-2404. doi:10.1023/a:1026665728213
2. Khullar SK, DiSario JA. Gastric outlet obstruction. *Gastrointest Endosc Clin N Am.* 1996;6(3):585-603.
3. Jeong SJ, Lee J. Management of gastric outlet obstruction: focusing on endoscopic approach. *World J Gastrointest Pharmacol Ther.* 2020;11(2):8-16. doi:10.4292/wjgpt.v11.i2.8
4. Kochhar R, Kochhar S. Endoscopic balloon dilation for benign gastric outlet obstruction in adults. *World J Gastrointest Endosc.* 2010;2(1):29-35. doi:10.4253/wjge.v2.i1.29
5. Solt J, Bajor J, Szabó M, Horváth OP. Long-term results of balloon catheter dilation for benign gastric outlet stenosis. *Endoscopy.* 2003;35(6):490-495. doi:10.1055/s-2003-39664
6. Lee M, Kubik CM, Polhamus CD, Brady CEIIIrd, Kadakia SC. Preliminary experience with endoscopic intralesional steroid injection therapy for refractory upper gastrointestinal strictures. *Gastrointest Endosc.* 1995;41(6):598-601. doi:10.1016/s0016-5107(95)70199-0
7. Paine E, Shen B. Endoscopic therapy in inflammatory bowel diseases (with videos). *Gastrointest Endosc.* 2013;78(6):819-835. doi:10.1016/j.gie.2013.08.023
8. Clarke JO, Sharaiha RZ, Kord Valeshabad A, Lee LA, Kalloo AN, Khashab MA. Through-the-scope transpyloric stent placement improves symptoms and gastric emptying in patients with gastroparesis. *Endoscopy.* 2013;45(suppl 2 UCTN):E189-E190. doi:10.1055/s-0032-1326400
9. Rodriguez J, Strong AT, Haskins IN, et al. Per-oral pyloromyotomy (POP) for medically refractory gastroparesis: short term results from the first 100 patients at a high volume center. *Ann Surg.* 2018;268(3):421-430. doi:10.1097/SLA.0000000000002927
10. Allemang MT, Strong AT, Haskins IN, Rodriguez J, Ponsky JL, Kroh M. How I do it: per-oral pyloromyotomy (POP). *J Gastrointest Surg.* 2017;21(11):1963-1968. doi:10.1007/s11605-017-3510-2

Chapter 32: Surgical Management of Gastroduodenal Perforation

Amy Rosenbluth and Givi Basishvili

DEFINITION

- **Gastroduodenal perforation**—full-thickness injury to the stomach wall or duodenum creating a communication between the gastric lumen and the peritoneal cavity. This communication leads to entry of air and gastric/intestinal contents into the peritoneal cavity and can lead to peritonitis, sepsis, and multi-organ failure. Most frequent locations include the anterior surface of the duodenal bulb, the gastric antrum, the lesser curvature of the stomach, and posterior duodenal bulb.[1,2]

DIFFERENTIAL DIAGNOSIS

- **Peptic ulcer disease (PUD):** It is the most common cause of gastroduodenal perforations. With the advent of medical proton pump inhibitor (PPI) therapy, this finding occurs in less than 10% of patients with PUD.[3] Risk factors for PUD include use of nonsteroidal anti-inflammatory drugs and smoking. *Helicobacter pylori* has been indicated in many PUD cases as an occult culprit and should be tested and treated if diagnosed.
    - Miscellaneous causes of PUD include alcohol use, cocaine use, steroid use, chemotherapy, prolonged fasting, high salt intake, Zollinger-Ellison syndrome, marginal ulcers, or post gastric bypass surgery.
- **Iatrogenic injury:** Upper endoscopy is the main cause of gastroduodenal perforation from iatrogenic source. Areas of biopsies/cauterization are at highest risk of perforation, as well as thinner parts of the lumen at the proximal stomach, or the lesser curve, which is least distensible. Although iatrogenic causes of duodenal perforations are rarer, they have been reported after endoscopy and laparoscopic cholecystectomy, with the second portion of the duodenum being the most common location.[4] Endoscopic interventions such as pyloromyotomy, stricture dilations, and removal of foreign bodies all increase the risk of endoscopy-associated perforation.
- **Malignancy:** Neoplastic etiology can cause perforation by direct invasion, obstruction causing increased pressure, or necrotic inflammation weaning the surrounding tissue. Reported incidence of gastric cancer–associated perforations is 0.4% to 6.0%.[5]
- **Trauma:** Both blunt and penetrating injuries can cause gastroduodenal perforations. Penetrating injuries involve the stomach in 5% to 10%[6,7] of cases and are commonly associated with gastric perforation as opposed to the duodenal perforation which is mostly associated with blunt injury causing shearing forces between the duodenum and its retroperitoneal attachments. Duodenal hematomas can also be found in blunt trauma which can cause subsequent gastric outlet obstruction and perforation.
- **Miscellaneous:** It includes duodenal diverticula, infections (rotavirus, norovirus, tuberculosis, *Ascaris lumbricoides*), ischemia, impacted stones/foreign bodies, autoimmune conditions (scleroderma, Crohn disease), and chemotherapy.

PATIENT HISTORY AND PHYSICAL FINDINGS

- **Subjective description:** Sudden onset of abdominal pain and distension. Additional symptoms can include fevers, chills, nausea, emesis, ileus, respiratory distress, chest pain, shoulder pain, hematemesis, or hematochezia.
- **History:** It is important to elicit any recent endoscopic procedures, operations, ingestion of foreign bodies, or esophageal testing undergone by the patient, use of anti-inflammatory agents, malignancy, smoking, immunosuppression, and unexplained weight loss.
    - *Note: Patient with immunosuppression or resent use of anti-inflammatory medications may have blunted physical examination findings and may have a delayed presentation.*
- **Physical examination:** Most common examination findings include abdominal distention, generalized abdominal tenderness which may include guarding, rigidity and peritonitis, tachycardia, and fever. Additional findings may include tachypnea, respiratory distress, and hypotension. Bowel sounds may be absent.

IMAGING AND OTHER DIAGNOSTIC STUDIES

- **Plain X-ray imaging:** This can be used to make a quick diagnosis of gastroduodenal perforation. Upright CXR and KUB can be used to identify pneumoperitoneum, depending on the amount of extraluminal air present.
- **Computed tomography imaging:** This is the most sensitive and specific modality for the diagnoses of gastroduodenal perforations. Computed tomography with PO and intravenous (IV) contrast is the preferred imaging of choice.[8]
    - Findings usually include pneumoperitoneum, extravasation of oral contrast, and free intra-abdominal fluid. Additional findings may include mesenteric air, discontinuity of hollow viscous wall, bowel wall thickening/edema, and mesenteric hematoma.

SURGICAL MANAGEMENT

Preoperative Planning

- Gastroduodenal perforations are managed with prompt surgical intervention.
    - Prior to proceeding to the operating room, the patient should be resuscitated IV fluids, broad-spectrum antibiotics should be initiated, and PPIs should be started.
    - Patient should be lined with a nasogastric tube, large bore IVs, and urinary catheter, and consideration should be given to central line as well as an arterial line in an unstable patient.
    - It is also important to identify the underlying cause of the gastroduodenal perforation as it guides the surgical intervention.
    - The decision of laparoscopic vs open surgical intervention is based on patient's hemodynamic stability, ability to tolerate pneumoperitoneum for laparoscopy, and experience of the surgeon.[9]

- Large-scale studies have shown no difference between open vs laparoscopic repairs in terms of complication rates, re-operations, or mortality.[10,11]
- Laparoscopic approach has shown to have lower surgical site infections, less postoperative pain, and shorter nasogastric tube duration.[12]
- Surgical management strategies include the following:
  - Primary repair—closure of defect with suture primarily.[13] Most used in setting of trauma.
  - Graham patch repair—closure of defect using omental flap without primary closure of defect. Employed in large perforations with friable surrounding edges.
  - Modified Graham patch repair—primary closure of defect, followed by placement of omental flap. Most optimal management strategy for small perforations with healthy surrounding mucosa.
  - Wedge resection—segmental resection of perforation. Used in setting of large perforation located along the greater curvature or in setting of suspected underlying malignancy.[14]
- Additional surgical interventions/reconstruction:
  - Pyloroplasty/vagotomy—rarely performed in setting of gastroduodenal perforation, indication for PUD refractory to medical management in stable patients.
  - Roux-en-y gastric bypass—resection of distal stomach/portion of duodenum, followed by gastrojejunostomy and jejunojejunostomy.
  - Billroth I—resection of distal stomach/proximal duodenum followed by gastroduodenostomy.
  - Billroth II—resection of distal stomach/proximal duodenum followed by gastrojejunostomy.

LAPAROSCOPIC MODIFIED GRAHAM PATCH REPAIR

Positioning

- Patient is positioned supine, with arms extended and available for further resuscitation.
- The patient should be secured with a strap going across the chest and hips, bearhugger going across the chest, and a foot board.
- The laparoscopic monitors are positioned at the head of the patient on each side, while the laparoscopic instruments and energy sources are located at the foot of the table.
- The surgeon stands on the right side of the patient. Alternative position includes prone with legs parted with the surgeon standing between the legs (**FIGURE 1**).[15]

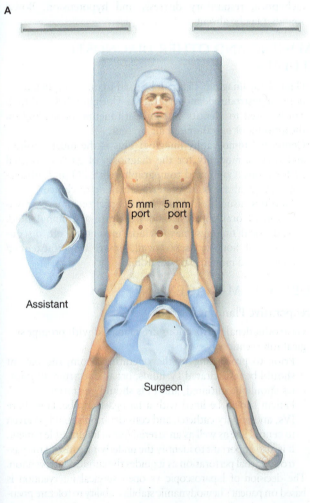
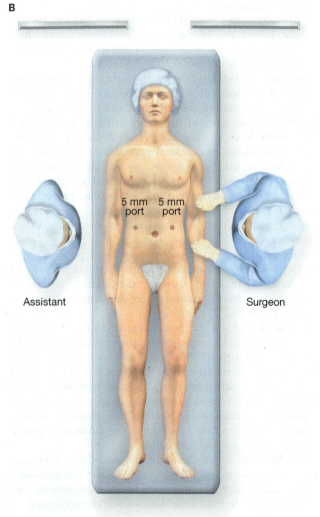

FIGURE 1 • Patient positioning for laparoscopic modified Graham patch repair.

Chapter 32 SURGICAL MANAGEMENT OF GASTRODUODENAL PERFORATION   277

ACCESS AND PORT PLACEMENT

- Access can be obtained via open Hasson technique via the umbilicus or using a Veress needle at Palmer point. Three trocars are placed in total, though more can be added if necessary. A 10-mm port in the umbilicus and 2 × 5-mm ports on either side are typically used.

DIAGNOSTIC LAPAROSCOPY AND PERITONEAL LAVAGE

- Diagnostic laparoscopy should be performed first, enteric contents should be suctioned, followed by a thorough irrigation of the abdominal cavity with several liters of saline.
- Once all the debris is removed, the defect in the gastroduodenal region should be identified and evaluated to assess the friability of surrounding tissue.

MANAGEMENT OF PERFORATION

- If the surrounding tissue around the perforation appears healthy and the defect is less than 5 mm, repair of the perforation should be performed using full-thickness large bites using a 2-0 permanent braided suture such as silk or Ethibond. The sutures should be interrupted and spaced approximately 2 mm apart (**FIGURE 2**).
- If suturing a duodenal perforation, bites should be taken in the direction of the duodenum to prevent narrowing the lumen.
- If a larger perforation is encountered, consideration should be given to patch repair without primary suture repair.
- Gastric ulcers have an increased association with malignancy and thus a biopsy of perforation margins should be performed.

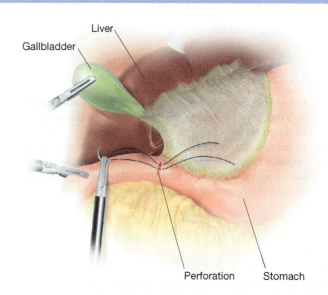

FIGURE 2 • Suture repair of a small defect using full-thickness large bites with permanent braided structure.

OMENTAL PATCH PLACEMENT

- An omental patch is sutured over the perforation to provide additional support to the repair. Care should be taken that the omentum is placed over the perforation in a tension-free manner to prevent separation from the repair (**FIGURE 3**).
- If necessary, part of the omental attachments to the transverse colon can be divided using electrocautery. Care should be taken to ensure that the omental flap used retains adequate blood supply after mobilization.
- Traditionally two interrupted sutures have been used to buttress the omentum in place over the area of perforation.

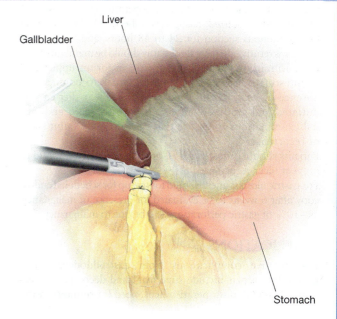

FIGURE 3 • Omental patch is sutured in a tension-free manner over the perforation to provide additional support.

LEAK TEST

- Following repair of the gastroduodenal perforation, the repair should be tested with insufflation for an air leak.
- Endoscopy should be utilized for the leak test as this will allow for evaluation of closure as well as the opportunity to obtain biopsies around the area of perforation for testing for *H. pylori* as well as for malignancy.

FINAL STEPS

- The peritoneal cavity should be thoroughly irrigated and suctioned one last time, nasogastric tube should be placed, and its position is confirmed laparoscopically.
- Fascia of the 10-mm port should be closed to prevent hernia formation.
- Drain placement is controversial and some studies have shown association with increased risk of infections without preventing abscess formation.[16] Alternatively, drain placement can be used to monitor for early leakage as the patient recovers and begins oral intake.

PEARLS AND PITFALLS

- To prevent progression of PUD to perforation, patients with PUD should be encouraged to take PPIs regularly and should be tested for underlying *H. pylori* infection.
- To prevent iatrogenic perforation during endoscopy, avoid excessive looping in the stomach, consider endoscopic ultrasound before resection of subepithelial lesions, and use submucosal fluid injection before resecting large lesions.
- Tension-free repair is key to prevent further tearing to already weakened tissue. If there is concern that primary repair would cause tension, or if the tissue appears friable, one should consider performing a Graham patch without primary repair.

POSTOPERATIVE CARE

- Postoperative care will vary depending on patient's clinical status, frailty, and degree of inflammatory response.[17]
- Broad-spectrum IV antibiotics should be continued for at least 3 to 4 days postoperatively, antifungal medications are controversial and should be based on intraoperative culture results,[18] PPIs should be utilized, nasogastric tube should be placed on low continuous suction for 24 to 48 hours, and until bowel functions return, adequate fluid status should be maintained.[19,20]
- Prior to initiating a diet, consideration for an upper gastrointestinal series can be given in order to confirm the absence of leak.[21] If no leak is notable, clear diet can be initiated and gradually advanced with frequent abdominal examinations to ensure that they do not exhibit signs of recurrence.
- Patients should be tested for *H. pylori* and treated if found to prevent ulcer recurrence.
- For gastric ulcers, patient should follow-up for scheduled endoscopy after 6 weeks to be evaluated for presence of malignancy, as ~10% of gastric perforations can be due to malignancy.[22]

COMPLICATIONS

- Postoperative complications from gastroduodenal ulcer perforation repair include superficial and deep space infections (3%-5%), postoperative ileus, need for re-intervention (2.5%-5.5%), gastric outlet obstruction secondary to stenosis, and mortality (4%-10%).[1,2,23,24]

REFERENCES

1. Sigmon DF, Tuma F, Kamel BG, Cassaro S. *Gastric perforation*. In: *StatPearls*. StatPearls Publishing; 2021.
2. Amini A, Lopez RA. *Duodenal perforation*. In: *StatPearls*. StatPearls Publishing; 2021.
3. Chung KT, Shelat VG. Perforated peptic ulcer—an update. *World J Gastrointest Surg*. 2017;9(1):1-12.
4. Machado NO. Duodenal injury post laparoscopic cholecystectomy: incidence, mechanism, management and outcome. *World J Gastrointest Surg*. 2016;8(4):335-344.
5. Lehnert T, Buhl K, Dueck M, et al. Two-stage radical gastrectomy for perforated gastric cancer. *Eur J Surg Oncol*. 2000;26(8):780-784.
6. Cardi M, Ibrahim K, Alizai SW, et al. Injury patterns and causes of death in 953 patients with penetrating abdominal war wounds in a civilian independent non-governmental organization hospital in Lashkargah, Afghanistan. *World J Emerg Surg*. 2019;14:51.
7. Naeem BK, Perveen S, Naeem N, et al. Visceral injuries in patients with blunt and penetrating abdominal trauma presenting to a tertiary care facility in Karachi, Pakistan. *Cureus*. 2018;10(11):e3604.
8. Furukawa A, Sakoda M, Yamasaki M, et al. Gastrointestinal tract perforation: CT diagnosis of presence, site, and cause. *Abdom Imaging*. 2005;30(5):524-534.
9. Mouly C, Chati R, Scotté M, Regimbeau J-M. Therapeutic management of perforated gastro-duodenal ulcer: literature review. *J Visc Surg*. 2013;150(5):333-340.

10. Bertleff MJ, Halm JA, Bemelman WA, et al. Randomized clinical trial of laparoscopic versus open repair of the perforated peptic ulcer: the LAMA Trial. *World J Surg.* 2009;33(7):1368-1373.
11. Druart ML, Van Hee R, Etienne J, et al. Laparoscopic repair of perforated duodenal ulcer. A prospective multicenter clinical trial. *Surg Endosc.* 1997;11(10):1017-1020.
12. Tan S, Wu G, Zhuang Q, et al. Laparoscopic versus open repair for perforated peptic ulcer: a meta analysis of randomized controlled trials. *Int J Surg.* 2016;33 Pt A:124-132.
13. Lo HC, Wu S-C, Huang H-C, et al. Laparoscopic simple closure alone is adequate for low risk patients with perforated peptic ulcer. *World J Surg.* 2011;35(8):1873-1878.
14. Kumar P, Khan HM, Hasanrabba S. Treatment of perforated giant gastric ulcer in an emergency setting. *World J Gastrointest Surg.* 2014;6(1):5-8.
15. Lagoo S, McMahon RL, Kakihara M, Pappas TN, Eubanks S. The sixth decision regarding perforated duodenal ulcer. *J Soc Laparoendosc Surg.* 2002;6(4):359-368.
16. Pai D, Sharma A, Kanungo R, Jagdish S, Gupta A. Role of abdominal drains in perforated duodenal ulcer patients: a prospective controlled study. *Aust N Z J Surg.* 1999;69(3):210-213.
17. Moller MH, Vester-Andersen M, Thomsen RW. Long-term mortality following peptic ulcer perforation in the PULP trial. A nationwide follow-up study. *Scand J Gastroenterol.* 2013;48(2):168-175.
18. Huston JM, Kreiner L, Ho VP, et al. Role of empiric antifungal therapy in the treatment of perforated peptic ulcer disease: review of the evidence and future directions. *Surg Infect.* 2019;20(8):593-600.
19. Soreide K, Thorsen K, Harrison EM, et al. Perforated peptic ulcer. *Lancet.* 2015;386(10000):1288-1298.
20. Gonenc M, Dural AC, Celik F, et al. Enhanced postoperative recovery pathways in emergency surgery: a randomised controlled clinical trial. *Am J Surg.* 2014;207(6):807-814.
21. Poris S, Fontaine A, Glener J, et al. Routine versus selective upper gastrointestinal contrast series after omental patch repair for gastric or duodenal perforation. *Surg Endosc.* 2018;32(1):400-404.
22. Tsujimoto H, Hiraki S, Sakamoto N, et al. Outcome after emergency surgery in patients with a free perforation caused by gastric cancer. *Exp Ther Med.* 2010;1(1):199-203.
23. Lee FY, Leung KL, Lai BS, et al. Predicting mortality and morbidity of patients operated on for perforated peptic ulcers. *Arch Surg.* 2001;136(1):90-94.
24. Sharma SS, Mamtani MR, Sharma MS, Kulkarni H. A prospective cohort study of postoperative complications in the management of perforated peptic ulcer. *BMC Surg.* 2006;6:8.

Chapter 33 Trauma Laparotomy

S. Ariane Christie and Andrew B. Peitzman

DEFINITION
- Trauma laparotomy encompasses a vast array of general surgery techniques, the details of which are covered comprehensively in other sections this book. This chapter will provide a framework for thinking through trauma laparotomy in the context of the overall treatment and resuscitation of the critically ill and often multiply injured patient. In particular, we will emphasize perioperative planning, intraoperative decision making, and taking a systematic, step-up approach to the repair of specific intra-abdominal injuries while balancing the patient's overall physiology and injury burden.

DIFFERENTIAL DIAGNOSIS
- Patients may require abdominal exploration for penetrating, blunt, blast, or combined trauma mechanisms. Common indications for trauma laparotomy include peritonitis, hemodynamic instability with positive Focused Assessment with Sonography for Trauma (FAST), positive diagnostic peritoneal aspirate (DPA), or computed tomography (CT) findings of free abdominal fluid without solid organ injury, penetrating injury extending through the fascia, or thoracoabdominal penetrating injury with trajectory concerning for diaphragmatic injury (laparoscopy is an option in these circumstances). The essential decision is whether the trauma patient requires laparotomy and not identification of specific organ injuries (**FIGURES 1** and **2**). Delay to hemorrhage control will result in avoidable morbidity and mortality.

PATIENT HISTORY AND PHYSICAL FINDINGS
- Regardless of injury mechanism or severity, trauma resuscitation follows the Advanced Trauma Life Support guidelines beginning with the primary survey and treatment of immediately life-threating conditions. Vascular access ideally consists of two large-bore intravenous (IV) catheters. Supradiaphragmatic IV access is preferred for abdominal

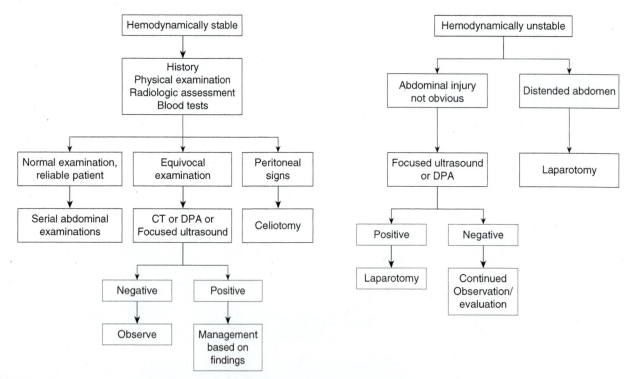

FIGURE 1 • Algorithm for management of blunt abdominal trauma. (Reprinted with permission from Peitzman AB, Yealy DM, Fabian TC, et al. *The Trauma Manual*. 5th ed. Wolters Kluwer; 2020:426. Figure 37.1.)

Penetrating Abdominal Trauma

```
                                    Penetrating Abdominal Trauma

    Unstable              Stable
    evisceration          no evisceration
    peritonitis           no diffuse tenderness
    unexaminable          reliable exam
         │         ┌──────────┼──────────┐
         │    Shotgun/blast  Stab      Gunshot
         │         │          │          │
         OR        OR      Linear US   CT w. IV contrast
                              │          │
                    ┌─────────┴─────┐    ├────────────┬──────────────┐
                 – Fascial      + Fascial Operative  No clear      Tangential /
                 penetration    penetration indication surgical injury subcutaneous
                     │              │        │          │              │
                 Wound          24 hr         OR      24 hr          Discharge
                 exploration    observation           observation
                     │
              ┌──────┴──────┐
          + Fascial     – Fascial
          penetration   penetration
              │             │
           24 hr         Discharge
           observation
```

FIGURE 2 • Algorithm for management of penetrating abdominal trauma. (Reprinted with permission from Britt LD, Peitzman AB, Barie PS, et al. *Acute Care Surgery*. 2nd ed. Wolters Kluwer; 2019:450. Algorithm 36.1.)

injury. With uncertain penetrating trajectory, obtain IV access above and below the diaphragm. Address hypotension rapidly with transfusion of whole blood[1,2] or a balanced 1:1:1 resuscitation strategy.[3,4] Additional resuscitation is guided by functional coagulation assays such as thromboelastography. The CRASH-2 trial was a randomized international clinical trial supporting early administration of tranexamic acid to patients at elevated risk of hemorrhagic shock. Notably, outcomes are best when tranexamic acid is administered within the first 3 hours of injury, ideally within the first hour.[5,6]

IMAGING AND OTHER DIAGNOSTIC STUDIES

- FAST is routinely performed in the trauma bay as part of the initial assessment and resuscitation of injured patients. Positive findings of fluid in the right upper quadrant, left upper quadrant, or pelvic windows are presumed to be blood until proven otherwise.
- If the patient is hemodynamically stable, obtaining cross-sectional imaging using multidetector CT provides valuable information regarding burden and severity of injury to guide operative strategy. However, unstable patients with clear operative indications should transfer to the operating room (OR) promptly and not be delayed to obtain cross-sectional imaging.[7]
- Patients with polytrauma and physiologic derangement require damage control planning and staged repair. Obtain consultation with neurosurgical, orthopedic, interventional radiology, and other services early.
- Most adjunctive tests and procedures beyond those performed in the ABCDE assessment are also better performed once the patient has been taken to the operating theater.

SURGICAL MANAGEMENT

Preoperative Planning

- The general operative strategy outlined here specifically addresses exploratory laparotomy for trauma. However, the following approach is equally applicable to any "crash" abdominal operation or emergency surgery. Acting in accordance with a few key principles greatly aids efficiency to gain and maintain control of complex injuries while minimizing collateral and iatrogenic injury. Plan for what you expect. Equally, anticipate and prepare for the unexpected.
- Conduct of the lead surgeon[8]
  - The comportment of the lead surgeon sets the tempo for the operating team and facilitates optimal communication and performance.
  - The lead surgeon should
    - Maintain situational awareness; quickly assess the OR when entering by obtaining a concise report from the other team members.
    - Control the room; maintain composure, communicate calmly. The commanding voice need not be the loudest. Request necessary actions or equipment in sequence, rather than issuing multiple requests at once. Be explicit to whom each request is made.
    - Encourage and reassure the team members; reserve constructive criticism for after the operation.
    - Perform deliberate, progressive maneuvers, without wasted movement or time.
    - Control bleeding rapidly, reconstruct deliberately. Control bleeding digitally; do not clamp or suture haphazardly. Repair correctly on the first attempt.

GENERAL OPERATIVE APPROACH

- The trauma laparotomy is systematic (**FIGURE 3**). The primary goals are to control hemorrhage and gastrointestinal contamination. Only after these goals are achieved should one begin a systematic search for all injuries.
- Recognize early when a patient requires damage control approach: either preoperatively or early in the laparotomy. Convey that decision to the entire OR team.[9,10]
- **Utilize a "step-up" approach**: Patients may have many intra-abdominal injuries. Begin with the most life-threatening; stabilize using the least invasive strategy. For bleeding, apply well-directed pressure. Packing may be effective damage control management of solid organ or pelvic bleeding. Although definitive repairs are tempting, hasty moves result in iatrogenic injury or "burning bridges" before the full extent of the problem is recognized. If conservative strategies fail to temporize the problem, proceed with stepwise escalation. Minor injuries should not distract from getting the patient off the operating table.[11,12]
- **Maintain a list of injuries**: Keep track of the patient's overall trauma burden to guide operative decisions. Definitive repair of an isolated bowel perforation is appropriate in a stable healthy patient but is poorly tolerated in an elderly patient with multiple injuries. Keep a mental (or physical) list of suspected and confirmed injuries and refer to this throughout the operation and resuscitation.[13]
- **Physiological embarrassment supersedes surgical repair.** Critically injured patients can withstand only a limited time for operative repair. Two hours has been suggested as a time benchmark, but physiologic embarrassment may occur sooner in patients with multiple injuries or shock, or in older or chronically ill patients. Do not truncate the operation until *surgical bleeding* is controlled. Temporize quickly and transfer the patient to the intensive care unit (ICU) to avoid the "deadly terrible triad" of acidosis, hypothermia, and coagulopathy. Keep track of operative time, physiologic metrics (blood transfused, temperature, pH, and thromboelastography), and clinical indicators of physiology such as "oozing" from the operative field (*medical bleeding*).[14]
- **Communication is essential**: Resuscitation and surgery require the coordinated interaction of a care team including the emergency room physicians and staff, anesthesia team, scrub and circulating nursing staff, blood bank, and surgeons and operative team. Without constant, ongoing communication, the patient will not have a successful outcome. Use a directed, closed-loop communication strategy with all members of the team empowered to share information and raise concerns.
  - Setting and instrumentation: The surgeon leads the resuscitative, nursing, and anesthesia teams in preparing the patient for a successful operation. Consider the operative setting and potential intraoperative adjuncts.
    - Where major vascular injury is expected, use a room with hybrid capabilities for digital subtraction angiography to expand options for bleeding control.
    - Call for endoscopy and bronchoscopy or proctoscopy equipment early.
    - Laparoscopy equipment is uncommonly indicated in trauma, and never when the patient is hemodynamically unstable.
  - A standard major basic set will suffice for most trauma laparotomies, with a major vascular set kept on hand. Also, have equipment available for median sternotomy or thoracotomy.
  - The set should include essential equipment only; keep instruments to the minimum required. If the likelihood of major vascular injury is high, the circulating staff should prepare heparin flushes, Fogarty balloons, and shunts of various sizes. A headlight and surgical loupes improve visualization and forestall delays. Consider monopolar and bipolar thermocoagulating instruments including Bovie electrocautery, LigaSure, Argon beam, and Aquamantys. Separate patient circuits and priming may be necessary to allow concomitant use. A list of standard equipment and recommended adjuncts for surgical laparotomy is given in **TABLE 1**.

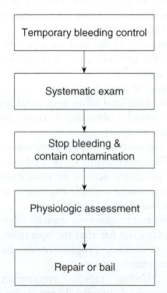

FIGURE 3 • Systematic approach to abdominal exploration for trauma.

Table 1: Instrumentation for Trauma Laparotomy	
Standard	**Major basic set**
Adjuncts	Major vascular set
	Self-retaining retractors: Balfour Thompson Bookwalter Omni
	Headlight Surgical loupes
	Proctoscope Vaginal speculae Endoscope Bronchoscope
	Thermocautery devices *(consider separate energy source)* LigaSure Aquamantys Argon beam

- Prepare to cross between body cavities during the operation, as injuries are often not fully delineated preoperatively (FIGURE 4). Drape from chin to knees and table to table laterally to allow extensile exposures and maximize reconstruction opportunities. A towel covering the genitals exposes the bilateral groins for potential REBOA (Resuscitative Endovascular Balloon Occlusion of the Aorta) access and the medial thighs for potential saphenous harvest. The patient's arms should be well padded and secured on arm boards abducted just under 90° to prevent neuropraxia. If there is a high suspicion of rectal or perineal injury, position the patient in lithotomy on an operating table with a removable or retractable footplate.

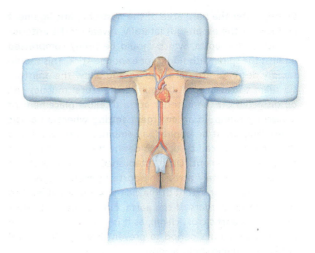

FIGURE 4 • Extensile exposures in trauma.

TRAUMA EXPLORATORY LAPAROTOMY: STEPS

Open the Abdomen

- Particularly in instances of severe injury and hemodynamic instability, induction should be postponed until the operating team is ready to make incision. We routinely prep and drape the patient prior to inducing anesthesia. Be ready with a #10 blade and two working suctions. The back table should have ready buckets for removal of clot, large handheld retractors, and a minimum of 20 to 30 laparotomy pads, rolled or unrolled according to the surgeon's preference.
- Make a midline incision with one pass of the knife from just below the xiphoid inferiorly to the lower abdomen and with a smooth transition around the umbilicus. A second pass of the knife should expose the linea alba, and a third the preperitoneal fat. In the unstable patient, do not be distracted by cauterizing subcutaneous and skin bleeding. In patients with intra-abdominal bleeding the peritoneum will often be dark and tented. This finding should be clearly communicated with the anesthesia team, as tamponade release may lead to hemodynamic instability and potential cardiac arrest. If possible, a large amount of uncross-matched blood product should be in the room and a rapid infusion system should be prepared before proceeding.
- The preperitoneal fat and peritoneum can be grasped with a forceps and opened with a Mayo scissors. The surgeon's nondominant hand should protect the intestine and other viscera, taking care to avoid injury to the liver, bowel, or bladder. The peritoneum should be opened completely for the length of the incision, regardless of the patient's physiologic response to tamponade release.

Stop Exsanguinating Hemorrhage

- As the surgeon is opening the abdomen, the assistant should help with counter-tension and begin evacuating clot. Once the peritoneum is fully opened, clot should be scooped into a bucket for removal from the field and liquid blood should be suctioned.
- The initial exploration should begin with the most compelling bleeding. The assistant should retract the sidewall, allowing the surgeon to tamponade any bleeding by packing laparotomy pads using a "hand-over-hand" approach. Once accomplished, the next quadrant should be addressed, proceeding in either a clockwise or counterclockwise fashion until all quadrants are packed and exsanguinating bleeding is controlled. Take care not to overpack and impair venous return. Special consideration should be taken in the right upper quadrant, where the surgeon may need to manually reconstitute the liver. With severe hepatic injury, compress the hemilobes of the liver together with your hands, then push the liver posteriorly to slow retrohepatic bleeding. If successful, then pack above and below the liver, restoring normal anatomy. Do not pack within the hepatic injury as this may exacerbate parenchymal bleeding. In the left upper quadrant, packing should similarly extend posterolaterally to the spleen. Take care to avoid iatrogenic injury to the liver, spleen, and other organs from forceful retraction or packing.
- If systematic packing fails to control the hemorrhage, a useful next step is to gently eviscerate the small bowel and reattempt packing. Effective packing will significantly attenuate bleeding from liver, spleen, mesentery, and retroperitoneal hematomas from blunt injury but will not stop hemorrhage from vascular lacerations. If specific bleeding vessels are visualized, targeted manual compression can control bleeding while preparations are made for vascular isolation, ligation, or repair. If major venous bleeding is identified within the abdomen, instruct the anesthesia team to stop any infusion through femoral or lower extremity intraosseous IV access.
- If the patient arrests or audible arterial bleeding is encountered, transition from packing to obtaining inflow control with supraceliac aortic compression. To accomplish this, the assistant should gently retract the left lobe of the liver to facilitate entry through the gastrohepatic ligament.

Bluntly enter the bare area of the gastrohepatic ligament and retract the esophagus laterally, revealing the anterior surface of the aorta, which should be firmly compressed against the spine with fingers or a sponge-stick. This should rapidly decrease arterial bleeding and allow the anesthesia team to resuscitate. If desired, the crural muscles can be dissected off the anterior aorta to allow placement of a vascular clamp. In an emergent setting where an aortic cross-clamp must be applied, a combination of blunt and sharp dissection can be used to define the periaortic space for clamp placement. Once established, confirm that the clamp is completely across the aorta by manually feeling that the posterior extent of the clamp continues at least to the posterior borders of the aorta. Finally, mark the start time of the aortic cross-clamp, as it is essential to unclamp within a 45-minute period to prevent irreversible visceral ischemia and metabolic acidosis.

- Increasingly, REBOA is utilized to gain rapid control of exsanguinating hemorrhage. Many centers routinely place REBOA in the resuscitation bay, particularly when the cause of bleeding is suspected to be a pelvic fracture. Our approach is (1) to prioritize prompt transfer of the hypotensive patient to the OR, (2) to routinely obtain femoral arterial access in all hypotensive patients either in the resuscitation bay or in the OR, and (3) to selectively utilize REBOA in the setting of a major pelvic fracture or zone I hematoma with a suspected vascular injury.

Perform a Systematic Examination of the Abdomen

- Once temporary hemorrhage control has been achieved, the next step in the trauma laparotomy is to perform a systematic survey to control other points of bleeding and identify and control sources of gross contamination.
- Exposure
  - Anatomic exposure can be optimized while the anesthesia team catches up on resuscitation efforts. Depending on the injury, it may be useful to extend the abdominal incision either cephalad to the xiphoid or caudally toward the symphysis pubis. Further exposure can be gained by excising the xiphoid process with a Mayo scissors or electrocautery.
  - To free up hands, place a self-retaining retractor. Retractor selection depends on both injury and surgeon comfort. The Bookwalter retractor is a good general abdominal retraction device, whereas the Thompson and Omni retractor systems are well suited for upper abdominal and liver injuries.
- Systematic examination of the abdomen
  - Begin removing abdominal packing starting from the least injured area and work toward the sites of the most severe injury. If removal results in hemorrhage, replace the packs until control is regained. Often, leaving packing in place is the most appropriate hemostatic option in an initial damage control laparotomy.
  - The abdominal cavity can be considered as two compartments separated by the transverse colon.
    - The supramesocolic compartment contains the stomach, spleen, liver, and gallbladder and is explored by gently retracting the transverse colon caudally.
    - The inframesocolic compartment contains the small bowel, colon and rectum, bladder, uterus, and pelvis and can be explored by gently retracting the transverse colon cephalad.
  - Careful visual inspection of all surfaces of the solid and hollow viscera and mesentery are required for adequate exploration. A two-person, hand-to-hand technique should be used to carefully inspect the small bowel and colon. In general, any structures that are found to have bruising or hematomas or those located close to a missile trajectory should be fully mobilized and carefully examined for injury.
  - Notable sites of missed intra-abdominal hollow viscus injury include the esophagogastric junction, the ligament of Treitz, the small bowel along the mesenteric border, the posterior stomach, the transverse colon, and the extraperitoneal rectum. Pancreatic or posterior diaphragmatic injury is also commonly missed. Missing injuries in these areas leads to considerable morbidity and may contribute to higher rates of mortality.
- Retroperitoneal exploration (FIGURE 5): In addition to the supramesocolic and inframesocolic intraperitoneal compartments, examine all three retroperitoneal compartments.
  - Zone I—The central/medial zone. All hematomas and injuries require surgical exploration regardless of mechanism. To evaluate, open the lesser sac by widely incising the gastrocolic ligament to

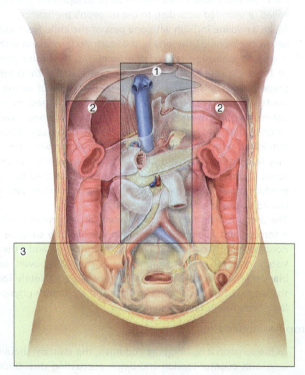

FIGURE 5 • Zones of the retroperitoneum. (Reprinted with permission from Peitzman AB, Yealy DM, Fabian TC, et al. *The Trauma Manual*. 5th ed. Wolters Kluwer; 2020:426. Figure 38.1.)

ensure that there is no hematoma overlying or underlying the pancreas. Suspected injury to the pancreas should be evaluated by visual inspection and mobilization for bimanual palpation.
- Zone II—The lateral retroperitoneal zone. Zone II injuries are managed differently based on mechanism. All penetrating injuries to zone II with hematomas should be surgically explored. Blunt injuries with *expanding* hematomas should be surgically explored, while those with stable hematomas can generally be observed.
- Zone III—The pelvic retroperitoneal zone. Management of pelvic retroperitoneal injuries also takes into account mechanism. Penetrating injuries should be explored. Blunt injuries are often amenable to endovascular intervention for angiographic management of bleeding, ideally in a hybrid OR.
- Surgical access to the retroperitoneum—In general, exposure of the retroperitoneum involves rotating overlying structures medially (**FIGURE 6**). The following specific approaches can be used to evaluate retroperitoneal structures:
- Left-to-right medial visceral rotation
  - This approach will expose zone I injuries to the suprarenal aorta and its visceral branches (eg, celiac artery, superior mesenteric artery, left renal artery) and can be extended to access the inframesocolic aorta and the aortic bifurcation with the left common iliac artery.
  - Begin by gently retracting the left colon toward the right to incise the white line of Toldt. Colonic mobilization is extended to the splenic flexure and continued lateral to the spleen. The dorsum of the surgeon's hand rests along the posterior abdominal musculature behind the spleen, left kidney, and pancreatic tail and provides anterior tension. Divide the avascular plane behind these organs, progressively rotating these structures medially to the diaphragmatic hiatus. Often, the hematoma in this region will have already performed much of the dissection maneuver. Alternatively, the left kidney may be left on the retroperitoneal musculature with the dissection plane proceeding anteriorly.
  - Potential pitfalls include iatrogenic splenic injury or avulsion of lumbar veins.
- Right-to-left visceral medial rotation
  - This approach will expose zone I injuries to right-sided structures, including the intrahepatic inferior vena cava (IVC), the right kidney, the right renal hilum, and the right common iliac artery and can be extended to the bilateral iliac structures.
  - There are three steps to this exposure.
    - Step 1: Kocherization of the duodenum and the hepatobiliary structures. Mobilize the right colon and hepatic flexure off the duodenum. Incise the peritoneum just lateral to the C-loop of the duodenum and begin to retract the duodenum and pancreatic head medially. Using a combination of blunt and sharp dissection free the avascular plane behind the common bile duct and the superior mesenteric vein (SMV) to reveal the IVC to the left renal vein. Avoid avulsion to the right gonadal vein as it dives into the IVC at this level.

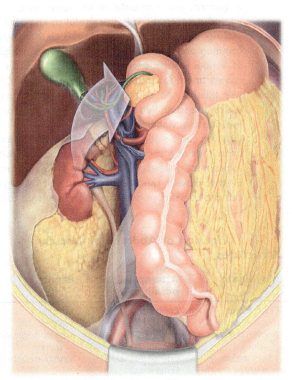

A. Right to left medial visceral rotation

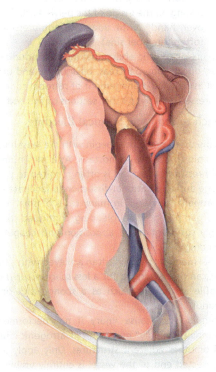

B. Left to right medial visceral rotation

FIGURE 6 • **A,** Right and **(B)** left medial visceral rotation.

- Step 2: Right colonic mobilization. Continue mobilizing proximally from the hepatic flexure by incising the white line of Toldt and medializing the right colon.
- Step 3: Superior-medial extension. Extend mobilization of the avascular plane behind the cecum and the distal ileum. Retract the small bowel toward the liver and incise the peritoneum along the small bowel mesentery from medial to the cecum to the ligament of Treitz. This will allow the small bowel, mesentery, and right colon to be retracted superiorly, revealing the widest exposure of the retroperitoneal vascular structures available. This exposure will gain access to the inframesocolic retroperitoneum and direct visualization of the infrarenal aorta, IVC, bilateral renal arteries and veins, bilateral common iliac arteries, third and fourth portions of the duodenum, and SMV.
- Potential pitfalls include injury to the right gonadal vein during kocherization and injury to the SMV at the root of the mesentery with undue traction or avulsion of the right colon vein off the SMV.
- Surgical treatment of pelvic hematoma: Temporize hemodynamically significant pelvic hematomas from blunt trauma with preperitoneal packing of the pelvic space.
  - Access the preperitoneum through the inferiormost aspect of a mid-line laparotomy or, ideally, through a separate incision above the symphysis pubis.
  - Dissect between the rectus and the peritoneum; avoid entering the peritoneal space. Bluntly dissect the avascular plane behind the rectus posterolaterally until the peritoneum is pushed medially and your knuckles are resting on the inside of the pelvis. Pack this space "hand over hand" until adequate compression is attained (often three per side).
- Repairs of specific abdominal injuries including the spleen, liver, duodenum, pancreas, biliary tree, and urinary tract as well as detailed management of retroperitoneal injuries are addressed directly in other sections of this text.

Approach to Stopping Surgical Bleeding

- As discussed previously, begin with the least invasive method possible to achieve hemostasis. At a minimum, direct manual pressure or packing is often required to prevent hemorrhage during additional dissection to facilitate safe definitive treatment. However, in many cases of small vessel, venous, or organ parenchymal bleeding, continued compression will apply sufficient tissue apposition and coagulation to stop bleeding.
- Initial manual control is often achieved with a hand or finger but can be exchanged for a less space-occupying and lower-profile instrument, such as a sponge-stick or a dissecting peanut.
- Clamping can cause injury if not performed judiciously. Clamping "blindly" may result in iatrogenic injury to the vessel or other adjacent structures. Only apply a clamp if the transected end of the vessel is entirely visible or the clamp can be passed cleanly around the vessel. Clamp application damages the endothelium; close clamps only to the setting necessary to stop bleeding.
- Although a basic surgical concept, suturing *well* on an actively bleeding vessel requires consideration and skill. Envision the axis along which the bleeding vessel runs. Place the initial needle pass on one side of the bleeding point, cross beneath the bleeding point without avulsion exiting the tissue several millimeters past the other side of the bleeding point. Gently hold up the suture to visualize the direction of ongoing bleeding relative to your suture. Place the next throw deep to this in the opposite direction, ideally creating a figure eight around the bleeding. Success is determined by pulling gently up upon the suture and surveying the results. Even if some bleeding persists, it is usually diminished, and another throw can be planned, again systematically in the direction toward the bleeding opposite the last throw.
- The importance of adequate exposure by the assistant during suturing cannot be overstated. Retraction should be maintained at all costs, and successful exposure may entail brief periods of allowing a vessel to bleed with well-targeted suctioning near, but without obstructing, the bleeding point. The suction itself is often best used as a combined suction device and retractor.
- Needle selection is also important. Take into consideration the suspected depth and location of the bleeding. Use a large, tapered needle such as a CT or SH needle. In a deep hole with a narrow aperture such as the pelvis, use a hemicircular needle such as an SH or CT-3 to allow smooth collection of the suture. With very deep bleeding and a narrow aperture consider using a UR-6 or tailor the needle carefully using two needle drivers.
- Vascular ligation
  - In general, any vein distal to the renal vessels can be ligated if necessary. Still, it is useful to know the general risk involved in ligation (**TABLE 2**). Sacrificing the common and external iliac veins portends a high risk of venous insufficiency. In these cases, consider four-compartment fasciotomy on the ipsilateral limb. Portal vein ligation can lead to massive intestinal edema and warrants a scheduled second-look laparotomy to examine intestinal viability.
  - Ligation can be performed in several ways. Clamping both ends of a vessel and tying around each with an appropriately sized silk tie remains the gold standard. Electric bipolar cautery devices such as the LigaSure can provide secure hemostasis of vessels up to 7 mm

Table 2: Ligation of Abdominal Vascular Structures

May ligate	Attempt repair if possible	Repair
Celiac artery	Common iliac artery	Aorta
Hypogastric artery	External iliac artery	Suprarenal IVC
Any vein below renal veins	Infrarenal IVC	Superior mesenteric artery
	Common iliac vein	Superior mesenteric vein
Inferior mesenteric artery	External iliac vein	
	Portal vein	
Inferior mesenteric vein	Proper hepatic artery	

in diameter. Notably, the LigaSure device does not function where staples or other metal clips have been deployed and may melt monofilament suture. Suture ligate or oversew arterial and high-pressure venous vessels. Finally, vascular staplers can control large and small vascular pedicles and can be maneuvered into difficult-to-access areas. Although beyond the scope of this chapter, vascular staplers facilitate good hemostasis with minimal dissection in hepatic resections.

- Named arteries and proximal veins should be repaired in the stable patient if possible. Begin by obtaining proximal and distal control with a combination of pressure, clamps, or obstructive balloons. Debride the vessel to healthy endothelium proximally and distally. Although systemic heparin is often not needed, a Fogarty catheter should always be passed proximally and distally until one clean Fogarty pass is performed without extracting clot. Dilute local heparin can also be infused.
- Depending on patient stability, proceed with shunting or definitive repair techniques.[15]
    - **Shunting**: Shunt vessels in unstable patients to maintain distal flow or when significant orthopedic reconstitution may change the geometric layout of the anastomosis. We typically use an Argyle shunt; however, any appropriately sized sterile plastic tubing can be passed from the proximal to distal ends and secured in place with a tie or a plastic band. In general, systemic heparinization is not necessary with arterial repairs as brisk flow remains the best anticoagulant. Shunting preserves perfusion and allows delayed repair when the patient has been stabilized.[16,17]
    - **Primary Repair**: Reserve primary repair for injuries where the vessel can be adequately mobilized to allow tension-free repair after debridement. Select a monofilament suture of appropriate size (for example, a 4-0 Prolene for aorta or IVC). Close partial defects transversely to avoid narrowing. Large venous repairs (such as the IVC) are tolerant of some narrowing, but attempt to maintain greater than 50% of the original lumen size. For smaller venous repairs, use an interrupted suture technique or a running technique leaving a slight air knot to allow for venous re-expansion. If it is not possible to perform a primary repair without tension or without significantly narrowing the lumen of the vessel, another approach should be considered.
    - **Patching**: Patch if a portion of the vessel wall remains uninjured but primary closure would result in significant narrowing of the vessel. Options for patch material include synthetic materials (such as Dacron), bovine pericardial patches, or portions of autologous vein cut to size. Patching decreases the risk of vessel narrowing but is more time consuming than primary repair.
    - **Interposition grafting**: Interposition grafting remains the gold standard for transected vessels where primary repair would lead to tension on the anastomosis. Options for conduit include synthetic materials such as PTFE and Dacron. However, synthetic materials should not be used where there is contamination from either enteric spillage or from the injury itself. In these instances, autologous vein is the conduit of choice. Options include the greater and lesser saphenous veins, the arm veins, the external jugular vein, and the internal iliac (or hypogastric) vein. Harvesting and repair can be time consuming. Shunt in the unstable or multiply injured patient. Where more conduit length is necessary, creating spiral vein grafts remains an option but this is beyond the scope of this chapter.

Contain Contamination

- The secondary objective of the trauma laparotomy is containment of gross contamination. Injured segments of hollow viscera should be identified and isolated.[18,19] Soft bowel clamps such as Doyen or intestinal clamps can be employed for temporary control and defects closed with a whip or baseball stitch. A GIA blue or purple load stapler can be used to contain spillage; black load staplers are similarly useful on the proximal stomach or other thick tissue. In patients who are stable, proceed with formal repair or resection and anastomosis. Unstable patients should be left in discontinuity and moved to the ICU for resuscitation.[20,21] Irrigation with warm sterile fluid should be performed to clear gross contamination. Neither copious irrigation nor antibiotic-impregnated fluid has been demonstrated to reduce surgical site infection rates.[22]

Physiologic Assessment and Planning

- Once bleeding has been controlled and contamination contained, make a physiologic assessment of the patient considering the overall burden of injury, time already spent on the operating table, blood products infused, and other needed procedures and operations.
- Physiologic criteria for damage control laparotomy in trauma include pH < 7.2, temperature <35 °C, and coagulopathy.[23] In many cases, the safest thing to do is to place a temporary abdominal closure and bring the patient to the ICU for the next steps in their care. Currently, there are many proprietary and bespoke methods to establish temporary abdominal closure.
    - Cut small perforations in a sterile, plastic, fluid impermeable drape to allow fluid egress, and place around the abdominal viscera. Place an overlying sponge or series of towels in the wound on top of the plastic drape. Place flat 19-Fr Jackson-Pratt drains over this layer and secure to the abdomen with Ioban drape or another adhesive fluid-impermeable dressing. Apply gentle wall or vacuum-monitored suction.[24,25]
    - The Abthera wound vac system is a proprietary system specifically designed to accommodate application to an open abdomen. To apply, a large premade plastic drape is tailored to the size of the abdominal cavity. Premade perforations in the drape allow passage of fluid while providing relative protection for the underlying bowel.

Definitive Closure

- Only leave the abdomen open when necessary. In stable patients with intra-abdominal injuries, primary fascial closure after all repairs have been completed is preferable at the index operation. Fascial closure should conform to general guidance regarding secure closure technique including 0.5-cm bites and distance from fascial edges, utilization of a 4:1 suture to wound length, and use of an absorbable synthetic suture. Large abdominal wall defects can be managed either in a single stage or multiple stages, depending on the patient's anatomy, associated comorbidities, and recovery of the surrounding injuries in a polytrauma patient.[26] With gross intraperitoneal contamination or profound hemorrhagic shock, the skin should not be closed.

PEARLS AND PITFALLS

Pearls	- Position the patient to allow extensile exposure and consider use of a hybrid room. - Decide early if the laparotomy will demand a damage control approach. - Keep a mental injury list. - Use a step-up approach to hemorrhage control. - Get the patient off the operating table before physiologic embarrassment.
Pitfalls	- Failure to communicate with the anesthesia and nursing teams. - Iatrogenic injuries from excessive force or retraction while opening and packing. - Failure to systematically examine the abdomen resulting in missed injuries. - Performing extensive repairs at the index operation in a critically ill patient.

POSTOPERATIVE CARE

- Wait 24 to 48 hours to return to the OR in critically ill patients, if possible. Wait to perform bowel anastomoses or ostomies until the patient no longer requires high-dose vasopressor support.
- Abdominal packing should be removed gently using copious warm fluid to minimize distraction of clot or iatrogenic injury to the viscera. If bleeding occurs, repack.
- Consider the need for future abdominal procedures prior to definitive closure; these may include feeding gastrostomy or jejunostomy creation, drain placement for pancreatic or duodenal injury, ileo- or colostomy creation to divert stool from perineal injuries, and on-table endoscopic retrograde cholangiopancreatography to access the biliary tree. A gastropexy for possible endoscopic gastrotomy at later time is also useful.

COMPLICATIONS

- The multiply injured and critically ill patient often receives massive fluid and blood product resuscitation leading to considerable fluid shifts and volume overload following injury. Furthermore, exposure to the environment with the open abdomen leads to intestinal swelling and third spacing, which may preclude early fascial closure. Premature closure can lead to abdominal compartment syndrome and relaparotomy. Monitor closely for signs and symptoms of compartment syndrome including oliguria, rising peak pressures, CO_2, difficulty ventilating, or new-onset respiratory failure. Measure bladder pressure as a vital sign. Critically, compartment syndrome can occur in patients with Abthera or other wound vacs or with skin-only closure. In all cases, the abdomen must be fully reopened to avoid morbidity.
- Options for interim closure of the abdomen include skin-only closure,[27,28] interposition of absorbable mesh or biologic mesh, and rarely closure by secondary intention. Generally, successful abdominal closure utilizes temporary closure, which combines a vacuum suction system and a method to maintain tension on the fascia (to avoid retraction). We plan repeated trips to the OR over the first week and progressive closure of the midline fascia to avoid the long-term risks of the open abdomen. In the patient on whom fascia cannot be closed, apply a split-thickness skin graft as soon as the tissue bed appears ready. Patients who survive their injuries may go on to have component separation and formal hernia repair months to years later.

REFERENCES

1. Murdock AD, Berséus O, Hervig T, Strandenes G, Lunde TH. Whole blood: the future of traumatic hemorrhagic shock resuscitation. *Shock*. 2014;41(suppl 1):62-69.
2. Strandenes G, BerséusO, Cap AP, et al. Low titer group O whole blood in emergency situations. *Shock*. 2014;41(suppl 1):70-75.
3. Holcomb JB, del Junco DJ, Fox EE, et al. The prospective, observational, multicenter, major trauma transfusion (PROMMTT) study: comparative effectiveness of a time-varying treatment with competing risks. *JAMA Surg*. 2013;148:127-136.
4. Holcomb JB, Tilley BC, Baraniuk S, et al. Transfusion of plasma, platelets, and red blood cells in a 1:1:1 vs a 1:1:2 ratio and mortality in patients with severe trauma: the PROPPR randomized clinical trial. *JAMA*. 2015;313:471-482.
5. CRASH-2 trial collaborators; Shakur H, Roberts I, Bautista R, et al. Effects of tranexamic acid on death, vascular occlusive events, and blood transfusion in trauma patients with significant haemorrhage (CRASH-2): a randomised, placebo-controlled trial. *Lancet*. 2010;376:23-32.
6. Li SR, Guyette F, Brown J, et al. Early prehospital tranexamic acid following injury is associated with a 30-day survival benefit: a secondary

analysis of a randomized clinical trial. *Ann Surg.* 2021;274(3):419-426. doi:10.1097/SLA.0000000000005002

7. Neal MD, Peitzman AB, Forsythe RM, et al. Over reliance on computed tomography imaging in patients with severe abdominal injury: is the delay worth the risk? *J Trauma.* 2011;70:278-284.
8. Moeng MS. *Visceral Trauma Surgery – Under Pressure—My Top 5 (Leadership) Tips to Regain Control in a Crisis.* 2021.
9. Stone HH, Strom PR, Mullins RJ. Management of the major coagulopathy with onset during laparotomy. *Ann Surg.* 1983;197:532-535.
10. Rotondo MF, Zonies DH. The damage control sequence and underlying logic. *Surg Clin.* 1997;77:761-777.
11. Sugrue M, D'Amours SK, Joshipura M. Damage control surgery and the abdomen. *Injury.* 2004;35:642-648.
12. Roberts DJ, Bobrovitz N, Zygun DA, et al. Indications for use of damage control surgery in civilian trauma patients: a content analysis and expert appropriateness rating study. *Ann Surg.* 2016;263:1018-1027.
13. Shapiro MB, Jenkins DH, Schwab CW, Rotondo MF. Damage control: collective review. *J Trauma.* 2000;49:969-978.
14. Moore EE, Burch JM, Franciose RJ, Offner PJ, Biffl WL Staged physiologic restoration and damage control surgery. *World J Surg.* 1998;22:1184-1190. discussion 1190-1191.
15. Davis TP, Feliciano DV, Rozycki GS, et al. Results with abdominal vascular trauma in the modern era. *Am Surg.* 2001;67:565-570. discussion 570-571.
16. Reilly PM, Rotondo MF, Carpenter JP, Sherr SA, Schwab CW. Temporary vascular continuity during damage control: intraluminal shunting for proximal superior mesenteric artery injury. *J Trauma.* 1995;39:757-760.
17. Ball CG, Feliciano DV. Damage control techniques for common and external iliac artery injuries: have temporary intravascular shunts replaced the need for ligation? *J Trauma.* 2010;68:1117-1120.
18. Behrman SW, Bertken KA, Stefanacci HA, Parks SN Breakdown of intestinal repair after laparotomy for trauma: incidence, risk factors, and strategies for prevention. *J Trauma.* 1998;45:227-231. discussion 231-233.
19. Torba M, Gjata A, Buci S, et al. The influence of the risk factor on the abdominal complications in colon injury management. *G Chir.* 2015;36:57-62.
20. Ott MM, Norris PR, Diaz JJ, et al. Colon anastomosis after damage control laparotomy: recommendations from 174 trauma colectomies. *J Trauma.* 2011;70:595-602.
21. Ordoñez CA, Pino LF, Badiel M, et al. Safety of performing a delayed anastomosis during damage control laparotomy in patients with destructive colon injuries. *J Trauma.* 2011;71:1512-1517. discussion 1517-1518.
22. Georgoff P, Perales P, Laguna B, et al. Colonic injuries and the damage control abdomen: does management strategy matter? *J Surg Res.* 2013;181:293-299.
23. Asensio JA, McDuffie L, Petrone P, et al. Reliable variables in the exsanguinated patient which indicate damage control and predict outcome. *Am J Surg.* 2001;182:743-751.
24. Barker DE, Green JM, Maxwell RA, et al. Experience with vacuum-pack temporary abdominal wound closure in 258 trauma and general and vascular surgical patients. *J Am Coll Surg.* 2007;204:784-792. discussion 792-793.
25. Brock WB, Barker DE, Burns RP. Temporary closure of open abdominal wounds: the vacuum pack. *Am Surg.* 1995;61:30-35.
26. Jernigan TW, Fabian TC, Croce MA, et al. Staged management of giant abdominal wall defects: acute and long-term results. *Ann Surg.* 2003;238:349-355. discussion 355-357.
27. Acker A, Leonard J, Seamon MJ, et al. Leaving contaminated trauma laparotomy wounds open reduces wound infections but does not add value. *J Surg Res.* 2018;232:450-455.
28. Seamon MJ, Smith BP, Capano-Wehrle L, et al. Skin closure after trauma laparotomy in high-risk patients: opening opportunities for improvement. *J Trauma Acute Care Surg.* 2013;74:433-439. discussion 439-440.

Chapter 34

Gastric and Small Bowel Injury: Primary Repair, Resection, Anastomosis, Wedge Resection

Alex Helkin and Carrie Sims

DEFINITION

- Gastric and small bowel injuries can be defined as direct damage to the organ resulting in contusion, hematoma, laceration, or completed transection requiring repair or reconstruction. Indirect injury may also occur to the mesentery or other vasculature, resulting in devascularized segments at risk for ischemia.

DIFFERENTIAL DIAGNOSIS

- Generating a differential diagnosis for trauma patients is focused on determining the most likely injuries based on the presenting mechanism.
- Abdominal stab wounds most commonly injure the liver, with small bowel being the second most likely organ to be injured. Estimates of incidence range from 30% to 80%, whereas in abdominal gunshot wounds, small bowel is the most likely organ to be injured.[1,2]
- Blunt hollow viscus injuries (HVIs) are rare compared to solid organ injuries, occurring in an estimated 5%-15% of blunt traumas. Small bowel injuries account for approximately 90% of HVI. High energy impacts and deceleration injuries, such as motor vehicle and bicycle accidents, falls, crush injuries, assaults, and the concussive force of explosions are the leading mechanisms of blunt HVIs.[3,4] The mobility and relatively elasticity of the bowel provides some protection. As a result, small bowel perforation is rare and occurs in only 1%-3% of blunt trauma.
- Blunt trauma resulting in gastric perforation is also uncommon, due to the stomach's thick walls, distensible nature, and relatively protected location in the abdomen. True gastric perforation from blunt trauma is estimated to occur with an incidence ranging from 0.02% to 1.7%. Anterior perforations are the most common.[5,6]
- Shear forces will localize to tethered points along the bowel including the ligament of Treitz, small bowel mesentery, ileocecal valve, and adhesions secondary to prior surgery. A full stomach or inappropriately place lap belt can also contribute to blunt gastric and small bowel injuries.

PATIENT HISTORY AND PHYSICAL FINDINGS

- Indications for laparotomy in search of gastric and small bowel injuries remain the same as in other instances of penetrating trauma. Hemodynamic instability, obvious evisceration or impalement, or peritonitis necessitate emergent progression to the operating room for exploration. Exploration is also indicated in hemodynamically stable patients with penetrating wounds suspected to violate the peritoneal cavity due to the likelihood of intra-abdominal injury.
- Indications for exploration in blunt trauma also include peritonitis, evidence of free intra-abdominal air on imaging, and hemodynamic instability with positive focused assessments with sonography (FAST). Patients who are hemodynamically stable and those with equivocal physical examinations on presentation provide a greater diagnostic challenge.

IMAGING AND OTHER DIAGNOSTIC FINDINGS

- Abdominal radiographs obtained in the trauma bay to evaluate for pelvic fracture may show air under the diaphragm indicative of bowel perforation. However, these films are typically taken with the patient supine, and absence of free intraperitoneal air does not rule out gastrointestinal injury.
- FAST examination performed in the trauma bay may demonstrate free intraperitoneal fluid; however, it is not sensitive for bowel injury.
- Computed tomography (CT) is the diagnostic modality of choice in hemodynamically stable patients. Although evidence of blunt HVI may be subtle, CT findings including mesenteric fat stranding, bowel wall thickening (4-5 mm), or mesenteric hematomas are suggestive of a small bowel injury.[7]
- Peritoneal free fluid in the absence of solid organ injury is the most commonly reported CT finding associated with blunt bowel injury; however, it remains nonspecific. Even in a large multicenter investigation, only 9% of patients with free peritoneal fluid and no solid organ injury on CT had true small bowel injury.[8]
- Blunt HVI is still possible even with negative CT (ie, no abnormal findings). Early reports have indicated a missed injury rate as high as 13%; however, newer studies have showed improvement to about a 4% missed injury rate, largely secondary to improved CT scan quality over the past 2 decades.[9]
- Providers should have a higher index of suspicion of blunt HVI in cases of high energy blunt trauma mechanisms, such as motor vehicle collisions, but also in relation to concomitant injuries such as thoracic or lumbar spine fracture, seat belt signs, direct abdominal wall injury, or evidence of other high shear force injuries, such as aorta dissection.
- Hemodynamically stable patients with equivocal physical examinations found to have free intraperitoneal fluid on CT should be admitted for monitoring and serial abdominal examinations. Repeat imaging or diagnostic laparoscopy may also be considered.

SURGICAL MANAGEMENT

Preoperative Planning

- Early identification and control of hemorrhage is the initial priority during trauma laparotomy, followed by the control of gastrointestinal contamination, identification of all injuries, and finally reconstruction.
- Early placement of a nasogastric tube by anesthesia providers can aid exposure by decompressing intraluminal air, fluid

contents, and to identify intraluminal bleeding. However, oftentimes trauma patients will have full stomachs of solid content, making it difficult to decompress the stomach by nasogastric tube.
- Broad-spectrum preoperative antibiotics are recommended with guidance from local antibiograms and antibiotic stewardship protocols.
- The role of diagnostic laparoscopy remains controversial in the evaluation of abdominal trauma. While contraindicated in the setting of hemodynamic instability, laparoscopic exploration may be useful in hemodynamically stable patients to rule out penetrating abdominal injuries or to evaluate abdominal pain following blunt injury. Evaluation of the gastrointestinal tract in its entirety, solid organs, and the diaphragm can be performed adequately, and repairs performed based on comfort and skill of the surgeon.[10]

POSITIONING

- Standard supine trauma positioning with arms extended for use during resuscitation should be used. Preparation with betadine or chlorhexidine/alcohol from chin to knees is the standard preparation for trauma patients and can facilitate additional procedures such as sternotomy or thoracotomy, if needed.

EXPOSURE

- Due to the intrathoracic abdominal location of the stomach, midline laparotomy beginning in the subxyphoid area is ideal for exploration of gastric and small bowel injuries and facilitates a complete abdominal exploration. Self-retaining retractors are crucial to maintain exposure, allowing for the examination of the entire stomach from gastroesophageal junction to pylorus.
- Caudal retraction of the transverse colon will aid in examining the anterior surface of the stomach, with care taken to avoid traction injuries to the greater curvature and underlying gastroepiploic arteries and arterial branches to the greater omentum.
- Division of the gastrohepatic ligament may be necessary to provide exposure to the lesser curvature and gastroesophageal junction. The vagus nerve or smaller braches, as well as an anomalous left hepatic artery may traverse this area and could be injured in the exposure.
- Additional exposure of proximal stomach injuries may be obtained by encircling the intra-abdominal esophagus with a Penrose drain to provide caudal traction.
- Exposure of the posterior stomach is an essential step in evaluating gastric injury, especially in penetrating injury mechanisms where through-and-through injuries are more likely to occur. We also recommend examination of the posterior stomach during exploration for blunt HVIs.
- The posterior stomach can be accessed by opening the avascular portion of the gastrocolic ligament, with care taken to avoid injury to the gastroepiploic vessels. The transverse colon is retracted caudally and the posterior gastropancreatic attachments carefully dissected to allow visualization as cranially as the lesser curvature.
- Accessing the posterior stomach in patients with a shortened transverse colon mesentery or a thick greater omentum may be facilitated by a lateral approach higher on the greater curvature by first ligating the short gastric vessels with an energy device.
- The small bowel examination, commonly called "running the bowel," should be performed from the duodenojejunal origin, at the ligament of Treitz, to the cecum. The ligament of Treitz can be located by lifting the transverse colon and tracing its mesentery posteriorly. A hand placed in the abdomen will palpate the left lateral border of the spine and moving anteriorly will locate the duodenojejunal junction coursing inferiorly, fixed at the ligament of Treitz. The bowel should be meticulously examined for injury on all surfaces including the associated mesentery.

INJURY GRADING

- Once gastric or small bowel injuries are identified, we recommend review of the American Association for the Surgery of Trauma (AAST) grading systems, to identify severity of injury and recommendations for reconstruction (**TABLES 1 and 2**).[11]

Table 1: AAST Stomach Injury Scale

Stomach injury scale

Grade[a]	Description of injury	ICD-9	AIS-90
I	Contusion/hematoma	863.0/0.1	2
	Partial thickness laceration	863.0/0.1	2
II	Laceration <2 cm in GE junction or pylorus	863.0/0.1	3
	<5 cm in proximal 1/3 stomach	863.0/0.1	3
	<10 cm in distal 2/3 stomach	863.0/0.1	3
III	Laceration >2 cm in GE junction or pylorus	863.0/0.1	3
	>5 cm in proximal 1/3 stomach	863.0/0.1	3
	>10 cm in distal 2/3 stomach	863.0/0.1	3
IV	Tissue loss or devascularization <2/3 stomach	863.0/0.1	4
V	Tissue loss or devascularization >2/3 stomach	863.0/0.1	4

[a]Advance one grade for multiple lesions up to grade III. GE, gastroesophageal. Reprinted with permission from Moore EE, Jurkovich GJ, Knudson MM, et al. Organ injury scaling. VI: Extrahepatic biliary, esophagus, stomach, vulva, vagina, uterus (nonpregnant), uterus (pregnant), fallopian tube, and ovary. J Trauma. 1995;39(6):1069-1070. Table 3.

Table 2: AAST Small Bowel Injury Scale

Grade[a]	Type of injury	Description of injury	ICD-9	AIS-90
I	Hematoma	Contusion or hematoma without devascularization	863.20	2
	Laceration	Partial thickness, no perforation	863.20	2
II	Laceration	Laceration <50% of circumference	863.30	3
III	Laceration	laceration ≥50% of circumference without transection	863.30	3
IV	Laceration	Transection of the small bowel	863.30	4
V	Laceration	Transection of the small bowel with segmental tissue loss	863.30	4
	Vascular	Devascularized segment	863.30	4

[a]Advance one grade for multiple injuries up to grade III.
Reprinted with permission from Moore EE, Cogbill TH, Malangoni MA, et al. Organ injury scaling, II: Pancreas, duodenum, small bowel, colon, and rectum. J Trauma. 1990; 30(11):1427-1429. Table 3.

GASTRIC INJURY

Primary Gastric Repair

- The stomach is a thick-walled, highly vascular organ, and as such, even long lacerations (>10 cm) can be primarily repaired without need for resection. In the setting of partial thickness injuries, hematomas should be opened to assess mucosal injury and repaired. We recommend two-layer closure with full-thickness 2-0 polyglactin 910 suture and a second 3-0 silk layer in the Lembert fashion to ensure hemostasis.

Wedge Gastric Resection

- Wedge resection of gastric trauma, such as isolated anterior or greater curvature stab wounds, may be performed as a primary repair instead of suture repair; however, little data exist to suggest superiority of either method in trauma. Staple height chosen should be appropriate for tissue thickness as guided by manufacturer instructions for the stapler chosen. We recommend staple heights of at least 1.5 mm to accommodate tissue thickness without ischemia.

Resection for Devastating Injury

- Gastric injuries resulting in tissue loss or devascularization are rare and typically associated with hemorrhagic shock due to solid organ and vascular injuries. Such injuries may require distal or total gastrectomy and a complex subsequent reconstruction dictated by the anatomy and viability of remaining bowel. These complex reconstructive surgeries should be deferred until the patient's physiology has normalized.

Intraoperative Leak test

- Intraoperative tests of gastric repairs are commonly conducted via insufflation of the stomach via nasogastric tube, or esophagogastroduodenoscopy, after filling the peritoneal cavity with saline. Leaks are indicated by bubbles emerging from the distended, submerged stomach. Alternatively, one ampule of methylene blue dye diluted into 200 cc saline may be administered via the nasogastric tube for identification of additional injuries or leaks in the current repair. This is commonly not necessary since the gastric repair is usually under no tension, due to its size and abundant vascular supply. The risk of leak is low as long as good technique is used.

SMALL BOWEL INJURY

Primary Small Bowel Repair

- For injuries less than 50% of the total circumference of the bowel, primary repair is often a viable option. We recommend two-layer closure with an inner layer of 3-0 polyglactin 910 suture consisting of full-thickness bites and a secondary layer utilizing silk suture in a Lembert fashion to cover the inner suture line. Care is taken to repair in a transverse fashion, so as not to narrow the bowel.

Resection

- Resection is advised for lacerations greater than 50% of the bowel circumference, complete transections, multiple injuries in close proximity (where primary closure would result in luminal narrowing or kinking), or devastating mesenteric injuries resulting in a devascularized segment.

Technique

- Create small window in mesentery of normal appearing bowel proximal and distal to injury (**FIGURE 1**).

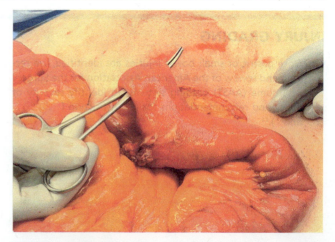

FIGURE 1 • Windows in the mesentery should be made close to the bowel with care taken to not injure either the bowel or vessels in the mesentery. The clamp can be left in place to assist guiding the stapler in place.

Chapter 34 GASTRIC AND SMALL BOWEL INJURY: PRIMARY REPAIR, RESECTION, ANASTOMOSIS, WEDGE RESECTION   293

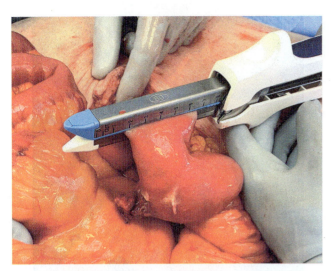

FIGURE 2 • A linear cutting stapler allows quick transection with control of enteric contents. Ensure that the staple load length is adequate for complete transection.

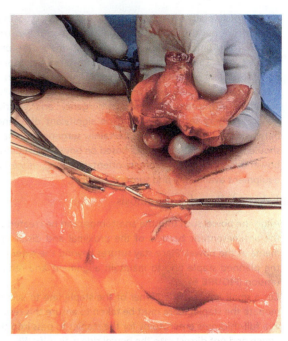

FIGURE 4 • Resected bowel segment with small edge of mesentery.

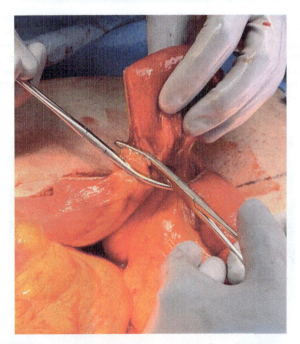

FIGURE 3 • For nononcologic resection such as during trauma, the mesentery may be taken close to the bowel as long as it is otherwise uninjured. Care must be taken to preserve the mesentery to the cut edges of bowel to provide adequate perfusion to the anastomosis. Here, the "clamp-and-tie" method is used; however, vessel-sealing energy devices are also acceptable.

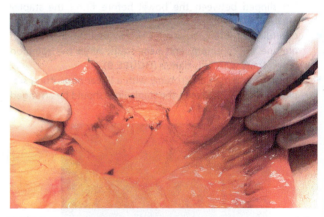

FIGURE 5 • The cut edges of bowel should be inspected for viability. Active bleeding from the staple line may be controlled with 3-0 polyglactin 910 suture. Cut edges with signs of ischemia (ie, dusky color or necrosis, or failure to hold staples) should be resected back to healthy appearing bowel.

- Apply stapler in a mesenteric to antimesenteric direction (or bowel clamps) and transect bowel (**FIGURE 2**).
- Ligate mesentery close to bowel with sequential clamps and ties or an energy device (**FIGURES 3** and **4**).
- Inspect the cut edges for viability (**FIGURE 5**).

ANASTOMOSIS

- Anastomoses in trauma surgery should follow the same principles as during elective surgery, with respect given to blood supply, tension, orientation, contamination, and condition of the bowel as well as overall condition of the patient. Patient with highly contaminated wounds, severe septic or hemorrhagic shock, acidosis, and associated coagulopathy may benefit from temporary abdominal closure and anastomosis after resuscitation.
- Consideration must be given to the total number of repairs and anastomoses to minimize opportunities for leaks and breakdown. In some cases, resection of a longer segment of bowel, incorporating multiple injuries, may be advantageous to serial repairs.

- The use of stapled vs handsewn small bowel anastomoses in trauma continues to be controversial, as no controlled trial specific to trauma patients has been performed. One prospective AAST multicenter trial, performed in emergency general surgery patients, demonstrated similar complication rates between stapled and handsewn anastomoses (12.5%), agreeing with prior data from emergency and elective general surgery settings showing no significant difference between the two techniques.[12] Certainly, surgeon judgment should dictate technique choice based on bowel wall edema, bowel size mismatch, mesentery orientation, etc., as well as equipment availability and surgeon comfort.

Stapled Small Bowel Anastomosis

- Align the bowel such that the anastomosis can be created on the antimesenteric borders of the proximal and distal segments of the bowel. Place stay sutures beyond the extent of the planned staple line to maintain alignment and reduce tension (**FIGURE 6**).
- Cut a small area off the corner of the staple line to accommodate the stapler. Care must be taken to ensure this results in a full-thickness enterotomy for the stapler to pass into the lumen and not dissect into the bowel side wall (**FIGURE 7**).
- Pass the stapler into the enterotomies, aligning the antimesenteric border inward and check to ensure that nothing has slipped between the bowel before firing the stapler (**FIGURE 8**).
- Carefully withdraw the stapler and inspect the interior staple line for continuity and hemostasis. Align the common enterotomy with Allis clamps (**FIGURE 9**).
- Close the common enterotomy with a linear noncutting stapler (**FIGURE 10**). Ideally, the staple lines should be arranged

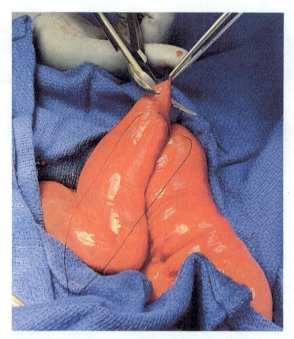

FIGURE 7 • Heavy curved scissors are used to cut the antimesenteric corner off the staple line from the proximal and distal bowel loops. The resulting enterotomies should be full thickness and allow a hemostat or other clamp to pass easily, or else introducing the staple could dissect along the bowel wall. The enterotomy should also not be too big, as this would allow enteric contents to spill into the field.

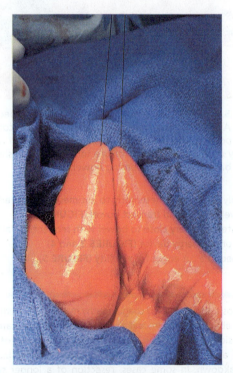

FIGURE 6 • Braided silk stay sutures placed on the antimesenteric wall near the cut edge of bowel and distally allow for easier alignment during anastomosis creation.

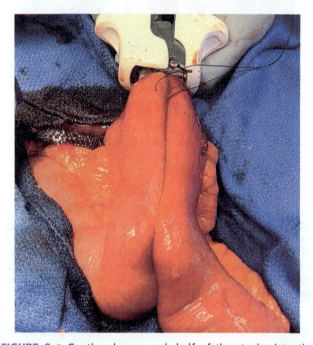

FIGURE 8 • Gently advance each half of the stapler into the enterotomies. Attention must be paid to the stapler angle to avoid perforating the bowel distally or misaligning the bowel before the anastomosis is created. The stay suture is useful here to uniformly advance the bowel up the stapler. The mesentery is then fanned out laterally to align the antimesenteric borders and ensure no bowel or other structures have slipped into the stapler trajectory.

Chapter 34 **GASTRIC AND SMALL BOWEL INJURY: PRIMARY REPAIR, RESECTION, ANASTOMOSIS, WEDGE RESECTION** 295

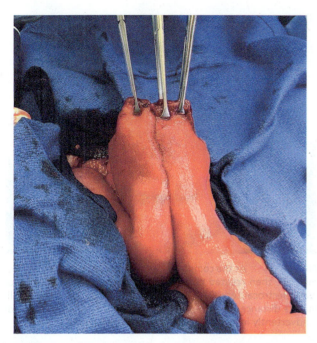

FIGURE 9 • After the stapler is withdrawn, a clamp or ringed forceps can be used to gently open and inspect the anastomosis for bleeding. A 3-0 polyglactin 910 suture could be used to internally suture ligate any active bleeding, should an area be found. After inspection, the common enterotomy is aligned with Allis or Babcock clamps with the staple line slightly offset to prepare for stapled transection.

so they do not cross, as leaks may arise. To prevent this potential complication, some operators will close the common enterotomy with a running layer of 3-0 polyglactin 910 suture and a second layer of interrupted 3-0 silk sutures.

- Inspect the staple lines for hemostasis (**FIGURE 11**).

Handsewn Anastomosis

- Align the bowel such that the anastomosis can be created on the antimesenteric borders of the proximal and distal small bowel segments. Place silk stay sutures beyond the extent of the planned anastomosis to maintain alignment and reduce tension (**FIGURE 12**).
- Place posterior row of interrupted silk seromuscular sutures (ie, Lembert sutures). It is critical to place these sutures at a 90° angle to the bowel wall in order to avoid skiving the tissue which can lead to ischemia and anastomotic breakdown (**FIGURE 13**).
- Create 4-5 cm parallel enterostomies. Care should be taken to create the enterostomies with reasonable distance from the posterior row such that those sutures are not incorporated into the posterior row of the anastomosis (**FIGURE 14**).
- Starting at the midpoint of the anastomosis, begin a bidirectional posterior layer of polyglactin 910 suture. Full-thickness bites are taken to align the mucosal layers and ensure the posterior silk suture line is excluded. Approaching the corners, we recommend transition to Connell sutures to avoid foreshortening when the suture is tightened (**FIGURE 15**). It is also critical to pull the suture through on the mucosal side in order to invert the serosa.

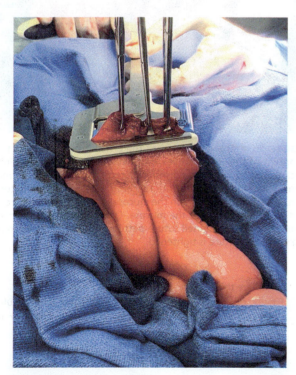

FIGURE 10 • A noncutting linear stapled is positioned just below the Allis clamps to close the common enterotomy. Cutting linear staplers may also be used, though leaks will occur if the staple lines are crossed.

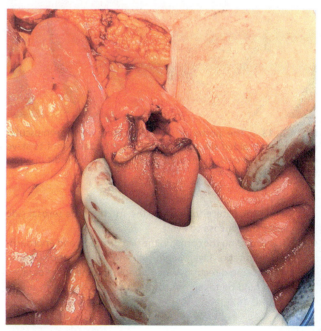

FIGURE 11 • Areas of active bleeding can be suture ligated with interrupted or "figure-of-eight" 3-0 polyglactin 910 sutures. Some operators will choose to oversew and imbricate the staple line with polyglactin 910 and a second layer of braided silk sutures in a Lembert pattern.

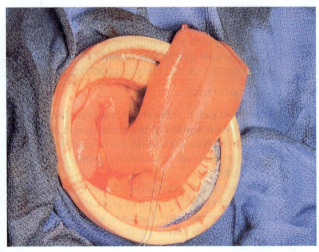

FIGURE 12 • The bowel is aligned, as above, with silk stay sutures placed near the bowel cut edge and again distally, approximately 6-7 cm to accommodate a 5-cm anastomosis. The anastomosis above is aligned in the antiperistaltic fashion, as in the stapled anastomosis in the prior example, but may be aligned in the isoperistaltic fashion, depending on which orientation is favorable and tension-free.

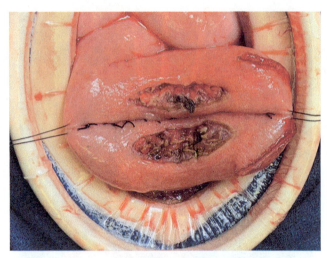

FIGURE 14 • At the completion of the posterior layer, enterotomies are then created parallel to the posterior layer, sharply or with electrocautery. Care should be taken to allow a few millimeters distance from the posterior layer of sutures, so it is not inadvertently incorporated in inner layer of suture.

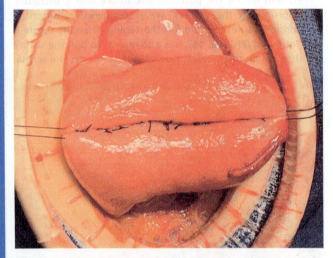

FIGURE 13 • The posterior wall is created with seromuscular interrupted braided silk sutures. Care must be taken not to skive on each needle pass, as an area of ischemia could result in anastomotic leak.

- Pulling the suture to advance the stitch on the serosal side causes the mucosa to evert.
- After rounding the corner in the first direction and approaching the anterior layer, begin suturing the posterior layer in the opposing direction. When completing the anterior layer, care should be taken not to grab the back wall with suture (**FIGURE 16**).

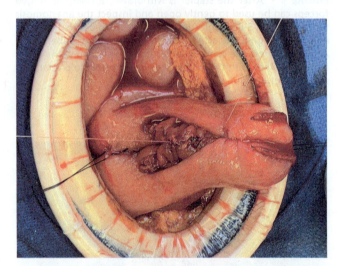

FIGURE 15 • The inner layer of the anastomosis begins at the midpoint of the enterotomies with two absorbable sutures. Full-thickness bites in a running fashion are performed in one direction toward the operator until reaching the corner. Each suture should be pulled through on the mucosal side to invert the serosa and allow apposition of the mucosa. Upon reaching the corner, transitioning to a Connell suture pattern will avoid foreshortening when the suture is tightened.

- Complete the anterior layer (**FIGURES 17** and **18**).
- Finally, perform anterior layer of interrupted seromuscular silk Lembert sutures to cover the polyglactin 910 layer to complete the anastomosis (**FIGURE 19**).

Chapter 34 GASTRIC AND SMALL BOWEL INJURY: PRIMARY REPAIR, RESECTION, ANASTOMOSIS, WEDGE RESECTION

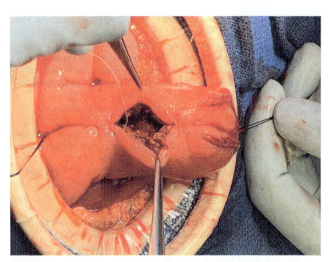

FIGURE 16 • The initial corner suture is progressed until it is rounded and advanced to the anterior bowel layer. The posterior layer is then completed with the remaining suture in the same fashion and transitioning to a Connell suture to round the corner. Again, care must be taken not to foreshorten the anastomosis.

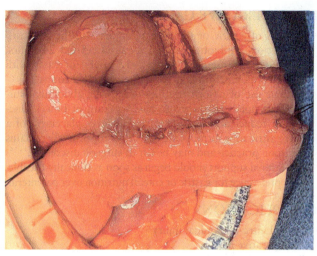

FIGURE 18 • The inner layer is completed by tying the two operating sutures together at the midpoint of the anastomosis.

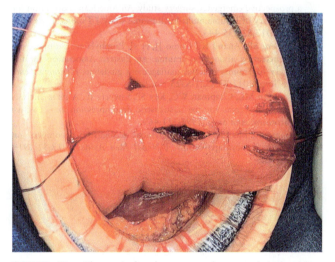

FIGURE 17 • The anterior layer may be completed with a Connell suture pattern or transitioned back to a simple running pattern. Be sure to examine each needle pass exiting and entering the mucosa to avoid inadvertently suturing to the back wall of the bowel.

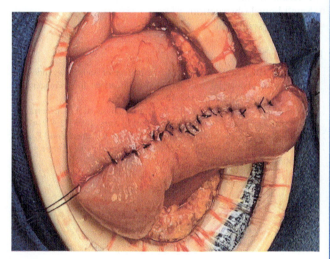

FIGURE 19 • The completed inner layer is imbricated with interrupted silk sutures in a Lembert pattern.

PEARLS AND PITFALLS

- CT is the diagnostic modality of choice for HVI; however, most findings are nonspecific and may be normal in 4% of patients with true injury.
- Blunt HVIs are present in 1%-3% of blunt trauma patients, with most (90%) occurring in the small bowel.
- Patients with deceleration injuries should raise suspicion for concomitant HVIs.
- Anterior gastric injuries necessitate dissection and examination of the posterior stomach.
- The decision for resection vs repair of small bowel injuries should aim to reduce the total number of repairs and anastomoses, while preserving bowel length.
- Superiority of stapled vs handsewn small bowel anastomosis remains controversial.

POSTOPERATIVE CARE

- In cases of gastric or small bowel injury with limited contamination, antibiotics are not required beyond 24 hours. Delayed presentation of injury (>12 hours) or cases with severe contamination may require an extended course.[13]
- Routine use of nasogastric tubes following abdominal surgery has not been shown to hasten return of bowel function or reduce anastomotic leaks. However, placement of a nasogastric tube intraoperatively or postoperatively remains common practice and may be left to surgeon discretion.[14,15]
- Nutritional support should begin as soon as clinically feasible, with preference for gastric or enteral nutrition over parenteral.

COMPLICATIONS

- Missed intra-abdominal injury
- Postoperative ileus
- Postoperative bleeding
- Anastomotic leak
- Intra-abdominal abscess
- Surgical site infection
- Enterocutaneous fistula
- Internal hernia
- Small bowel obstruction
- Short gut syndrome

REFERENCES

1. Bloom MB, Ley EJ, Liou DZ, et al. Impact of body mass index on injury in abdominal stab wounds: implications for management. *J Surg Res.* 2015;197(1):162-166.
2. Salim A, Teixeira PGR, Inaba K, et al. Analysis of 178 penetrating stomach and small bowel injuries. *World J Surg.* 2008;32:471-475.
3. Mathonnet M, Peyrou P, Gainant A, Bouvier S, Cubertafond P. Role of laparoscopy in blunt perforations of the small bowel. *Surg Endosc.* 2003;17(4):641-645.
4. Watts DD, Fakhry SM. Incidence of hollow viscus injury in blunt trauma: an analysis from 275,557 trauma admissions from the East multi-institutional trial. *J Trauma.* 2003;54(2):289-294.
5. Tejerina Alvarez EE, Holanda MS, López-Espadas F, Dominguez MJ, Ots E, Díaz-Regañón J. Gastric rupture from blunt abdominal trauma. *Injury.* 2004;35(3):228-231. doi:10.1016/s0020-1383(03)00212-2. PMID: 15124787.
6. Oncel D, Malinoski D, Brown C, et al. Blunt gastric injuries. *Am Surg.* 2007;73:880-883.
7. Atri M, Hanson JM, Grinblat L, et al. Surgically important bowel and/or mesenteric injury in blunt trauma: accuracy of multidetector CT for evaluation. *Radiology.* 2008;249(2):524-533.
8. Livingston DH, Lavery RF, Passannante MR, et al. Free fluid on abdominal computed tomography without solid organ injury after blunt abdominal injury does not mandate celiostomy. *Am J Surg.* 2001;182:6-9.
9. Fakhry SM, Allawi A, Ferguson PL, et al. Blunt small bowel perforation (SBP). *J Trauma Acute Care Surg.* 2019;86:642-650.
10. Bain K, Meytes V, Chang GC, Timoney MF. Laparoscopy in penetrating abdominal trauma is a safe and effective alternative to laparotomy. *Surg Endosc.* 2019;33(5):1618-1625.
11. Moore EE, Jurkovich GJ, Knudson MM, et al. Organ injury scaling. VI: Extrahepatic biliary, esophagus, stomach, vulva, vagina, uterus (nonpregnant), uterus (pregnant), fallopian tube, and ovary. *J Trauma.* 1995;39:1069-1070.
12. Bruns BR, Morris DS, Zielinski M, et al. Stapled versus hand-sewn: a prospective emergency surgery study. An American Association for the Surgery of Trauma multi-institutional study. *J Trauma Acute Care Surg.* 2017;82:435-443.
13. Goldberg SR, Anand RJ, Como JJ, et al. Prophylactic antibiotic use in penetrating abdominal trauma: an Eastern Association for the Surgery of Trauma practice management guideline. *J Trauma Acute Care Surg.* 2012;73:S321-S325.
14. Cheatham ML, Chapman WC, Key SP, Sawyers JL. A meta-analysis of selective versus routine nasogastric decompression after elective laparotomy. *Ann Surg.* 1995;221:469.
15. Sapkota R, Bhandari RS. Prophylactic nasogastric decompression after emergency laparotomy. *J Nepal Med Assoc.* 2013;52(191): 437-442.

Chapter 35: Operative Management of Duodenal Injury

David I. Hindin and David A. Spain

DEFINITION

- Both penetrating and blunt injuries to the duodenum are rare. Overall, less than 2% of all abdominal traumas involve duodenal injury, and among patients who receive a laparotomy following abdominal trauma, a duodenal injury is appreciated in less than 2% of patients with stab wounds, 5% to 6% of patients with blunt trauma, and 10% to 11% of patients with gunshot wounds.[1,2]
- Despite the rarity of these injuries, duodenal trauma remains the subject of much focus, in part due to the risk of associated major vascular injury, as well as the challenges presented by the complexity of pancreaticoduodenal anatomy. Injuries to the duodenum are most commonly graded by using the AAST Organ Injury Scale (**TABLE 1**).[3]

PATIENT HISTORY AND PHYSICAL FINDINGS

- As with all trauma patients, the initial assessment and management should follow the established protocols defined by the American College of Surgeons Advanced Trauma Life Support (ATLS) guidelines.[4] The patient's airway should be assessed and, if necessary, secured. Breathing, ventilation, and adequate oxygenation must all be confirmed. Hemodynamic status should be evaluated, with consideration that in the earliest stages of hemorrhagic shock, tachycardia may be present in the absence of hypotension.
- Relevant information to collect for blunt trauma patients includes the mechanism of injury (deceleration vs assault), whether the patient sustained a handlebar-type injury, and the estimated speed at impact. Among patients presenting after motor vehicle collisions, additional pertinent details include whether the patient was wearing a seatbelt at the point of impact, whether there was airbag deployment in the vehicle, and whether the patient had to be manually extricated from the vehicle following the incident. If the patient was seated in the driver's seat, information regarding the status of the steering wheel (ie, whether this was damaged during the collision) can also be useful.
- Among patients arriving to the trauma bay after sustaining stab wounds, information about the size and length of knife involved may be helpful. For patients who have sustained gunshot wounds, any available details regarding the direction and source of gunfire may be useful in seeking to understand potential missile trajectories and their associated injuries.
- During physical examination, the surgeon should seek to determine whether the patient exhibits frank peritoneal signs, whether there is evidence of abdominal bruising or abrasion (including the so-called "seatbelt sign"), and for patients of penetrating trauma, whether there is obvious visible violation of fascia. Other more subtle findings may include isolated right upper quadrant tenderness or tenderness localized to the epigastrium.
- A thorough accounting should be made of all stab wounds or gunshot wounds, taking care to recognize that penetrating trauma which is not immediately overlying the abdomen (including the back, chest, and legs) may ultimately result in an intra-abdominal trajectory. Among hemodynamically

Table 1: Duodenum Organ Injury Scale

Grade[a]	Type of injury	Description of injury	AIS-90
I	Hematoma	Involving single portion of duodenum	2
	Laceration	Partial thickness, no perforation	3
II	Hematoma	Involving more than one portion	2
	Laceration	Disruption <50% of circumference	4
III	Laceration	Disruption 50%-75% of circumference of D2	4
		Disruption 50%-100% of circumference of D1, D3, D4	4
IV	Laceration	Disruption >75% of circumference of D2	5
		Involving ampulla or distal common bile duct	5
V	Laceration vascular	Massive disruption of duodenopancreatic complex	5
		Devascularization of duodenum	5

AIS, abbreviated injury score; D1, first portion of duodenum; D2, second portion of duodenum; D3, third portion of duodenum; D4, fourth portion of duodenum.
[a]Advance one grade for multiple injuries up to Grade III.
Reprinted with permission from Moore EE, Cogbill TH, Malangoni MA, et al. Organ injury scaling II: pancreas, duodenum, small bowel, colon, and rectum. J Trauma. 1990;30:1427-1429. Table 2.

- stable patients with an odd number of gunshot wounds, it is a helpful practice to briefly gather plain films within the trauma bay to determine the location of retained missiles.
- A key determination during the physical examination is whether to proceed directly to the operating room or not. Penetrating trauma patients who are hemodynamically unstable should be brought directly to the operating room for exploration, as should those with frank abdominal tenderness or obvious fascial violation. Among hemodynamically stable patients who have sustained penetrating trauma, lack abdominal tenderness, and have unclear fascial violation, computed tomography (CT) imaging may be obtained, with variable use of oral and per-rectum contrast, before determining whether to proceed to diagnostic laparoscopy.
- A point-of-care ultrasound (focused assessment with sonography in trauma, or FAST) examination may be helpful in determining the presence of intra-abdominal fluid and the role for operative exploration in hemodynamically unstable blunt trauma patients. Among hemodynamically unstable blunt trauma patients who have an equivocal FAST examination, some clinicians may elect to perform a diagnostic peritoneal lavage in determining whether to proceed to operative exploration.

IMAGING AND OTHER DIAGNOSTIC STUDIES

- The majority of traumatic duodenal injuries following penetrating trauma are discovered at the time of laparotomy: often, these patients have not undergone preoperative imaging. However, among penetrating trauma population with duodenal injuries that are captured on CT, a variety of findings may suggest the diagnosis. It should be noted that whenever possible, CT imaging for patients with potential duodenal injury should include both oral and intravenous (IV) contrast.
- A duodenal hematoma may be suggested by the presence of isolated wall thickening. In the case of perforation, oral contrast extravasation may be observed either into the retroperitoneum or the general intraperitoneal space. Extravasation of IV contrast may be seen as well, immediately adjacent to the site of injury. Due to the partially retroperitoneal nature of the duodenum, injury may be exhibited as isolated retroperitoneal air—or, in contrast, free air within the abdomen.[5]
- CT findings consistent with blunt duodenal injury may include the above findings, as well as wall thickening or a "coiled spring" sign suggestive of intramural hematoma within D2 or D3. These injuries can also be associated with a flexion/distraction fracture of L1-L2 (so-called "Chance fracture") which may be seen on imaging, as well.[6,7]
- With the exception of frank extravasation of contrast from the duodenum, no imaging finding is pathognomonic for duodenal injury; a high index of suspicion is therefore paramount.

SURGICAL MANAGEMENT

- The patient is positioned supine on the operating room table. Broad-spectrum antibiotics are administered. Anesthesia is induced, and the patient is intubated. A Foley is placed. Both arms are left out, and the patient is prepped and draped from the chin to knees in standard trauma fashion. Some practitioners advocate lithotomy positioning if a rectal injury is suspected.
- A generous midline incision is carried out from xiphoid to pubis. A Bookwalter or other self-retraining retractor is inserted. All four quadrants of the abdomen are packed with rolled laparotomy pads. Zones of the retroperitoneum are assessed for overt injury or hematoma. Laparotomy pads are gradually removed from each quadrant, evaluating for bleeding after each quadrant before proceeding to the next.
- In patients with concern for duodenal injury, exposure of the duodenum (inframesocolic Zone I) is carried out, typically beginning with a right medial visceral rotation, or Cattell-Braasch maneuver.[8] The colon is mobilized along the white line of Toldt, followed by the hepatic flexure. Right colon and small bowel are mobilized medially. A Kocher maneuver is now performed to fully expose the duodenum (FIGURE 1).
- At this point, an assessment of overall injury burden and the patient's hemodynamic status is carried out, in addition to evaluation of the specific duodenal injury. For patients with hemodynamic instability, ongoing transfusion and/or pressor requirement, significant base deficit, or multiple comorbid injuries, a damage control procedure with temporary abdominal closure is performed and the patient is transferred to intensive care unit (ICU) for further resuscitation.
- For patients with isolated injury to the duodenum, a variety of techniques may be used depending on injury grade, surgeon preference, and patient anatomy. These techniques include primary repair, resection and anastomosis, pyloric exclusion, jejunal serosal patch, and use of a jejunal Roux limb.

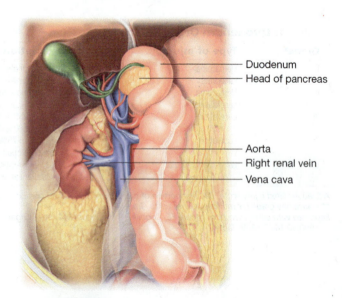

FIGURE 1 • Right medial visceral rotation.

PRIMARY REPAIR

- Patients with Grade II (laceration <50% of circumference) injuries and some Grade III injuries (laceration of 50%-75% of circumference of D2, or 50%-100% of circumference of D1, D3, D4) may be amenable to primary repair.
- An inner layer of interrupted, 3-0 absorbable suture is used to close the defect in transverse fashion. This is followed with an outer layer of interrupted 3-0 silk suture. One layer closure using 3-0 PDS is an option as well. Some surgeons also advocate mobilizing a flap of omentum to cover this repair.[7] In distal D2 or proximal D3 injuries, it is critical to ensure the major papilla has not been involved with the injury. For these defects, the papilla should be palpated and examined for injury prior to addressing the defect. In situations when it is difficult to locate the papilla, some surgeons will perform an open cholecystectomy and pass a small catheter through the common bile duct (via the cystic duct) to aid in localizing the papilla.

RESECTION AND ANASTOMOSIS

- For injuries distal to D3 and D4 that are not amenable to primary repair, resection and anastomosis may be considered.
- An intestinal load GIA stapler is used (two rows of titanium staples, closed staple size 1.5 mm) to divide proximal and distal to the defect.
- Intervening mesentery is divided with a vessel-sealing device, completing the resection.
- The ends are brought side by side. A seromuscular fixation stitch is used along the adjacent antimesenteric borders.
- A small corner of the staple line along each antimesenteric border is now excised from each end.
- Another intestinal load GIA stapler is now inserted and fired, creating a common channel. A TIA stapler can be used to complete the anastomosis or it can be oversewn (**FIGURE 2**).

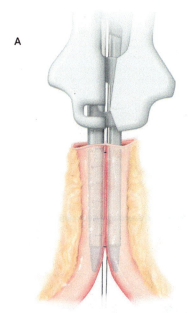
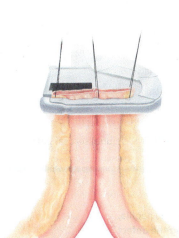

FIGURE 2 • Duodenal anastomosis following resection. **A,** A GIA stapler is inserted and fired, creating a common channel. **B,** A TIA stapler is shown completing the anastomosis.

JEJUNAL SEROSAL PATCH

- In defects of the duodenum that have too much tissue loss to consider primary repair but are not amenable to resection and anastomosis, a jejunal serosal patch can be a useful option.[9]
- The defect is debrided to healthy tissue. An adjacent loop of distal jejunum is now brought antecolic and positioned to lie adjacent to the defect. Interrupted, serosa-to-serosa sutures are used to close the defect.
- Typically, a drain is left adjacent to this repair. Jejunal serosal patches are less commonly performed in recent years, with a Roux limb of jejunum (see section that follows) increasingly being used to address similar defects (**FIGURE 3**).

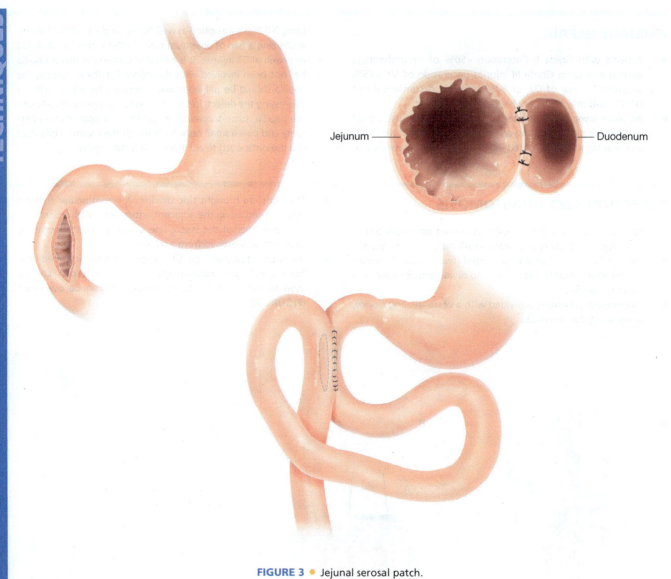

FIGURE 3 • Jejunal serosal patch.

JEJUNAL ROUX LIMB REPAIR

- For a large duodenal defect that does not involve the papilla, but is not amenable to primary repair, addressing the defect with a jejunal Roux limb is increasingly gaining popularity. This is also seen as a useful adjunct to address narrowing of the duodenum caused by a primary repair carried out at the index damage control laparotomy.[2]
- Edges of the duodenal defect are debrided to healthy tissue. A 40-cm Roux limb of jejunum is created and passed through a defect in the transverse mesocolon. The hood of this Roux limb is now brought over the duodenal defect. A two-layer, side-to-end duodenojejunostomy is carried out, using 3-0 absorbable suture for the inner mucosal layer and an outer layer of interrupted 3-0 silk. An end-to-side jejunojejunostomy is now performed, once again with an inner layer of 3-0 absorbable suture and an outer layer of interrupted, 3-0 silk (FIGURE 4).

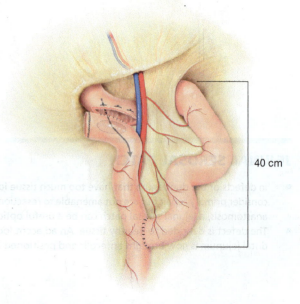

FIGURE 4 • Roux-en-y duodenojejunostomy.

PYLORIC EXCLUSION

- Pyloric exclusion is considered when an existing duodenal repair is felt to be at risk for narrowing or potential breakdown (and risk for subsequent duodenal fistula). In these scenarios, a pyloroplasty may be performed, along with a diverting gastrojejunostomy.
- A portion of the greater curvature of the stomach is cleared of tissue and the overlying short gastric vessels or branches of gastroepiploic vessels are divided. A dependent gastrotomy is carried out and the pyloric muscle is grasped with babcocks and pulled toward the gastrotomy. A series of #1 polypropylene sutures are used to oversew the pylorus. In an alternative stapled approach, the pylorus may instead be closed by firing a single staple load (typically a TA-50) across the pylorus, followed by gastrojejunostomy creation (see section that follows).
- Next, a loop of jejunum is brought antecolic and positioned to lie adjacent to the gastrotomy. If the pylorus was closed with a stapled approach, a gastrostomy is made along the greater curvature of the stomach. A gastrojejunostomy is created, with an inner layer of 3-0 resorbable suture and an outer layer of 3-0 silk suture. The site of the duodenal repair is drained widely. Some surgeons elect to leave a drain adjacent to the

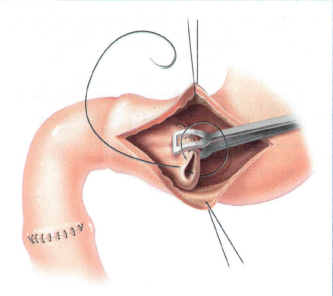

FIGURE 5 • Pyloric exclusion.

gastrojejunostomy, as well (**FIGURE 5**). A second option for pyloric exclusion is to fire a TA-30 stapler distal to the pylorus

FEEDING JEJUNOSTOMY TUBE

- As described in the previous secions, the initial operation for some patients with duodenal trauma may be a damage control procedure with temporary abdominal closure only.
- At the time of definitive repair however, a feeding jejunostomy tube is frequently placed.

PEARLS AND PITFALLS

Pearls	■ For any major duodenal repair, enteral access must be a consideration. Whether this is a feeding jejunostomy, a nasogastric tube, etc., a surgeon should not leave the operating room following definitive repair without a plan in place for enteral access. ■ Less is often better. In general, the minimum repair is typically the safest. When an isolated duodenal injury is amenable to primary repair, for instance, this is often the best approach. ■ In contrast, a complex repair, such as a trauma pancreaticoduodenectomy, should almost never be attempted in the acute setting.
Pitfalls	■ Inadvertently narrowing the duodenum during primary repair. ■ Inadequate drainage of duodenal repair. ■ Not securing enteral access at time of definitive repair. ■ Doing too much: in an unstable patient, the focus should be on damage control with prompt transfer to the ICU for further resuscitation. ■ Attempting a complex reconstruction in the acute setting leads to increased risk of morbidity and mortality.

POSTOPERATIVE CARE

- Postoperatively, patients are kept NPO on IV fluids, with a nasogastric tube in place until demonstrated return of bowel function.

COMPLICATIONS

- Missed enterotomy
- Missed pancreatic injury
- Risk of duodenal leak and fistula

REFERENCES

1. Malhotra A, Biffl WL, Moore EE, et al. Western trauma association critical decisions in trauma: diagnosis and management of duodenal injuries. *J Trauma Acute Care Surg*. 2015;79(6):1096-1101.
2. Feliciano DV. Abdominal trauma revisited. *Am Surg*. 2017;83(11):1193-1202.
3. Moore EE, Cogbill TH, Malangoni MA, et al. Organ injury scaling II: pancreas, duodenum, small bowel, colon, and rectum. *J Trauma*. 1990;30:1427-1429.
4. Henry S. *ATLS Advanced Trauma Life Support, 10th Edition Student Course Manual*. 10th ed. American College of Surgeons; 2018.
5. Jayaraman MV, Mayo-Smith WW, Movson JS, Dupuy DE, Wallach MT. CT of the duodenum: an overlooked segment gets its due. *Radiographics*. 2001;21 Spec No:S147-S160.
6. LeBedis CA, Anderson SW, Soto JA. CT imaging of blunt traumatic bowel and mesenteric injuries. *Radiol Clin North Am*. 2012;50(1):123-136.
7. Scalea TM, Feliciano DV. *The Shock Trauma Manual of Operative Techniques*, 2nd ed. Pancreas and Duodenum Injuries: Techniques. Springer, 2021; Vol 13: 339-351.
8. Cattell RB, Braasch JW. A technique for the exposure of the third and fourth portions of the duodenum. *Surg Gynecol Obstet*. 1960;111:378-379.
9. McKittrick JE. Use of a serosal patch in repair of a duodenal fistula. clinical application of an experimental method. *Calif Med*. 1965;103(6):433.

Chapter 36 Antrectomy

Sherif R. Z. Abdel-Misih

DEFINITION

- Antrectomy by definition is surgical removal of the antrum of the stomach. From a clinical and practical standpoint, antrectomy involves surgical resection of the distal aspect of the stomach, also often referred to as distal gastrectomy. Appreciating the surgical anatomy and physiology of the stomach is important to understanding the technical aspects of and indications for antrectomy, respectively.
- The antrum resides in the distal aspect of the stomach extending from below the incisura angularis to the pylorus. The antrum contains mucus-secreting cells as well as the G cells importantly. The G cells are responsible for gastrin secretion, which is a peptide hormone serving as a major contributor to the secretion of hydrochloric acid in the stomach.
- Antrectomy is now generally reserved for complicated peptic ulcer disease (PUD) refractory to medical management as well as for neoplasms limited to the distal stomach.
- Reconstruction is undertaken to reestablish gastrointestinal (GI) continuity.
  - This is most commonly done with Billroth I, Billroth II, or Roux-en-Y reconstruction.
  - The Billroth I reconstruction establishes GI continuity through a gastroduodenostomy.
  - Billroth II reconstruction does so through a loop gastrojejunostomy.
  - Roux-en-Y reconstruction employs a Roux limb with anastomosis to the remnant stomach and a jejunojejunostomy anastomosis between the alimentary channel (from the stomach) and the biliopancreatic limb to create the common channel. It is uncommonly used with antrectomy and often utilized with bariatric surgery and subtotal/total gastrectomy.

DIFFERENTIAL DIAGNOSIS

- Antrectomy with reconstruction is largely utilized to address complicated PUD refractory to medical management and neoplasms of the distal stomach (**TABLE 1**).

Peptic Ulcer Disease

- The development of ulcers has been attributed to overuse of nonsteroidal anti-inflammatory drugs (NSAIDs), *Helicobacter pylori* infection, pathologic conditions like Zollinger-Ellison syndrome (gastrinoma) responsible for acid hypersecretion, or malignancy-associated ulcers (**TABLE 2**).
- Epigastric pain is a common presenting symptom for PUD, but also common to other GI and surgical pathology warranting thorough assessment of a broad differential diagnoses list that includes biliary (cholecystitis, symptomatic cholelithiasis, cholangitis, choledocholithiasis) pathology, pancreatitis, gastritis, Mallory-Weiss tear, as well as GI neoplasms, which will be discussed subsequently.

Neoplasms

- The stomach has wide range of neoplasms associated with it, both benign and malignant, which may warrant surgical intervention including antrectomy. These include gastric adenocarcinoma, gastrointestinal stromal tumors (GISTs), leiomyoma, neuroendocrine tumors (carcinoid), lymphoma, mucosa-associated lymphoid tissue, and other rare tumors (ie, schwannoma). Neoplasms located in the distal stomach or antrum may mimic symptoms and signs of PUD including abdominal pain, satiety, bleeding, nausea/vomiting (associated with obstruction), dysphagia, and anemia. Patients may selectively benefit from antrectomy with or without regional lymphadenectomy as clinically or oncologically indicated.

PATIENT HISTORY AND PHYSICAL FINDINGS

- A thorough history and physical examination is prudent to assess and detail patient history, symptoms, and signs. Patients with PUD commonly present with abdominal (epigastric) pain due to the effects of acid on the gastric mucosa typically described as burning in nature. Pain is sometimes transiently ameliorated with meals, but typically returns. Other associated chronic symptoms of nausea, vomiting, and early satiety may develop due to the chronic inflammatory state associated with untreated PUD and may contribute to weight loss over time.
- Given the risk factors outlined previously, it is important to direct questions to elicit the use of specific medications (including NSAIDs, immunosuppressive drugs, and steroids) as well as medical history of *H. pylori*, Zollinger-Ellison syndrome (gastrinoma), or other contributing modifiable

Table 1: Indications for Antrectomy

Peptic ulcer disease
Recalcitrant—Persistent disease refractory to medical management
Perforation—Antral (distal) ulcer
Bleeding—Type I, II, or III gastric ulcer
Obstruction—Inflammation-associated gastric outlet or duodenal obstruction

Neoplasm
Benign—Polyp, leiomyoma, lipoma, schwannoma
Malignant—Distal adenocarcinoma, neuroendocrine tumor (carcinoid), gastrointestinal stromal tumor

Table 2: Risk Factor to Peptic Ulcer Disease

Risk factors

Helicobacter pylori infection
Medications (nonsteroidal anti-inflammatory drugs, aspirin)
Zollinger-Ellison syndrome/gastrinoma
Smoking
Alcohol
Stress (surgery, chronic illness, etc)

risk factors like smoking and alcohol. Understanding the etiology will direct the treatment team toward the appropriate medical management and surgical intervention when warranted. Importantly, there are complications of PUD including bleeding, obstruction, and perforation that may warrant emergency medical and surgical intervention so it is important to determine this early and triage acuity appropriately.
- Bleeding associated with PUD may present in a chronic, indolent fashion with anemia noted on routine blood work sometimes accompanied by generalized fatigue and weakness. Alternatively, PUD-associated bleeding may present acutely with hematemesis or melena with associated hemodynamic instability warranting resuscitative management including blood transfusion and sometimes requires urgent endoscopic or surgical intervention to address. Ulcer associated perforation leads to acute onset of notable abdominal pain secondary to peritonitis due to peritoneal contamination from gastric contents extruded via the perforation.
- Obstruction associated with PUD has typical obstructive symptoms of epigastric pain, nausea, vomiting, early satiety, and weight loss.
- As indicated previously, there are numerous types of neoplasms, both benign and malignant, that are associated with the stomach. Irrespective of neoplastic potential, these may present with symptoms or as incidental radiographic findings given the increasing use of imaging diagnostics. Gastric neoplasms commonly present with symptomatology similar to those discussed with PUD. Epigastric (abdominal) pain and discomfort are common and are often associated with GI complaints of nausea, vomiting, and early satiety due to the sometimes obstructive effects of the neoplasm. When there is neoplastic involvement of the antrum and particularly the prepyloric area, patients develop gastric outlet obstructive symptoms that are often accompanied by notable, sometimes rapid weight loss. Malignant neoplasms not uncommonly have associated bleeding due to mucosal friability or ulceration as in PUD, but often can be difficult to manage endoscopically sometimes warranting antrectomy with regional lymphadenectomy and reconstruction.
- Neoplasm may also be asymptomatic.

IMAGING AND OTHER DIAGNOSTIC STUDIES

- Endoscopy is vital to assessment of the esophagus, stomach, and proximal duodenum to determine the etiology and management of patients presenting with dyspepsia symptomatology guided by recommendations by the *American Society for Gastrointestinal Endoscopy*.[1] They identify several high-risk or *alarm features* that should be considered in the management of patients with dyspepsia symptoms (TABLE 3). With these alarm features in mind, treatment and surveillance can be tailored to the individualized patient (TABLE 4).
- Endoscopic evaluation allows for visualization and documentation of the foregut assessing for inflammatory conditions, neoplasms, and ulcers while also providing therapeutic options (FIGURE 1A-C).
- Findings of gastritis, duodenitis, and peptic ulcers will typically prompt initiation of proton pump inhibitors as well as *H. pylori* drug therapy when warranted. It is generally

Table 3: ASGE Alarm Features for Dyspeptic Patients

Age ≥ 50 y
Family history of foregut malignancy in first-degree relative
GI bleeding and/or iron deficiency anemia
Dysphagia or odynophagia
Persistent vomiting
Weight loss
Abnormal imaging

ASGE, American Society for Gastrointestinal Endoscopy.

Table 4: ASGE Endoscopic Guidelines for Dyspepsia

Age ≥ 50 y with alarm features and new-onset dyspepsia: Initial endoscopy
Age < 50 y without alarm features: Test and treat (*Helicobacter pylori* testing and PPI)
Age < 50 y without alarm features and negative *H. pylori*: PPI trial
H. pylori–negative refractory to PPI therapy: Initial endoscopy

ASGE, American Society for Gastrointestinal Endoscopy; PPI, proton pump inhibitor.

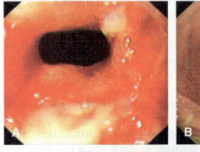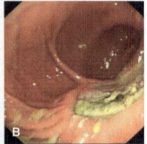
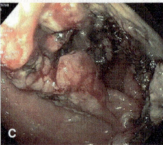

FIGURE 1 • A and B, Endoscopic image of partial pyloric obstruction due to chronic inflammation. B, Endoscopic image of large gastric ulcer with central cratering. C, Endoscopic image of an ulcerated, fungating antral cancer.

accepted to pursue *H. pylori* testing in all patients with PUD given the association. With the association of malignancy, most gastric ulcers should undergo biopsy with exceptions or individualized decisions made in appropriate clinical circumstances when the etiology appears benign (ie, NSAID related).
- In the case of neoplasms and malignancy, in addition to conventional esophagogastroduodenoscopy (EGD) for diagnostic purposes, endoscopic ultrasound (EUS) is another diagnostic tool for consideration as part of neoplastic or oncologic workup.[2] EUS provides additional clinical staging information related to the tumor itself (T stage) as well as local nodal status (N stage), which helps determine whether this is a localized malignancy (cTis or cT1a), locoregional (cT1b-cT4a, cM0), or metastatic

(cT4b, cM1) (**TABLE 5**). Only patients with locoregional disease would be considered for antrectomy. In addition to staging, EUS provides important biopsy capabilities distinct from EGD, including sonographic-guided fine-needle aspiration or fine-needle biopsy. This is especially important with uncommon neoplasms distinct from adenocarcinoma like GIST, neuroendocrine tumors, leiomyoma, and schwannoma (**FIGURE 2**).

Table 5: TNM Staging of Gastric Cancer

Primary tumor (T stage)	Regional lymph nodes (N stage)	Distant metastasis (M stage)
T0 No evidence of tumor	N0 No regional node metastasis	M0 No distant Metastasis
Tis Carcinoma *in situ*, intraepithelial tumor without invasion of lamina propria, high-grade dysplasia	N1 Metastasis in 1-2 nodes	M1 Distant metastasis
T1 Tumor invades the lamina propria or muscularis mucosae	N2 Metastasis in 3-6 nodes	
T1a Tumor invades the lamina propria or muscularis mucosae	N3 Metastasis in ≥7 nodes	
T1b Tumor invades the submucosa	N3a Metastasis in 7-15 nodes	
T2 Tumor invades the muscularis propria	M3b Metastasis in ≥16 nodes	
T3 Tumor penetrates the subserosal connective tissue without invasion of the visceral peritoneum or adjacent structures		
T4 Tumor invades the serosa (visceral peritoneum) or adjacent structures		
T4a Tumor invades the serosa (visceral peritoneum)		
T4b Tumor invades the adjacent structures/organs		

Used with the permission of the American College of Surgeons. Amin MB, Edge SB, Greene FL, et al. (eds.) *AJCC Cancer Staging Manual.* 8th ed. Springer; 2017.

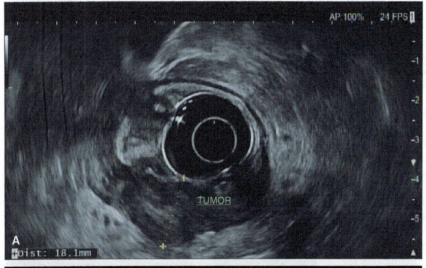
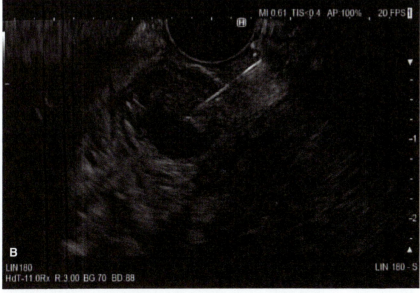

FIGURE 2 • **A,** Endoscopic ultrasound image of an antral tumor (labeled). **B,** Endoscopic ultrasound image with fine-needle biopsy (FNB) undertaken of a leiomyoma.

- Imaging plays a selective role in the management of those diseases warranting antrectomy. In the case of straight forward PUD, imaging is not necessarily required.
- In advanced PUD or with suspected neoplasms or malignancy, imaging is essential when considering surgical intervention to provide insights on extent of PUD-associated inflammation as well as information relevant to potential malignancy (**FIGURES 3** and **4**).
- With suspected malignancy, cross-sectional imaging, most commonly with CT scan with intravenous and oral contrast, is helpful to determine the extent of tumoral involvement especially as it may relate to contiguous structures as well as aid in clinical staging by highlighting associated perigastric or mesenteric adenopathy in addition to visceral, systemic, or peritoneal metastases. CT of the chest/abdomen/pelvis with contrast to complete radiographic staging workup is prudent and helpful. Subsequent imaging considerations include fluorodeoxyglucose–positron emission tomography/CT if clinically indicated and if no apparent metastatic disease by CT scan in order to assess for occult metastatic disease.

SURGICAL MANAGEMENT

Preoperative Planning

- Following thorough diagnostic workup, preoperative medical assessment, and informed consent detailing the planned surgical intervention with the associated risks, benefits, alternatives, and anticipated recovery, surgical intervention can be pursued.
- The indication and acuity may affect the preoperative and perioperative approach to care. In an elective setting as in antrectomy undertaken for a gastric neoplasm, or gastric outlet obstruction, it is reasonable to consider utilization of enhanced recovery after surgery (ERAS) protocols.
- For surgery in bleeding cases, the associated higher acuity requires timely care and surgical management as in other surgical emergencies.
- Appropriate IV access/lines placed by anesthesia, nasogastric tubes, and urinary catheters are placed to decompress the stomach and monitor fluid status, respectively.
- All patients receive preoperative antibiotics in an appropriately timed fashion prior to surgery to decrease perioperative infectious risk and complications.
- Chemoprophylaxis (heparin subcutaneously) for deep venous thrombosis and venous thromboembolism (VTE) may be considered for preoperative or intraoperative administration.

Positioning

- In the operating room, patients are most commonly positioned supine with arms out or tucked as appropriate for an open approach. With improved technology and surgeon skill sets, minimally invasive surgical approaches have had increasing use in foregut-directed surgical interventions, and a split-leg patient position with foot

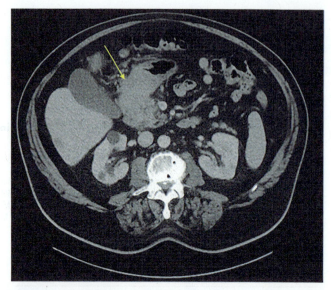

FIGURE 3 • CT scan demonstrating notable inflammation (*arrow*) of the distal stomach and proximal duodenum that could be secondary to both peptic ulcer disease and neoplastic processes. Note the proximity of the gallbladder infundibulum.

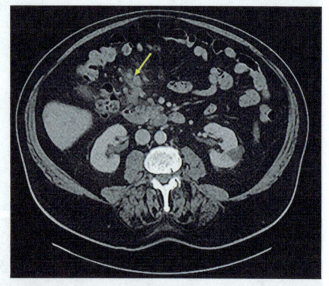

FIGURE 4 • CT scan demonstrating perigastric adenopathy (*arrow*) along the left gastric vasculature consistent with metastatic disease from a gastric adenocarcinoma.

boards to facilitate a reverse Trendelenburg positioning is helpful.
- Given the prevalent use of self-retaining retractors for operative exposure (abdominal wall or liver retraction), positioning should be mindful of the need for attachment of such retractors.

- For an open approach, a midline supraumbilical incision is generally undertaken to access the abdomen (**FIGURE 5**). Once accessed, the falciform ligament is taken down from the abdominal wall to facilitate placement of a self-retaining retractor to optimize exposure as well as abdominal exploration to assess for additional pathology particularly with an oncologic surgical indication.
- With planned antrectomy, the distal stomach is then mobilized by dividing the gastrocolic ligament providing access to the lesser sac. This allows dissection to proceed proximally and distally along the greater curvature by continuing to take down the gastrocolic ligament using electrocautery, vessel sealer device, or traditional surgical ligature technique. This should be carried out proximally enough to comfortably allow for adequate mobilization for proximal gastric transection and future reconstruction. During this dissection, it is important to be cognizant of the gastroepiploic arcade arising from the left and right gastroepiploic vasculature and coursing along the greater curvature of the stomach (**FIGURE 6A**). The right gastroepiploic vasculature courses between the first part of the duodenum and the pancreas with the right gastroepiploic artery arising from the gastroduodenal artery and the right gastroepiploic vein draining into the superior mesenteric vein.
- For antrectomy and the distal transection, it is necessary to ligate the right gastroepiploic vasculature with whatever technique one is comfortable with. It is important to be meticulous with traction and dissection of these vessels to avoid undesirable, bothersome bleeding. With lesser sac access, it is important to deepen dissection into the lesser sac by elevating the stomach cranially and anteriorly to facilitate dividing the typically avascular attachments between the posterior stomach and anterior pancreatic capsule (**FIGURE 6B**). With the stomach elevated and the dissection along the greater curvature carried out sufficiently, attention can be turned to the cranial dissection along the lesser curvature.

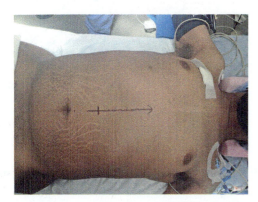

FIGURE 5 • Midline upper abdominal incision.

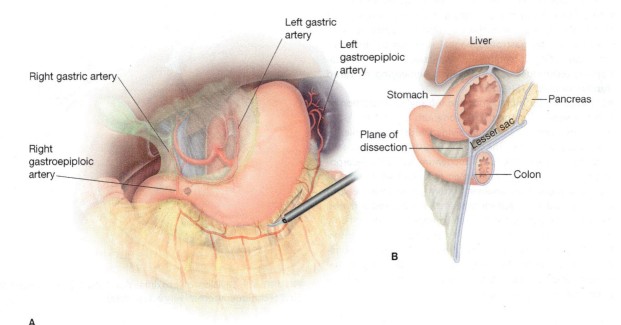

FIGURE 6 • **A,** Dissection of the gastrocolic ligament along the greater curvature of the stomach to gain access to lesser sac. The gastroepiploic vessels should be identified and either preserved or ligated as appropriate based on patient-specific needs. **B,** Sagittal view of the upper abdomen demonstrating plane of dissection to gain access to lesser sac via the gastrocolic ligament and relationship of the pancreas warranting deep dissection into lesser sac to elevate the stomach away from the pancreas.

- It is helpful to open the pars flaccida to carry out the lesser omental dissection caudally toward the suprapyloric area and also toward the incisura angularis as part of preparation for future transection.
- It is important to be aware of the right gastric artery that typically arises from the common hepatic artery as it courses to supply the lesser curvature vascular arcade in combination with the left gastric artery. Identification and ligation of the right gastric artery allows safer dissection around the pylorus and duodenal bulb (first portion of the duodenum) to facilitate distal transection when ready.
- It is sometimes necessary or helpful to proceed with a Kocher maneuver, particularly in the setting of notable inflammation or for oncologic reason to elevate and/or medialize the gastroduodenal junction to facilitate the pyloric and proximal duodenal dissection.
- With the stomach and proximal duodenum mobilized and the related vasculature in mind, it is appropriate to proceed with ligation of the gastroepiploic vasculature near the pylorus at the level of the infrapyloric region if for benign reason or pursue high ligation closer to the pancreas if for oncologic reason. It is necessary to divide again along the greater curvature at the planned proximal transection line.
- With vasculature controlled and ligated, it is then appropriate to proceed with proximal transection of the stomach. The line of transection to assure adequate antrectomy is commonly accepted to be from the incisura angularis (also several centimeters proximal to the commonly referred to "crow's foot" that represents the terminal branches of anterior vagus along the lesser curvature innervating the antrum) directed toward a point that is about two-thirds the way along the greater curvature from the gastroesophageal junction to the pylorus. Transection is commonly undertaken with surgical stapling techniques, particularly with emerging powered staplers available (**FIGURE 7**).
- After appropriate suprapyloric and infrapyloric dissection to create a window around the duodenum beyond the pylorus, the duodenum can also be divided with linear stapler or sharply as preferred by the surgeon (**FIGURE 8**). It is prudent to assure that the adequate duodenum has been incorporated in the antrectomy specimen to ensure while uncommon that there is no retained antrum which could lead to recurrent PUD. Not necessarily needed, nor advised, a frozen section can be checked at the distal margin to confirm if only the duodenum is present. Prior to any stapling or transection, it is prudent to assure that the typically placed nasogastric tube has been adequately withdrawn into the proximal stomach or distal esophagus to ensure it is not errantly incorporated into any staple line.

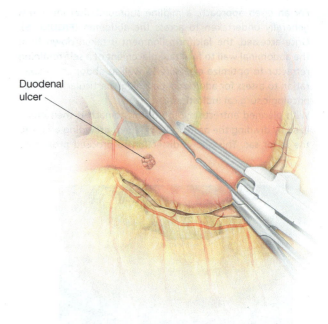

FIGURE 7 • Proximal transection of stomach using linear stapler.

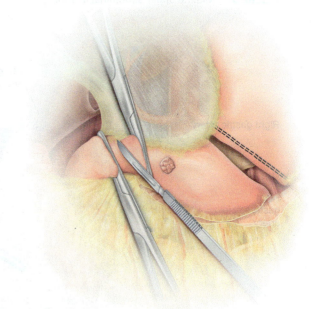

FIGURE 8 • Division of proximal duodenum (with scalpel; stapled technique alternatively acceptable).

RECONSTRUCTION

- There are several reconstruction options to consider to establish GI continuity after antrectomy. This includes Billroth I (gastroduodenostomy), Billroth II (loop gastrojejunostomy), and Roux-en-Y reconstructions. We will discuss each approach separately.
- A Billroth I reconstruction involves reestablishment of GI continuity through anastomosis of the remnant stomach to the proximal duodenum.

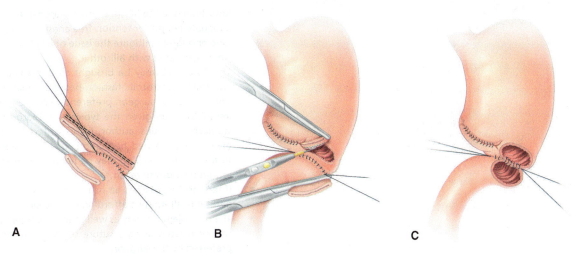

FIGURE 9 • Two-layer handsewn Billroth I (gastroduodenostomy). **A,** Interrupted seromuscular (3-0 silk) sutures used for posterior outer layer. **B,** Gastrotomy created by removing greater curvature staple line using electrocautery. **C,** After opening the duodenum (bowel clamp removal or removing staple line if duodenum transected with stapler), the inner layer is undertaken by utilizing two 3-0 polydioxanone sutures run circumferentially starting from the middle of the posterior inner layer. An anterior outer layer of 3-0 silk interrupted seromuscular sutures utilized to complete the anastomosis.

- Given the long staple line of the proximal gastric transection site, oversewing the staple line not planned to be incorporated into the reconstruction is reasonable with running or interrupted Lembert technique.
- As in all GI anastomoses, it is important to assure there is no tension as well as good vascularity for reconstruction. Hence, it is important to assure an adequate Kocher maneuver and mobilization of the duodenum and the remnant stomach undertaken to provide adequate tension-free reach. If necessary, the remnant stomach can be further mobilized by dividing the gastrocolic and gastrohepatic ligament further as needed. Should there be an issue with reach or tension, it is important to consider an alternative reconstruction option.
- Vascular assessment has improved with the advent of indocyanine green (ICG) fluorescence angiography. This adjunct allows operative assessment of the adequacy of the vascular supply to the intestinal tract of interest for reconstruction.[3]
- The gastroduodenostomy is commonly undertaken with anastomosis of the greater curvature of the remnant stomach to the duodenum. This can be pursued using a traditional single-layer suture technique using 3-0 silk (or alternatives) sutures preferred by the author, but two-layer suture and stapled techniques are acceptable alternative approaches (FIGURE 9). This can be undertaken using and end-to-end anastomosis stapler with the anvil purse stringed into the duodenum and the stapler placed through an anterior gastrotomy. The stapler trocar can be deployed through the posterior stomach or at the staple line along the greater curvature of the stomach. The stapler can be synced to the anvil with creation of the anastomosis and the anterior gastrotomy closed with suture or stapler techniques.
- A Billroth II reconstruction is a reconstruction option with a loop gastrojejunostomy with many modifications (sutured/stapled, ante/retrocolic, ante/retrogastric, isoperistaltic/antiperistaltic) that have been developed with variations that are appropriate and without data to date suggesting a clear superior approach (FIGURE 10).
    - The gastrojejunostomy should be constructed with a short afferent limb (less than 20 cm) to decrease the likelihood of developing afferent loop syndrome (ALS).
    - The duodenal stump also warrants acknowledgment with this reconstruction approach. With healthy, vascularized duodenum, a single-layer suture closure or staple (± reinforced staple loads) technique is typically sufficient, but with duodenal inflammation, it may be necessary to consider closure in multiple layers, buttress (omentum), tube duodenostomy, and/or surgical drainage.
    - This authors favor an infracolic anastomotic position (not pictured) by pexying the stomach to the defect in the transverse mesocolon. With the gastrojejunostomy lying below the transverse mesocolon, this helps limit afferent/efferent limb kinking in addition to issue of mesocolic herniation.
- A Roux-en-Y reconstruction is an alternative option that may be considered.
    - The technical aspects of this worth noting relate to Roux limb length. Unlike for bariatric surgical indication where a long Roux limb is of benefit for weight loss, a

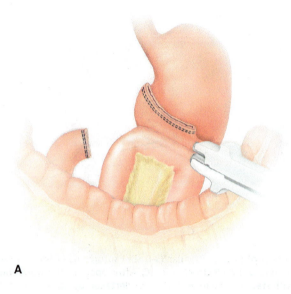

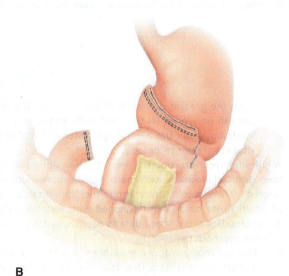

Roux limb of 40 to 50 cm is often reasonable to provide adequate length for tension-free anastomosis as well as long enough to mitigate the issue of alkaline bile reflux often associated with Billroth II.

- The Roux limb may be brought to the stomach in an antecolic or retrocolic fashion based on anatomic considerations and surgeon preference. With length being less of an issue given the typically still large remnant stomach size, this author favors antecolic approach given the decreased herniation risk. An omental split to the transverse colon may be helpful to decrease the required length to reach.
- If tension-free reach is an issue, a retrocolic approach is a suitable alternative affording easier reach.
- The gastrojejunostomy as well as the jejunojejunostomy can be created using a suture or stapler technique as preferred by the surgeon.
- Following meticulous reconstruction after antrectomy without any surgical issues or concerns, it is the view of this author that it is not necessary or advisable to utilize routine surgical drainage based on numerous studies not supporting routine drainage for other GI diseases.[4]

FIGURE 10 • **A,** Billroth II reconstruction demonstrating a retrogastric, retrocolic loop gastrojejunostomy using linear stapler technique. **B,** Common enterotomy for stapler insertion oversewn with suture technique. With retrocolic placement, the transverse mesocolic defect should be closed to prevent intestinal herniation. With retrocolic reconstruction, this author favors an infracolic anastomotic position (not pictured) by pexying the stomach to the rent in the transverse mesocolon. With the gastrojejunostomy lying below the transverse mesocolon, this helps prevent afferent/efferent limb kinking as well as herniation.

MINIMALLY INVASIVE APPROACH

- As minimally invasive surgery has become more pervasive and adopted for surgery for both benign and malignant disease, there has been increasing use of these approaches for antrectomy for the indications discussed. Laparoscopy and robot-assisted approaches are reasonable options for well-selected patients by those surgeons and teams comfortable and facile with these techniques. Patient factors including previous surgery, comorbidities, body habitus, and patient/surgical acuity should be considered as they may contribute to the difficulty and need for conversion. Patient condition is of utmost importance because patients with hemodynamic instability, peritonitis, chronic symptoms/signs (inflammation in setting of PUD or obstruction), and pathologic inflammation may not tolerate pneumoperitoneum.
- Minimally invasive techniques utilized in many foregut operations (antireflux, bariatric, etc) provide surgeons with many of the requisite techniques to consider for antrectomy. As is typical of a minimally invasive foregut-directed operation, the patient is positioned and well secured with the legs abducted in a split-leg position with foot boards to allow for safe reverse Trendelenburg positioning. This allows for the surgeon or assistant to be positioned between the patient's legs to facilitate ergonomic and ideal instrument handling. Commonly, a four- or five-port laparoscopic approach can be utilized with a liver retractor selectively used to retract the left lateral segment of the liver anteriorly for minimally invasive approach.
- With the continued expansion of robotic-assisted surgery, a robotic approach may be pursued, commonly utilizing the DaVinci Xi platform. For antrectomy, four 8-mm robotic ports are utilized with one or two assistant ports to further facilitate this approach.
- Similar to the open approach described, the techniques for dissection, mobilization, resection, and reconstruction translate well to the minimally invasive approach.

PEARLS AND PITFALLS

Indication	▪ Refractory or complicated (perforation, hemorrhage, obstruction) PUD and distal gastric neoplasms
Operative planning	▪ EGD/EUS essential to assess type of pathology, extent, and potential therapeutic options (surgical, endoscopic, medical) ▪ Open, laparoscopic, and robotic approach options based on patient selection and surgeon (team) skill set ▪ Oncologic indication warrants thorough staging workup (imaging ± EUS) ▪ Detailed understanding of vascular anatomy and controlled ligation limits bothersome bleeding
Exposure/dissection/ mobilization	▪ Minimally invasive surgical cases and approaches optimized by appropriate patient positioning and liver retractor ▪ Extent of dissection dictated by indication (oncologic may require regional lymphadenectomy) and reconstruction plan (to facilitate tension-free anastomoses) ▪ Inflammation related to the pathology (PUD particularly) may distort normal anatomy leading to difficult dissection and meticulous care to avoid injury to vital structures (pancreas, middle colic vessels, common hepatic artery, and common bile duct)
Gastric mobilization	▪ Adequate dissection of gastrocolic ligament important for stomach mobilization and transection ▪ Be mindful of gastroepiploic vasculature along greater curvature and especially right gastroepiploic vessels as they arise between the duodenum and pancreas with risk of avulsion or injury, particularly with extensive inflammation or neoplasia
Lines of transection	▪ Adequate antrectomy achieved proximally with line of transection from incisura angularis to about two-thirds the way from GE junction to pylorus ▪ Status of duodenum (healthy vs inflamed) should be considered in transection technique utilized to lessen risk of duodenal stump leak ▪ Ensure nasogastric tube withdrawn to proximal stomach or distal esophagus to avoid interference with intestinal transection
Reconstruction	▪ Billroth I, II, and Roux-en-Y viable options with acceptable outcomes without statistically significant demonstrable advantage ▪ BI: Adequate mobilization needed (Kocher maneuver and proximal gastric mobilization) to facilitate tension-free reach ▪ BII: Short afferent limb (<20 cm) decreases likelihood of ALS; omental split helps facilitate antecolic reconstruction if length or reach is an issue; with retrocolic reconstruction, recommend inframesocolic anastomotic position by pexying the stomach to the mesocolon to minimize torsion/kinking and herniation of small bowel ▪ "Angle of sorrow" (where the stomach meets the duodenum or jejunal end of the staple line) felt to be the area of risk and commonly managed with a U-stitch or triple seromuscular stitch to imbricate the anterior and posterior stomach over the corner ▪ ICG is a useful surgical adjunct to assess vascularity prior to and after reconstruction

POSTOPERATIVE CARE

- Patient surgical indication, acuity, comorbidities, and immediate postoperative status will dictate the appropriate triage and care of patients undergoing antrectomy.
- Those patients undergoing urgent/emergent antrectomy may have a guarded condition postoperatively with higher acuity needs warranting surgical intensive care unit or intermediate care unit.
- Those patients undergoing elective antrectomy should be considered for institution-specific ERAS protocols and otherwise be triaged to the surgical ward.
- An orogastric/nasogastric tube is commonly utilized in surgery, but may be considered for removal intraoperatively, at the conclusion or the procedure, or on postoperative day (POD) 1 per surgeon preference.
- Routine postoperative care should be pursued including pulmonary toilet, deep vein thrombosis/VTE prophylaxis, early mobilization, and early initiation of oral intake (POD 0/1) as determined by the surgeon.

COMPLICATIONS

- Overall, the outcomes associated with antrectomy are excellent with very low risk of recurrent (1%-2%) PUD and oncologic outcomes dictated by biology assuming appropriate oncologic management and operative approach. However, there are short-term operative as well as long-term functional complications associated with antrectomy worth noting.
- Short-term surgical complications are typical of most GI surgical interventions.
    - Importantly, irrespective of reconstruction approach, anastomotic leak, while uncommon, is still a potential source of major morbidity affecting overall outcomes and is the reason for meticulous attention during the reconstruction.

Table 6: Postgastrectomy Reconstruction and Unique Associated Complications or Technical Issues

Reconstruction method	Complications/issues
Billroth I	Tension, duodenal status, or oncologic reasons may limit option
Billroth II	Bile reflux gastritis/esophagitis, remnant gastritis, afferent loop syndrome, dumping syndrome, anemia
Roux-en-Y	Roux stasis, more demanding (two anastomoses)

- Delayed gastric emptying is a common functional complication and issue in patients undergoing distal gastrectomy with potential negative impact on patient quality of life.[5]
- With the robust gastric blood supply and required operative control and ligation needed, operative and postoperative bleeding is important to monitor for.
- There are also long-term complications related to antrectomy and the reconstruction approach used that warrant mention (**TABLE 6**).
  - ALS is constellation of symptoms and signs in the postoperative period classically described after Billroth II reconstruction in an acute or chronic form. Symptoms include sudden upper abdominal pain with associated nausea and emesis that localized epigastric tenderness. Uncommonly, patients may present with jaundice due to secondary biliary obstruction. A chronic ALS may present months to years after surgery with similar symptoms including weight loss due to food aversion as well as bilious emesis that relieves symptoms. This often requires surgical management either with a Braun enteroenterostomy (afferent to efferent limb bypass) or conversion to Roux-en-Y reconstruction.
  - Reflux gastritis and esophagitis is associated with Billroth I and particularly Billroth II reconstructions, with resulting symptoms of burning epigastric pain due to bile reflux into the stomach and sometimes esophagus. This physiologic issue if significant enough may warrant surgical conversion to Roux-en-Y reconstruction to mitigate it.
  - Dumping syndrome is another physiologic functional condition more commonly associated with Billroth II reconstruction. Dumping syndrome manifests in two forms, early and late, based on the onset of the symptoms and signs related to meals. Early dumping syndrome results in onset of abdominal pain, cramps, and diarrhea within 10 to 30 minutes after eating. Late dumping syndrome typically develops symptoms 1 to 3 hours after eating. The symptoms and signs include nausea, vomiting, cramps, diarrhea, dizziness, and tachycardia with late dumping syndrome also having flushing and hypoglycemia. The syndrome is thought to be secondary to the effects of a hyperosmolar sugar load that rapidly transits to the duodenum with the effects of the pylorus. Fortunately, this can often be managed with lifestyle modification focusing on changes in diet and nutrition to smaller, frequent meals and limiting simple sugars. Surgical conversion to Roux-en-Y may be utilized in patients refractory to medical management.
  - Postgastrectomy anemia is a long-term issue related to the surgical resection and reconstruction with the associated physiologic and nutritional derangements. With the reconstruction, particularly Billroth II and Roux-en-Y, there are issues of B_{12} and iron malabsorption that can occur due to lack of intrinsic factor and the lack of gastric acid production to convert dietary iron to the absorbed form for the duodenum that is bypassed, respectively. For this reason, it is necessary to be vigilant with follow-up for anemia and nutritional recommendations (B_{12} supplementation, oral iron, etc) to avoid it.[6]

REFERENCES

1. ASGE Standards of Practice Committee; Shaukat A, Wang A, et al. The role of endoscopy in dyspepsia. *Gastrointest Endosc*. 2015;82(2):227-232.
2. Valero M, Robles-Medranda C. Endoscopic ultrasound in oncology: an update of clinical applications in the gastrointestinal tract. *World J Gastrointest Endosc*. 2017;9(6):243-254.
3. Degett TH, Andersen HS, Gogenur I. Indocyanine green fluorescence angiography for intraoperative assessment of gastrointestinal anastomotic perfusion: a systematic review of clinical trials. *Langenbeck's Arch Surg*. 2016;401(6):767-775.
4. Wang Z, Chen J, Su K, Dong Z. Abdominal drainage versus No drainage post-gastrectomy for gastric cancer. *Cochrane Database Syst Rev*. 2011;(8):CD008788.
5. Kim DH, Yun HY, Song YJ, et al. Clinical features of gastric emptying after distal gastrectomy. *Ann Surg Treat Res*. 2017;93(6):310-315.
6. Lim CH, Kim SW, Kim WC, et al. Anemia after gastrectomy for early gastric cancer: long-term follow-up observational study. *World J Gastroenterol*. 2012;18(42):6113-6119.

Chapter 37 Subtotal Gastrectomy for Cancer

Anthony M. Villano, Patrick G. Jackson, and Waddah B. Al-Refaie

DEFINITION
- Subtotal gastrectomy is removal of 70% to 80% of the distal stomach, including the pylorus. This is only performed for distal tumors, whereby a 5-cm proximal margin can be obtained, with the advantage of achieving a gastric remnant of reasonable size and thus reservoir function.

DIFFERENTIAL DIAGNOSIS
- The presenting symptoms of gastric cancer are generally nonspecific, which leads to delays in diagnosis and advanced disease at presentation.
- Benign etiologies within the differential include gastroesophageal reflux disease (GERD), peptic ulcer disease (PUD), gastritis, and gastric bezoar.
- Other considerations, though less likely, include gastrointestinal (GI) stromal tumor, gastric lymphoma, esophageal neoplasm (leiomyoma, adenocarcinoma), and extrinsic compression (pancreatic neoplasm, metastatic perigastric lymphadenopathy).

PATIENT HISTORY AND PHYSICAL EXAMINATION FINDINGS

Presentation
- The presenting symptoms of gastric cancer are nonspecific and overlap with many common, benign conditions such as GERD or PUD. Unfortunately, this often leads to delays in diagnosis and advanced presentation.
- The most common presenting symptoms of gastric cancer are epigastric pain, weight loss, anorexia, anemia, and early satiety.
  - The pain of gastric cancer is often constant, nonradiating, and not altered by meals. These characteristics help distinguish it from more common etiologies such as peptic ulcer disease.
  - Less common symptoms include dysphagia, persistent emesis, and hematemesis/melena. These are associated with advanced disease and large primary tumors. A particularly worrisome symptom is progressive abdominal distention, which may signify underlying malignant ascites.
- Special attention must be paid to weight loss, as it signifies a potential need for preoperative nutritional optimization. Preoperative malnutrition is a significant independent predictor of postoperative morbidity,[1,2] and persistent malnutrition has been associated with worse long-term survival.[3] The surgeon should have a low threshold to place a nutrition consultation and initiate supplemental nutrition to facilitate weight gain.
  - Preoperative rehabilitation (or "prehabilitation") with a structured exercise and nutrition program has continued to gain traction. Prehabilitation may carry even greater importance with growing utilization of perioperative chemotherapy for gastric cancer, which may worsen preoperative malnutrition. Neoadjuvant therapy has been observed to increase the odds of malnutrition by over twofold.[4]
  - A structured exercise/nutrition program improved functional performance status both pre- and postoperatively among 62% of patients in a recent randomized trial.[5] Such improvements may allow more patients to complete both surgery and their intended perioperative adjuvant therapy.
- Severe gastric outlet obstruction, with the inability to tolerate anything by mouth, is an ominous presenting symptom which warrants immediate management. Initial attention should be focused on gastric decompression (most often via nasogastric [NG] tube placement), intravenous (IV) fluid resuscitation, and correction of electrolyte abnormalities.
  - Management of gastric outlet obstruction secondary to gastric cancer should take place in a multidisciplinary fashion. Next steps are determined by a multifactorial assessment of the patient's performance status, the stage and extent of disease present, and the intent of oncologic treatment (curative or palliative).
  - In the setting of potentially curative treatment, we recommend initial staging with imaging (see "Imaging Studies and Staging Evaluation"). As most patients in this situation would go on to receive neoadjuvant chemotherapy, establishment of enteral feeding access distal to the obstruction is a crucial next step. Most commonly this takes the form of a feeding jejunostomy. These can be placed at the time of initial staging laparoscopy or at the time of admission.

Physical Findings
- The physical examination, in conjunction with a detailed history, is critical to the preoperative assessment and can quickly allow the clinician to ascertain the patient's overall performance status. A poor performance status may affect the patient's candidacy for surgery and/or adjuvant therapies.
- Simple observations such as how the patient traverses the room (transitions to and from the examination table, ambulation, balance, etc) and their general body habitus can quickly give the surgeon a general sense of the patient's physical fitness.
- Physical examination findings of poor nutrition such as cachexia, pallor, poor skin turgor, sunken eyes, and bitemporal wasting are critical and signify a need to initiate preoperative supplemental nutrition.
- Particular attention to the abdominal, lymph node, and rectal examinations will provide clues to potential metastatic disease.
  - Signs of advanced disease include supraclavicular lymphadenopathy, a palpable abdominal mass, hepatomegaly, severe abdominal distention, a fluid wave, or palpable metastases in the cul-de-sac (known as "Blumer shelf").

IMAGING AND OTHER DIAGNOSTIC STUDIES

Laboratory Tests

- Important laboratory values to obtain in every patient undergoing subtotal gastrectomy for cancer include a hemoglobin (to assess for anemia), basic metabolic panel (with attention to electrolytes and renal function), liver enzymes (elevation may suggest occult metastatic disease), and albumin/prealbumin (markers of nutrition).
- There are no specific tumor markers for gastric cancer, unlike adenocarcinomas of the colon or rectum. However, CEA and CA-125 may be obtained as changes in these markers throughout the course of treatment if initially elevated (pre/post systemic therapy and postoperatively) can have prognostic value.

Imaging Studies and Staging Evaluation

- The initial step in the workup of gastric cancer is most frequently an upper endoscopy (**esophagogastroduodenoscopy, EGD**).
  - The preoperative EGD will provide critical information with respect to the location of the primary tumor (cardia, fundus, antrum, greater or lesser curvature), size of the primary tumor, and extent of disease (**FIGURE 1A** and **B**).
  - A critical maneuver in the evaluation of gastric cancer is insufflation of the stomach, which will aid in identification of *linitis plastica* or *diffuse-type* gastric cancer. As the name suggests, patients with *linitis plastica* will have a stiff stomach which is difficult to distend with air owing to diffuse infiltration of signet ring cells throughout the gastric wall. These patients are often not amenable to subtotal gastrectomy and must undergo a total gastrectomy.
  - Biopsy of the primary tumor is generally also performed at the initial EGD to obtain tissue for histologic diagnosis.
- **Endoscopic ultrasound (EUS)** is routinely employed to assess the T-stage and N-stage of the primary tumor.
  - T-stage is dictated by the depth of invasion into the gastric wall. This is of critical importance, as invasion into the submucosa (T1b) is associated with a significant risk of lymph node invasion and necessitates gastrectomy as the intervention of choice. Very select T1a lesions which are small (<2 cm), well to moderately differentiated, without lymphovascular invasion may be amenable to advanced endoscopic resection; however, the indications for this approach continue to evolve.[6,7]
  - EUS is highly accurate for the purpose of T-staging. Discrimination between T1 and T2 on EUS was found to have a sensitivity and specificity of 0.85 (95% CI 0.78-0.91) and 0.90 (95% CI 0.85-0.93), respectively, in a large meta-analysis.[8]
  - EUS may also provide valuable information regarding locoregional lymph node involvement, and suspicious nodes may be biopsied via fine needle aspiration.
- Pretherapy cross-sectional imaging via **computed tomography (CT)** or **magnetic resonance imaging (MRI) of the chest, abdomen, and pelvis** adds significant value to the staging workup by providing additional information regarding the primary tumor and ruling out distant metastatic disease (**FIGURE 2A**).
  - Lymphadenopathy should be carefully noted. If within the field of operative resection (see "Surgical Management"), bulky lymphadenopathy should not preclude a patient from surgical intervention. Distant lymph nodes, however, should raise appropriate hesitation in offering a resection.
- **Positron emission tomography (PET)-CT** scanning has evolved as an additional noninvasive approach to rule out distant metastatic disease.
  - Approximately 50% of gastric cancers are fluorodeoxyglucose-avid, and as such this will not be useful in all patients. Those with signs or symptoms suggestive of occult metastatic disease may benefit from the addition of PET-CT into the staging workup.
- **Staging laparoscopy** is the final step in the complete workup for gastric cancer. Landmark series from the 1990s which

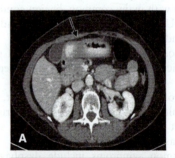
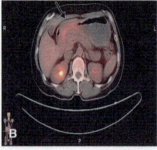

FIGURE 2 • Cross-sectional imaging in the form of computed tomography (CT) and CT/positron emission tomography (PET) evaluates locoregional and distant metastases. **A,** CT scan in a patient with gastric cancer demonstrating thickening of the gastric antrum with nodularity in the gastrocolic ligament suggestive of direct spread to the transverse colon. **B,** PET/CT corroborated with CT scan to suggest involvement of the gastrocolic ligament. No metastatic disease was observed.

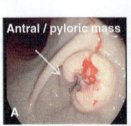
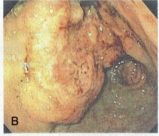

FIGURE 1 • Esophagogastroduodenoscopy provides anatomic information and allows for biopsy. **A,** Biopsy-proven poorly differentiated adenocarcinoma with signet cell features in the antral/prepyloric region of stomach. **B,** Fungating adenocarcinoma of the distal third of the stomach in a 75-year-old man who presented with iron deficiency anemia.

assessed the utility of staging laparoscopy in gastric cancer identified that 23% to 37% of gastric cancer patients harbored subradiographic, occult peritoneal metastases which would preclude curative resection.[9,10] Similar rates of occult metastatic disease persist in more modern gastric cancer cohorts.[11]

- Staging laparoscopy is typically performed prior to the initiation of perioperative chemotherapy (or definitive surgery if an upfront surgical approach is planned).
- The addition of peritoneal cytology remains controversial; however, those with positive peritoneal cytology in the absence of gross carcinomatosis have poor survival outcomes similar to those with gross peritoneal metastases.[12] Owing to this fact, it is our practice to routinely employ peritoneal cytology with staging laparoscopy to identify additional patients that may be spared unnecessary surgery.
- In line with the American College of Surgeons Cancer Surgery Standards and NCCN guidelines, we routinely perform staging laparoscopy prior to the initiation of neoadjuvant therapy or definitive operation for clinical stage T1b disease (or greater).

SURGICAL MANAGEMENT

- The most critical oncologic components of subtotal gastrectomy are margin-negative resection along with an adequate lymphadenectomy. All aspects of the operation are conducted with these two basic tenets in mind.

Preoperative Planning

- **Preoperative nutrition:** As aforementioned, patients with gastric cancer may be afflicted with severe malnutrition. Preoperative placement of a feeding nasojejunal or jejunostomy tube may be necessary, especially throughout neoadjuvant treatment if that is employed. This can be placed at staging laparoscopy.
- **Evaluation of functional status:** The history and physical examination as detailed earlier will identify patients who may not be candidates for curative treatment. Those who are borderline may require aggressive physical therapy in conjunction with nutritional supplementation to "prehabilitate" for surgery. Rarely, admission to the inpatient setting is required to accomplish these goals.
- **Restaging after neoadjuvant therapy:** Repeat imaging is recommended after completion of neoadjuvant treatment to assess response. Consideration may be given to repeat EGD and/or staging laparoscopy to further assess burden of tumor and finalize operative plans. Subtotal gastrectomy may become feasible after dramatic responses to neoadjuvant treatment.
- **Preoperative antibiotics:** Second-generation cephalosporins are routinely employed for prophylaxis.
- **Deep venous thrombosis (DVT) prophylaxis:** All patients should have a lower extremity sequential compression device applied during the procedure. As gastric cancer patients represent a high-risk population for venous thromboembolism, we routinely administer preoperative subcutaneous heparin and continue heparin/low molecular weight heparin throughout hospitalization unless contraindicated. At some centers, 30 days postdischarge prophylaxis is also offered.

Positioning

- The patient is placed in supine position with both arms out at 90°. Pressure points are carefully padded. The patient is prepped from the nipples to the upper thigh.

STAGING LAPAROSCOPY

- The peritoneal cavity is entered at the umbilicus either by an open technique or via establishment of pneumoperitoneum with a Veress needle and subsequent port placement. A 30° scope is inserted and one to two additional 5-mm ports on the left or right side of the abdomen are placed for manipulation of tissues, biopsy of suspicious lesions, and aspiration of peritoneal washings.
- A complete survey of the peritoneal cavity for metastatic disease is performed, including the diaphragm, liver, spleen, pelvis, small bowel, large bowel, parietal peritoneum, and omentum. If suspicious disease is observed, it is biopsied and sent for frozen section. In the setting of biopsy-proven peritoneal disease, gastrectomy should not be performed and definitive resection should be aborted to pursue systemic therapies. However, selective palliative surgical procedures may be indicated, for example, in bleeding or obstructing cancers that cannot be palliated by endoscopic measures. These decisions need to be individualized based on the patient's presentation, performance status, extent of metastatic burden, and projected survival.
- **Peritoneal cytology:** 200 to 500 mL of normal saline is instilled into the abdominal cavity and allowed to dwell for 5 to 7 minutes. During this time, the patient is gently rocked from left to right to maximize capture of occult cells. After dwelling, the fluid is aspirated with a suction device which has a mechanism to trap the sample.
- If the staging laparoscopy is negative for peritoneal spread of the disease, operative resection is performed.

EXPLORATORY LAPAROTOMY

- The abdomen is entered through a midline incision extending from the xiphoid process to just below the umbilicus. A bilateral subcostal incision, approximately 2 cm below the costal margin, also provides excellent exposure. During entry into the abdomen, the falciform ligament should be preserved as it can be used to buttress the duodenal closure.
- A second careful exploration of the peritoneal cavity with palpation is performed to confirm the absence of peritoneal or metastatic disease. The liver is examined for any suspicious nodules.

MOBILIZATION OF THE GREATER CURVATURE OF THE STOMACH

- First, the transverse colon is separated from the greater omentum in an avascular plane (FIGURE 3). The stomach and the greater omentum are reflected superiorly, and the transverse colon is reflected inferiorly. The plane of fusion between the greater omentum and the transverse mesocolon is identified as a faint white line. This plane is incised with electrocautery to enter the lesser sac. This plane is advanced proximally and distally along the transverse colon until the greater omentum is freed. Formal omentectomy is classically described but is provider-dependent owing to emerging data that metastasis to the omentum is infrequent and omentectomy does not alter local recurrence or overall survival, even in locally advanced cases.[13,14]
- The dissection proceeds to the proximal greater curvature of the stomach using either clamps and ties or an energy device, such as Harmonic or LigaSure. When performing a subtotal gastrectomy, this dissection should stop prior to the short gastric arteries as they provide the blood supply to the proximal gastric remnant.

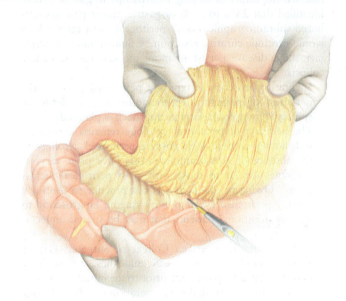

FIGURE 3 • Division of the greater omental attachments to the transverse colon. Transection of the avascular plane between these two structures provides access to the transverse mesocolon and the lesser sac.

DUODENAL MOBILIZATION AND TRANSECTION

- The hepatic flexure of the colon is mobilized by dividing the avascular attachment of the right colon to the retroperitoneum along the white line of Toldt and reflecting it inferomedially. The separation of the greater omentum from the transverse mesocolon is completed to the hepatic flexure if not already performed. Cranial reflection of the stomach and caudal tension on the transverse colon will expose the gastrocolic trunk of Henle. The gastrocolic trunk is classically formed by the confluence of right gastroepiploic vein, the right superior colonic vein, and the anterior-superior pancreaticoduodenal vein and drains into the superior mesenteric vein (FIGURE 4), although anatomic variants do exist. The right gastroepiploic vein can be divided at its junction with the gastrocolic trunk, or the entire gastrocolic trunk can be divided with a single fire of a vascular stapler. At this stage, the right gastroepiploic artery is divided at its origin from the gastroduodenal artery at the infraduodenal level. The infrapyloric nodes, located adjacent to the origin of gastroduodenal artery, are mobilized with the specimen (FIGURE 5).
- The lesser curvature is mobilized by dividing the lesser omentum as close to the liver as possible to preserve any lymph nodes which should remain with the specimen (FIGURE 6). If a replaced or accessory left hepatic artery is identified, it should be temporarily ligated, and the perfusion of the left lobe of the liver should be assessed prior to transecting the vessel. The dissection is carried distally to the portal triad. The right gastric artery is identified as arising from the common hepatic artery and is divided at its origin to include its associated lymphatic tissue with the specimen. The duodenum is circumferentially dissected about 2 to 3 cm distal to the pylorus, encircled with a Penrose drain, and divided with either a stapler or in between straight bowel clamps

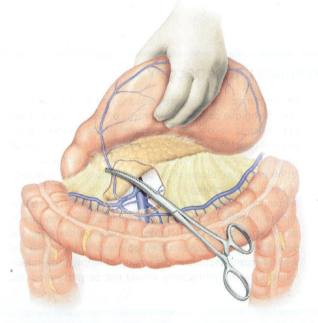

FIGURE 4 • Ligation of the right gastroepiploic vein. The right gastroepiploic vein is ligated at its junction with the colonic veins. Alternatively, the gastrocolic trunk can be divided with a single fire of a vascular stapler load.

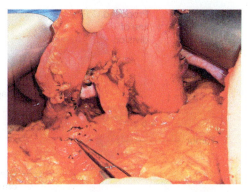

FIGURE 5 • Dissection of the infrapyloric nodal packet at the level of right gastroepiploic vessels.

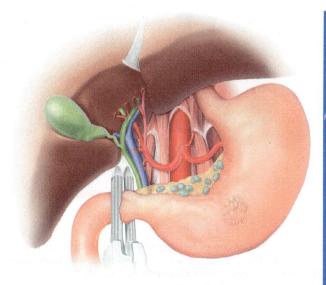

FIGURE 7 • Division of duodenum. The duodenum is encircled with a Penrose and divided with a blue gastrointestinal anastomosis (GIA) stapler load. Care is taken to avoid injury to portal vein, bile duct, and hepatic artery.

(FIGURE 7). Care is taken not to injure the bile duct, hepatic artery, or portal vein when encircling the duodenum. The duodenal staple line is oversewn with 3-0 silk Lembert sutures and can be buttressed with the falciform ligament (Moossa patch). However, in the setting of extensive inflammation, consideration should be given to dividing the duodenum between two straight bowel clamps and suture closure of the duodenal stump.

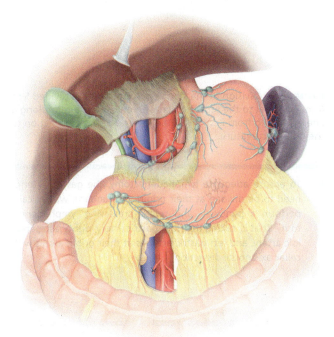

FIGURE 6 • Mobilization of the lesser curvature of the stomach. The lesser omentum is divided as close to the liver as possible. Presence of a replaced or accessory left hepatic artery is carefully sought.

GASTRIC TRANSECTION

- The gastrectomy specimen, now disconnected distally, is lifted anteriorly. The left gastric artery is identified, suture ligated, and divided at its origin (FIGURE 8). The areolar tissue associated with the left gastric artery is mobilized with the specimen.
- Next, the stomach is divided about 4 to 6 cm proximal to the primary cancer (FIGURE 9). Our preference is to use several green loads of a gastrointestinal anastomosis (GIA) stapler.
- We send the resected specimen in separate containers in the following manner: (1) stomach with a marking stitch on the proximal end, (2) greater omentum, (3) infrapyloric nodal packet, and (4) lesser curvature nodal packet with a long stitch on the left gastric artery. The operating surgeon should communicate with the pathologist to orient them to the specimen and indicate the proximal and distal margins for frozen section assessment.

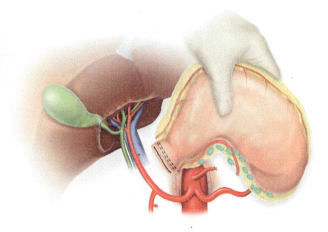

FIGURE 8 • Division of left gastric artery. The stomach is lifted anteriorly, the left gastric artery is identified, and then suture ligated. The lymph node packet along the left gastric artery is mobilized along with the specimen.

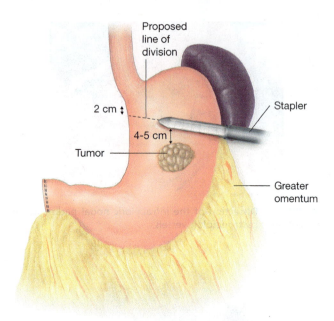

FIGURE 9 • Division of the stomach. The stomach is divided 5 to 6 cm proximal to the most proximal extent of the tumor along a line extending from 2 cm distal the gastroesophageal junction to the greater curvature.

LYMPHADENECTOMY

- Current NCCN guidelines state that the gastric resection should include the regional lymphatics. Namely, the perigastric lymph nodes and those along the named vessels of the celiac axis (left gastric artery, common hepatic artery, celiac artery, and splenic artery, ie, a D2 dissection) with the goal of obtaining at least 16 lymph nodes for adequate staging.[15]

- To ensure adequate lymphadenectomy, the gastric arteries need to be divided at their origin. By standard, we typically perform a pancreas- and spleen-preserving lymphadenectomy. That is, taking the right gastric artery, right gastroepiploic artery, and left gastric arteries at their origin along with celiac axis nodal dissection.

RECONSTRUCTION

- Restoration of GI continuity can be achieved by performing a Billroth II gastrojejunostomy or Roux-en-Y gastrojejunostomy. Our preference is Roux-en-Y gastrojejunostomy as it is associated with less alkaline (bile) reflux gastritis.
- **Roux-en-Y reconstruction**: While awaiting frozen section on the gastric margins, we proceed with the reconstruction. A loop of jejunum at least 30 cm distal to the ligament of Treitz that reaches the gastric pouch without tension is identified. The jejunum is divided at this point with a blue GIA stapler. The staple line on the end of the Roux limb is oversewn with 3-0 silk stitches in Lembert fashion. The Roux limb needs to be at least 40 cm (ie, from level of stomach to the jejunojejunostomy). Our preference is a retrocolic configuration for the Roux limb. As such, a defect is created in the transverse mesocolon to the left of the middle colic vessels (**FIGURE 10**). We then confirm that the Roux limb can easily reach the stomach without tension. Our preference is to first perform a stapled side-to-side anastomosis between the biliopancreatic limb and the jejunum. Our rationale behind this order of reconstruction is to allow for an easier reconstruction of this anastomosis away from the transverse mesocolon defect. Stay sutures are placed between the biliopancreatic limb and the jejunum. Enterotomies are made in the biliopancreatic limb and the jejunum. One limb of the blue GIA stapler is introduced into the biliopancreatic limb and the other in the jejunum. The blue load is fired and the common

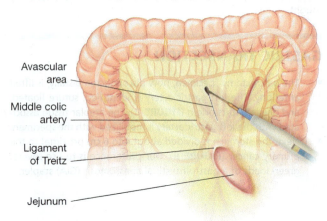

FIGURE 10 • Creation of the defect in transverse mesocolon. A defect is created in the transverse mesocolon to the left of middle colic veins. The Roux limb is delivered to the gastric remnant in a retrocolic fashion.

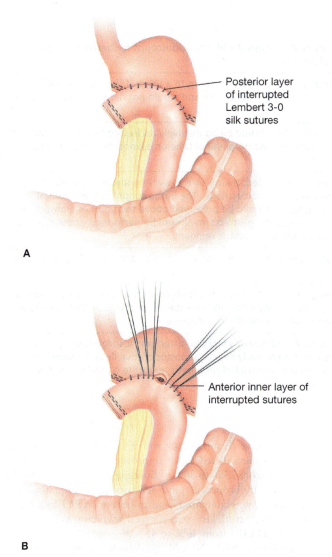

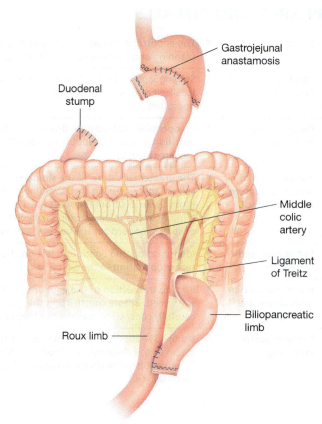

FIGURE 11 • Construction of two-layered handsewn gastrojejunal anastomosis. **A,** A series of posterior layer of interrupted 3-0 silk sutures is placed. **B,** Anterior inner layer also consists of interrupted 4-0 absorbable full-thickness stitches. Prior to completion of the anterior layer, an NG tube is advanced into the afferent limb of the jejunum. Following completion of the inner layer of the two-layered anastomosis, an anterior layer of interrupted 3-0 silk is placed.

- enterotomy is closed either in a handsewn fashion or with a single fire of GIA or thoracoabdominal stapler.
- Next, the Roux limb is navigated through the defect in the transverse mesocolon. A two-layered side-to-side handsewn anastomosis is created between the anterior surface of the gastric pouch and the Roux limb. A posterior layer of

FIGURE 12 • Final anatomy after completion of the gastrojejunal anastomosis.

interrupted 3-0 silk seromuscular (Lembert) sutures is placed (**FIGURE 11A**). Two opposing enterotomies are made on the stomach and the antimesenteric border of the Roux limb. The length of the opening along the jejunum should be shorter than that made in the stomach as the opening in the small bowel tends to expand. Next, an inner posterior layer of full-thickness interrupted 3-0 silk (or absorbable) sutures is placed, followed by an anterior layer of interrupted 3-0 silk (or absorbable) full-thickness sutures (**FIGURE 11B**). Prior to completion of anterior layer, the anesthesiologist advances the NG tube into the afferent limb of the jejunum. Following completion of the inner layer of the two-layered anastomosis, an anterior layer of interrupted 3-0 silk seromuscular (Lembert) sutures is placed (**FIGURE 12**). Alternatively, the surgeon can perform this anastomosis as a stapled anastomosis. We favor the handsewn anastomosis as it is consistent with our academic mission of training residents in complex intestinal reconstruction techniques. The Roux limb is sutured to the transverse mesocolon to prevent herniation of small bowel through this defect.

CLOSURE

- The abdomen is irrigated and the fascia closed with a running number 1 absorbable monofilament suture. The skin is closed with staples or running subcuticular absorbable suture.

PEARLS AND PITFALLS

Diagnostic studies	▪ The endoscopy should be performed or personally discussed with the endoscopist for better operative planning and intraoperative localization of the tumor.
Staging laparoscopy	▪ Staging laparoscopy is critical to avoid nontherapeutic laparotomy. Up to a third of the patients with localized disease on imaging will have occult peritoneal metastases and would not derive benefit from an operation.
Preoperative nutrition	▪ Preoperative malnutrition drives poor outcomes. This should be aggressively addressed by a structured nutrition program or supplemental enteral nutrition (via nasojejunal tube or jejunostomy placed at staging laparoscopy).
Mobilization of greater curvature of the stomach	▪ The greater curvature of the stomach should be mobilized, taking care to avoid unnecessary traction on splenic adhesions and thus avoiding splenic injury and hemorrhage. The blood supply to the proximal gastric pouch is from the short gastric arteries, which should be preserved above the point of transection. If injury to the spleen requires a splenectomy, then total gastrectomy should be performed as the removal of spleen jeopardizes the vascular supply to the proximal gastric remnant.
Left gastric pedicle dissection	▪ Identification and ligation of left gastric artery/vein should be done with care to avoid bleeding or venous tear propagating to the portal vein.
Reconstruction of gastrointestinal continuity	▪ Prior to transection of the jejunum, its ability to reach the predicted location of the anastomosis should be confirmed. Before constructing the gastrojejunal anastomosis, the orientation of the Roux limb should be carefully checked to prevent twisting or undue tension on the anastomosis.
Delayed gastric emptying	▪ Up to 15%-20% of the patients demonstrate delayed gastric emptying after gastric surgery. Early recognition of this diagnosis, and not mistaking vomiting or early satiety as postoperative ileus, is important. Treatment is supportive with gastric decompression and trial of prokinetic agents (e.g., metoclopramide or erythromycin).

POSTOPERATIVE CARE

- **General management:** Similar to other intra-abdominal operation, patients with subtotal gastrectomy should undergo a regimen of aggressive pulmonary hygiene, early ambulation, and physical therapy. Careful attention should be paid to the volume status, electrolytes, and input/output balance.
- **DVT prophylaxis:** We start patients on DVT prophylaxis within 24 hours after completion of the procedure unless contraindicated.
- **NG tube:** We keep the NG tube until 2 to 3 days postoperatively. If the tube gets dislodged accidently, we do not replace it. If replacement of an NG tube is necessary, it should be performed under fluoroscopy to avoid accidental disruption of the anastomosis by a blindly placed NG tube.
- **Nutrition:** A clear liquid diet is initiated on postoperative day 3 or 4 and advanced as tolerated. We consult a dietitian to educate patients on issues related to postgastrectomy diet. This new diet is a significant lifestyle modification for patients and dehydration is a common issue which should be monitored for.

OUTCOMES

- **Prognosis:** A 5-year survival based on the 8th edition of the AJCC TNM staging system is 81% for stage IA, 68.4% for stage IB, 59.3% for stage IIA, 46.3% for stage IIB, 34.7% for stage IIIA, 23.4% for stage IIIB, 12.3% for stage IIIC, and 5.6% for stage IV.[16]
- Survival outcomes in gastric cancer have improved over time as a result of more effective chemotherapeutic regimens. In the landmark MAGIC trial, the implementation of perioperative chemotherapy with ECF (epirubicin, cisplatin, and fluorouracil) led to an improvement in 5-year overall survival from 23% to 36%.[17] Building upon this, the FLOT4 regimen (fluorouracil plus leucovorin, oxaliplatin, and docetaxel) was compared head-to-head with ECF in a recent randomized trial. Five-year survival was improved even further by FLOT4 from 36% to 45%.[18]
- Compliance with NCCN guidelines (complete staging, adequate lymphadenectomy, and perioperative receipt of adjuvant treatment) improves survival outcomes. A recent assessment of national compliance identified a median overall survival benefit if all three criteria were met (45.5 months compliant vs 32.0 months noncompliant).[19]
- Quality-of-life outcomes are an underappreciated and significant aspect of postoperative care for gastric cancer patients. Patients should be counseled appropriately prior to surgery so that expectations are clear. Over half of patients self-report significant impairment in global quality of life immediately following surgery, with most improving to baseline by 6 months postoperatively.[20] Proximal and total gastrectomy are associated with worse patient reported outcomes as compared to distal/subtotal gastrectomy, especially with respect to reflux symptoms and nausea.[20,21]

COMPLICATIONS

Early Complications

- **Pulmonary complications**
    - Pulmonary complications are frequent after upper abdominal surgery and include atelectasis, aspiration, pneumonia, and pulmonary embolism. Patients who undergo

subtotal gastrectomy are at particular risk for aspiration if delayed gastric emptying develops. Among the elderly or frail, aspiration can be a devastating complication that can lead to death. Good pulmonary toilet, early mobilization, elevation of the head of the bed, close attention to fluid balance, and early initiation of DVT prophylaxis are paramount to minimizing these occurrences.

- **Postoperative bleeding**
  - **Presentation:** Postoperative bleeding can be intraluminal or intraperitoneal. Intraluminal bleeding presents with fresh blood in the NG tube, melena, downtrending serial hemoglobin, and potentially hemodynamic instability. Bleeding from the anastomosis is the major cause of the intraluminal bleeding and usually occurs around postoperative days 5 to 7. Intraperitoneal bleeding presents with hypotension, tachycardia, downtrending hemoglobin, and abdominal distension. Intraperitoneal bleeding usually presents in the first 12 to 24 hours following surgery. Unrecognized splenic injuries in the form of capsular tears or inadequate control of short gastric vessels are the major causes of postoperative intraperitoneal bleeding following subtotal gastrectomy.
  - **Management:** Intraluminal bleeding can generally be managed by supportive measures in the form of correction of coagulopathy and volume resuscitation. The vast majority originate from the anastomosis and will resolve on their own. Bleeding that causes hemodynamic compromise or does not respond to supportive measures requires careful endoscopic therapeutic measures. Reoperation for bleeding not controlled with endoscopy is rare. Intraperitoneal bleeding requires volume resuscitation and correction of coagulopathy. Patients with hemodynamic compromise or who do not immediately respond to supportive measures (suggestive of ongoing bleeding) should return promptly to the operating room for definitive control of the bleeding source. Particular attention to the spleen, short gastric vessels, and ligated main branches of the celiac trunk will swiftly identify the source in most cases.
- **Anastomotic leak**
  - **Presentation:** The overall incidence of anastomotic leak after subtotal gastrectomy with gastrojejunostomy is significantly less as compared to esophagojejunostomy after total gastrectomy and occurs in less than 2% of patients. Anastomotic leak presents with intra-abdominal sepsis, leading to fevers, tachycardia, and leukocytosis. Unexplained tachycardia in the immediate postoperative period should always raise the suspicion of unrecognized leak.
  - **Management:** When anastomotic leak or intra-abdominal sepsis is suspected, a CT scan of the abdomen and pelvis with oral and IV contrast is performed. The anastomotic leak can be further characterized with a Gastrografin swallow study if cross-sectional imaging does not visualize the source. Most leaks can be managed by making the patient nil-per-os (NPO), starting parenteral nutrition, and performing percutaneous drainage of any intra-abdominal collection to create a controlled fistula. Weekly Gastrografin swallow studies can document when the leak is healed. Rarely is surgical intervention required. Reoperating beyond 5 to 7 days postoperatively is fraught with complications and is generally a futile exercise. If surgical intervention is pursued, small leaks can be closed primarily and buttressed with an omental patch. Larger leaks may require a revision of the anastomosis with wide drainage and placement of a jejunostomy tube for enteral feeding access.
- **Duodenal stump blowout**
  - **Presentation:** Duodenal stump blowout is a dreaded complication of gastrectomy and is fortunately uncommon. It can present in various ways, from localized abscess to intra-abdominal sepsis. Overzealous dissection of the duodenum leading to its devascularization, chronic scarring of the duodenum complicating its closure, and obstruction of the biliopancreatic limb are potential etiologies.
  - **Management:** A CT scan will demonstrate an abscess or free air in the right upper quadrant and will not contain oral contrast. Cross-sectional imaging will rule out afferent/efferent limb obstruction, which can be an underlying etiology. A percutaneous drain to generate a controlled fistula is the initial step in management. A contrast study through the drain will confirm connection with duodenum. Management is largely through supportive measures including NPO, parenteral or enteral nutrition, and replacement of fluid losses. A percutaneous transhepatic duodenal diversion can assist with closure of the leak by diverting the bile and pancreatic effluent away from the fistula.[22] Operative management might be required if the fistula does not close. If the duodenal blowout presents as an acute abdomen, then exploratory laparotomy, placement of a tube duodenostomy, and wide drainage of right upper quadrant is performed.
- **Delayed gastric emptying**
  - **Presentation:** Disruption of normal vagally mediated mechanisms of gastric function with surgical resection leads to delayed gastric emptying. Delayed gastric emptying presents as nausea, vomiting, bloating, hiccups, and continued high NG tube output in the presence of antegrade bowel function. The diagnosis is clinical and can be confirmed by slow emptying of the stomach on a contrast study or nuclear medicine gastric emptying study.
  - **Management:** Treatment is largely supportive and includes gastric decompression with NT tube and trial of promotility agents such as metoclopramide (up to 10 mg three times per day) and/or erythromycin (up to 250 mg four times per day). Chronic, unremittent delayed gastric emptying is a challenging problem to manage. In rare circumstances, if symptoms are severe and persistent, the intervention of choice is completion total gastrectomy with esophagojejunostomy.

Delayed Complications
- **Alkaline (bile) reflux gastritis**
  - **Presentation:** Contact of gastric mucosa with biliary contents causes alkaline reflux gastritis and presents as epigastric pain unrelieved by antacids, nausea, and bilious emesis. The diagnosis is clinical and one of exclusion. It is more common with Billroth I or II reconstructions and less common with Roux-en-Y reconstruction. Anastomotic ulceration, afferent and efferent loop syndrome, and disease of the gallbladder or pancreas must be ruled out. Endoscopy demonstrates hyperemic gastric mucosa with

biliary staining, which supports the diagnosis. Bile reflux can be further documented using a hepatobiliary iminodiacetic acid (HIDA) scan.
- **Management:** Alkaline reflux gastritis does not respond well to medical therapy. However, a trial of medical therapy with cholestyramine, sucralfate, or antacids is still warranted. Surgical treatment involves diverting duodenal contents away from the stomach by converting a Billroth II to a Roux-en-Y gastrojejunostomy with a 45-cm to 60-cm Roux limb. An alternative approach is the performance of a Braun enteroenterostomy (ie, a side-to-side jejunojejunostomy diverting effluent of the afferent limb past the stomach).

- **Afferent and efferent loop syndrome**
  - **Presentation:** Afferent or efferent loop syndrome occurs due to obstruction of the afferent or the efferent loop when a Billroth II reconstruction has been used to restore GI continuity. This can present as an acute problem if the obstruction is complete or as a chronic problem due to partial obstruction. The potential causes are numerous and include internal herniation, volvulus, or kinking at the anastomosis. Acute afferent limb obstruction is the most common cause of duodenal stump blowout and is a surgical emergency. Patients present with severe epigastric and right upper quadrant pain associated with nausea and vomiting. Physical examination may reveal an intra-abdominal mass, and CT scan of the abdomen reveals the diagnosis. When the afferent limb is partially blocked, then it presents as chronic afferent loop syndrome where patients complain of postprandial abdominal pain with nausea and projectile vomiting, which typically does not contain food and relieves the pain. Diagnosis is clinical and is complemented with endoscopy and upper GI fluoroscopy studies. Obstruction of the efferent loop is less common and presents as abdominal pain, nausea, and bilious vomiting with food particles in it. The diagnosis can be confirmed by Gastrografin study, which shows a holdup in the passage of contrast into the efferent limb. Potential causes include retroanastomotic hernia, adhesions, and stricture.
  - **Management:** Acute afferent loop syndrome is an emergency and requires immediate operative exploration. If the duodenum and afferent limb are viable, then addressing the etiology may include shortening the redundant afferent limb, reducing internal herniation, closing the mesenteric defects, or revision of the gastrojejunal anastomosis. In the case of chronic afferent loop syndrome, conversion of a Billroth II gastrojejunostomy to a Roux-en-Y anastomosis addresses the problem. Surgery is usually required for efferent loop obstruction and involves correction of the underlying source of obstruction.

- **Nutritional consequences:** Gastrectomy is associated with specific mineral and vitamin deficiencies as described below.
  - **Iron deficiency:** Iron deficiency is the most common cause of anemia after gastrectomy. Iron malabsorption, decreased intake, and increased losses from friable mucosa are reasons for iron deficiency. The duodenum and proximal jejunum are also responsible for the majority of iron absorption from the GI tract, thus reconstruction bypasses the major physiologic sites of iron uptake. Daily supplementation of 150 to 300 mg/d in divided doses should be provided.
  - **Vitamin B_{12} deficiency:** Reduction in production of intrinsic factor and decrease in stomach acidity (decreasing absorption of vitamin B_{12}) underlie vitamin B_{12} deficiency. Daily supplementation of 100 μg of oral vitamin B_{12} or a monthly 1 mg intramuscular vitamin B_{12} injection is recommended following subtotal gastrectomy.
  - **Other mineral and vitamin supplementation:** Decreased oral intake and decreased absorption due to decreased gastric acid secretion can contribute to folate deficiency, thus supplementation of folate is also recommended. Supplementation of vitamin D and calcium is also recommended after gastric surgery.

REFERENCES

1. Zhou J, Hiki N, Mine S, et al. Role of prealbumin as a powerful and Simple index for predicting postoperative complications after gastric cancer surgery. *Ann Surg Oncol.* 2017;24(2):510-517. doi:10.1245/s10434-016-5548-x
2. Hennessey DB, Burke JP, Ni-Dhonochu T, et al. Preoperative hypoalbuminemia is an independent risk factor for the development of surgical site infection following gastrointestinal surgery: a multi-institutional study. *Ann Surg.* 2010;252(2):325-329. doi:10.1097/SLA.0b013e3181e9819a
3. Fujiya K, Kawamura T, Omae K, et al. Impact of malnutrition after gastrectomy for gastric cancer on long-term survival. *Ann Surg Oncol.* 2018;25(4):974-983. doi:10.1245/s10434-018-6342-8
4. Martin L, Jia C, Rouvelas I, et al. Risk factors for malnutrition after oesophageal and cardia cancer surgery. *Br J Surg.* 2008;95(11):1362-1368. doi:10.1002/bjs.6374
5. Minnella EM, Awasthi R, Loiselle SE, et al. Effect of exercise and nutrition prehabilitation on functional capacity in esophagogastric cancer surgery: a randomized clinical trial. *JAMA Surg.* 2018;153(12):1081-1089. doi:10.1001/jamasurg.2018.1645
6. Draganov PV, Wang AY, Othman MO, et al. AGA institute clinical practice update: endoscopic submucosal dissection in the United States. *Clin Gastroenterol Hepatol Off Clin Pract J Am Gastroenterol Assoc.* 2019;17(1):16-25.e1. doi:10.1016/j.cgh.2018.07.041
7. Pimentel-Nunes P, Dinis-Ribeiro M, Ponchon T, et al. Endoscopic submucosal dissection: European society of gastrointestinal endoscopy (ESGE) guideline. *Endoscopy.* 2015;47(9):829-854. doi:10.1055/s-0034-1392882
8. Mocellin S, Pasquali S. Diagnostic accuracy of endoscopic ultrasonography (EUS) for the preoperative locoregional staging of primary gastric cancer. *Cochrane Database Syst Rev.* 2015;2015(2):CD009944. doi:10.1002/14651858.CD009944.pub2
9. Burke EC, Karpeh MS, Conlon KC, et al. Laparoscopy in the management of gastric adenocarcinoma. *Ann Surg.* 1997;225(3):262-267. doi:10.1097/00000658-199703000-00004
10. Lowy AM, Mansfield PF, Leach SD, et al. Laparoscopic staging for gastric cancer. *Surgery.* 1996;119(6):611-614. doi:10.1016/s0039-6060(96)80184-x
11. de Graaf GW, Ayantunde AA, Parsons SL, et al. The role of staging laparoscopy in oesophagogastric cancers. *Eur J Surg Oncol.* 2007;33(8):988-992. doi:10.1016/j.ejso.2007.01.007
12. Allen CJ, Newhook TE, Vreeland TJ, et al. Yield of peritoneal cytology in staging patients with gastric and gastroesophageal cancer. *J Surg Oncol.* 2019;120(8):1350-1357. doi:10.1002/jso.25729
13. Jongerius EJ, Boerma D, Seldenrijk KA, et al. Role of omentectomy as part of radical surgery for gastric cancer. *Br J Surg.* 2016;103(11):1497-1503. doi:10.1002/bjs.10149
14. Ri M, Nunobe S, Honda M, et al. Gastrectomy with or without omentectomy for cT3-4 gastric cancer: a multicentre cohort study. *Br J Surg.* 2020;107(12):1640-1647. doi:10.1002/bjs.11702
15. Ajani JA, D'Amico TA, Bentrem DJ. National comprehensive cancer network. Gastric Cancer (Version 3.2020)https://www.nccn.org/professionals/physician_gls/pdf/gastric.pdf. 2020. Accessed March 5, 2021.

16. In H, Solsky I, Palis B, et al. Validation of the 8th edition of the AJCC TNM staging system for gastric cancer using the national cancer database. *Ann Surg Oncol.* 2017;24(12):3683-3691. doi:10.1245/s10434-017-6078-x
17. Cunningham D, Allum WH, Stenning SP, et al. Perioperative chemotherapy versus surgery alone for resectable gastroesophageal cancer. *N Engl J Med.* 2006;355(1):11-20. doi:10.1056/NEJMoa055531
18. Al-Batran SE, Homann N, Pauligk C, et al. Perioperative chemotherapy with fluorouracil plus leucovorin, oxaliplatin, and docetaxel versus fluorouracil or capecitabine plus cisplatin and epirubicin for locally advanced, resectable gastric or gastrooesophageal junction adenocarcinoma (FLOT4): a randomized phase 2/3 trial. *Lancet.* 2019;393(10184):1948-1957. doi:10.1016/S0140-6736(18)32557-1
19. Thiels CA, Hanson KT, Habermann EB, et al. Integrated cancer networks improve compliance with national guidelines and outcomes for resectable gastric cancer. *Cancer.* 2020;126(6):1283-1294. doi:10.1002/cncr.32660
20. Karanicolas PJ, Graham D, Gönen M, et al. Quality of life after gastrectomy for adenocarcinoma: a prospective cohort study. *Ann Surg.* 2013;257(6):1039-1046. doi:10.1097/SLA.0b013e31828c4a19
21. Hu Y, Vos EL, Baser RE, et al. Longitudinal analysis of quality-of-life recovery after gastrectomy for cancer. *Ann Surg Oncol.* 2021;28(1):48-56. doi:10.1245/s10434-020-09274-z
22. Zarzour JG, Christein JD, Drelichman ER, et al. Percutaneous transhepatic duodenal diversion for the management of duodenal fistulae. *J Gastrointest Surg.* 2008;12(6):1103-1109. doi:10.1007/s11605-007-0456-9

Chapter 38 Minimally Invasive Total Gastrectomy

Elliot Newman and Marcovalerio Melis

DEFINITION

- The indications for minimally invasive total gastrectomy (MITG) do not differ from the indications for open gastrectomy and include both benign and malignant diseases.
- Gastric malignancies (adenocarcinomas, neuroendocrine tumors, gastrointestinal stromal tumors [GISTs], and other submucosal neoplasms) account for the single largest indication for gastric resection and will be the focus of this chapter.
- MITG performed for malignancies should follow the same standard oncologic principles generally followed during open resections.
- For adenocarcinomas, gastric resection should be extended proximally for 5 to 6 cm from the gross tumor margins. If adequate proximal margin cannot be achieved by a partial gastrectomy, a total gastrectomy is indicated. Randomized trials have shown that total gastrectomy offers no oncologic value over a distal gastrectomy, as long as a negative margin can be obtained.[1,2] Appropriate extent of lymphadenectomy for gastric adenocarcinoma in the western population is a topic of great debate, and beyond the scope of the present chapter. In our practice, we usually perform a D2 lymph node dissection. A meta-analysis has shown that MITG for gastric adenocarcinoma is safe and associated with reduced overall morbidity.[3] Comparative studies with long-term follow-up are still lacking, but available evidence suggests that oncologic outcomes are comparable after either MITG or open distal gastrectomy.
- For GISTs, gastric resection follows different oncologic principles. A lymph node dissection is not required, and surgery is considered curative as long as the resection margins are negative. Therefore, more limited resections (eg, wedge resections) are appropriate for GIST. Partial gastrectomies may still be required for large tumors or when the pylorus is involved.
- Occasionally, GISTs located near the gastroesophageal junction may also require a total gastrectomy to achieve negative resection margins.
- While decreasing in frequency, complications of peptic ulcer disease (bleeding, gastric outlet obstruction, failure of medical treatment) are still significant indications for distal gastrectomy. The same technique described in this chapter may be used for benign pathologies, omitting the lymphadenectomy.

IMAGING AND OTHER DIAGNOSTIC STUDIES

- Following the diagnosis of gastric adenocarcinoma, accurate clinical staging is necessary.
- CT scan of the chest abdomen and pelvis will evaluate for metastatic disease.
- Positron emission tomography/CT is recommended if no metastatic disease is detected by the CT.
- Endoscopic ultrasound will evaluate depth of tumor invasion and possible lymph node metastases.
- Diagnostic laparoscopy should be considered for locally advanced tumors (eg, T3 or N+) to rule out subradiographic peritoneal dissemination and obtain peritoneal washing for cytologic examination.
- Endoscopic dissection with negative margins can be considered as adequate therapy for Tis or T1a tumors (invasion of the lamina propria or muscularis mucosae) if the tumor is well or moderately differentiated with diameter ≤2 cm, in absence of ulceration and lymphovascular invasion (strongest risk factor for presence of lymph node metastases).
- Perioperative chemotherapy should be considered for any gastric adenocarcinoma stage T2N0M0 or greater, as recommended by National Comprehensive Cancer Network guidelines.

SURGICAL MANAGEMENT

Preoperative Planning

- The choice of minimally invasive vs open techniques should be at the discretion of the surgeon.
- Regardless of the technique, the primary goals of the operation are the same: resection of the cancer with negative margins, lymphadenectomy for staging, and restoration of intestinal continuity.
- The patient should be medically optimized for surgery. Special attention needs to be given to malnourished patients.
- Preoperative nutritional panels are mandatory and occasionally the placement of a preoperative feeding jejunostomy is warranted. Consider preoperative tube feedings in patients with significant weight loss or other evidence of malnutrition, especially if candidates for neoadjuvant treatment.
- Insist on smoking cessation to reduce postoperative pulmonary and wound complications.
- Consider a preoperative liquid protein diet to improve steatohepatitis in obese patients.
- Perioperative antibiotic should be given within 30 minutes prior to the initial skin incision.

Chapter 38 MINIMALLY INVASIVE TOTAL GASTRECTOMY

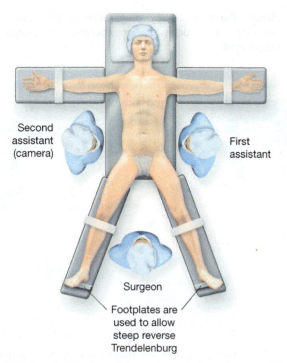

FIGURE 1 • Positioning of the patient on the operative table for laparoscopic-assisted total gastrectomy.

- Deep vein thrombosis prophylaxis with calf length pneumatic compression devices and subcutaneous heparin should be instituted prior to induction of anesthesia.
- General anesthesia may be supplemented with epidural analgesia and/or injection of local anesthetics in the transversus abdominis plane block.
- The bladder is decompressed with a Foley catheter.
- An orogastric or a nasogastric tube is inserted.
- Use an operating room table that may accommodate very steep reverse Trendelenburg position.
- For either robotic or laparoscopic-assisted gastrectomy, the preferred position is supine split leg with footplate attachments to prevent patient migration. The footplates should be snugly placed with the toes pointing slightly outward. Pad pressure points along arms and legs and secure the knees in the locked position. Use pillow cases or folded sheets and 2-in silk tape to keep the knees from buckling (**FIGURE 1**).
- Upper extremities can be secured on arm rests, or tucked to the patient's sides, as per surgeon's preference.
- Prior to prepping and draping, check the positioning by manipulating the bed in all of the positions that will be used during the operation.

ACCESS AND PORT PLACEMENT FOR LAPAROSCOPIC-ASSISTED TOTAL GASTRECTOMY

- Place a 10-mm trocar at the umbilicus with the usual Hassan technique. In obese patients or with an unusually low umbilicus, or for tumors located in the proximal stomach, the camera port may need to be more cephalad, often 2 or 3 finger-breadth above the umbilicus and left to the midline. The umbilical trocar is generally used for the camera.
- Establish a 15-mm Hg pneumoperitoneum and perform a diagnostic laparoscopy to rule out peritoneal or hepatic metastases. If metastatic lesions are suspected, they should be biopsied and sent for frozen section prior to committing to gastrectomy. If ascites is present, washings should be performed.
- Place the patient in steep reverse Trendelenburg position and insert the trocars under direct visualization and in a direction that minimize torque. Our typical port setup is shown in **FIGURE 2**.

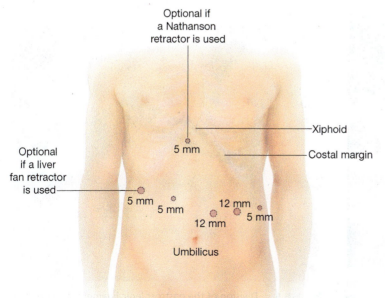

FIGURE 2 • Port placement for laparoscopic total gastrectomy. Depending on surgeon's preference for liver retraction, a 5-mm port can be placed either at the epigastrium for a Nathanson retractor or in the lateral right upper quadrant for a snake retractor.

- Retract the liver with a subxiphoid Nathanson retractor. Stiff or floppy livers are best lifted up with a snake retractor from the patient's right side.
- Identify the neoplasm by visualization or by instrument palpation. If unsuccessful, intraoperative endoscopy is encouraged.

ACCESS AND PORT PLACEMENT FOR ROBOTIC-ASSISTED TOTAL GASTRECTOMY

- The four robotic ports are placed, equally spaced, along a transverse line at the level of the umbilicus or slightly above, with port 1 just to the right of the mid-clavicular line, and port 4 in correspondence of the left colon gutter. These are all 8-mm ports, except for port 2, which is a 12-mm port to allow use of the robotic stapler (FIGURE 3).
- A laparoscopic 5-mm port placed as lateral as possible under the right rib cage is used for a liver retractor.
- A laparoscopic 12-mm assistant port is placed caudally to the robotic ports 2 and 3.
- We typically use port 3 for the camera.

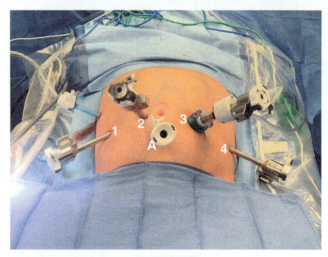

FIGURE 3 • Port placement for robotic-assisted total gastrectomy. The robotic port 3 is cannulated through a 12-mm laparoscopic port that we used to access the peritoneal cavity.

DISSECTION OF THE GREATER CURVE

- Retract the transverse colon and the greater omentum caudally.
- Access the lesser sac by entering the gastrocolic ligament in an avascular area.
- Extend the dissection of the gastrocolic ligament distally toward the pylorus and cephalad toward the spleen. We typically use a vessel sealing device for this part.
- Continue the dissection of the gastrocolic ligament along the upper third of the greater curvature staying lateral to the gastroepiploic arcade. Then divide the gastrosplenic ligament including the short gastric vessels. This portion of the dissection is greatly facilitated by retracting the stomach toward the patient's feet and rolling the greater curvature anteriorly toward the abdominal wall in order to expose the back wall of the stomach (FIGURE 4).
- By performing the dissection of the greater curvature lateral to the gastroepiploic arcade, the lymph nodes along the gastroepiploic vessels (stations 4d and 4sb) are included in the specimen.
- In order to expose the lesser cavity in its entirety, divide the avascular posterior gastropancreatic adhesions that are almost

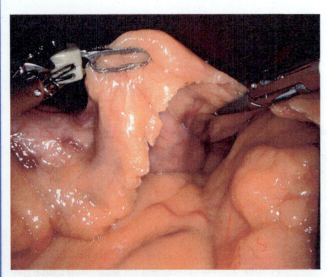

FIGURE 4 • After division of the gastrocolic ligament, dissection is *continued* using the vessel-sealing device across the gastrosplenic ligament including the short gastric vessels.

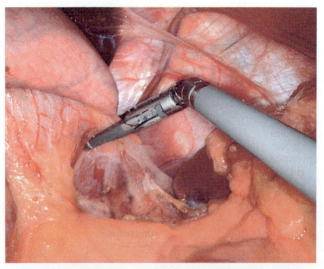

FIGURE 5 • Division of the gastrosplenic ligament is completed, exposing the left crus.

always present between the posterior wall of the stomach and the anterior surface of the pancreas. Division of those adhesions will also facilitate anterior retraction of the stomach.
- Next, continue the dissection more cranially along the greater gastric curvature, until all of the short gastric vessels are divided and the fundus is completely mobilized. At this time, the left crus and the hiatus with the distal esophagus should be visualized (**FIGURE 5**). Elevating the underside of the stomach toward the abdominal wall and to the patient's right will facilitate exposure of the hiatus.
- Using the hook (preferred for robotic assisted) or the ultrasonic dissector (preferred for laparoscopic assisted), divide the lateral portion of the phrenoesophageal ligament and expose the fibers of the left crus.

ANTRAL DISSECTION

- Firm anterior retraction of the stomach aids in the duodenal dissection. While retracting the antrum toward the abdominal wall, separate the posterior wall of the duodenum off the anterior surface of the pancreatic head. The gastroduodenal artery marks the limit of this pancreaticoduodenal dissection.
- Identify the origin of the right gastroepiploic artery. This is usually a direct continuation of the gastroduodenal artery caudally emanating from the inferior edge of the pancreas. Use the lower border of the pancreas as a guide for where to divide the right gastroepiploic artery (**FIGURE 6**).
- Sweep the lymphatic tissue around the right gastroepiploic vessels (infrapyloric nodes, station 6) toward the specimen. Now divide the right gastroepiploic vessels between clips or using a vascular load stapler. If clips have been used in proximity of the vessels, take great care to ensure they are not included in the stapler line.
- Retract the duodenum caudally. Incise the peritoneum over the hepatoduodenal ligament. Visualize the right gastric artery at its takeoff from the common hepatic. Sweep the lymphatic tissue around the right gastric artery toward the specimen. This maneuver clears the suprapyloric lymph nodes (station 5). Once the right gastric artery is dissect free, doubly clip and divide it. The first portion of the duodenum is then cleared of any residual filmy adhesions. Alternatively, identification and division of the right gastric artery can be completed after transection of the duodenum.

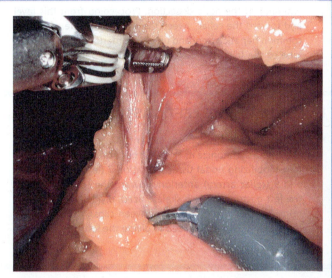

FIGURE 6 • With the antrum retracted anteriorly toward the abdominal wall, the right gastroepiploic vessels are identified and dissected at the inferior edge of the pancreas.

DIVISION OF THE DUODENUM

- Remove nasogastric tubes and even esophageal temperature probes from the patient's mouth to prevent inadvertent inclusion in the jaws of the stapler.
- Make sure adequate length of duodenum is mobilized to easily allow placement of a linear stapler across the first portion of the duodenum, just distal to the pylorus.
- A linear stapler is placed close to the level of the duodenal dissection to avoid the pyloric ring and minimize duodenal ischemia (**FIGURE 7**). We use a blue load for the robotic stapler and a purple load for the laparoscopic stapler. Before firing, make sure once again that any esophageal/gastric tube has been removed and that the portal structures are excluded from your stapler line.
- Make every attempt to divide the duodenum in one firing. The duodenum should easily fit in the jaws of a 60-mm linear stapler. If the operating surgeon encounters difficulties in encompassing the duodenum win a single 60-mm stapler, one should verify the stapler is positioned distal to the pylorus. Carefully inspect for integrity the duodenal staple line. We routinely oversew the duodenal staple line with a running 2-0 barbed suture.

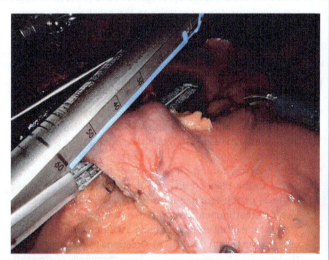

FIGURE 7 • The duodenum is divided using a robotic Endo GIA stapler.

DISSECTION OF THE HEPATODUODENAL LIGAMENT

- Retract the stomach anteriorly to expose the upper edge of the pancreas. Incise the peritoneum overlying the common hepatic artery.
- The hepatic artery node, which usually lies at the take-off of the gastro-duodenal artery, is a good landmark for the lateral limit of the node dissection. Proceeding from this level and toward the celiac, sweep the lymphoid tissue off of the common hepatic artery and up to the inferior edge of the left lobe of the liver. This way, lymph nodes along the common hepatic (station 8), proper hepatic (station 12), and splenic (station 11) arteries are removed en bloc with the specimen.
- Be mindful of IVC and portal vein, which can be injured if dissection is carried on posterior to the hepatic artery. Our preference is to use the hook to clear those vessels by the lymph node–bearing tissue. The assistant may facilitate this dissection by retracting caudally the upper edge of the pancreas using a "cigar" or a laparoscopic Q-tip.
- During the dissection of those lymph node stations, the coronary vein and the left gastric artery are usually encountered. Divide the coronary vein in between clips or using a vessel sealing device.

DIVISION OF THE LEFT GASTRIC ARTERY

- Once the celiac anatomy is evident, dissect the left gastric artery and skeletonize its takeoff from the celiac trunk, therefore mobilizing nodal tissue of station 7 (left gastric artery) and 9 (celiac artery) anteriorly toward the specimen. Once the left gastric pedicle is skeletonized, divide it at its origin, using a vessel sealing device between clips. Alternatively, a vascular stapler may be used to divide the left gastric artery.
- We do not routinely include the peritoneum covering the anterior surface of the pancreas in our dissection.
- We do not routinely perform a splenectomy or a distal pancreatectomy, since in the western literature, potential benefits of a complete dissection of the lymph nodes in station 11 is outweighed by a significant increase in postoperative morbidity (specifically pancreatic leaks) without measurable effect in long-term survival.

DISSECTION OF THE INTRA-ABDOMINAL ESOPHAGUS

- Division of the left gastric artery will increase exposure to the hiatus.
- Have the assistant retract the stomach down and to the patient's left. This will improve exposure of the right crus.
- Free the gastroesophageal junction from the hiatus by dissecting up the right crus.
- Divide the phrenoesophageal ligament and proceed through the connective tissue posterior to the esophagus to extend the dissection toward the left crus.
- Divide the right and left vagus nerves when identified.
- The gastroesophageal junction is now dissected circumferentially. Guide a 2-cm wide Penrose drain around the esophagus. Secure the two ends of the Penrose together with either a linear stapler or an Endoloop, leaving little space between the drain and the esophageal wall.
- The assistant may now use the Penrose drain to retract the esophagus caudally and increase exposure of the hiatal region. Complete the dissection of the lower esophagus using a combination of blunt dissection and vessel sealer device.

PROXIMAL DIVISION

- With the assistant pulling on the Penrose to retract the stomach caudally, complete (if necessary) the mobilization of the intra-abdominal esophagus using the hook and/or the vessel-sealing device.
- Place two stay sutures on each side of the esophagus, proximally to the planned division. Those sutures will facilitate retrieval of the esophagus, as it will likely retract into the lower mediastinum after transection of the distal esophagus.
- Transect the distal esophagus using a 3.5-mm linear stapler of appropriate length (FIGURE 8). Occasionally, you may need a thicker load if the esophagus has been chronically obstructed.
- The stump of the excised portion of esophagus may be submitted for frozen section examination to assure a microscopically negative margin.
- Place the specimen in an Endo Bag and keep it away from the working area. We typically place the specimen above the liver.
- Obtain hemostasis.

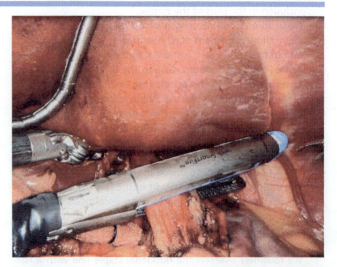

FIGURE 8 • The distal esophagus is divided using a robotic Endo GIA stapler.

RECONSTRUCTION WITH STAPLED ESOPHAGOJEJUNOSTOMY

- Our choice for the reconstruction is a Roux-en-Y esophagojejunostomy in a retrocolic fashion.

Side-to-Side Esophagojejunostomy

- Identify the ligament of Treitz by lifting in cranial direction the mesentery of the transverse colon. Create a window in an avascular portion of the transverse colon mesentery (usually to the patient left of the middle colic artery) through which you then deliver the proximal jejunum to the upper abdomen. Select an appropriate site on the antimesenteric side of the jejunum for the esophagojejunostomy. Make sure it can easily reach the esophageal stump without tension.
- Divide the jejunum with linear stapler just proximal to the site selected for the anastomosis. Divide the corresponding mesentery with the vessel sealer.
- Make a small enterotomy in the mid portion of the esophageal staple line.
- Make a small enterotomy about 7 to 8 cm distal to the stapled line of the Roux limb. Insert the thick jaw of a GIA stapler in the enterotomy and use it to align the Roux limb under the esophagus. Insert the thin jaw of the GIA in the esophagus. Exposure of the distal esophagus is facilitated by gentle tension on the stay sutures previously placed.
- We use a 60-mm stapler to achieve a 30- to 40-mm anastomosis and do not necessarily introduce the entire device into the bowel. Alternatively, you can use a 45-mm stapling device.
- Create a side-to-side esophagojejunostomy by firing the Endo GIA (FIGURE 9). Make sure that nasogastric tubes and/or temperature probes are removed prior to engaging the stapler.
- Close the common enterotomy with a running 2-0 barbed suture in a single layer. Perform an air leak test by asking the anesthesiologist to insufflate air through a nasogastric or orogastric tube.

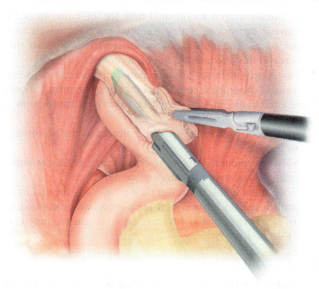

FIGURE 9 • One jaw of linear stapler is introduced in the jejunal limb and used to align the jejunum to the posterior side of the esophagus. The second jaw is then inserted into the esophagus, and the stapler is fired to create the anastomosis.

Side-to-Side Jejunojejunostomy

- The jejunojejunostomy is typically created 40 to 50 cm distal to the esophagojejunostomy.
- Use stay sutures to secure in a side-to-side fashion the stapled end of the biliopancreatic limb to the alimentary limb of the jejunum, just caudal to the transverse colon and avoiding any tension.
- Make a small enterotomy in the antimesenteric side of each limb.
- Insert the jaws of a 3.5-mm GIA stapler in the enterotomies. Make sure that no mesentery or other loops of bowel are caught in the stapler prior to firing.
- Once the stapler is fired, the staple line is inspected for bleeding.
- Close the remaining anastomotic defect using a 2-0 barbed suture in a running fashion.

CLOSING

- Complete a final inspection of all staple lines and vascular pedicles for hemostasis and well-formed staples. Bleeding points and areas of malformed staples should be oversewn with absorbable suture.
- Closed suction drainage is optional.
- Abdominal fascia is closed for all port sites larger than 5 mm.

POSTOPERATIVE CARE

- We usually keep a nasojejunal tube for 24 hours in order to avoid distension of the proximal jejunum, which may compromise the integrity of the anastomosis. Whether this decreases the leak rate has not been proven.
- Immediately after surgery, the patient is instructed to use incentive spirometry, cough, and take deep breaths. Patients are encouraged to stay out of bed and ambulate within 6 hours from surgery.
- Prophylactic antibiotics are not indicated in the postoperative period.
- Unless an epidural catheter is used for analgesia, the Foley catheter is removed in postoperative day 1.
- If the patient is able to protect their airway and the abdomen is not distended, clear liquids are allowed on postoperative day 1, and then diet is advanced to a postgastrectomy diet as tolerated.

OUTCOMES

- Minimally invasive total gastrectomy is a safe and effective treatment of gastric cancer.
- Available evidence shows no major differences in morbidity, mortality, number of nodes harvested, or disease-free survival.
- The addition of a D2 dissection elevates this operation to a higher difficulty level.
- Oncologic principles and safety are paramount and should not be sacrificed for a less invasive approach.

COMPLICATIONS

- The postoperative complications observed after minimally invasive total gastrectomy generally are comparable with those of an open procedure.
- *Intraoperative*
  - Bleeding
  - Splenic injury
  - Iatrogenic enterotomy
- *Early postoperative*
  - Esophagojejunal leak
  - Duodenal leak
  - Bleeding
- *Late postoperative*
  - Dumping
  - Afferent limb syndrome
  - Malnutrition
  - Anastomotic stricture

REFERENCES

1. Bozzetti F, Marubini E, Bonfanti G, Miceli R, Piano C, Gennari L. Subtotal versus total gastrectomy for gastric cancer: five year survival rates in a multicenter randomized Italian trial. *Ann Surg*. 1999;230:170-178.
2. Gouzi JL, Huguier M, Fagniez PL, et al. Total versus subtotal gastrectomy for adenocarcinoma of the gastric antrum: a French prospective controlled study. *Ann Surg*. 1989;209:162-166.
3. Zorcolo L, Rosman AS, Pisano M, et al. A meta-analysis of prospective randomized trials comparing minimally-invasive and open distal gastrectomy for cancer. *J Surg Oncol*. 2011;104:544-551.

Chapter 39 Robotic/Minimally Invasive Distal Gastrectomy

Sharona B. Ross, Harel Jacoby, Cameron Syblis, Iswanto Sucandy, and Alexander S. Rosemurgy

DEFINITION

- Distal gastrectomy is indicated for both malignant and benign conditions. Gastric malignancies comprise a majority of the indications, which include adenocarcinoma (most common), gastrointestinal stromal tumor (GIST), neuroendocrine tumor, and lymphoma (rarely). Benign conditions constitute a minority of the indications for surgery and include benign tumors, complications of peptic ulcer disease, and trauma. This chapter focuses on distal gastrectomy for adenocarcinoma.
- Distal gastrectomy is an optimal surgical procedure for middle or lower-third gastric cancer in early and locally advanced stages. Compared with total gastrectomy, it offers better short-term and long-term outcomes.[1]
- The robotic system offers several advantages compared with the "open" and traditional laparoscopic approaches including better view by magnified and stable three-dimensional visualization, improved articulation with seven degrees of freedom, more precise vascular dissection, easy ambidextrous suturing, and better surgeon ergonomics.[2] Its application in gastric surgery has been increasing steadily and may soon become the preferred approach for most gastric operations.[3-6]
- Robotic/minimally invasive distal gastrectomy (RDG) should follow the same oncological principles as the open approach. Perioperative chemotherapy is indicated for any gastric adenocarcinoma staged cT2N0M0 or greater.
- D2 lymphadenectomy is the standard of care for resectable gastric cancer according to the National Comprehensive Cancer Network (NCCN) guidelines, with a goal of harvesting at least 16 or greater lymph nodes. For GIST, lymph node dissection is not required.[7]

IMAGING AND OTHER DIAGNOSTIC STUDIES

- Patients should complete accurate clinical staging following upper endoscopy with biopsy confirming malignancy.
- Chest/abdomen/pelvis computed tomography (CT) with oral and intravenous (IV) contrast.
- 18 F-fluorodeoxyglucose-positron emission tomography (FDG-PET)/CT evaluation to rule out metastatic disease and if clinically indicated.
- Endoscopic ultrasound if early-stage disease is suspected or if early vs locally advanced disease needs to be determined.
- Diagnostic laparoscopy should be considered in selected operations.

SURGICAL MANAGEMENT

Preoperative Planning

- All patients should undergo a comprehensive preoperative assessment regarding their functional status and medical condition.
- Patients should complete cardiac clearance and additional consults, as needed.
- All patients complete blood workup including complete blood count (CBC), comprehensive metabolic panel (CMP), and coagulation function.
- Patients undergo preoperative counseling for Enhanced Recovery After Surgery (ERAS) protocol to achieve early recovery and improved outcomes.
- Special attention needs to be given to malnourished patients. Patients may need to be consulted with a nutritionist and may need total parenteral nutrition if stenting is not an option. Feeding jejunostomy is not recommended due to the potential risk of cancer implants at the J-tube site.
- Provide counseling on smoking cessation to reduce postoperative pulmonary and wound complications.
- IV antibiotics should be given within 30 minutes prior to the initial skin incision.
- Deep vein thrombosis prophylaxis with calf length pneumatic compression devices should be instituted prior to induction of anesthesia.
- The bladder is decompressed with a Foley catheter.
- A nasogastric tube is inserted.

Positioning

- The patient lies supine in a reverse Trendelenburg position. Legs are attached to the table with a belt on the pelvis.
- The left arm is secured by Kerlix gauze wrapped around the armboard. The right arm is extended. Arm extension gives the anesthesiologist(s) access to the arm and does not encumber the robot docking. This is particularly true with the Da Vinci Xi platform (Intuitive Surgical Inc, Sunnyvale, CA).
- The robot is docked from the right side of the patient. The scrub tech stands on the left and the first assistant on the right side of the patient (**FIGURE 1**).
- We use integrated table motion that enables dynamical positioning of the patient while the surgeon operates.

SECTION VIII SURGERY OF THE STOMACH AND DUODENUM

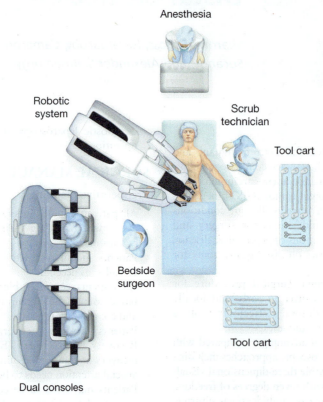

FIGURE 1 Operating room setup.

STEP 1: ACCESS AND PORT PLACEMENT

- We begin the operation with a small incision at the umbilicus. This incision is just large enough to accommodate an 8-mm robotic trocar. Once pneumoperitoneum is established diagnostic laparoscopy is undertaken and then the additional trocars are placed under videoscopic visualization.
- To best maintain pneumoperitoneum, it is our routine to utilize the AirSeal insufflation system (Conmed Corporation, Utica, NY).
- We place an 8-mm trocar at the level of the umbilicus just to the right of the right midclavicular line. A 12-mm trocar, to accommodate the 45 mm EndoWrist Stapler (Intuitive Surgical Inc, Sunnyvale, CA), is placed at the level of the umbilicus in the left midclavicular line. An 8-mm trocar is placed along the left anterior axillary line just cephalad to the umbilicus. A 5-mm trocar to accommodate the AirSeal Access Port (Conmed Corporation, Utica, NY) is placed along the right anterior axillary line at or near the right costal margin for the liver retractor (**FIGURE 2**).
- An additional 2- to 3-cm incision is made, between and slightly caudal to the umbilical port and the right midclavicular line port, for an Applied GelPoint (Applied Medical, Rancho Santa Margarita, CA) (**FIGURE 3**).
- The bed is placed in 10° to 20° (depending on BMI) reverse Trendelenburg and 5° tilted to the left.

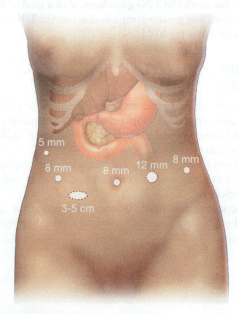

FIGURE 2 Port placement.

Chapter 39 ROBOTIC/MINIMALLY INVASIVE DISTAL GASTRECTOMY   335

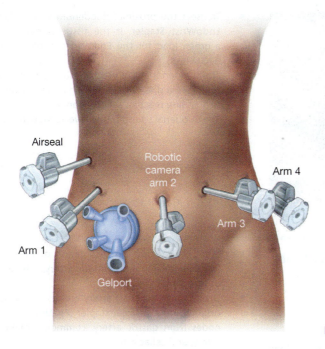

FIGURE 3 • Port placement.

STEP 2: GASTRIC MOBILIZATION ALONG THE GREATER AND LESSER CURVATURE
(▶ VIDEO 1)

- Arms setup:
  - Arm 1: Fenestrated bipolar or bowel grasper
  - Arm 2: Camera
  - Arm 3: Monopolar scissors, hook cautery, or vessel sealer
  - Arm 4: Bowel grasper
  - Bedside assistant: Laparoscopic bowel grasper, suctioning device
- Begin the operation by dissecting, ligating, and dividing the right gastroepiploic artery and vein, found caudal to the pylorus, and the right gastric artery, found just along the cephalad edge of the duodenum along the common hepatic artery.
- Next, with the beside surgeon retracting the stomach in the cephalad direction and the transverse colon in the caudal direction by arm 4, the gastrocolic omentum is divided.
- This dissection is done dorsal to the gastroepiploic vessels, in order to include all perigastric lymph nodes with the specimen. Omentectomy is also included.

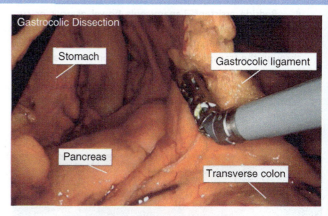

FIGURE 4 • Gastrocolic dissection.

- The lesser sac is then entered, and the dissection is carried along the greater curvature up to the spleen where the left gastroepiploic vessels are divided using the vessel sealer (FIGURE 4).
- Preserve the proximal short gastric vessels to enable adequate perfusion to the remnant stomach, for distal gastrectomy.
- Complete the mobilization of the posterior wall of the stomach with the division of gastropancreatic attachments.

STEP 3: DUODENAL DISSECTION AND TRANSECTION (▶ VIDEO 2)

- Arms setup:
  - Arm 1: Fenestrated bipolar bowel grasper
  - Arm 2: Camera
  - Arm 3: Monopolar scissors, vessel sealer, or blue load robotic stapler
  - Arm 4: Bowel grasper
  - Bedside assistant: Laparoscopic Bowel Grasper, Suctioning Device
- While the stomach is retracted further toward the abdominal wall using arm #4 (robotic bowel grasper), continue dissection along the greater curvature toward the distal stomach and the proximal duodenum.
- Complete the dissection of the superior and inferior border of the duodenum. The supra- and subpyloric nodes are taken with the gastric resection in-continuity.

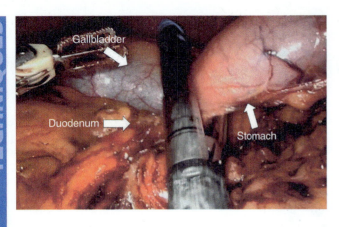

- Transect the proximal duodenum with a 45-mm blue load EndoWrist Stapler. If the tissue is significantly thickened a green load for the EndoWrist Stapler should be utilized (**FIGURE 5**).
- The duodenal margin should have a frozen section analysis to ensure a disease-free margin and to ensure that the transection line is across the duodenum.
- The duodenal stump is then oversewn with the V-lock suture.

FIGURE 5 • Gastric transection.

STEP 4: PROXIMAL GASTRIC TRANSECTION AND D2 LYMPHADENECTOMY

- Arms setup:
  - Arm 1: Fenestrated bipolar
  - Arm 2: Camera
  - Arm 3: Monopolar scissors, vessel sealer, or green load robotic stapler
  - Arm 4: Bowel grasper
  - Bedside assistant: Laparoscopic bowel grasper or suctioning device
- Open the gastrohepatic ligament and dissect the mesentery through the transparent gastrohepatic omentum along the lesser curvature of the stomach utilizing the vessel sealer. The mesentery is divided to commensurate with a proposed gastric division near the incisura or wherever the cancer dictates.

- Identify the common trifurcation of the celiac artery that includes the common hepatic artery, splenic artery, and left gastric artery.
- Divide the left gastric artery and its lymph node basin at its origin using a vascular stapler (**FIGURE 6**, ▶ **Video 3**). Take nodes from gastric artery, common hepatic artery, splenic artery, and celiac artery.
- Complete modified D2 lymphadenectomy along the common hepatic artery, celiac trunk, and proximal splenic artery.
- If it is necessary to sacrifice an accessory left hepatic artery, do so without hesitation to promote the oncologic quality of the operation.
- Transect the mesentery near the incisura and prepare for transection of the proximal stomach.
- Transect the stomach with a green load EndoWrist stapler. Prior to the transection, it is very important to communicate with the anesthesiologist to pull the nasogastric tube back into the esophagus (▶ **Video 4**, **FIGURE 7**).

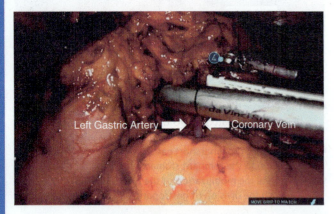

FIGURE 6 • Ligation of left gastric artery and coronary vein.

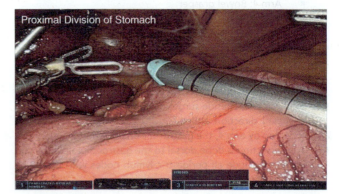

FIGURE 7 • Proximal division of stomach.

STEP 5. SPECIMEN REMOVAL

- Extract the resected gastric specimen along with the regional lymph nodes through the Applied GelPoint utilizing a laparoscopic specimen retrieval bag.
- Label both proximal and distal margins for frozen section analysis to exclude microscopic involvement and document duodenum with distal margin.

STEP 6. GASTROJEJUNAL ANASTOMOSIS
(▶ VIDEO 5)

- Arm Setup:
  - Arm 1: Needle Driver
  - Arm 2: Camera
  - Arm 3: Needle Driver
  - Arm 4: Bowel Grasper
  - Bedside assistant: Laparoscopic Bowel Grasper or Suctioning Device
- Given a gastric remnant of acceptable size, a Billroth II reconstruction is preferred to reestablish gastrointestinal tract continuity. However, if after resection the gastric reservoir is small, a Roux-en-Y gastrojejunostomy should be constructed.
- The transverse colon is elevated in the cephalad direction, and the proximal jejunum is identified distal to the ligamentum of Treitz. An experienced bedside assistant can greatly facilitate this step.
- At approximately 30 to 40 cm distal to the ligamentum of Treitz, the proximal jejunum is brought up to the gastric pouch in an antecolic fashion.
- It is our preference to perform a side-to-side gastrojejunostomy anastomosis using the robotic blue load stapler. First, fix the jejunum to the stomach using a V-Loc suture. Next, make an enterotomy to the antimesenteric part of the jejunum and on the posterior wall of the stomach. Then, use two 45-mm blue load staplers to perform a side-to-side anastomosis (FIGURE 8).
- Suture the common enterotomy using two 6-in 3-0 V-Loc sutures. Start at the 3-o'clock position outside-in on the jejunum and inside-out on the stomach. When reaching halfway with the first suture take a second V-Loc suture and start at the 9-o'clock position. Suturing should begin outside-in on the stomach and inside-out on the jejunum. The sutures should be across from each other when they are tied (FIGURE 9).
- Alternatively, the anastomosis can be undertaken in a single-layer end-to-side hand-sewn fashion.

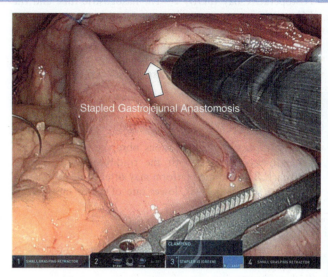

FIGURE 8 • Stapled gastrojejunal anastomosis.

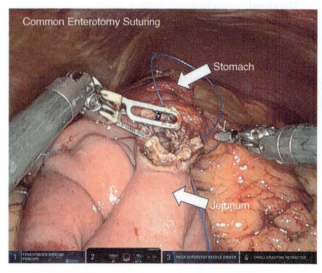

FIGURE 9 • Common enterotomy suturing.

STEP 7: CLOSING

- Final inspection of the operative field is completed to confirm that the anastomosis looks viable, nontwisted, and tension-free.
- Irrigate the operative field with local anesthesia.
- Abdominal port incisions are closed along fascial layers with Maxon sutures, and the skin is approximated with Vicryl sutures and Steri-Strips.

POSTOPERATIVE CARE

- Immediately after their operation the patient is instructed to frequently use the incentive spirometer, cough, and take deep breaths.
- Patients are encouraged to ambulate within 6 hours from their operation.
- Physical therapy is ordered twice a day.
- Pain is controlled with IV ketorolac and Tylenol, oral Celecoxib, and oral gabapentin.
- Prophylactic antibiotics are not indicated in the postoperative period.
- CBC and CMP are taken daily.

- Postoperative day (POD) 1—The nasogastric tube and the Foley catheter are removed.
- Clear liquid diet is started a few hours after the nasogastric tube is removed if patient is not nauseous.
- POD 2—Diet is advanced to full liquid diet.
- POD ¾—The patient is discharged with a follow-up at the clinic in 1 to 2 weeks.

COMPLICATIONS

- The postoperative complications observed after RDG are generally comparable with the traditional laparoscopic approach. The robotic platform may offer some advantages including less blood loss, lower rate of major morbidities, and faster recovery.[3-5]
- Intraoperative:
  - Bleeding
  - Splenic injury
  - Iatrogenic enterotomy
- Early postoperative:
  - Gastrojejunal anastomotic leak
  - Duodenal stump leak
  - Bleeding
  - Delayed gastric emptying
- Late postoperative:
  - Dumping
  - Afferent limb syndrome
  - Marginal ulcer
  - Bile reflux gastritis
  - Malnutrition

OUTCOMES

- Utilization of the robotic system does not change the nature of gastric operations, only the approach and the morbidity associated with it.
- To appropriately utilize the robotic platform the surgeon must undergo a learning curve starting with minor procedures and gradually reach the more challenging procedures as gastrectomy with D2 lymphadenectomy.
- The robotic platform facilitates and, in our opinion, reduces morbidity of gastric surgery.

REFERENCES

1. Li Z, Bai B, Xie F, et al. Distal versus total gastrectomy for middle and lower-third gastric cancer: a systematic review and meta-analysis. *Int J Surg*. 2018;53:163-170.
2. Giulianotti PC, Coratti A, Angelini M, et al. Robotics in general Surgery: personal experience in a large community hospital. *Arch Surg*. 2003;138:777-784.
3. Rosemurgy A, Ross S, Bourdeau T, Sucandy I. Robotic gastrectomy. In: Novitsky Y, Ballecer C, Belyansky I, eds. *Atlas of Robotic General Surgery*. Elsevier; 2021.
4. Park JM, Kim HI, Han SU, et al. Who may benefit from robotic gastrectomy?: a subgroup analysis of multicenter prospective comparative study data on robotic versus laparoscopic gastrectomy. *Eur J Surg Oncol*. 2016;42:1944-1949.
5. Guerrini GP, Esposito G, Magistri P, et al. Robotic versus laparoscopic gastrectomy for gastric cancer: the largest meta-analysis. *Int J Surg*. 2020;82:210-228.
6. Lu J, Zheng CH, Xu BB, et al. Assessment of robotic versus laparoscopic distal gastrectomy for gastric cancer: a randomized controlled trial. *Ann Surg*. 2021;273:858-867.
7. National Comprehensive Cancer Network. *Gastric Cancer (Version 4.2021)*. 2021. Accessed December 2021. https://www.nccn.org/professionals/physician_gls/pdf/gastric.pdf

Chapter 40 Proximal Gastrectomy

Sushanth Reddy and Martin J. Heslin

DEFINITION
- Proximal gastrectomy is defined as a procedure to remove the upper third to one-half of the stomach and the distal portion of the esophagus. This is a procedure to remove cancers or premalignant lesions in the gastroesophageal (GE) junction or the distal esophagus. Proximal gastrectomy is usually used in conjunction with systemic chemotherapy and/or external beam radiation for malignant lesions in this area.

PATIENT HISTORY AND PHYSICAL FINDINGS
- Patients typically present with difficulty swallowing, dysphagia, upper gastrointestinal (GI) bleeding, or reflux symptoms, especially in the setting of unexplained weight loss. Initial diagnostic evaluation typically includes an esophagogastroduodenoscopy with biopsy showing malignancy.
- A thorough history and physical examination should be performed prior to surgery. Particular attention should be paid to cardiac and pulmonary comorbidities and nutritional status. Risk factors for cancer including acid reflux disease, history of Barrett esophagus, and tobacco use should be identified.
- Patients who have disease in the proximal to midesophagus should not undergo proximal gastrectomy.[1] These patients should be considered for either an Ivor Lewis (Chapter 16) or transhiatal esophagectomy (Chapter 15). Patients with cancers in the proximal stomach should be evaluated for a total gastrectomy (Chapter 41).
- All patients with cancer should undergo staging prior to consideration for surgery.
- Patients with high-grade dysplasia or T1 tumors without lymph node metastases should be considered for endoscopic management before consideration of surgery. Patients with advanced tumors (T2 or greater) or those with lymph node involvement should be considered for either upfront (neoadjuvant) chemotherapy alone or in conjunction with radiation therapy.[2,3] Those patients who are nutritionally depleted should have a feeding jejunostomy tube placed prior to initiating therapy.[4]
- Following completion of chemotherapy and radiation therapy, patients should be restaged. The presence of distant metastases is a contraindication for surgery.
- The period of upfront therapy allows for optimization of cardiac and pulmonary comorbidities prior to surgery.

IMAGING AND OTHER DIAGNOSTIC STUDIES
- All patients should undergo staging evaluation prior to surgery. Endoscopic ultrasound is used to identify tumor depth (T stage) and regional lymph node metastases (N stage). Computed tomography (CT) scan or positron emission tomography scan is used to identify distant metastases. The liver is the most common site of distant metastases for adenocarcinoma and squamous cell carcinoma (the two most common tumor histologies).
- Staging should be repeated after the completion of upfront chemotherapy or chemoradiation therapy prior to surgery.
- The celiac axis anatomy should be carefully studied prior to surgery to look for anomalies. Specific attention should be paid toward an accessory or replaced left hepatic artery within the gastrohepatic ligament.

SURGICAL MANAGEMENT

Preoperative Planning
- Many patients with gastric or esophageal malignancy have comorbid conditions related to age or tobacco use. These patients should undergo optimization of their comorbidities prior to surgery.
- Anesthesia should consider placement of an arterial monitoring catheter and/or a central venous catheter. During hiatal dissection, the heart may be compressed and invasive monitoring can be useful in guiding resuscitation in the operating room.
- A nasogastric (NG) tube will be placed during the operation. It may not be possible to pass an NG tube prior to removal of the tumor (if it is obstructing). The surgeon should have good communication with anesthesia in regard to NG tube position as it will be manipulated through the operation.

Positioning
- The patient is positioned with both arms at 90° with the torso. This will facilitate with exposure by spreading the lower ribs laterally. Alternatively the right arm can be tucked to the patient's side to aid in attachment of the self-retaining retractor device to the operating room table. If a feeding jejunostomy tube has already been placed, the tube should be prepped into the sterile field.

DIAGNOSTIC LAPAROSCOPY

- The abdomen is entered through the supraumbilical midline and a laparoscope placed (Chapter 39). The entire abdomen should be evaluated with specific attention to the liver and the peritoneal surfaces for the presence of metastatic disease. Any suspicious lesions should be biopsied and sent for frozen section analysis in the pathology. The presence of metastatic disease is a contraindication for surgical resection.

MOBILIZATION OF THE STOMACH

- A formal laparotomy is performed and a self-retaining retractor is placed. Excision of the xiphoid process may be used to aid with retraction (this allows for wider retraction of the costal margin).
- The lesser sac is entered along the avascular plane that separates the gastrocolic omentum from the transverse mesocolon. The dissection should proceed away from the greater curve of the stomach to avoid injury to the right gastroepiploic artery. The right gastroepiploic artery will be the primary blood supply of the residual stomach (FIGURE 1). The right gastric artery can be spared to keep the gastric conduit well vascularized. Mobilization of the stomach is usually sufficient for resection and reconstruction for a proximal gastrectomy without the need for ligation of the right gastric artery and a Kocher maneuver to mobilize the duodenum (needed for transhiatal esophagectomy [see Chapter 15] or Ivor Lewis esophagectomy [see Chapter 16]).
- The left lateral section of the liver is mobilized to expose the lesser curve of the stomach and the esophageal hiatus. The left triangular ligament is incised. This is avascular. The falciform ligament may also be incised to aid with visualization of the left triangular ligament (FIGURE 2). The ligament need not be mobilized to its confluence with the falciform to avoid injury to the left hepatic vein. The gastrohepatic ligament is divided. This structure is typically also avascular, but attention should be paid for any accessory or replaced left hepatic artery (FIGURE 3). This will allow exposure of the esophageal crura.
- The gastrosplenic ligament is divided between clamps and ties. The *vasa brevia* are individually dissected and divided between ties. Alternative strategies for division of this structure would include an advanced energy device or an articulating 45-mm stapler with vascular loads.
- The distal esophagus is circumferentially freed using a combination of sharp and blunt dissection. A Penrose drain is placed around the esophagus to aid with retraction (FIGURE 4). The Penrose drain can be used to retract the esophagus to expose the diaphragmatic hiatus and aid with lower mediastinal dissection. The hiatal attachments of the esophagus are taken down with an advanced energy device. The hiatus should be opened to facilitate dissection of the esophagus. During this dissection, it may be necessary to put pressure on the heart to free the mediastinal attachments of the esophagus. The proximal extent of the tumor and the length of the intra-abdominal esophagus will dictate the amount of mediastinal dissection necessary.

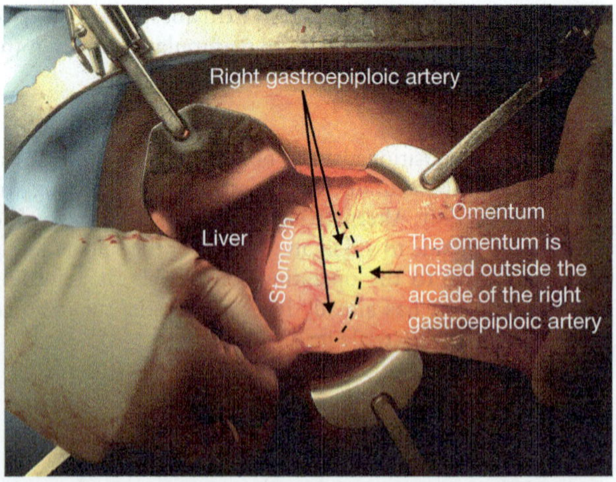

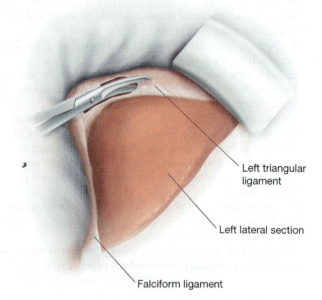

FIGURE 2 • The left lobe of the liver is mobilized. The falciform ligament has already been divided and the left triangular ligament is being incised. Both of these structures are avascular. The falciform ligament should be divided near the liver. As dissection proceeds cephalad, the falciform will divide into the right and left triangular ligaments when dissection is closer to the liver. If dissection is closer to the abdominal wall, division of the falciform will lead into the hepatic venous confluence. Injury to one of these vessels can lead to catastrophic blood loss.

FIGURE 1 • The greater curve of the stomach is mobilized. Care is taken to stay outside the right gastroepiploic artery as this is the vascular pedicle of the gastric conduit. This portion of the gastrocolic omentum is typically avascular, although small blood vessels may be encountered requiring ligation. The vasa brevia should be ligated as dissection proceeds cephalad.

Chapter 40 PROXIMAL GASTRECTOMY 341

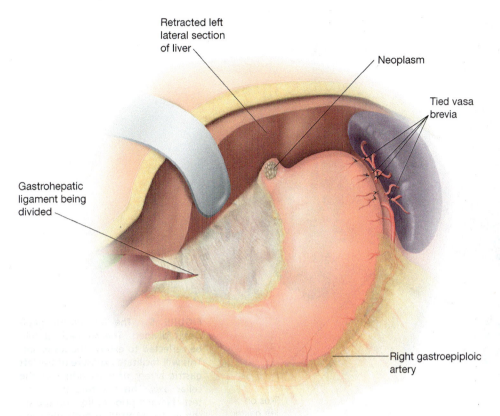

FIGURE 3 • The lesser curve of the stomach is mobilized. By mobilizing the left lobe of the liver, the left lateral section can be retracted to expose the gastrohepatic ligament. This is also typically avascular. Attention should be given in case there is an accessory or replaced left hepatic artery. This can usually be seen on preoperative contrast CT scans. By opening the gastrohepatic ligament, the diaphragmatic crura can be visualized.

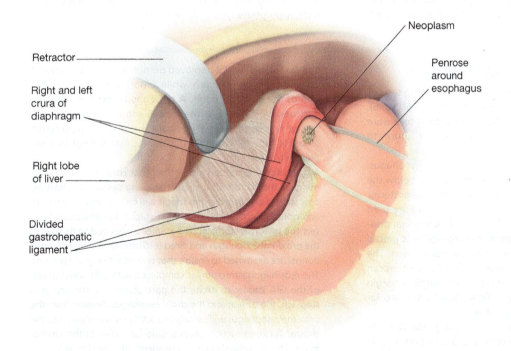

FIGURE 4 • The distal esophagus and gastroesophageal junction are dissected. Once the stomach's greater and lesser curves have been mobilized, this dissection can be performed bluntly. In patients who have undergone preoperative radiation therapy, scarring in this region can make dissection difficult. A Penrose drain is placed around the esophagus. This drain allows the esophagus to be manipulated in all directions to aid with transhiatal dissection. A sufficient length of esophagus should be mobilized into the abdomen so that the proximal esophageal margin is grossly clear from the tumor. A high-energy device can be used to aid with distal esophageal mobilization (minimizing blood loss seen with blunt or cautery dissection).

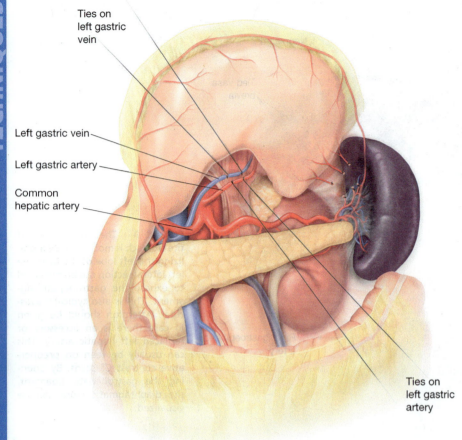

FIGURE 5 • The left gastric pedicle is divided. The stomach should be reflected to expose the lesser sac. This will facilitate exposure of the left gastric artery near its origin at the celiac axis. This structure should be test clamped prior to ligation (pulses should be assessed in both the common hepatic and splenic arteries). Ligation of the left gastric artery near its origin will facilitate with lymphadenectomy (for patients with malignancy).

- With the stomach reflected anteriorly, the left gastric vessels are ligated (FIGURE 5). Prior to ligation, the left gastric artery is test clamped to make sure that flow remains in both the common hepatic artery and the splenic artery. The left gastric artery is ligated at its root off the celiac trunk to facilitate appropriate lymphadenectomy.

GE RESECTION AND RECONSTRUCTION

- Using the NG tube as a guide, place two purse-string sutures in the esophagus proximal to the neoplasm (FIGURE 6). These will be an alternating horizontal mattress to ensure complete donuts after stapling. Do not allow the sutures to go through the NG tube.
- Anesthesia should retract the NG tube into the esophagus. Partially divide the esophagus with electrocautery below the purse-string sutures and above the neoplasm. The posterior wall of the esophagus and the purse-string sutures are used to keep the proximal esophagus in an intra-abdominal position. The anvil of a circular linear stapling device is placed in the esophagus and the purse-string sutures are tied. The division of the esophagus is completed. The GE junction can now be delivered extracorporally. A proximal surgical margin is sent for frozen section analysis. Typically, a 25-mm circular stapler will be sufficient for reconstruction.
- Multiple firings of the gastrointestinal anastomosis (GIA) linear stapler are used to both resect the proximal stomach while tubularizing the remaining stomach for the reconstruction. The first staple load is deployed perpendicular to the greater curvature of the stomach while ensuring adequate perfusion of the gastric conduit. A pulse should be present in the gastroepiploic artery at the chosen site of transection. The stapler is fired sequentially toward the lesser curve, creating a gastric tube (FIGURE 7). The stomach should not be completely transected.
- A gastrotomy is created along the lesser curve to allow placement of the handle of a circular stapling device. This gastrotomy should be positioned so that it will be resected as part with additional firings of the GIA linear stapler to completely transect the proximal stomach. The stapler is attached to its anvil in the proximal esophagus and fired (FIGURE 8). The anastomotic donuts are examined to ensure that two intact rings are present. The esophagogastrectomy is completed with additional firings of the GIA stapler to excise the gastrotomy site, the proximal stomach, the tumor, and the distal esophagus. Tension from the proximal esophagus will usually retract the anastomosis into the thorax. A closed suction drain should be placed at the anastomosis. The NG tube should be advanced into the stomach.

Chapter 40 PROXIMAL GASTRECTOMY 343

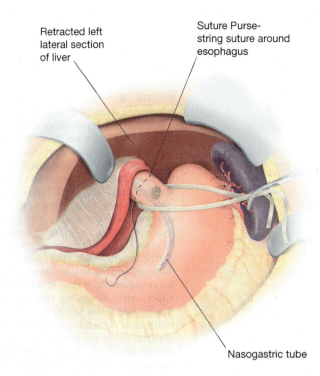

FIGURE 6 • The resection margins are planned. The proximal resection margin can be grossly approximated based on the tumor's location. Two purse-string sutures are placed on the esophagus just above the planned proximal margin. The NG tube can be used as a guide to ensure the sutures are transmural (as the needle meets resistance from the NG tube, it should be rotated away from the tube). The suture should not pass through the NG tube. After the sutures are placed, the NG tube should be retracted into the esophagus above the sutures. The anterior wall of the esophagus is then transected, and the anvil of a 25-mm circular stapler is placed into the esophagus. The sutures are tied to keep the anvil in place. The posterior wall of the esophagus is then divided. The distal esophagus and stomach can now be delivered extracorporally. An esophageal margin should be sent for frozen section to ensure negative resection margins (this can be taken from the distal esophagus above the tumor).

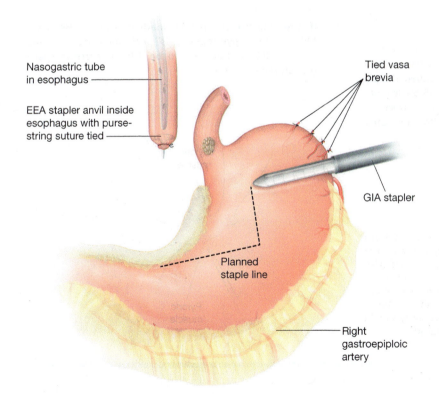

FIGURE 7 • A gastrointestinal anastomosis (GIA) stapler is then used to begin gastric transection. The first staple load should be horizontally across the stomach just below the vasa brevia (to a portion of the stomach with vascular supply from the right gastroepiploic artery). Subsequent staple loads should be fired in a manner to create a gastric tube for the esophagogastrostomy anastomosis. EEA, end-to-end anastomosis.

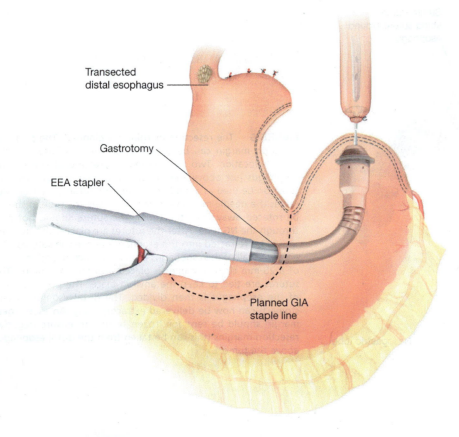

FIGURE 8 • Prior to completing the gastric resection, a gastrotomy is made in the lesser curve in a portion of the stomach that will be transected with the gastrointestinal anastomosis stapler. The handle of the circular stapler is inserted to create an end-to-side esophagogastrostomy. The handle is opened so that it can dock with the anvil in the proximal esophagus. This stapler is fired to create an end-to-side esophagogastric anastomosis. The stapler is removed and the anastomotic donuts are retrieved. Both donuts should be intact. After removing the circular stapler, additional firings of the gastrointestinal anastomosis stapler are used to complete the gastric transection along the lesser curve. The nasogastric tube is then advanced into the gastric conduit and secured at the nose. A closed suction drain is left in proximity of the anastomosis. EEA, end-to-end anastomosis; GIA, gastrointestinal anastomosis.

PYLOROMYECTOMY

- The pylorus is identified by palpation and the presence of the vein of Mayo. Stay sutures are placed at the 12- and 6-o'clock positions. The pylorus muscle is opened sharply and a piece of the muscle is removed with a 15-blade knife to the level of the mucosa without entering the GI tract.
- The pyloromyectomy is closed transversely with interrupted sutures (FIGURE 9).

- If the mucosa is opened inadvertently, a Heineke-Mikulicz–type pyloroplasty is performed instead (see Chapter 30). A drain should be left in Morrison space (hepatorenal recess).[5]

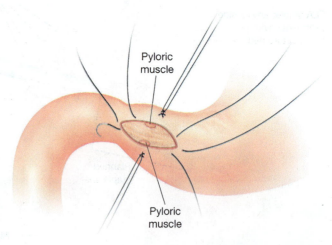

FIGURE 9 • A pyloromyectomy is performed. First, stay sutures are placed at the 6- and 12-o'clock positions (to ligate the vein of Mayo). The serosa and submucosa of the pylorus are incised with a knife. The mucosa should not be entered. In most patients, the pyloric muscle can be visible after sharp transection. The pyloromyectomy should be closed transversely with interrupted sutures. If the mucosa is opened, a Heineke-Mikulicz pyloroplasty should be performed. A closed suction drain should be placed.

FEEDING JEJUNOSTOMY

- If a jejunal feeding tube has not already been placed, one should be created at this time (Chapter 39).[4]

PEARLS AND PITFALLS

Workup	▪ The nutritional status of the patients should be assessed prior to proximal gastrectomy with strong consideration of a feeding jejunostomy tube prior to attempting proximal gastrectomy. ▪ Careful preoperative and intraoperative staging should take place to assure that there is no distant metastatic disease. ▪ Patients with comorbid conditions should undergo optimization of their cardiopulmonary status prior to proximal gastrectomy.
Mobilization	▪ Care should be taken to avoid injury to the right gastroepiploic artery when entering the lesser sac through the gastrocolic omentum. ▪ While mobilizing the lesser curve of the stomach, attention should be paid for a replaced left hepatic artery. ▪ The left gastric artery should be test clamped prior to ligation in case there is a celiac axis anomaly. ▪ A phrenic vein typically courses just anterior to the esophageal hiatus and may need to be ligated to facilitate opening the hiatus and exposure of the distal esophagus.
Postoperative care	▪ The NG tube should not be manipulated or replaced blindly. ▪ Most postoperative leaks can be managed with drainage alone or with endoscopic stenting. ▪ Many patients will have symptoms of reflux requiring prolonged use of proton pump inhibitors.
Nutrition	▪ The feeding jejunostomy tube should be left in place until the patient can demonstrate adequate oral intake to maintain nourishment—especially if the patient will undergo adjuvant therapy. ▪ If the patient does not have a feeding jejunostomy placed prior to operation, there should be one placed in all cases of a proximal gastrectomy because leaks and delayed gastric emptying are two major complications.

POSTOPERATIVE CARE

- Most patients have medical comorbidities related to advanced age and tobacco use. Intensive care unit care with special attention to aspiration precautions should be considered for the immediate postoperative period.
- The NG tube should remain in place until a contrast esophagogastrogram is performed. If the NG tube is inadvertently removed, it should not be blindly replaced.
- On postoperative days 4 to 5, the anastomosis should be studied with a contrast esophagogastrogram. A water-soluble contrast agent should be used initially followed by barium to evaluate for anastomotic leaks. After a successful swallow study, the patient may begin oral nutrition.
- The operative drain should be removed only after the patient starts an oral diet without clinical evidence of an anastomotic leak.
- The feeding jejunostomy tube should be left in place to supplement nutrition until the patient reliably demonstrates adequate oral intake to maintain nourishment.[4]

OUTCOMES

- Reflux esophagitis and anastomotic strictures are present in up to 40% of patients undergoing proximal gastrectomy.[6]
- The overall survival for patients undergoing proximal gastrectomy is similar to other gastric resections and is heavily dependent on tumor stage (5-year survivorship: stage I, 75% to 90%; stage II, 49%; stage III, 13% to 33%; stage IV, 11%).[7]

COMPLICATIONS

- If a leak identified after the swallow study, the patient's clinical condition should direct therapy. Patients who are demonstrating evidence of sepsis should undergo urgent source control and resuscitation. With advances in endoscopy, this can usually be accomplished with a covered stent excluding the area of leak, clips to close the defect, or endoscopic vacuum assisted closure.[8] If surgically placed drains are not sufficient, percutaneous drainage using CT- or ultrasound-guided techniques may be needed.
- Most small leaks in clinically stable patients will resolve with conservative measure (keeping the patient NPO with jejunal enteral nutrition). A contrast esophagogastrogram should be repeated prior to initiating oral nutrition.
- If advanced endoscopic techniques are not available, consider early reoperative intervention. Options can include wide drainage or conversion to an Ivor-Lewis or transhiatal esophagectomy. However, the majority of the time, simply widely draining the region and controlling abdominal sepsis is the primary focus of early reoperative surgery for leaks.

REFERENCES

1. An JY, Youn HG, Choi MG, et al. The difficult choice between total and proximal gastrectomy in proximal gastric cancer. *Am J Surg.* 2008;196(4):587-591.
2. Al-Batran S-E, Homann N, Pauligk C, et al. Perioperative chemotherapy with fluorouracil plus leucovorin, oxaliplatin, and docetaxel versus fluorouracil or capecitabine plus cisplatin and epirubicin for locally advanced, resectable gastric or gastro-oesophageal junction adenocarcinoma (FLOT4): a randomised, phase 2/3 trial. *Lancet.* 2019;393(10184):1948-1957.

3. Macdonald JS, Smalley SR, Benedetti J, et al. Chemoradiotherapy after surgery compared to surgery alone for adenocarcinoma of the stomach or gastroesophageal junction. *N Engl J Med.* 2001;345(10):725-730.
4. Llaguna OH, Kim HJ, Deal AM, et al. Utilization and morbidity associated with placement of a feeding jejunostomy at the time of gastroesophageal resection. *J Gastrointest Surg.* 2011;15(10):1663-1669.
5. Nakane Y, Michiura T, Inoue K, et al. Role of pyloroplasty after proximal gastrectomy for cancer. *Hepatogastroenterology.* 2004;51(60):1867-1871.
6. Wen L, Chen XZ, Wu B, et al. Total vs. proximal gastrectomy for proximal gastric cancer: a systematic review and meta-analysis. *Hepatogastroenterology.* 2012;59(114):633-640.
7. Kim JH, Park SS, Kim J, et al. Surgical outcomes for gastric cancers in the upper third of the stomach. *World J Surg.* 2006;30(10):1870-1876.
8. Raju GS, Tarcin O. Endoscopic management of anastomotic esophageal leaks. *Tech Gastrointest Endosc.* 2006;8(2):66-71.

Chapter 41 Total Gastrectomy for Cancer

Anthony M. Villano, Jennifer F. Tseng, and Waddah B. Al-Refaie

DEFINITION
- Total gastrectomy is removal of the stomach in its entirety including the gastroesophageal (GE) junction. This is typically performed for patients with proximal gastric cancer, including Siewert type II and III GE junction cancers, in whom a subtotal gastrectomy with 4- to 6-cm proximal margin does not leave a reasonable gastric remnant. Even though proximal gastrectomy is widely performed in Asia and select US cancer centers for proximal gastric tumors, proximal gastrectomy has not gained wide adoption in Western centers and thus total gastrectomy is generally employed.

DIFFERENTIAL DIAGNOSIS
- Please see Chapter 37 for an overview of the differential diagnosis for gastric cancer.

PATIENT HISTORY AND PHYSICAL EXAMINATION FINDINGS

Presentation
- The presenting symptoms of gastric cancer are nonspecific and overlap with many common, benign conditions such as gastroesophageal reflux disease (GERD) or peptic ulcer disease. Unfortunately, this often leads to delays in diagnosis and advanced presentation.
- The common presenting symptoms for gastric cancer are previously reviewed in Chapter 37.
- Special attention must be paid to weight loss, as it signifies a potential need for preoperative nutritional optimization. This is even more paramount for total gastrectomy, wherein oral tolerance of food postoperatively may pose significant challenges. Measures to optimize patients prior to surgery are reviewed thoroughly in Chapter 37.
- Severe gastric inlet obstruction, with the inability to tolerate anything by mouth, is an ominous presenting symptom which warrants immediate management.
  - Hydration with intravenous (IV) fluids and correction of electrolyte abnormalities (which can be severe) are the initial steps in management.
  - Gastric inlet obstruction secondary to gastric cancer should be managed among a multidisciplinary team. Assessment of the patient's performance status, the stage and extent of disease present, and the intent of oncologic treatment (curative or palliative) will guide next steps.
  - In the setting of potentially curative treatment, we recommend initial staging with imaging (see "Imaging Studies and Staging Evaluation"). As most patients in this situation would go on to receive neoadjuvant chemotherapy, establishment of enteral feeding access distal to the inlet obstruction is a crucial next step. Most commonly this takes the form of a feeding jejunostomy. These can be placed at the time of initial staging laparoscopy or at the time of admission. Stenting of the gastric inlet or GE junction can be helpful during the preoperative therapy phase. However, for prolonged periods, it is generally not well tolerated and mired by stent migration.

Physical Findings
- The physical examination findings for patients who require a total gastrectomy for cancer are similar to those who require subtotal gastrectomy; please see Chapter 37.

Laboratory Tests
- Please see Chapter 37 for a full review of necessary laboratories prior to gastrectomy.
- Among these, preoperative nutritional markers (albumin/prealbumin) carry even greater significance in total gastrectomy owing to the challenges of maintaining adequate nutrition in the postoperative setting.

Imaging Studies and Staging Evaluation
- The imaging and staging evaluation for gastric cancer is reviewed in Chapter 37. (See also **FIGURES 1-3**.)
- **Esophagogastroduodenoscopy** (EGD) is a particularly important aspect of staging in patients who may require total gastrectomy. Careful communication with the performing endoscopist (if not the primary surgeon) should aim to delineate the proximal extent of cancer.
  - The surgeon should have a clear idea of the proximal extent of mucosal changes prior to proceeding to the operating room, as this will guide the need for total gastrectomy vs potential esophagogastrectomy.

SURGICAL MANAGEMENT
- The most critical oncologic components of total gastrectomy are margin-negative resection along with an adequate lymphadenectomy. All aspects of the operation are conducted with these two basic tenets in mind.
- As important as the conduct of the operation is the multidisciplinary care of gastric cancer patients. We strongly favor neoadjuvant chemotherapy for patients with proximal gastric tumors in all indicated cases that require total gastrectomy and perform staging laparoscopy before initiation of neoadjuvant therapy.
  - Particularly for total gastrectomy, the resultant challenges in nutrition and high risk of postoperative complications make receipt of postoperative therapy difficult to tolerate. Neoadjuvant therapy ensures at least a portion of systemic therapy is delivered.
- We selectively place a feeding jejunostomy during staging laparoscopy, especially in persons who are elderly, frail, have suboptimal performance status, or present with malnutrition.

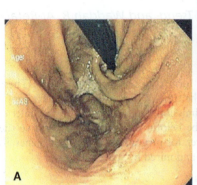 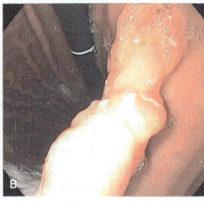 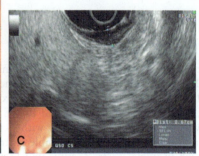

FIGURE 1 • Endoscopy and endoscopic ultrasound (EUS) are critical for the diagnosis and staging of gastric cancer. **A,** Endoscopic findings in a 68-year-old man who presented with iron deficiency anemia and anorexia. An ulcerated adenocarcinoma of the proximal third of the stomach was discovered. **B,** A retroflexed endoscopic view of T2 gastric adenocarcinoma in the gastric fundus. **C,** EUS provides accurate preoperative T staging of the primary tumor.

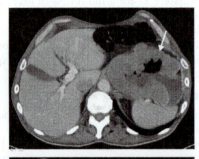
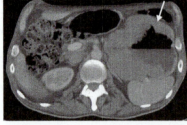

FIGURE 2 • Cross-sectional imaging with computed tomography (CT) or MRI evaluates for **(A)** distant metastatic disease and **(B)** bulky adenopathy. Seen here is an abdominal CT scan of a patient with known high-grade neuroendocrine tumor. No liver metastases were noted. Note diffuse nodular heterogeneous thickening of the stomach (*white arrow*).

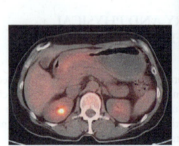 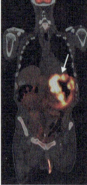

FIGURE 3 • Positron emission tomography (PET) scan may help in the evaluation of distant metastasis. Left image demonstrates mild uptake in the distal stomach. PET scan in a patient with known high-grade neuroendocrine tumor (right image) demonstrates hypermetabolic activity (*white arrow*) in the stomach but no distant organs. This patient required total gastrectomy for complete disease clearance.

Preoperative Planning

- Preoperative nutrition: Patients requiring total gastrectomy are at exceptionally high risk of malnutrition. Preoperative placement of a feeding nasojejunal or jejunostomy tube should be seriously considered, especially throughout neoadjuvant treatment.
- Evaluation of functional status: The history and physical examination as detailed above will identify patients who may not be candidates for curative treatment. Those who are borderline may require aggressive physical therapy in conjunction with nutritional supplementation to "prehabilitate" for surgery. Rarely, admission to the inpatient setting is required to accomplish these goals.
- Restaging after neoadjuvant therapy: Repeat imaging is recommended after completion of neoadjuvant treatment to assess response. Consideration may be given to repeat EGD and/or staging laparoscopy to further assess burden of tumor and finalize operative plans. Subtotal gastrectomy may become feasible after dramatic responses to neoadjuvant treatment.
- Preoperative antibiotics: Second-generation cephalosporins are routinely employed for prophylaxis.
- Deep venous thrombosis prophylaxis: All patients should have a lower extremity sequential compression device applied during the procedure. As gastric cancer patients represent a high-risk population for venous thromboembolism, we routinely administer preoperative subcutaneous heparin and continue heparin/low molecular weight heparin throughout hospitalization unless contraindicated. Also, 30-day postdischarge prophylaxis is offered at some centers.

Positioning

- The patient is placed in supine position with both arms out at 90°. Pressure points are carefully padded. The patient is prepped from the shoulders to the upper thigh to include the left chest in the event left thoracotomy is necessary to complete the operation.

STAGING LAPAROSCOPY

- The peritoneal cavity is entered at the umbilicus either by an open technique or via establishment of pneumoperitoneum with a Veress needle and subsequent port placement. A 30° scope is inserted and one to two additional 5-mm ports on the left or right side of the abdomen are placed for manipulation of tissues, biopsy of suspicious lesions, and aspiration of peritoneal washings.
- A complete survey of the peritoneal cavity for metastatic disease is performed, including the diaphragm, liver, spleen, pelvis, small bowel, large bowel, parietal peritoneum, and omentum. If suspicious disease is observed, it is biopsied and sent for frozen section. In the setting of biopsy-proven peritoneal disease, gastrectomy should not be performed and definitive resection should be aborted to pursue systemic therapies. However, selective palliative surgical procedures may be indicated, for example, in bleeding or obstructing cancers that cannot be palliated by endoscopic measures. These decisions need to be individualized based on the patient's presentation, performance status, extent of metastatic burden, and projected survival given the magnitude of the procedure itself on future quality of life and recovery.
- **Peritoneal cytology**: 200 to 500 mL of normal saline is instilled into the abdominal cavity and allowed to dwell for 5 to 7 minutes. During this time, the patient is gently rocked from left to right to maximize capture of occult cells. After dwelling, the fluid is aspirated with a suction device which has a mechanism to trap the sample.
- **Feeding jejunostomy**: If one is to be placed pretherapy, it is critical to place the enterotomy remote from the expected site of Roux limb formation. Ideally, this enterotomy can be incorporated into a future anastomosis or it can be resected entirely.

EXPLORATORY LAPAROTOMY AND LIVER MOBILIZATION

- In open cases, the abdomen is entered through a midline incision extending from the xiphoid process to just below the umbilicus. A bilateral subcostal incision, approximately 2 cm below the costal margin, also provides excellent exposure. During entry into the abdomen, the falciform ligament should be preserved as it can be used to buttress the duodenal closure.
- A second careful exploration of the peritoneal cavity with careful palpation is performed to confirm the absence of peritoneal or metastatic disease.
- For better access and visualization of the GE junction, we typically mobilize the left liver by dividing the left triangular ligament.

MOBILIZATION OF THE GREATER CURVATURE OF THE STOMACH

- First, the transverse colon is separated from the greater omentum in an avascular plane (**FIGURE 4**). The stomach and the greater omentum are reflected superiorly, and the transverse colon is reflected inferiorly. The plane of fusion between the greater omentum and the transverse mesocolon is identified as a faint white line. This plane is incised with electrocautery to enter the lesser sac. This plane is advanced proximally and distally along the transverse colon until the greater omentum is freed. Formal omentectomy is classically described but is provider-dependent owing to emerging data that metastasis to the omentum is infrequent and omentectomy does not alter local recurrence or overall survival, even in locally advanced cases.[1,2]
- Proceeding from the patient's right to left side, the hepatic flexure of the colon is mobilized by dividing the avascular attachment of the right colon to the retroperitoneum along the white line of Toldt and reflecting it inferomedially. The separation of the greater omentum from the transverse mesocolon is completed to the hepatic flexure if not already performed. Cranial reflection of the stomach and caudal tension on the transverse colon will expose the gastrocolic trunk of Henle. The gastrocolic trunk is classically formed by the confluence of right gastroepiploic vein, the right superior right colonic vein, and the anterior-superior pancreaticoduodenal vein and drains into the superior mesenteric vein (**FIGURE 5**), although anatomic variants do exist. The right gastroepiploic vein is divided at its junction with the gastrocolic trunk, or the gastrocolic trunk can be

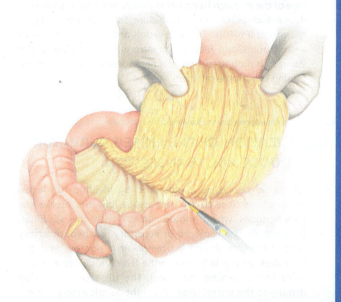

FIGURE 4 • Division of the greater omental attachments to the transverse colon. Transection of the avascular plane between these two structures provides access to the transverse mesocolon and the lesser sac.

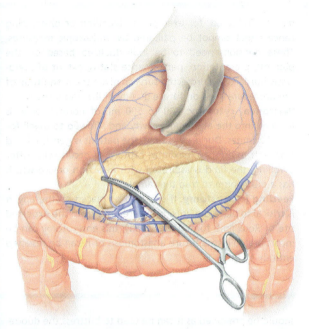

FIGURE 5 • Ligation of the right gastroepiploic vein at its confluence with gastrocolic trunk. Alternatively, the gastrocolic trunk can be divided with the single fire of a vascular stapler.

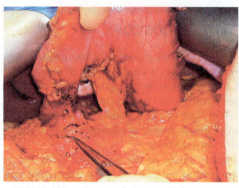

FIGURE 6 • Dissection of the infrapyloric nodal packet at the level of right gastroepiploic vessels.

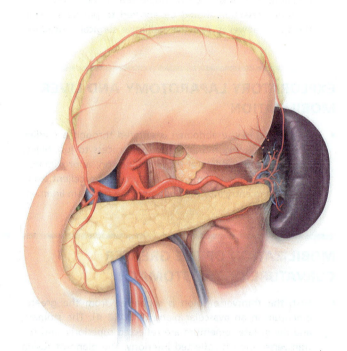

FIGURE 7 • Division of the short gastric arteries. The short gastric arteries are divided between ligatures or using bipolar energy devices. Care is taken to avoid iatrogenic splenic injury.

- divided with a single fire of a vascular stapler. At this stage, the right gastroepiploic artery is divided at its origin from the gastroduodenal artery at the infraduodenal level. We recommend additional time spent when performing this dissection in obese patients given the potential difficulty in identifying this artery. The infrapyloric nodes, located adjacent to the origin of gastroduodenal artery, are mobilized with the specimen (**FIGURE 6**).
- The dissection proceeds proximally along the greater curvature of the stomach using either clamps and ties or an energy device, such as Harmonic or LigaSure, to divide the short gastric vessels (**FIGURE 7**). These vessels are divided carefully to avoid troublesome bleeding or iatrogenic splenic injury. The stomach is mobilized from the phrenoesophageal ligament, freeing it from the left crus.

MOBILIZATION OF THE LESSER CURVATURE AND DUODENAL TRANSECTION

- The lesser curvature is mobilized by dividing the lesser omentum as close to the liver as possible to preserve any lymph nodes which should remain with the specimen (**FIGURE 8**). If a replaced or accessory left hepatic artery is identified, it should be temporarily ligated, and the perfusion of the left lobe of the liver should be assessed prior to transecting the vessel. The dissection is carried distally to the portal triad. The right gastric artery is identified as arising from the common hepatic artery and is divided at its origin to include its associated lymphatic tissue with the specimen. The duodenum is circumferentially dissected about 2 to 3 cm distal to the pylorus, encircled with a Penrose drain, and divided with either a stapler or in between straight bowel clamps (**FIGURE 9**). Care is taken not to injure the bile duct, hepatic artery, or portal vein when encircling the duodenum. The duodenal staple line is oversewn with 3-0 silk Lembert sutures and can be buttressed with the falciform ligament (Moossa patch). However, in the setting of extensive inflammation, consideration should be given to dividing the duodenum between two straight bowel clamps and suture closure of the duodenal stump.
- The gastrectomy specimen, now disconnected distally, is lifted anteriorly. The left gastric artery is identified, suture ligated, and divided at its origin (**FIGURE 10**). The areolar tissue associated with the left gastric artery is mobilized with the specimen.

Chapter 41 TOTAL GASTRECTOMY FOR CANCER   351

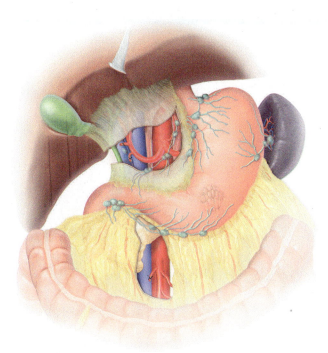

FIGURE 8 • Division of the lesser omentum. The lesser omentum is divided as close to the liver as possible. Presence of a replaced or accessory left hepatic artery arising from the left gastric artery is carefully sought for to prevent injury.

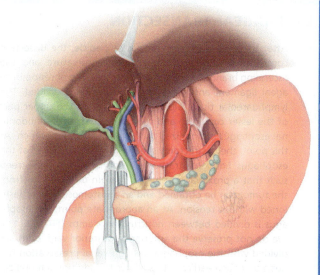

FIGURE 9 • Division of the duodenum. The duodenum is circumferentially dissected, encircled with a Penrose, and divided with a gastrointestinal anastomosis (GIA) stapler using a blue or green load.

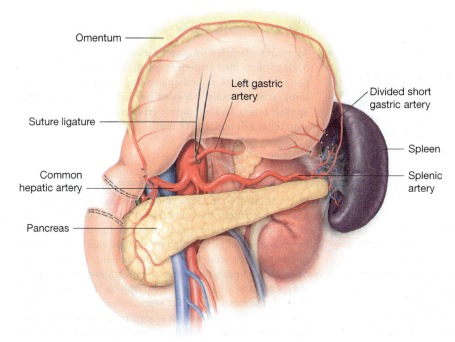

FIGURE 10 • Division of the left gastric artery. The left gastric artery is divided at its origin. The lymphatic tissue surrounding the origin of the left gastric artery is mobilized with the specimen.

ESOPHAGEAL TRANSECTION

- After the division of the left gastric pedicle, the dissection continues proximally along the lesser curvature and the ascending branch of the left gastric artery. The phrenoesophageal ligament anterior to the GE junction is divided. The lymphoareolar tissue along and anterior to the upper part of the lesser curvature and the right aspect of the abdominal esophagus is mobilized to the left with the specimen. At this point, the gastrectomy specimen is only anchored at the esophagus. Enough intrathoracic esophagus should be freed such that a proximal esophageal margin of 4 to 5 cm from the tumor can be obtained and an anastomosis can be fashioned without tension. At an appropriate point, the esophagus is divided between noncrushing clamps (**FIGURE 11**). We do not preserve the anterior or posterior vagi; both are divided with the esophagus, though vagal preservation has been described earlier.[3,4] This allows for additional mobilization of the distal esophagus into the abdomen.

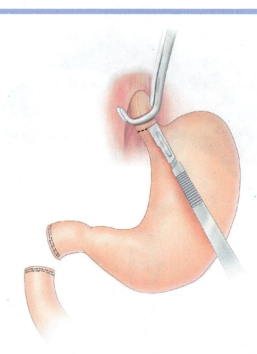

FIGURE 11 • Division of the esophagus. The esophagus is divided at least 5 cm proximal to the most cranial aspect of the gastric tumor.

SPECIMEN PROCESSING

- The operating surgeon is encouraged to deliver the specimen to orient the pathologist with the details of the resection and to perform frozen section assessments of the proximal and distal margins. We typically send the resected specimen in separate containers in the following manner: (1) stomach with a marking stitch on proximal end, (2) greater omentum if included in the resected specimen, (3) infrapyloric nodal packet, and (4) lesser curvature nodal packet with a long stitch on the left gastric artery.
- Once the frozen section of the proximal margin returns negative for malignancy, we proceed with restoration of intestinal continuity. In the meantime, we complete our lymphadenectomy.

LYMPHADENECTOMY

- Current NCCN guidelines state that the gastric resection should include the regional lymphatics. Namely, the perigastric lymph nodes and those along the named vessels of the celiac axis (left gastric artery, common hepatic artery, celiac artery, and splenic artery, ie, a D2 dissection) with the goal of obtaining at least 16 lymph nodes for adequate staging.[5]
- To ensure adequate lymphadenectomy, the gastric arteries need to be divided at their origin. By standard, we typically perform a pancreas- and spleen-preserving lymphadenectomy. That is, taking the right gastric artery, right gastroepiploic artery, and left gastric arteries at their origin along with celiac axis nodal dissection.

RECONSTRUCTION

- After total gastrectomy, intestinal continuity is restored by Roux-en-Y esophagojejunostomy. The length of the Roux limb from the esophagojejunal anastomosis to jejunojejunal anastomosis should be 40 to 60 cm to avoid alkaline reflux esophagitis.
- **Construction of the Roux limb**: A loop of jejunum distal to the ligament of Treitz that will reach the transected esophagus without any tension is identified. Jejunum at this point is divided with a blue gastrointestinal anastomosis (GIA) stapler. The staple line on the end of the Roux limb is oversewn with 3-0 silk stitches in Lambert fashion. The Roux limb needs to be at least 40 cm (ie, from level of esophagojejunostomy to the jejunojejunostomy). A defect is created in the transverse mesocolon to the left of the middle colic vessels (**FIGURE 12**). We then test that the Roux limb can easily reach the esophagus in a retrocolic orientation without tension. Our preference is to first perform the stapled side-to-side anastomosis between the biliopancreatic limb and the jejunum. Our rationale behind this order is to allow for an easier reconstruction of this anastomosis away from the mesenteric defect, which is typically the case once the Roux limb has been passed through the mesocolic defect and esophagojejunostomy has been done. Stay sutures are placed between the biliopancreatic limb and the jejunum and enterotomies for insertion of the limbs of stapler are made. One limb of the blue GIA stapler is introduced into the biliopancreatic limb and the other in the jejunum. The blue load is fired and the common enterotomy is closed either in a handsewn fashion or with a single fire of GIA or thoracoabdominal stapler.

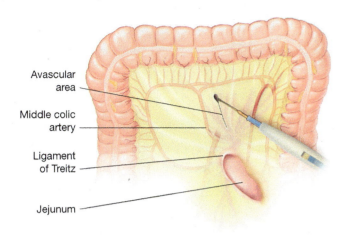

FIGURE 12 • Creation of the defect in the mesocolon. A defect is created in the mesocolon to the left of middle colic vessels. The Roux limb is passed through this defect in a retrocolic fashion.

- Next, the Roux limb is passed through the mesocolic defect to the left of middle colic vessels, and esophagojejunal anastomosis is performed.
- **Creation of the anastomosis**: The esophagojejunal anastomosis can be fashioned either in a handsewn or stapled fashion. Herein we describe both; however, we favor the handsewn anastomosis as it is consistent with our academic mission of training residents in complex intestinal anastomosis techniques. Ultimately, the optimal technique is the one which the operating surgeon is most comfortable as to minimize technical error and complications.
    - Some surgeons choose to fashion a small jejunal pouch as part of the esophagojejunal anastomosis. There are various available techniques, with the most popular being a J-pouch configuration. This is accomplished by creating a small loop of jejunum (10-15 cm) at the most proximal aspect of the alimentary Roux limb. Enterotomies are created in each limb and a common channel is created with a single firing of a GIA stapler.
    - Two meta-analyses of available randomized, controlled trials comparing pouch formation to no pouch formation cite several potential benefits to a pouch, including less frequent dumping syndrome and reflux, improved nutrition markers (albumin, prealbumin) at 2 years, and quality-of-life scores both early (6 months) and late (2 years).[6,7]
    - Given mixed findings in available data, the choice to include a pouch is provider-dependent. The authors do not routinely include a pouch.
- **Handsewn esophagojejunostomy**: Two seromuscular stay sutures, passing through the 3- and 9-o'clock positions on the esophagus and antimesenteric aspect of Roux limb, are placed to keep the esophagus and the Roux limb approximated while the anastomosis is created. We prefer a single-layer end-to-side anastomosis. An enterotomy is made on the antimesenteric border of the Roux limb with electrocautery. The opening in the jejunum is kept smaller than that of the esophagus because the jejunal opening tends to stretch larger. A stay stitch on the anterior lip of the esophagus helps to keep the lumen open, thus facilitating the anastomosis. First, the posterior layer of equally spaced interrupted full-thickness 3-0 silk (or absorbable) sutures is placed (**FIGURE 13A**). Special attention should be given to

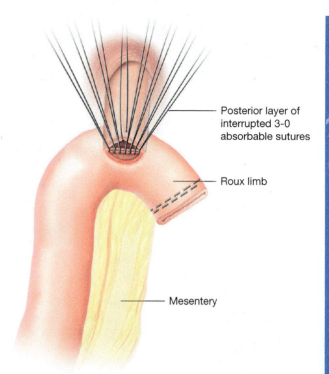

A Handsewn esophagojejunal anastomosis posterior layer

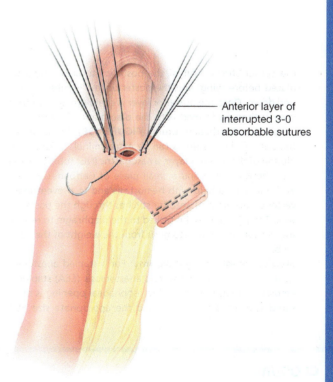

B Handsewn esophagojejunal anastomosis anterior layer

FIGURE 13 • Handsewn esophagojejunal anastomosis. An end-to-side anastomosis is created between the esophagus and the Roux limb. An enterotomy, smaller than that of the opening in the esophagus, is made along the antimesenteric border of the Roux limb. First, the **(A)** posterior layer of interrupted absorbable sutures is placed followed by **(B)** anterior layer of sutures.

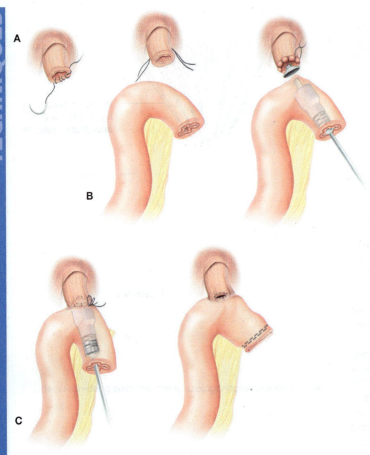

FIGURE 14 • Stapled esophagojejunal anastomosis. **A**, A purse string is placed at the end of esophagus with 2-0 Prolene. **B**, The anvil of the end-to-end anastomosis (EEA) stapler is introduced into the esophagus and the purse string is tied. **C**, The EEA stapler is introduced into the Roux limb through the end of the jejunum and directed toward the antimesenteric border of the Roux limb. The pin of the EEA stapler is now opened with counterclockwise rotation of the knob and brought out through the point on the antimesenteric border of the Roux limb where the anastomosis is planned. This pin is attached to the anvil, the stapler is closed, and subsequently fired. The donuts are checked for completeness and integrity.

the corner stitches. All of the posterior sutures should be placed before tying, and the posterior row is subsequently tied down. Once the posterior layer is complete, the anterior layer is then performed with the placement of interrupted 3-0 silk (or absorbable) sutures (**FIGURE 13B**). The knots on the anterior layer sutures can be extraluminal. Before completion of the anterior layer, a nasogastric (NG) tube is passed into the Roux limb and a small piece of Gelfoam is placed in the lumen to help with hemostasis and to prevent inadvertent placement of anterior stitches through the posterior wall. The jejunum can be tacked to the diaphragm to reduce the tension on the anastomosis from the weight of the Roux limb.

- **Stapled esophagojejunostomy**: For a stapled anastomosis (**FIGURE 14**), an end-to-end anastomosis (EEA) stapler is employed. First, the size of the esophageal opening is measured with calibrated sizers and the appropriate size EEA stapler is chosen. In general, a 25-mm EEA stapler is used for the esophagojejunostomy. A purse string is placed at the end of esophagus with a 2-0 Prolene (**FIGURE 14A**). The anvil of the EEA stapler is now introduced into the esophagus and the purse string is tied (**FIGURE 14B**). Next, the EEA stapler is introduced into the Roux limb preferably through the end of the jejunum or through an opening created in the Roux limb and directed toward the antimesenteric border of the Roux limb (**FIGURE 14C**). The pin of the EEA stapler is now opened with counterclockwise rotation of the knob and brought out through the predetermined site on the antimesenteric border of the Roux limb where the anastomosis is planned. This pin is attached to the anvil, the stapler is closed, and it is fired. The donuts are checked for completeness and integrity. If the stapler was inserted through the blind end of the jejunum, this can be stapled close or handsewn after the anastomosis is created.

CLOSURE

- After the restoration of gastrointestinal continuity, a feeding jejunostomy is placed distal to the jejunojejunal anastomosis. The patient may already have a feeding jejunostomy if one was placed during staging laparoscopy before neoadjuvant therapy.
- Prior to abdominal wall closure, we typically ensure absence of kinks, twists, or tension in the Roux-en-Y reconstruction.

PEARLS AND PITFALLS

Mobilization of the greater curvature	• The short gastric vessels should be carefully divided to avoid troublesome bleeding or iatrogenic splenic injury.
Dissection of the infrapyloric region	• The origin of the right gastroepiploic artery from the gastroduodenal artery should be carefully dissected, especially in the obese patients, due to difficulty in identifying this vessel.
Dissection of the GE junction	• Proximal mobilization of the esophagus should yield at least 2 cm of intra-abdominal length to allow for a tension-free anastomosis.
Construction of esophagojejunal anastomosis	• The esophagojejunal sutures should be full thickness to ensure a robust anastomosis. Special care should be taken for the corner sutures, which are a classic site of anastomotic leak.
Feeding jejunostomy tube	• If the feeding jejunostomy tube is placed during the staging laparoscopy, the surgeon should be cognizant of the need of constructing a Roux limb for the restoration of gastrointestinal continuity at the time of definitive surgery. Thus, the loop of jejunum just distal to the ligament of Treitz, which would be used for fashioning the Roux limb, should not be used for the placement of jejunostomy tube.
Duodenal stump closure	• Meticulous attention should be paid to closure of the duodenal stump, which is classically performed in two layers. The authors favor buttressing with the falciform ligament.

POSTOPERATIVE CARE

- The authors recommend establishing multidisciplinary, standardized postoperative care pathways as these have been shown to improve objective outcomes and unify nursing care.[8]
- Similar to other major abdominal operations, patients who undergo total gastrectomy require close attention to hemodynamics, fluid/electrolyte status, pain management, and pulmonary toilet.
- We increasingly use analgesic blocks (epidural, paravertebral blocks) in the care of these patients with anecdotal success in minimizing opioid requirements.
- The NG tube is typically left to suction and is removed on postoperative day 1. If the NG tube accidently comes out, it should not be replaced due to the concern for anastomotic disruption. If NG tube needs to be replaced (this is rare), it should be done under fluoroscopic guidance.
- If the patient does not demonstrate any signs or symptoms of anastomotic leak by days 5 to 7, then they are initiated on a clear liquid diet and advanced to a postgastrectomy diet as tolerated. Postgastrectomy diet consists of six small meals instead of three large meals. Most patients with time are able to liberalize their food choices as well as portion size.
  - A consultation to nutrition should be placed upon initiation of diet. A proportion of patients will require continued supplemental enteral feeding via their jejunostomy. Providing education to the patient regarding expected lifestyle changes is paramount to optimizing their postoperative recovery.

OUTCOMES

- Oncologic outcomes specific to gastric cancer are similar between distal and total gastrectomy. Please see Chapter 37 for a detailed discussion.
- Quality-of-life outcomes are an underappreciated and significant aspect of postoperative care for gastric cancer patients. Proximal and total gastrectomies are associated with worse patient reported outcomes as compared to distal/subtotal gastrectomy, especially with respect to reflux symptoms and nausea.[9,10]
  - Patients should be counseled appropriately prior to surgery so that expectations are clear. Over half of patients self-report significant impairment in global quality of life immediately following surgery, with most improving to baseline by 6 months postoperatively.[10]

COMPLICATIONS

- Morbidity/mortality rates for total gastrectomy are significant. Realistic counseling with the patient is critical to manage postoperative expectations.
- American College of Surgeon NSQIP data have demonstrated an overall complication rate of 36%, reoperation rate of 10%, and 4.7% 30-day mortality.[11] These national rates are comparable to those at high-volume centers, highlighting the significant physiologic challenges of total gastrectomy irrespective of experience with the operation.[12,13]
- The high complication rate is partially attributable to the baseline comorbid status and poor nutrition of this patient population. Complete removal of the stomach only serves to worsen these conditions and predisposes to further insult. As a result, seemingly small complications often lead to severe physiologic insult or beget additional complications.
  - Age > 70, dependent functional status, preoperative weight loss, and hypoalbuminemia are all independently associated with postoperative complications following total gastrectomy.[11]

Early Complications
- Anastomotic leak

- **Presentation:** Leak rates of 4% to 14.7% have been reported for esophagojejunal anastomosis.[11-13] This complication presents around postoperative days 6 to 14 (mainly between day 5 and 8) and is heralded by unexplained fevers, tachycardia, and systemic inflammatory response.
- **Management:** When suspected, a Gastrografin swallow (followed by use of thin barium if needed) is used to evaluate for a leak. A computed tomography (CT) scan with oral and IV contrast to evaluate for drainable intra-abdominal collections should be obtained. Most leaks can be managed by making the patient NPO, administering broad-spectrum antibiotics, and performing percutaneous drainage of any intra-abdominal collection to create a controlled fistula. Endoscopically placed stents may be considered; however, literature specific to gastric cancer is sparse. Success in the majority of cases, when managed in a multidisciplinary fashion, has been observed post-esophagectomy[14] and bariatric surgery.[15] Subsequent Gastrografin swallow studies will document when the leak is healed. Rarely is surgical intervention required.
- **Postoperative bleeding**
  - **Presentation:** Postoperative bleeding can be intraluminal or intraperitoneal. Intraluminal bleeding presents with fresh blood in the NG tube, melena, downtrending serial hemoglobin, and potentially hemodynamic instability. Bleeding from the anastomosis is the major cause of the intraluminal bleeding and usually occurs around postoperative days 5 to 7. Intraperitoneal bleeding presents with hypotension, tachycardia, downtrending hemoglobin, and abdominal distension. Intraperitoneal bleeding usually presents in the first 12 to 24 hours following surgery. Unrecognized splenic injuries in the form of capsular tears or inadequate control of short gastric vessels are the major causes of postoperative intraperitoneal bleeding following total gastrectomy.
  - **Management:** Intraluminal bleeding can generally be managed by supportive measures (correction of coagulopathy and volume resuscitation). The vast majority originate from the anastomosis and will resolve on their own. Bleeding that causes hemodynamic compromise or does not respond to supportive measures requires careful endoscopic intervention. Reoperation for bleeding not controlled with endoscopy is rare. Intraperitoneal bleeding is more ominous and often requires surgical intervention. Patients with hemodynamic compromise or who do not immediately respond to supportive measures (suggestive of ongoing bleeding) should return promptly to the operating room. Particular attention to the spleen, short gastric vessels, and ligated main branches of the celiac trunk will identify the source in most cases.
- **Duodenal stump blowout**
  - **Presentation:** Duodenal stump blowout is a dreaded complication of gastrectomy and is fortunately uncommon. It can present in various ways, from localized abscess to intra-abdominal sepsis. Overzealous dissection of duodenum leading to its devascularization, chronic scarring of the duodenum complicating its closure, and obstruction of the biliopancreatic limb are potential etiologies.
  - **Management:** A CT scan will demonstrate an abscess or free air in the right upper quadrant and will not contain oral contrast. Cross-sectional imaging will rule out afferent/efferent limb obstruction, which can be an underlying etiology. A percutaneous drain to create a controlled fistula is the initial step in management. A contrast study through the drain will confirm connection with the duodenum. Management is largely through supportive measures including NPO, parenteral or enteral nutrition, and replacement of fluid losses. A percutaneous transhepatic duodenal diversion can assist with closure of the leak by diverting the bile and pancreatic effluent away from the fistula.[16] Though uncommon, operative management might be required if the fistula does not close. If the duodenal blowout presents as an acute abdomen, then exploratory laparotomy, placement of a tube duodenostomy, and wide drainage of right upper quadrant are performed.

Delayed Complications

- **Anastomotic stricture**
  - **Presentation:** Patients may present with structure any time, even many years after the initial operation. Symptoms may be vague, such as dull chest pain after meals or discomfort resembling GERD. Dysphagia indicates severe stenosis.
  - **Management:** The differential diagnosis for anastomotic stricture includes postoperative edema, fibrosis/scarring, and local cancer recurrence. The diagnostic workup starts with contrast study followed by endoscopy with biopsy. Dysphagia secondary to edema will resolve with no interventions. Benign strictures can be managed by endoscopic or fluoroscopic balloon dilation. There is an increasing role of self-expanding metal stent for this condition. If the stricture is due to recurrent cancer, then the patient should be restaged and managed accordingly.
- **Nutritional deficiencies**
  - **Iron deficiency:** Postgastrectomy patients need to be on iron supplementation as the duodenum is the primary site of iron absorption and is bypassed. Also, the loss of gastric acidity impairs the conversion of ferric iron to the more absorbable ferrous form; 150 to 300 mg/d of elemental iron in three divided doses is recommended.
  - **Vitamin B_{12} deficiency:** Patients with total gastrectomy will develop vitamin B_{12} deficiency if not supplemented. Reduction in intrinsic factor and loss of gastric acidity impairs its absorption. Oral vitamin B_{12} (up to 100 μg/d) or monthly intramuscular vitamin B_{12} is recommended.
  - Supplementation of folate, calcium, and vitamin D is also recommended.

REFERENCES

1. Jongerius EJ, Boerma D, Seldenrijk KA, et al. Role of omentectomy as part of radical surgery for gastric cancer. *Br J Surg.* 2016;103(11):1497-1503. doi:10.1002/bjs.10149
2. Ri M, Nunobe S, Honda M, et al. Gastrectomy with or without omentectomy for cT3-4 gastric cancer: a multicentre cohort study. *Br J Surg.* 2020;107(12):1640-1647. doi:10.1002/bjs.11702
3. Tomita R, Fujisaki S, Tanjoh K, et al. Operative technique on nearly total gastrectomy reconstructed by interposition of a jejunal J pouch with preservation of vagal nerve, lower esophageal sphincter, and pyloric sphincter for early gastric cancer. *World J Surg.* 2001;25(12):1524-1531. doi:10.1007/s00268-001-0163-8

4. Tomita R, Tanjoh K, Fujisaki S. Total gastrectomy reconstructed by interposition of a jejunal J pouch with preservation of hepatic vagus branch and lower esophageal sphincter for T2 gastric cancer without lymph node metastasis. *Hepatogastroenterology.* 2004;51(58):1233-1240.
5. Ajani JA, D'Amico TA, Bentrem DJ. *National Comprehensive Cancer Network. Gastric Cancer (Version 3.2020).* 2020. Accessed March 5, 2021. https://www.nccn.org/professionals/physician_gls/pdf/gastric.pdf
6. Gertler R, Rosenberg R, Feith M, et al. Pouch vs. no pouch following total gastrectomy: meta-analysis and systematic review. *Am J Gastroenterol.* 2009;104(11):2838-2851. doi:10.1038/ajg.2009.456
7. Syn NL, Wee AI, Shabbir AA, et al. Pouch versus no pouch following total gastrectomy: meta-analysis of randomized and nonrandomized studies. *Ann Surg.* 2019;269(6):1041-1053. doi:10.1097/SLA.0000000000003082
8. Cassidy MR, Rosenkranz P, McCabe K, et al. I COUGH: reducing postoperative pulmonary complications with a multidisciplinary patient care program. *JAMA Surg.* 2013;148(8):740-745. doi:10.1001/jamasurg.2013.358
9. Hu Y, Vos EL, Baser RE, et al. Longitudinal analysis of quality-of-life recovery after gastrectomy for cancer. *Ann Surg Oncol.* 2021;28(1):48-56. doi:10.1245/s10434-020-09274-z
10. Karanicolas PJ, Graham D, Gönen M, et al. Quality of life after gastrectomy for adenocarcinoma: a prospective cohort study. *Ann Surg.* 2013;257(6):1039-1046. doi:10.1097/SLA.0b013e31828c4a19
11. Bartlett EK, Roses RE, Kelz RR, et al. Morbidity and mortality after total gastrectomy for gastric malignancy using the American College of surgeons national surgical quality improvement program database. *Surgery.* 2014;156(2):298-304. doi:10.1016/j.surg.2014.03.022
12. Selby LV, Vertosick EA, Sjoberg DD, et al. Morbidity after total gastrectomy: analysis of 238 Patients. *J Am Coll Surg.* 2015;220(5):863-871.e2. doi:10.1016/j.jamcollsurg.2015.01.058
13. Li SS, Costantino CL, Mullen JT. Morbidity and mortality of total gastrectomy: a comprehensive analysis of 90-Day outcomes. *J Gastrointest Surg.* 2019;23(7):1340-1348. doi:10.1007/s11605-019-04228-7
14. Liang DH, Hwang E, Meisenbach LM, et al. Clinical outcomes following self-expanding metal stent placement for esophageal salvage. *J Thorac Cardiovasc Surg.* 2017;154(3):1145-1150. doi:10.1016/j.jtcvs.2017.03.051
15. Jaruvongvanich V, Matar R, Storm AC, et al. Endoscopic management of refractory leaks and fistulas after bariatric surgery with long-term follow-up. *Surg Endosc.* 2021;35(6):2715-2723. doi:10.1007/s00464-020-07702-5
16. Zarzour JG, Christein JD, Drelichman ER, Oser RF, Hawn MT. Percutaneous transhepatic duodenal diversion for the management of duodenal fistulae. *J Gastrointest Surg.* 2008;12(6):1103-1109. doi:10.1007/s11605-007-0456-9

Chapter 42: Surgical Management of Injuries to the Cervical Esophagus

James P. Byrne and Patrick M. Reilly

DEFINITION

- Injury to the cervical esophagus is defined as injury to the esophagus in the neck due to blunt or penetrating trauma. Anatomically, the cervical esophagus extends from the cricopharyngeus muscle, which forms the upper esophageal sphincter, to the sternal notch. Esophageal injuries, including those in the neck, are described along a spectrum of organ injury severity (**TABLE 1**).[1] While these injuries are relatively rare, morbidity and mortality are high particularly if diagnosis is delayed. Therefore, early recognition is a cornerstone of effective management.

DIFFERENTIAL DIAGNOSIS

- Trauma to the neck presents a unique challenge due to proximity of several critical structures in a confined anatomic region. These include aerodigestive structures (trachea and esophagus), carotid artery and jugular vein, and the spinal column including spinal cord and vertebral arteries. Multiple concomitant injuries are commonly present and it is often difficult to determine which structures are involved from mechanism or physical examination alone. High degree of suspicion for esophageal injury must be maintained.

PATIENT HISTORY AND PHYSICAL FINDINGS

- Injuries to the cervical esophagus are most commonly caused by penetrating mechanisms (60%-90%),[2,3] two-thirds of which are due to firearm injury.
- Rapid evaluation of the ABCs in keeping with ATLS should be prioritized.
- An early logroll with careful inspection of the head and neck (in addition to the rest of the body) must be performed to identify penetrating wounds. Where feasible, wounds should be marked with radio-opaque markers (eg, taped paperclips) for X-ray identification to aid in determining trajectories (**FIGURE 1**).
- Where hard signs of airway injury are present (respiratory distress, hemoptysis, or bubbling from wounds), early intubation should be performed with a surgeon at standby to perform a surgical airway procedure if required.
- Where there are hard signs of vascular injury (expanding hematoma or active bleeding), direct finger pressure should be applied. Adjunctive maneuvers such as placing a Foley catheter into the wound followed by insufflation of the balloon can help to achieve temporary hemostasis.
- While dysphagia, odynophagia, bloody secretions, or subcutaneous emphysema could reflect esophageal injury, these findings are not pathognomonic and are neither sensitive nor specific.

IMAGING AND OTHER DIAGNOSTIC STUDIES

- Plain film X-rays: These are an essential adjunct to the primary survey in the trauma bay. In patients with gunshot wounds, X-rays should encompass the body compartments at risk for injury. For patients with gunshot wounds to the neck we advocate obtaining X-rays of the head (so-called "big head"), neck, and chest. Retropharyngeal air or pneumomediastinum raise concern for esophageal injury and warrant further investigation (**FIGURE 1**).
- Computed tomographic angiography (CTA): CTA has become the diagnostic modality of choice in patients with

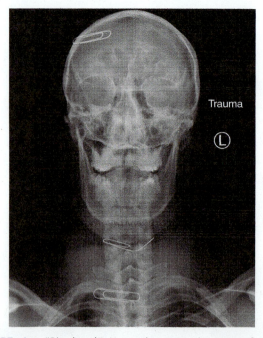

FIGURE 1 • "Big head" X-ray demonstrating use of radio-opaque markers (in this case, paperclips) to mark gunshot wounds. Closed paperclips denote anterior injuries, while bent paperclips denote posterior injuries. No retained projectiles are seen. Findings in this patient are clearly concerning for transcervical trajectory. Gas in the deep tissue planes of the neck raise concern for aerodigestive injury. The scalp wound was tangential and did not penetrate the skull.

Table 1: Grading of Esophageal Injuries

Grade	Description of injury
I	Contusion/hematoma or partial thickness laceration
II	Laceration <50% circumference
III	Laceration >50% circumference
IV	Segmental loss or devascularization <2 cm
V	Segmental loss or devascularization >2 cm

Advance one grade for multiple injuries up to grade III

Chapter 42 SURGICAL MANAGEMENT OF INJURIES TO THE CERVICAL ESOPHAGUS

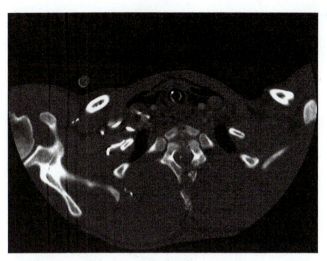

FIGURE 2 • Computed tomographic angiography of the neck of patient with anterior cervical gunshot wound. Extensive subcutaneous emphysema and gas in the paratracheal and paraesophageal spaces raise high concern for tracheal and esophageal injuries. Combined with trajectory showing cervical spinal column injury, operative exploration was clearly indicated.

neck trauma where immediate operative exploration is not indicated by hemodynamic instability or hard signs. CTA should be performed in all stable patients with penetrating injuries to the neck, with the rare exception of asymptomatic patients with trajectories that are clearly low risk. In patients with penetrating injury, CTA is highly sensitive (100%) and specific (97.5%) for aerodigestive and vascular injury (**FIGURE 2**).[4] However, sensitivity for detecting esophageal injury might be lower in stab wounds.[5] In patients with blunt trauma, CTA is indicated based on history of trauma to the neck, external signs of injury (such as seatbelt sign), or the presence of soft signs such as nonexpanding hematoma, dysphonia, dysphagia, odynophagia, or subcutaneous emphysema.
- Esophagography: Gastrografin or thin barium esophagography is a helpful imaging modality in stable patients where CTA is nondiagnostic for esophageal injury. Patients undergoing esophagography must be able to sit up and follow instructions to swallow contrast material. The decision to pursue esophagography must also take into consideration the timing and availability of this resource since the diagnosis of esophageal injury should not be delayed.
- CT esophagography: It is possible to evaluate the cervical esophagus with contrast esophagography using CT. This can be challenging, however, requiring an alert patient capable of following instructions to swallow a bolus of contrast with precise timing while supine. Therefore, this test is often not useful in the acute phase of care, and more reliable diagnostic approaches, such as flexible endoscopy, are favored.
- Flexible esophagoscopy: Esophagoscopy is a resource that can be readily mobilized to the bedside or the operating room (OR) in real time. In one series of patients with esophageal injuries, predominantly in the neck, flexible esophagoscopy diagnosed the injury with a sensitivity of 96%.[6] Therefore, esophagoscopy is an extremely helpful modality in patients where there is diagnostic uncertainty and esophagography is not readily available.

SURGICAL MANAGEMENT

Indications
- Patients with hard signs of aerodigestive or vascular injury require operative exploration.
- In patients with esophageal injury identified on CTA, esophagography, or flexible esophagoscopy, prompt surgical intervention is the safest decision to avoid the increased morbidity and mortality associated with delays in treatment.

Preoperative Planning
- Early communication with the OR and anesthesia teams is essential prior to transporting the patient to the OR. Information regarding the patient history and current status, the planned operation and positioning, expected blood loss, and transfusion requirements should be given.
- Specific equipment needs should be relayed. These might include flexible endoscope and bronchoscope, vascular shunts, and feeding tubes not typically stored in the OR.

Positioning
- The patient is positioned on the operating table supine with arms out. A rolled sheet or inflatable support is placed transversely under the patient's upper back to hyperextend the neck. The bed is placed in reverse Trendelenburg or flexed at its midpoint to elevate the patient's head, neck, and chest.
- Where there is concern for unstable cervical spinal column injury, which is unlikely in the setting of penetrating trauma, the decision to limit neck extension while maintaining inline stabilization is made in selected patients.
- The patient should be prepped and draped from the chin to the knees. Access to the chest is important should proximal arterial injury in the neck or thoracic vascular injury necessitate median sternotomy or thoracotomy. At least one lower extremity should be prepped to allow for harvest of a saphenous vein graft. Prepping the abdomen reserves the option of placing a gastrostomy tube if long-term need for enteral access is predicted.

SKIN INCISION

- The incision of choice for suspected injury to the cervical esophagus is a left-sided oblique cervical incision (**FIGURE 3**). This incision follows a line along the anterior border of the sternocleidomastoid muscle (SCM) from the mastoid to the sternal notch. This approach is chosen because the esophagus in the neck lies to the left of midline posterior to the trachea.
- Depending on the burden of injury suspected, extension of this incision across the midline into a modified collar incision, or into bilateral oblique incisions, might be required for adequate exposure of associated injuries.

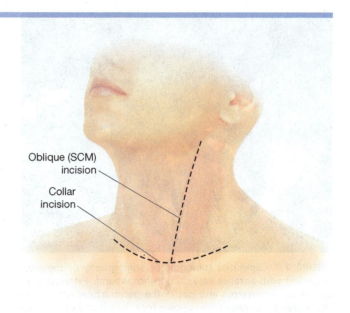

FIGURE 3 • Depiction of incisions for surgical exposure of the neck. The esophagus is best exposed through a left oblique incision, along the anterior border of the sternocleidomastoid muscle (SCM). Where broader exposure to the bilateral neck is required, the collar incision or bilateral oblique incisions can be used.

EXPOSURE AND EVALUATION OF THE ESOPHAGUS

- Through a left-sided oblique cervical incision, the platysma is divided and the SCM is retracted laterally. This exposes the underlying strap muscles and carotid sheath (**FIGURES 4** and **5**).
- Omohyoid, the lateral-most strap muscle belly, is divided to provide exposure of the deep structures in the neck.
- The carotid sheath is retracted laterally with SCM, while trachea with thyroid gland are retracted medially, to expose the length of the esophagus in the neck. A blunt Weitlaner self-retaining retractor can be placed to maintain this exposure (**FIGURE 6**).

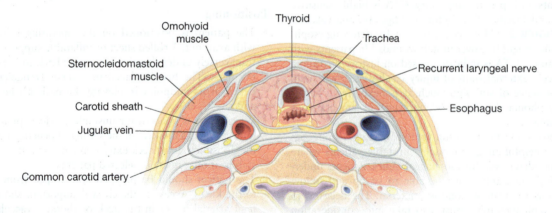

FIGURE 4 • Cross section of the neck at the level of C6 or C7. The relationship between the sternocleidomastoid and strap muscles, the carotid sheath, and the trachea and esophagus is shown.

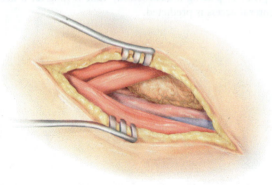

FIGURE 5 • Left oblique neck incision with retraction of the sternocleidomastoid muscle laterally exposes sternothyroid and omohyoid strap muscles and the carotid sheath. The omohyoid must be divided to provide access to the trachea and esophagus.

Chapter 42 SURGICAL MANAGEMENT OF INJURIES TO THE CERVICAL ESOPHAGUS   361

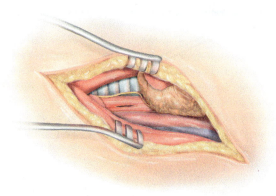

FIGURE 6 • With omohyoid divided, a blunt Weitlaner retractor is used to retract sternocleidomastoid muscle laterally to expose the trachea and esophagus.

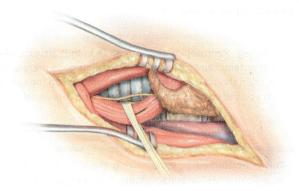

FIGURE 7 • After bluntly separating the esophagus from the anterior surface of the spinal column, a Penrose drain is placed around it for the purpose of mobilization and inspection.

- The recurrent laryngeal nerve should be identified running in the tracheoesophageal groove with the purpose of protecting it during further dissection.
- A nasogastric tube (NGT) should be gently passed to aid in palpating the esophagus.
- Blunt finger dissection posterior to the esophagus can now be performed to separate it from the prevertebral fascia and anterior surface of the vertebral column. The prevertebral fascia may need to be incised first. With a hooked finger, the esophagus is mobilized circumferentially. Care to avoid injury to the overlying trachea is critical.
- A Penrose drain is placed around the esophagus for manipulation. With this control the surgeon can now inspect the length of mobilized esophagus for injury (FIGURE 7).
- Areas of questionable injury or hematoma should be gently explored with Metzenbaum scissors.
- If there remains question of injury, the cervical esophagus can be tested for leak. The NGT is withdrawn to the level of the esophagus in the neck. The esophagus is occluded

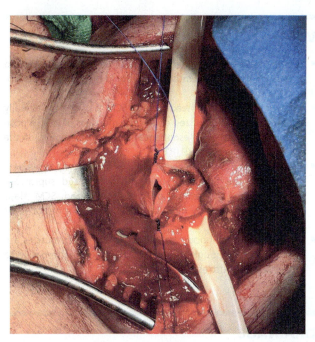

FIGURE 8 • Esophageal injury exposed through left oblique neck incision. Penrose is in place. The thyroid is cranial (right in picture) and the trachea to the right (top of picture) of the injury. The edges of the mucosal defect are seen well exposed with use of stitches placed at the apices of the planned closure.

distally at the thoracic outlet. With the neck incision filled with saline, the esophagus is gently insufflated with air via the NGT by the anesthesia team. Bubbling indicates a full-thickness injury. Alternatively, methylene blue dye injected by NGT can be used to identify full-thickness perforation.

Esophageal Repair

- Once an injury is identified, care must be taken to delineate the full extent of the mucosal defect. This might require enlarging the muscular defect to achieve. Devitalized tissue is debrided.
- Repair is performed in a two-layer tension-free fashion.
- The inner mucosal layer is approximated using a 3-0 absorbable suture (eg, Maxon, PDS, or Vicryl).
- The outer muscular layer is closed using 3-0 nonabsorbable suture (eg, silk).
- Using the long tail of suture from the apex of the injury, the margins of the defect can be brought outward under subtle tension to better expose the edges of the injury and make placement of suture bites easier (FIGURE 8).
- The inner layer should carefully reapproximate the mucosal edges to achieve water-tight closure in running fashion. This is particularly important to the integrity of the repair because the esophagus lacks serosa.
- The outer layer of the repair reapproximates the muscular layer over the inner repair in running or interrupted fashion.

VASCULARIZED MUSCLE FLAP

- In the setting of concomitant injuries to the trachea or carotid artery, a vascularized muscle flap should be positioned to separate the repairs.
- Use of the sternal head of the SCM has been classically described. The mobilized end of the muscle is placed in position to separate the esophageal repair from repairs of the trachea or carotid (FIGURE 9).
- Because the SCM receives blood supply at multiple levels from the occipital, superior thyroid, and suprascapular arteries, variations of well-vascularized SCM flaps can be fashioned by mobilizing the muscle from above or below.
- In young or well-nourished patients, the strap muscles are often robust enough to provide an adequate alternative to the SCM for buttressing repairs.

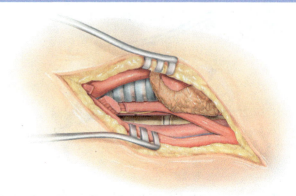

FIGURE 9 • If needed after repair of concomitant tracheal and esophageal injuries, the sternal head of the sternocleidomastoid muscle can be separated from its insertion and mobilized as a vascularized muscle flap. This is placed between the tracheal and esophageal repairs as a buttress.

DRAINAGE

- Because leak rates are high, a drain should be placed adjacent to the repair and exiting the skin away from the surgical incision at the base of the neck.
- Open (eg, Penrose) or closed (eg, Jackson-Pratt or Blake) drain systems can be used depending on surgeon preference.
- The drain should not be left in direct contact with the carotid artery out of concern for risk of erosion into the vessel.

DAMAGE CONTROL

- Where injury to the esophageal wall is too extensive, or local sepsis due to a delayed diagnosis makes primary repair not feasible, a cervical esophagostomy should be created.
- This is performed by exteriorizing the site of perforation as a "blowhole" esophagostomy, loop esophagostomy, or double-barreled esophagostomy.

ENTERAL ACCESS FOR NUTRITION

- We recommend leaving an NGT in place at the time of surgery, initially for gastric decompression, but also to allow for feeding in the early postoperative period. This tube should be bridled to the nasal septum before leaving the OR (this can be done tying the large-bore NGT to a small-bore feeding tube bridle using 0 silk suture). Clear signage in plain view should be left at the bedside in the intensive care unit (ICU) stating that only the surgical team should manipulate this tube.
- Open surgical gastrostomy tube placement is reasonable if a patient is expected to be unable to eat for a prolonged period. Examples are patients with complex esophageal injuries, concomitant tracheal or spinal cord injuries, or anticipation of prolonged mechanical ventilation.

PEARLS AND PITFALLS

Indications for surgery	• Hemodynamically unstable patients and those with hard signs of aerodigestive or vascular injury should undergo urgent operative exploration, bypassing CT scan.
Incision	• The left-sided oblique incision provides the best exposure of the cervical esophagus. • If exposure is difficult, do not struggle. Extend the incision across the midline into a "modified collar" incision or bilateral oblique incisions for better exposure.
Mobilization of the esophagus	• Finger dissection is used to separate the esophagus from the anterior surface of the spinal column. A hooked finger is then used to mobilize the esophagus along its full length in the neck. • This step is easiest with an NGT present.

Identifying the injury	▪ If suspicion for injury exists, persistence is required to thoroughly evaluate the cervical esophagus. ▪ Inspect the full circumference of the esophagus and examine areas of hematoma. ▪ Test for full-thickness perforation by distending with air or using methylene blue dye. ▪ Use flexible endoscopy. ▪ Where a single penetrating injury is seen, examine for a paired through-and-through injury.
Muscle flaps	▪ The SCM receives blood supply from multiple levels and can therefore be mobilized in either direction to achieve a tension-free flap. ▪ Strap muscles are a viable alternative if sized and placed appropriately.
Enteral access for nutrition	▪ Always consider need for durable access for feeding. ▪ Leave an NGT. ▪ Bridle the NGT to the nasal septum yourself before leaving the OR. This can be done using a bridle designed for a small-bore feeding tube (Dobhoff tube). The large-bore NGT is tied to the bridle using an 0 silk tie. ▪ Leave a sign in the ICU stating that this tube should be manipulated only by the surgical team.

POSTOPERATIVE CARE

- Postoperative care begins in the ICU. Due to a high frequency of concomitant injuries (75%), patients remain mechanically ventilated for a median of 4 days. Median ICU length of stay is 6 days.[2]
- Patients with esophageal repair should remain nil per os (NPO) in the early postoperative period. We recommend that patients remain NPO for 7 days. A contrast esophagogram on day 7 is performed to evaluate for signs of leak (**FIGURE 10**). If this study is negative, the patient can be advanced to oral intake.
- Enteral feeding, by NGT or gastrostomy tube, should begin early while the patient is NPO.
- Drains left at the time of surgery should be monitored for volume and character of output. These are removed after the patient has progressed to oral intake and output is negligible.

COMPLICATIONS

Leak

- The most frequent complication specific to cervical esophageal injury is leak, most often following attempted primary repair. In one multi-institutional study, the rate of leak following intervention for cervical esophageal injury was approximately 29%.[3] Half of leaks were uncontained and all required subsequent intervention. One-fifth of leaks persisted despite subsequent intervention. An important predictor of esophageal injury-related complications such as leak is delayed recognition and treatment,[7] reinforcing that high index of suspicion and expeditious treatment are essential.

Infectious Complications

- Patients with cervical esophageal injuries are high risk for septic complications, due to breakdown of repair or failure of drainage, often in the setting of multiple injuries. Infectious complications of some kind (eg, pneumonia, mediastinitis, sepsis, esophageal fistula) arise in 14%-37% of patients.[2,3]

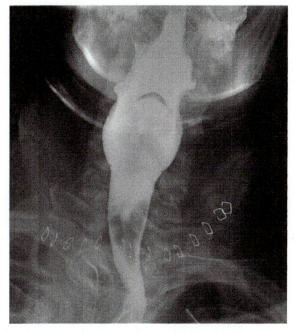

FIGURE 10 • Barium swallow on postoperative day 7 following primary repair of a cervical esophageal injury. No leak is seen.

Mortality

- While lower than mortality observed following thoracic esophageal injury (13%), mortality following cervical esophageal injury remains relatively high (8%-9%).[2,3]

REFERENCES

1. Moore EE, Jurkovich GJ, Knudson MM, et al. Organ injury scaling. VI: Extrahepatic biliary, esophagus, stomach, vulva, vagina, uterus (nonpregnant), uterus (pregnant), fallopian tube, and ovary. *J. Trauma*. 1995;39(6):1069-1070.
2. Aiolfi A, Inaba K, Recinos G, et al. Non-iatrogenic esophageal injury: a retrospective analysis from the National Trauma Data Bank. *WJES*. 2017;19(12):19. doi:10.1186/s13017-017-0131-8

3. Raff LA, Maine RG, Jansen J, et al. Contemporary management of traumatic cervical and thoracic esophageal perforation: the results of an Eastern Association for the Surgery of Trauma multi-institutional study. *J Trauma Acute Care Surg.* 2020;89(4):691-697.
4. Inaba K, Branco BC, Menaker J, et al. Evaluation of multidetector computed tomography for penetrating neck injury: a prospective multicenter study. *J Trauma Acute Care Surg.* 2012;72(3):576-584.
5. Gonzalez RP, Falimirski M, Holevar MR, Turk B. Penetrating zone II neck injury: does dynamic computed tomographic scan contribute to the diagnostic sensitivity of physical examination for surgically significant injury? A prospective blinded study. *J. Trauma.* 2003;54(1):61-64.
6. Arantes V, Campolina C, Valerio SH, et al. Flexible esophagoscopy as a diagnostic tool for traumatic esophageal injuries. *J. Trauma.* 2009;66(6):1677-1682.
7. Asensio JA, Chahwan S, Forno W, et al. Penetrating esophageal injuries: multicenter study of the American Association for the Surgery of Trauma. *J. Trauma.* 2001;50(2):289-296.

Chapter 43 Gastrostomy

Erin E. Devine, David I. Hindin, and Carla M. Pugh

DEFINITION

- A gastrostomy tube (G-tube) is a transcutaneous enteral access device that passes into the lumen of the stomach.
- The primary function of G-tubes is nutrition, though they are also used for decompression and in some cases gastropexy.
- G-tubes can be temporary or permanent, depending on the underlying etiology, though they are typically left in for at least 8 weeks.
- For patients unable to swallow, G-tube feeding is often the preferred form of nutrition because it most closely mimics the physiology and hormonal response of normal feeding. Additionally, patients with a G-tube can be bolus fed, which allows then to disconnect from the pump and improves quality of life.
- Open, laparoscopic, and percutaneous approaches can be used to place G-tubes. The approach typically depends on patient factors, as well as surgeon experience and resources.

PATIENT HISTORY AND PHYSICAL FINDINGS

- Pertinent history includes the indication for enteral access, hemodynamic stability, functional status of the gastrointestinal (GI) tract, past GI surgical history, planned upcoming surgical procedures, and expected duration of need for enteral access.
- Pertinent physical examination findings include abdominal scars and abdominal wall anatomy, including abdominal wall thickness (this may also be apparent on preoperative imaging; see below). These are considerations in determining the best approach and counseling patients about the likelihood of converting to a laparoscopic or open approach.

Indications

- Functional inability to eat or swallow
  - Dysphagia (eg, stroke patients)
  - Altered head and neck anatomy (eg, facial trauma, laryngectomy, glossectomy)
  - Altered mental status (eg, traumatic brain injury, subarachnoid hemorrhage)
- Inability to meet nutritional needs
  - Obstruction (eg, esophageal atresia, achalasia, malignancy along the pharynx or esophagus)
  - Anorexia (changes in taste, nausea, reduced appetite, early satiety)
  - Increased metabolic demand (burns, trauma, cancer)
  - Fatigue and muscle weakness (high-level spinal cord injury, acquired or inborn musculoskeletal disorders)

Contraindications

- Esophageal cancer: Tube gastrostomy may pose challenges for eventual construction of gastric conduit.
- Hemodynamic instability: Patients who are hemodynamically unstable should not undergo tube gastrostomy placement.

Alternatives

- Feeding jejunostomy tubes are preferred in patients undergoing esophageal reconstruction with a planned gastric conduit or in patients who have undergone prior total gastrectomy.
- Gastrojejunostomy tubes are preferred in patients who can tolerate distal enteral feeding (small bowel), but require proximal gastric decompression.
- KEO feeding (nasoduodenal) tubes are preferred in patients who require a feeding tube for less than 6 to 8 weeks, or who are hemodynamically unstable. These tubes can be placed in the stomach or postpylorically in the duodenum or jejunum.
- Total parenteral nutrition (TPN) should be considered in patient who do not have a functioning GI tract, such as patients with high intestinal losses (high ileostomy output, short gut syndrome) or chronic dysmotility disorders.

IMAGING AND OTHER DIAGNOSTIC STUDIES

- Routine imaging and diagnostic studies are not indicated for most G-tube placements, although patients often have abdominal imaging available and these images can be helpful in surgical planning.

SURGICAL MANAGEMENT

Preoperative Planning

- Patients must be NPO (nothing by mouth) a minimum of 6 hours prior to gastrostomy placement.
- Prophylactic antibiotics should be given within 30 minutes of skin incision.
- Prior to the procedure, patients should rinse with an antiseptic mouthwash.

Positioning

- For endoscopic and open G-tube placement, patients are positioned supine on the operating room table.
- For planned laparoscopic G-tube placement, the patient is typically positioned supine, with the right arm tucked.

PERCUTANEOUS ENDOSCOPIC GASTROSTOMY TUBE

Equipment

- Percutaneous endoscopic gastrostomy (PEG) tube kit—there are several available.
- Standard adult or pediatric endoscope with an external display.

Transillumination for Tube Site Selection

- The endoscopist stands at the patient's head and the surgeon stands scrubbed in at the patient's abdomen. Room lights should be dimmed and the endoscopist advances the endoscope to the patient's stomach.
- The stomach is insufflated and the endoscope advanced. A visual survey is carried out to fully evaluate for occult pathology.
- A polypectomy snare is advanced, typically 2 cm beyond the tip of the scope.
- Transillumination is carried out as follows: the scope is directed toward the anterior gastric wall, 2 to 3 cm distal to the gastroesophageal junction (GEJ). Whenever possible, we increase our light source to maximum brightness and reduce ambient lights in the room to a minimum. The skin along the abdominal wall is examined to choose the portion of maximal transillumination. Often, we find it helpful to palpate the abdominal wall to better confirm this portion. Secondary confirmation is achieved by endoscopically visualizing a dimpling of the gastric wall during abdominal wall palpation.
- After determining the area on the abdominal wall with the brightest transillumination, we confirm that this is a minimum of 2 to 3 cm beyond the costal margin, as any closer can make the G-tube uncomfortable for the patient (**FIGURE 1**).
- The site is marked, either with a pen or with indentation from plastic needle cap.
- Local anesthesia is used to infiltrate the skin and eventual tract for the G-tube.

Additional Assurance of Site Selection—Optional Technique (Foutch Reference)

- A 10-mL syringe is filled with several milliliter of saline and attached to a small-gauge needle.
- The needle is advanced perpendicularly through the chosen location on the abdominal wall, visualizing the site with the endoscope, while drawing back on the syringe.
- Saline in the syringe is examined for bubbles throughout this process.
- If bubbles are visualized before the needle is endoscopically noted within the stomach, this suggests the needle tip is in the colon.
- If bubbles are visualized simultaneously in the syringe as the needle tip is seen endoscopically entering the stomach, this suggests safe positioning in the stomach (**FIGURE 2**).

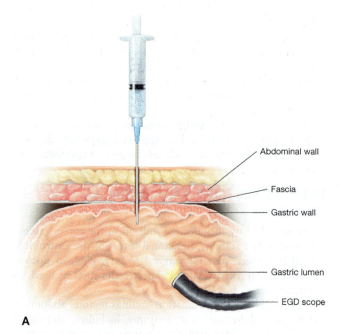

A

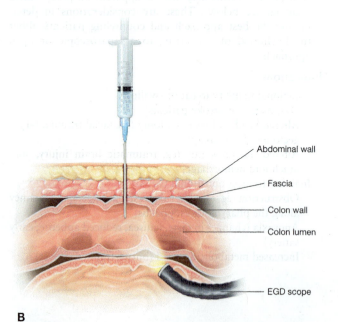

B

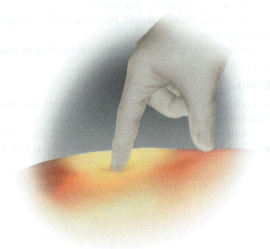

FIGURE 1 • Palpation and transillumination of the abdominal wall.

FIGURE 2 • **A,** Bubbles are seen at the same time as the endoscopist sees the needle, confirming intragastric positioning and excluding intervening bowel. **B,** Bubbles are seen before the needle is seen by the endoscopist, suggesting bowel between the stomach and abdominal wall. EGD, esophagogastroduodenoscopy.

- Potential pitfall: One must take care not to compress the tissue between the stomach and the skin with too much force as this can compress a portion of the bowel, allowing a through-and-through passage across the lumen without visualizing bubbles.

Tube Placement

- Once a safe site is selected and marked, the skin is infiltrated with local anesthetic.
- Using an 11 blade, an approximately 0.5-cm skin incision is carried out.
- The polypectomy snare previously prepared by the endoscopist is advanced; its loop is centered over the area of mucosa identified during abdominal wall site selection (FIGURE 3).
- Next, the needle with the angiocath is firmly advanced through the abdominal wall at the selected site, into the stomach, and through the snare loop under direct endoscopic visualization.
- The needle is withdrawn, leaving the angiocath in place (FIGURE 4A).
- The looped or stiff wire is next advanced through the angiocath (either push or pull method—see below) (FIGURE 4B).
- The snare is tightened firmly around the wire once several centimeters have been passed through.
- Keeping the polypectomy snare snug around the wire, the endoscope is fully withdrawn, pulling more of the wire through the abdominal wall into the stomach, through the esophagus, and out the mouth.
- The next steps follow either a "push" or a "pull" technique.

Pull Technique

- The looped wire that exited the mouth is now closed over the external end of the PEG tube (FIGURE 5).
- The surgeon pulls on the portion of wire exiting the abdominal wall, causing the PEG tube to advance back down through the esophagus and into the stomach.
- The endoscopist keeps the polypectomy snare cinched around half of the button of the PEG, allowing the endoscope to easily follow the PEG tube into the stomach (FIGURE 6).
- The surgeon should then see the tapered end of the PEG tube beginning to exit the abdominal wall. Additional force may be applied perpendicular to the abdominal wall to pull the tube through (FIGURE 7).
- The tube is further pulled through the abdominal wall under direct endoscopic view until the bumper is seen resting loosely against the gastric mucosa.
- The position of the bumper is confirmed endoscopically and the gastric wall examined for signs of bleeding.
- The surgeon should note the thickness of the abdominal wall and secure the bolster.

Push Technique

- This technique requires a stiffer guidewire than the pull technique.
- The endoscopist inserts the G-tube over the guidewire.
- The surgeon and the endoscopist hold tension on the guidewire while the G-tube is advanced into the stomach by the endoscopist.
- Next, the tube is pushed until the tapered end can be grasped by the surgeon at the bedside.

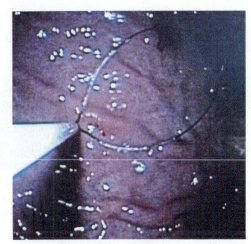

FIGURE 3 • The snare is positioned against the mucosa where the needle is intended to pass.

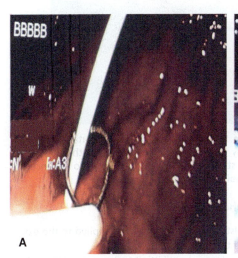

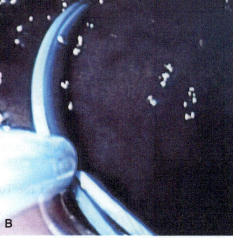

FIGURE 4 • A, The surgeon advances the needle and angiocath into the stomach in the center of the snare. The needle is removed. B, The wire is passed through the angiocath and the snare is then tightened around the wire.

SECTION VIII SURGERY OF THE STOMACH AND DUODENUM

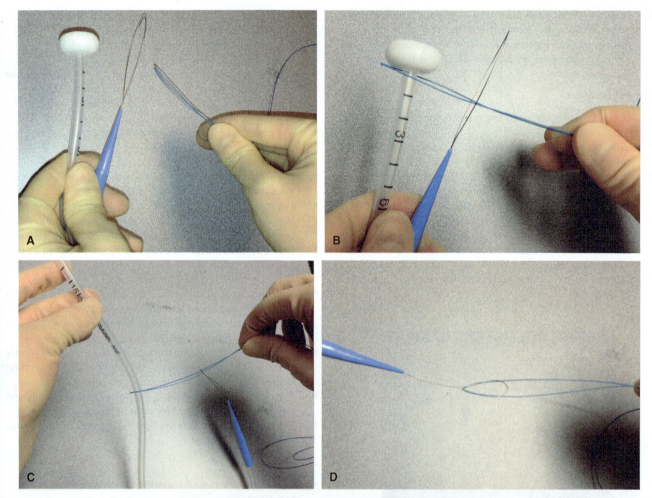

FIGURE 5 • With the looped wire exiting the patient's mouth, the tapered end of the percutaneous endoscopic gastrostomy (PEG) tube is secured to the wire. There is often a wire loop on the PEG to facilitate this attachment. Pass the wire through the loop **(A)** and around the button end of the tube **(B)**. Pull the rest of the tube through the wire **(C)** so that they are now secured together **(D)**.

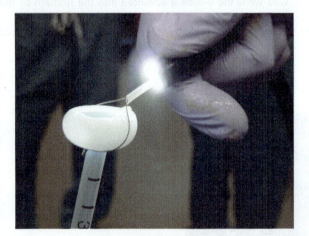

FIGURE 6 • Optionally, tighten the snare around half of the percutaneous endoscopic gastrostomy flange to facilitate prompt scope reentry into the stomach.

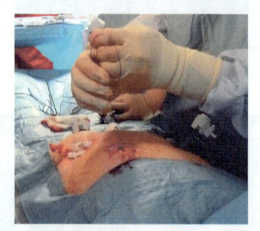

FIGURE 7 • Once the tapered end of the percutaneous endoscopic gastrostomy (PEG) is seen exiting through the abdominal wall, the surgeon steady pulls toward the ceiling to advance the PEG tube to its final position.

- The surgeon pulls the tube until the bumper rests loosely against the gastric mucosa, again applying force perpendicular to the abdominal wall.
- The endoscopist visualizes for good position of the button and hemostasis.

Securing the Tube

- The outer bolster provided in the kit is applied to the external portion of the G-tube.
- The bolster is advanced until it is 2 to 3 mm above the skin.

- It is key to avoid compressing the abdominal wall between the bumper and bolster (**Figure 8**), as this can cause necrosis of the tissue and lead to abdominal wall infection, tube extrusion, or the stomach to fall away from the abdominal wall.
- Antibiotic ointment may be to the interface of the tub where it meets the skin, although this is optional.
- The tube is cut to a manageable length and secured with an adapter to allow a sealed connection for feeding or drainage. Alternatively, a cap can be applied to prevent leakage.
- Immediately postoperatively, the tube is connected to a gravity bag to allow for drainage and to decompress gas that was insufflated during the procedure. This also decreases the risk of reflux during extubation.

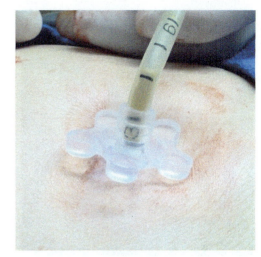

FIGURE 8 • The bolster is advanced so that it is just touching and depressing the skin.

OPEN G-TUBE PLACEMENT

Equipment
- A standard laparotomy tray is set up.
- Both a 22 Fr Foley catheter and dedicated G-tube from a laparoscopic kit may be used. Additionally, there are gastrostomy-jejunostomy tubes that allow jejunal feeding and simultaneous gastric decompression.

Incision
- A 4-cm upper midline incision is carried out to expose the stomach (**FIGURE 9**).
- Extraperitoneal fat and falciparum ligament are swept to the right to expose the left upper quadrant.
- To aid in retraction and protect the wound, a small wound protector can be used.

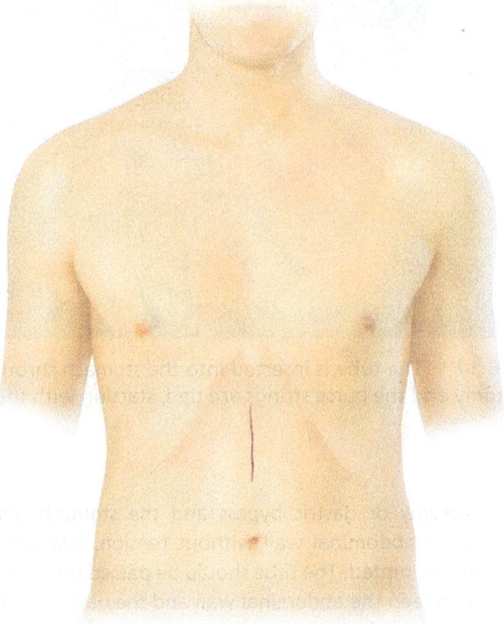

G-tube and Placement
- The planned site of the G-tube is marked with cautery. The preferred location is the anterior surface of the mid portion of the stomach (**FIGURE 10**).
- Two purse-string stitches are created around the planned G-tube site with 3-0 absorbable monofilament on a taper needle. The diameter of the first circle should be about 1 cm; the second should be approximately 2 cm (**FIGURE 11**).
- The G-tube's exit site is now chosen on the abdominal wall, with a trajectory passing through the left rectus muscle. It should be at about the level of the planned gastrotomy and at least 2 cm from the costal margin for patient comfort.
- Linea alba is grasped with a Kocher and the abdominal wall is elevated. A small 5-mm incision is made with an 11 blade. A fine clamp is passed from the peritoneum through the rectus muscle and the 5-mm skin incision (**FIGURE 12**).
- Now, the end of the G-tube catheter is grasped and brought back through the abdominal wall, taking care not to damage

FIGURE 9 • Open gastrostomy tube incision.

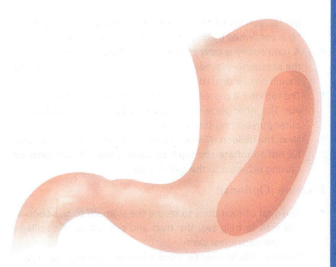

FIGURE 10 • Preferred location of gastrostomy on the anterior surface of the stomach.

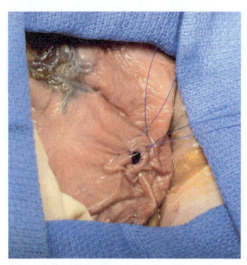

FIGURE 11 • Using nonabsorbable suture, the surgeon places a double purse-string stitch around the enterotomy site. The inner circle should be about 1 cm in diameter and the outer should be about 2 cm in diameter.

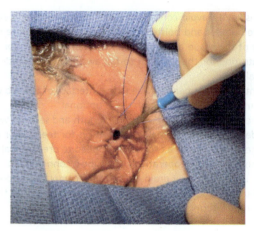

FIGURE 13 • Cautery is used to create a gastrotomy at the center of the purse string.

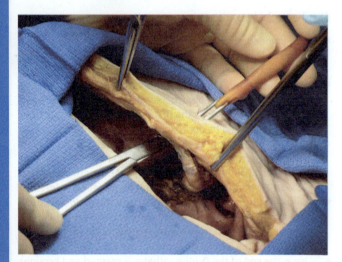

FIGURE 12 • The left linea alba is grasped and retracted medially.

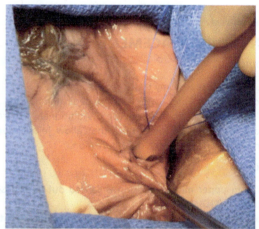

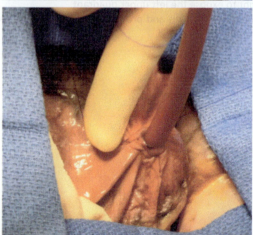

FIGURE 14 • The tube is inserted into the stomach through the gastrotomy and the purse strings are tied, starting with the inner circle.

- the balloon tip of the catheter. The integrity of the balloon tip is confirmed by inflating with sterile water (not saline).
- A gastrotomy is now created using cautery in the center of the previously placed purse-string stitches (**FIGURE 13**). This should not be dilated.
- The catheter is passed through the gastrotomy into the stomach. The inner purse-string stitch is tied first, followed by the outer purse-string stitch (**FIGURE 14**).
- Next, the balloon is inflated with 10 mL sterile water. Be careful not to inflate too tight to avoid closing the catheter or causing ischemia to the gastric wall.

Fixation (Optional)

- The goal of fixation is to secure the stomach to the abdominal wall to help seal the tract and prevent gastric spillage into the peritoneal cavity.
- Fixation should only be done when the stomach can reach the abdominal wall. In cases where the patient had a prior gastrectomy or gastric bypass and the stomach does not reach the abdominal wall without tension, dilation should not be attempted. The tube should be passed through omentum between the abdominal wall and the gastrotomy to aid in formation of a healthy tract.

- Four sutures are placed through the serosal layer of the stomach and the peritoneum of the abdominal wall. Without tying initially, place 3-0 absorbable monocryl sutures starting with the lateral stitch, then superior, inferior, and medial stitch around the G-tube tract. The sutures are now tied down in the order they were placed, relaxing retraction on the abdominal wall.
- Ensure the stomach is not under too much tension or twisted before tying sutures down.

Closure

- Closure is carried out in the standard fashion.
- The tube is secured with a 3-0 nylon suture to prevent dislodgement of the tube.
- This may also be secured with a bolster if provided with a manufactured G-tube. Again, it is critical to ensure the bolster is not too tight.

LAPAROSCOPIC G-TUBE

Equipment and Port Placement

- A commercially available laparoscopic G-tube kit is typically used. This chapter will describe the Flexiflo Lap G by Abbott Nutrition; however, the steps are similar to other commercially available tubes. Be sure to read the package insert if using a different tube to find pearls for success.
- A standard laparoscopic setup with a 5-mm, 0° or 30° laparoscope and a single 5-mm port is used. A single periumbilical port for the camera is sufficient as long as there are no adhesions that need to be taken down and the stomach can be sufficiently insufflated by anesthesia via orogastric tube. If there are adhesions or the stomach cannot be insufflated, additional ports may be required.
- T-fasteners may be used to provide traction for the stomach while the tract is being dilated when a single port is used. They are not needed when additional ports are placed for adhesions or stomach manipulation.

Laparoscopy

- The abdomen is entered using a 5-mm periumbilical port for the laparoscope. If adhesions are seen or additional retraction is needed for the stomach, two additional ports may be placed to triangulate the stomach (FIGURE 15).

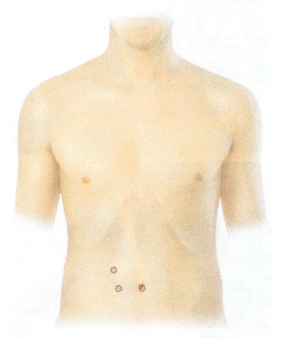

FIGURE 15 • Port placement for laparoscopic gastrostomy tube.

- Adhesions may need to be taken down for adequate visualization.
- Stomach may be guided into position using instruments or additional gastric insufflation via nasogastric tube.

Tube Placement

- A site on the left upper quadrant of the abdominal wall is selected where the G-tube should enter. This should be at least 2 cm from the costal margin for patient comfort. The abdominal wall is palpated under laparoscopic visualization in order to select a safe place where the stomach meets the abdominal wall. If it is placed too close to the GEJ or in the antrum, there is a risk of obstructions, so avoid these areas. The preferred location is the anterior mid body closer to the greater curvature (FIGURE 10).
- The tube site is marked on the skin, along with two points 2 cm away in all four directions for the T-fasteners.
- The needle loaded with a T-fastener is advanced through the abdominal wall at the most superior marking, angling slightly toward the center mark. This is passed into the peritoneal cavity.
- The needle is directed to the desired gastrotomy site that lines up with the skin incision. It is now advanced into the stomach up to the double line marking. The T-fastener is deployed by pressing the plunger on the needle (FIGURE 16). Clamp the T-fastener tail 1 to 2 cm from the skin.
- This process is now repeated to deploy the remaining T-fasteners at the marked locations.
- At this point, the anesthesia team should be asked to deflate the stomach slightly. The anterior wall of the stomach should be visible as it falls away from the abdominal wall with the four T-fasteners creating a diamond shape with the tube insertion site in the middle.
- A 5-mm skin incision is made at the marked location on the skin.
- The 18-gauge needle with a 40 mL slipped-tip syringe is directed through the abdominal wall and into the peritoneal cavity.
- The needle is passed into the stomach at the center of the diamond created by the T-fasteners under direct visualization of the laparoscope (FIGURE 17). These T-fasteners can aid in creating traction on the stomach to help guide the needle (FIGURE 18).
- Air is insufflated into the stomach to ensure the needle tip is intraluminal.
- A wire is passed through the needle and removes the needle.
- Serially dilate the tract, ensuring that the stomach is just off the abdominal wall so there is direct visualization of the dilators passing into the lumen of the stomach (FIGURE 19).
- The smallest dilator is inserted back in once the tract is adequately dilated.

372 SECTION VIII SURGERY OF THE STOMACH AND DUODENUM

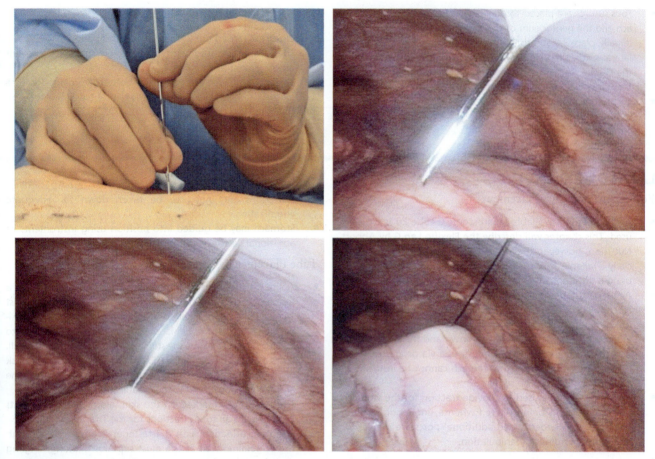

FIGURE 16 • The sequence of steps for T-fastener placement is shown here. The needle should be inserted to the double black bar before deployment of the T-fastener.

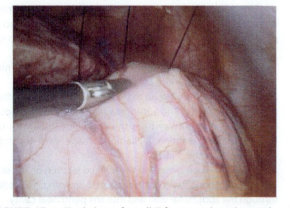

FIGURE 17 • Final view after all T-fasteners have been placed.

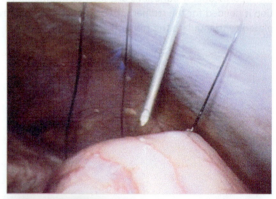

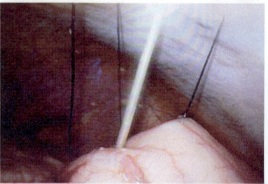

FIGURE 18 • The large-bore needle is directed into the stomach through the center of the T-fasteners.

Chapter 43 **GASTROSTOMY** 373

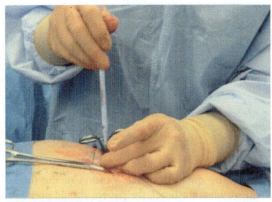

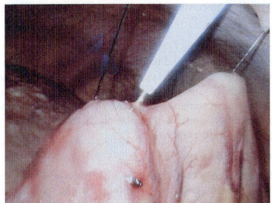

FIGURE 19 • The dilator is passed over the wire though the abdominal wall and into the stomach.

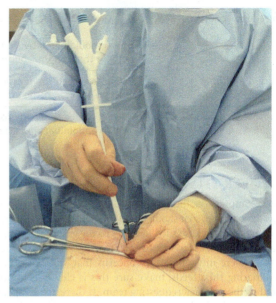

FIGURE 20 • The smallest dilator is inserted into the gastrostomy tube and two are guided over the wire through the tract and into the stomach. The wire and dilator are removed together leaving the tube in place.

- The G-tube is passed over the smallest dilator. Dilator and wire together are now removed together, leaving the G-tube in place (**FIGURE 20**).
- The balloon is inflated using 18 to 20 mL of sterile water.
- Pull back so that the stomach rests gently against the abdominal wall. The outer flange is advanced to rest gently on the skin. Avoid too much pressure between the balloon and the flange to prevent tissue injury and abdominal wall or gastric necrosis (**FIGURE 8**).
- T-fasteners are left in place and secured with small white cotton bolsters, also being careful not to put too much pressure on the tissue. These can be removed after 2 weeks by cutting the sutures below the bolsters (**FIGURE 21**).

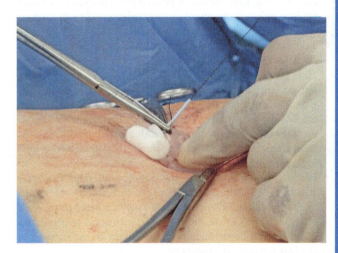

FIGURE 21 • The T-fasteners are gently retracted so that the stomach is secured against the abdominal wall and crimped into place.

PEARLS AND PITFALLS

Indications	■ Ensure that a G-tube fits the needs of the patient. ■ Ensure the patient is stable for the procedure. G-tube placement is elective, and there are alternatives (TPN, KEO tube feeds) in unstable patients.
Preprocedure planning	■ Take a thorough surgical history. ■ Be prepared to convert to laparoscopic or open in patients at risk of requiring these approaches. ■ Ensure you can darken the room adequately for transillumination when preforming a PEG.
Patient positioning	■ Position the patient supine and tuck the right arm if performing a laparoscopic approach. ■ Expose the entire abdomen.

Tube site selection	• The G-tube should pass through the skin at least 2 - 3 cm from the costal margin for patient comfort. • There should be no tension or rotation of the stomach—it should like up well with the G-tube coming through the abdominal wall.
Securing the tube	• Avoid too much compression of the skin and soft tissue between the bolster and the bumper since this can result in tissue injury and necrosis.
Postprocedure care	• Keep the tube to gravity for a few hours to decompress the stomach after the procedure. • Use an abdominal binder to secure the tube and prevent early dislodgement of the tube.

POSTOPERATIVE CARE

- For decompression, the G-tube should be kept to a gravity bag. There is no sump, so it should not be hooked up to wall suction, as doing so may cause suction injury to the gastric mucosa.
- Practices vary as to when to start postoperative tube feeds. If there were intraoperative concerns that warrant a delay in initiating tube feeds, make sure this is clearly communicated to the primary requesting team. If there are no specific concerns, tube feeds can be safely started as early as 4 hours after the tube is placed.
- Tube feeds should start at a low rate (10-20 mL/h) and should be increased by 10 mL about every 6 to 8 hours until the goal rate is reached. For patients requiring long-term tune feeding, tube feeds can be converted to cycled or bolus feeds to improve quality of life for patients and to disconnect them from the feeding tube pump.
- Take care to protect the new G-tube from inadvertent injury or dislodgement, which can require a trip back to the operating room.
- For patients in the hospital, keep a Foley catheter at bedside that nursing can replace in the newly formed tract if the G-tube is displaced to temporize. Patients with altered mental status may require an abdominal binder, mitts, or sometimes even restraints to protect from inadvertent dislodgement of the G-tube.
- For patients going home, the patient and their caregiver should get education on proper tube care and troubleshooting. They should also be given a Foley catheter to place in the tract if the G-tube dislodges and instructed to present to an emergency department (ED) right away if that happens in the first 6 weeks after surgery.

COMPLICATIONS

Clogged Tube

- Clogged G-tubes occur frequently and can almost always be resolved by flushing the tube. A small diameter syringe will generate more pressure so the smallest syringe that can create a seal with the tube should be used. Additionally, colas can be used to clear G-tubes since the carbonation and acidity of the drink helps clear it out. The cola should be left in the tube for an hour or more to help break down the clog.

Dislodged Tube

- In the first 6 weeks postoperative, it is critical that patients and families are taught how to replace the G-tube should it fall out. They should be discharged with a spare G-tube to replace or a Foley catheter that can temporize the tract and prevent it from closing.
- If there is any question of the location of the tube (pain, discomfort when flushing), the patient should present to the ED or clinic to confirm the location of the tube before using.

Stoma Leakage

- Leakage around the G-tube site can be irritating to the surrounding skin and lead to skin breakdown. Good tube site care is important to prevent this and can be burdensome to patients. G-tube exchange (often done by interventional radiology) can sometimes improve the leakage from around the tube. Occasionally, the tube needs to be removed and replaced at a different site.

Fractured Tube

- A fractured tube can be sealed with a waterproof tape (duct tape, Tegaderm, electrical). It should then be replaced at the next clinic visit. It is within about 6 weeks of surgery, the tube may need to be exchanged by GI, IR, or the surgeon over a guidewire.

Tube Site Infections

- Tube site infections may present as redness, swelling, and pain around the tube site. Simple tube site infections can be treated with a course of antibiotics to cover skin flora.
- Abdominal wall abscesses are less common than tube site wound infections. If present, they should be treated with incision and drainage. If there is associated cellulitis, then a course of antibiotics may also be indicated to cover skin flora.
- Rarely, the G-tube needs to be removed to allow a tube site infection to heal.

Tube Placed Through Another Piece of Bowel

- If discovered acutely and the patient requires a G-tube for their care, the patient should be taken back to the operating room for repair of the intestinal injury and placement of an open G-tube.
- If discovered later, the tube can be removed if the patient no longer requires it, though there will be a potential need for repair and gastroenteric fistulas may form. Many of these fistulas will close on their own.
- Colocutaneous fistulas can form following through-and-through injuries to the colon (typically during PEG placement). This requires removal of the G-tube to allow the tract to heal (at least 1 month).

Gastric Outlet Obstruction

- Overinflating the balloon or positing the G-tube too near the GEJ or antrum can cause gastric outlet obstruction. Often, deflating the balloon will relieve the obstruction. If the balloon is not secure against the gastric wall, it is also possible that it can float to the pylorus and cause obstruction. Tightening the balloon gently may also relieve the obstruction.

Abdominal Wall Necrosis

- Abdominal wall necrosis can be caused by a G-tube bumper and fastener that are too tight, compressing the skin and soft tissue of the abdominal wall and the gastric wall. In severe cases, this can lead to necrotizing fasciitis requiring antibiotics and emergent surgery for debridement.
- See **FIGURES 22-25** for additional details.

Buried Bumper Syndrome

- Buried bumper syndrome occurs when the internal bolster burrows into the gastric wall. This can be the result of compression of the gastric wall between the bumper and the external fastener. Buried bumper syndrome can be complicated by GI bleeding, perforation, peritonitis, and intra-abdominal or abdominal wall abscess. These complications can be life threatening. This requires removal and replacement of the G-tube.

Tumor Seeding

- Tumor seeding can occur during PEG placement when it passes oral or pharyngeal tumors and seeds the abdominal wall. This requires a surgical and oncology consult.

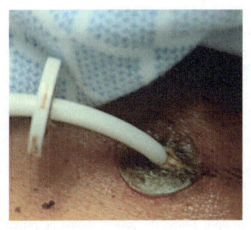

FIGURE 22 • Gastrostomy tube site wound on postoperative day 5 with a small amount of tissue necrosis.

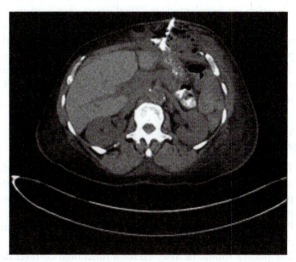

FIGURE 24 • CT imaging on postoperative day 9 showing oral contrast extravasating along the anterior abdominal wall and multilocular fluid and gas.

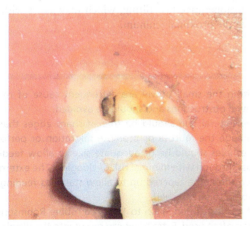

FIGURE 23 • Gastrostomy tube site on postoperative day 8. Intraoperative findings would include an excoriated gastrostomy site and necrosis of the anterior rectus sheath and subcutaneous tissue.

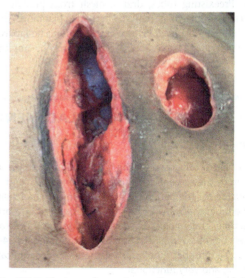

FIGURE 25 • Photo of postoperative wound following debridement.

Chapter 44 Feeding Jejunostomy

Kelsey B. Montgomery and John R. Porterfield Jr.

DEFINITION

- A jejunostomy tube (J-tube) is a flexible soft tube that connects the intraluminal jejunum with the outside world through the abdominal wall. The main function is to provide long-term access to the proximal gastrointestinal (GI) tract for enteral nutrition when oral intake is not possible or inadequate.
- A J-tube can be placed through an open or a laparoscopic approach. Often, it is placed in conjunction with a larger operation (eg, esophagectomy, total gastrectomy) when it is anticipated that the patient will not progress to adequate oral intake in a timely fashion or if it is preferred for the patient to be nil per os (NPO) to protect a new anastomosis during the early postoperative course. The J-tube affords the advantage of early enteral nutrition even when the upper GI tract cannot be used.

PATIENT HISTORY AND PHYSICAL FINDINGS

- The history and physical examination should focus on the indication for enteral access, hemodynamic stability of the patient, current functional status of the GI tract, and previous abdominal surgeries.
- Patients who are hemodynamically unstable generally should not undergo elective J-tube placement.
- The patient should be assessed for a functional GI tract distal to the ligament of Treitz (LOT) and should not have evidence of mechanical bowel obstruction, adynamic ileus, GI ischemia, or peritonitis.
- A thorough surgical history is imperative prior to J-tube placement. Preexisting tubes, drains, mesh from previous hernia repairs, or stomas may require alternative planning. An extensive abdominal surgical history may prohibit safe laparoscopic J-tube placement, and an open technique may be employed.

IMAGING AND OTHER DIAGNOSTIC STUDIES

- Radiologic workup is generally not necessary for J-tube placement. However, it is often the case that patients have had abdominal imaging for other reasons that may provide valuable information including previous surgical procedures or unexpected anatomic findings.

SURGICAL MANAGEMENT

Preoperative Planning

- The patient should be NPO for a minimum of 6 hours prior to the procedure.
- Antibiotics should be given within 30 minutes of incision to reduce the incidence of abdominal wall infection around the tube site. First-generation cephalosporins are our preference when not contraindicated by the patient's known allergies.
- Generally, the jejunostomy tube will exit the patient's abdomen in the left upper quadrant (LUQ). As mentioned previously, preexisting tubes, drains, implanted mesh, and stomas may require tube site adjustment.

Positioning

- For an open J-tube, the patient should be placed in the supine position. Usually, this procedure is done in addition to a larger procedure and thus the patient is already positioned accordingly.
- For a laparoscopic J-tube, the patient should be positioned supine with the right arm tucked to allow for adequate room for the surgeon and assistant to both work comfortably on the right side.
- It is important to be certain the patient is secured to the bed for intraoperative bed tilting, which may assist with exposure of the proximal jejunum.

TECHNIQUES

OPEN JEJUNOSTOMY TUBE PLACEMENT

Equipment

- The type of tube used for the feeding jejunostomy is decided upon by the surgeon to optimize the longevity, comfort, and function for the patient. There are many commercially available tubes that vary widely in features, availability, and cost.
- If a tube is being placed as part of a larger procedure and will likely be removed within 6 to 8 weeks, a standard 14-French (Fr) "red rubber Robinson" catheter is economical, time tested, and very functional.
- The most important tube characteristics are that it should be soft, pliable, and preferentially not containing a balloon unless it is a small balloon, less than 5 mL, and specifically designed to be placed within the jejunum. Balloon catheters within the small bowel are a frequent cause of recurrent bowel obstructions and should be avoided.
- The enteral end should be free of sharp edges that could damage the mucosa or promote migration or perforation. The holes should be of adequate size to allow feedings to pass through with minimal risk of clogging. The external portion should be tapered up to allow standard feeding pump tubing to be attached.
- At our institution, a 12- to 18-Fr red rubber Robinson catheter is often used. Extra holes can be cut into the distal portion to allow tube feeds to flow with less resistance. These holes may be created by folding the tube over and cutting the corner of the fold (**FIGURE 1**). Alternatively, the tube from a laparoscopic jejunostomy kit can be used (Flexiflo Lap J laparoscopic jejunostomy kit by Abbott Nutrition).

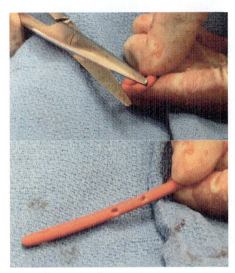

FIGURE 1 • Cutting extra holes in a red Robinson tube will reduce resistance of flow to the tube feeds.

Incision

- If the open J-tube placement is being performed as a standalone operation, the incision should be centered in the midline at the level of the LOT.
- The supraumbilical vertical midline incision should be carried through the linea alba with enough length to locate the LOT, mobilize 20 to 30 cm of jejunum, and allow for fixation of the jejunal segment to the peritoneum of the abdominal wall around the tube exit site. If there are minimal adhesions, this incision may be kept relatively small, 5 to 7 cm, and the majority of the operation can be done on eviscerated jejunum (**FIGURE 2**).
- A limitation of an incision that is too small is that it may prove difficult to fix the bowel to the abdominal wall through the small incision. Exposure of this step should not be compromised in any way to avoid lengthening the incision.

Mobilization of Jejunum

- Once the peritoneal cavity has been entered, the omentum and transverse colon are retracted cephalad to expose the small bowel. A segment of small bowel is chosen in the LUQ and traced proximally until the LOT is identified.
- Once the LOT is identified, the small bowel is examined all the way to the ileocecal valve to ensure no occult pathology, obstruction, or torsion is present.
- The tube insertion site is chosen where the tube will pass through the abdominal wall. This will generally be in the LUQ. The surgeon must ensure the chosen segment of jejunum will reach the parietal surface of the abdominal wall without any tension or torsion. Lysis of adhesions may be needed to make sure the jejunum can reach the abdominal wall without tension.
- Placement of atraumatic clamps on the left side of the fascia allows the abdominal wall to be retracted anteriorly for exposure of tube placement. While keeping retraction, a strong fine clamp is passed from inside the abdomen through the point chosen in the abdominal wall. A 3-mm skin incision, at the clamp exit site, is created, and the tube

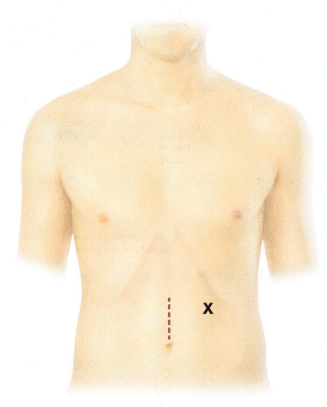

FIGURE 2 • Open incision diagram with tube exit site marked.

is grasped and the distal end is pulled through the abdominal wall into the peritoneal cavity. Both ends of the tube are clamped together and positioned out of the way (**FIGURE 3**).

Enterotomy and Placement of the Jejunostomy Tube

- A segment of jejunum approximately 30 cm from the LOT is chosen as the site for the J-tube placement. This portion of jejunum can be eviscerated for the next steps if a smaller incision has been used. Using a 3-0 nonabsorbable or absorbable suture, place an approximately 4-mm purse-string suture in a box formation on the antimesenteric side of the small bowel (**FIGURE 4**). A double purse-string stitch may be used for additional security (**FIGURE 5**).
- At this point, it is essential to confirm the proximal and distal ends of the jejunum and to ensure the orientation is maintained through the entire procedure.
- Using cautery, create a small enterotomy in the center of the purse-string suture. It is helpful to grasp the bowel by the mesentery during this step. Inadvertent cautery injury to the opposite side of the small bowel can be avoided by cutting the serosa and muscularis with the cautery but "popping" into the lumen with a fine clamp (**FIGURE 5**).
- Place the distal end of the feeding tube through the enterotomy into the lumen and direct it distally. The catheter is advanced until at least 10 cm is intraluminal. It can be advanced further if there is an excessive amount of tubing left externally (**FIGURE 6**).
- Tie down the purse-string suture, taking care not to overtighten and occlude the tube (**FIGURE 7**).
- The tube entry site is then imbricated using a three-point triangular technique (**FIGURE 8**).

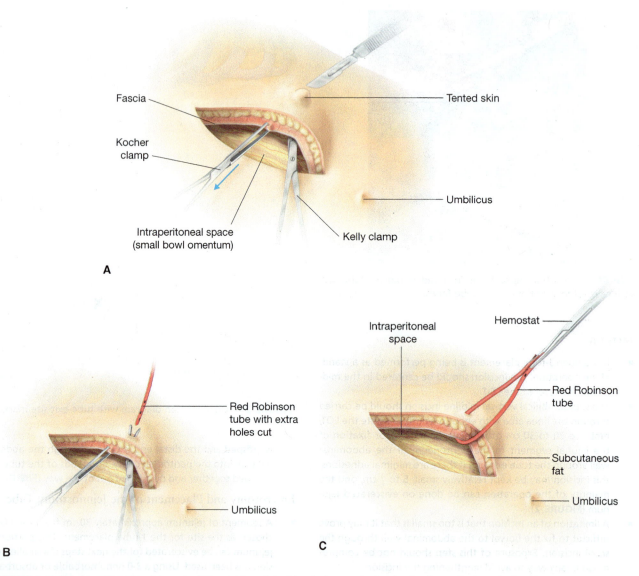

FIGURE 3 • Facial retraction anterior and midline with stab incision being made for the feeding tube. **A,** A kelly clamp is used to guide skin incision. **B,** After extending the clamp, a red Robinson tube is grasped and brought into the abdominal cavity. **C,** The tube is secured in place using a hemostat.

- Next, a Witzel tunnel is created. Starting at the enterotomy, the small bowel is imbricated over the feeding tube using interrupted 3-0 absorbable suture on a taper needle (**FIGURE 9**) for a distance of about 5 cm. These are seromuscular bites spaced approximately 5 to 10 mm apart, ensuring the tube is not exposed. Care should be taken not to place the bites too far from the tube, as this will draw more bowel into the Witzel tunnel and narrow the jejunal lumen (**FIGURE 10**).
- The jejunal segment must now be secured to the parietal peritoneum. This will allow the formation of a tract so that if the tube is inadvertently removed, it can be replaced without reentering the abdomen. This should be done in a way that the bowel is flush with the abdominal wall. Four "tacking" sutures of absorbable 3-0 suture can be placed around the tube exit site. The first is placed lateral to the tube, away from the operating surgeon. A seromuscular bite is taken and then a bite of peritoneum is taken at the corresponding location in the abdominal wall (**FIGURE 11**). Start with the lateral (furthest) suture first, then superior, inferior, and finally medial. Secure each suture with a clamp after it is placed, and do not tie until they are all appropriately placed.
- Once all four sutures have been placed, it is best to tie them in the order they were placed (**FIGURE 12**). An additional tacking suture may be placed 5 to 10 cm distally to secure a longer segment of bowel to the abdominal wall. This may help prevent torsion on the bowel around a single fixed point. The small bowel should now be adherent to the LUQ abdominal wall (**FIGURE 13**).
- The external portion of the tube should be secured to the skin using a 2-0 nonabsorbable monofilament suture (**FIGURE 14**).
- The abdomen is then closed in layers.
- The tube may be capped or placed to gravity drainage via a bag. Covering the tube with a dressing and tape or abdominal binder will help prevent it from being inadvertently dislodged during patient movement.

Chapter 44 FEEDING JEJUNOSTOMY 379

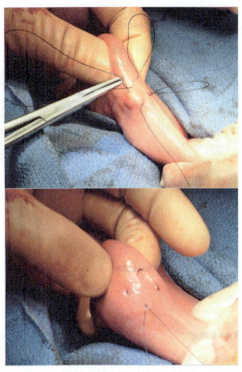

FIGURE 4 • Placement of purse-string stitch on antimesenteric jejunum.

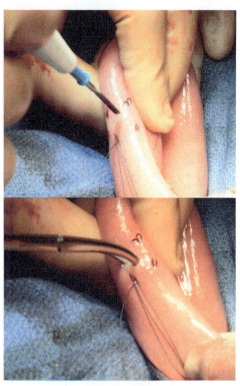

FIGURE 5 • The enterotomy is made with a cautery and then a hemostat is used to "pop" into the lumen. Note the double purse-string stitch used.

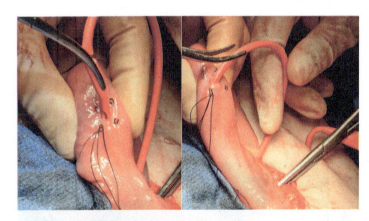

FIGURE 6 • Directing end of feeding tube into distal jejunum.

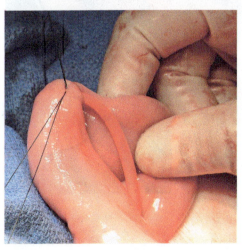

FIGURE 7 • Tying down purse string to secure the feeding tube.

380 SECTION VIII SURGERY OF THE STOMACH AND DUODENUM

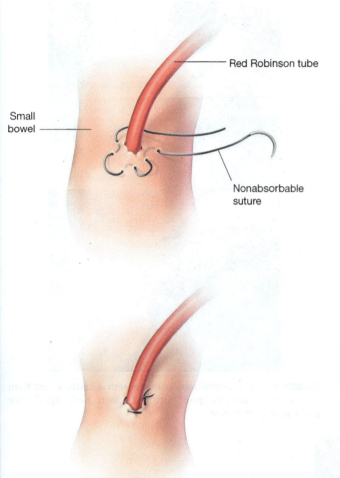

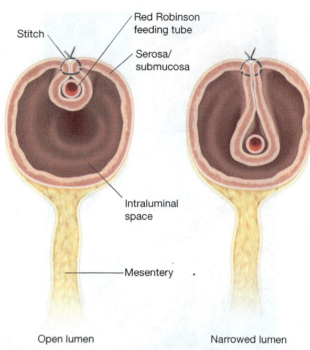

FIGURE 10 • Cross section of Witzel tunnel. The **left** shows the correct placement of sutures with adequate lumen diameter. The **right** shows a narrowed lumen from suture bites placed too far from the tube.

FIGURE 8 • Triangle stitch to imbricate the tube entry site.

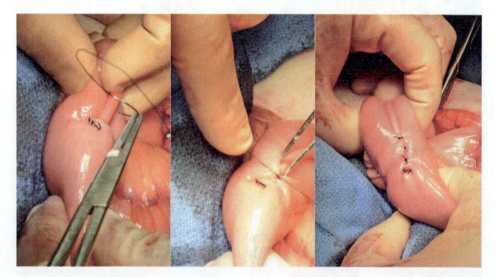

FIGURE 9 • Creation of the Witzel tunnel.

Chapter 44 FEEDING JEJUNOSTOMY

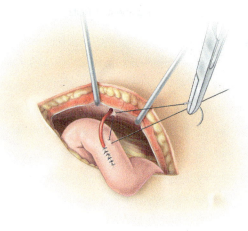

FIGURE 11 • Placement of first tacking suture.

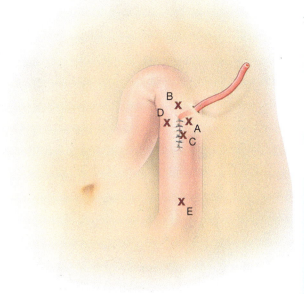

FIGURE 12 • Final appearance of bowel attached to the abdominal wall. The sutures should be placed in order from A to E.

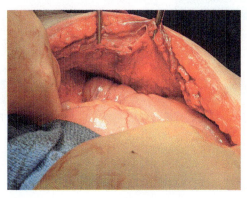

FIGURE 13 • Final view of small bowel fixed to abdominal wall after the four tacking sutures have been placed. Note the feeding tube is not visible.

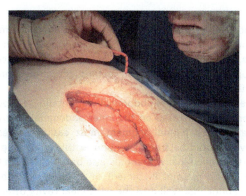

FIGURE 14 • Securing the external portion of the tube to the abdominal wall.

LAPAROSCOPIC JEJUNOSTOMY

Equipment and Port Placement

- Several commercially available laparoscopic jejunostomy kits are available. We use the Flexiflo Lap J laparoscopic jejunostomy kit by Abbott Nutrition. This section will describe J-tube placement using this kit. The steps described can be modified for other kits, and the package inserts for each kit should be read as they often contain pertinent pearls for success.
- A standard laparoscopic setup including a 5-mm 0° or 30° laparoscope and three 5-mm ports is used.
- Port placement should triangulate toward the proposed tube exit site in the LUQ (FIGURE 15). The J-tube site should be at least two fingerbreadths below the left costal margin at approximately the midclavicular line.

Jejunal Mobilization

- Once the ports are placed, the abdomen should be inspected to rule out occult pathology or evidence of a distal obstruction.
- The upper port should be used to retract the colon and omentum cephalad. The middle port is used for the camera. The lower port should be used to expose the small bowel.
- To identify the LOT, the transverse colon is retracted anteriorly as the patient is placed in Trendelenburg position and the mesentery of the transverse colon is followed toward its origin. The proximalmost portion of the jejunum can be seen exiting the retroperitoneum at the LOT. Alternatively, if this exposure is unable to be obtained, the small bowel may be followed in the LUQ until the LOT is reached (FIGURE 16).

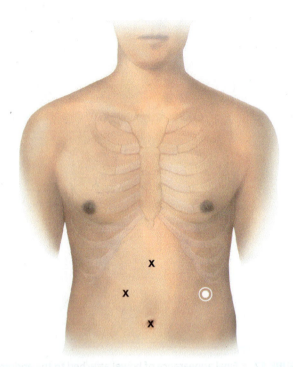

FIGURE 15 • Port placement diagram for laparoscopic J-tube. The tube site is represented by the target.

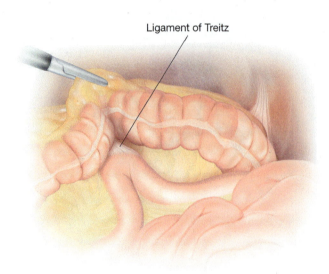

FIGURE 16 • The small bowel is followed in the LUQ to the LOT.

- Once the proximal jejunum is convincingly identified, it should be traced distally 20 to 30 cm to identify the tube site. Once the tube site is identified, it is essential to keep the proper orientation of the bowel throughout the completion of the procedure.
- The tube site on the abdominal wall should be chosen by identifying the area on the inner abdominal wall where the selected jejunal segment most easily reaches. The bowel should be free of tension at this point. The point on the abdominal wall should also be at least 2 cm below the costal margin. Placement of a fine needle through the abdominal wall into the peritoneal cavity often facilitates identifying and maintaining the best placement (**FIGURE 17**).

Tube Placement

- The T-fasteners supplied in the kit are placed next. They are placed in a diamond configuration around the tube entry site, marked with the fine needle. They should be placed 2 cm from the needle at the skin level, pass through the fascia, and exit approximately 1 cm from the needle in the peritoneal cavity (**FIGURE 18**).
- Alternatively, the J-tube can be secured by placing intracorporal 3-0 absorbable sutures with seromuscular bites through the jejunum in a similar diamond configuration.
- To start, the assistant grasps the chosen segment of jejunum and pulls it to the tube site, holding it in proper orientation. The first T-fastener is passed through the superior point of the diamond. Once intra-abdominal, the needle/T-fastener is advanced through the bowel wall. It is easy to inadvertently pass the needle through the posterior wall of the bowel at this point. The assistant should orient the bowel so that the

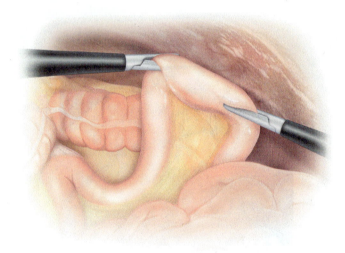

FIGURE 17 • There should be no tension when the small bowel is retracted toward the chosen area on the abdominal wall. A needle can be placed through the abdominal wall to easily mark the area from the peritoneal cavity.

mesenteric side is as far from the needle as possible during placement.
- The needle should be advanced to the 2-cm (double) mark and then deployed (**FIGURE 19**). Pull back on the fastener to ensure the bowel catches, retract it to the abdominal wall, and then apply a clamp to the external portion of the suture to keep the bowel in position.
- The next three T-fasteners are placed in a similar manner. The far lateral one should be deployed after the superior one, followed by the inferior, and then finally the medial fastener.
- If intracorporal sutures are used, as the first three sutures are placed they are sequentially passed through the abdominal wall with a Carter-Thomason device using the same hole through the skin but three separate entry points through the peritoneum

Chapter 44 **FEEDING JEJUNOSTOMY** 383

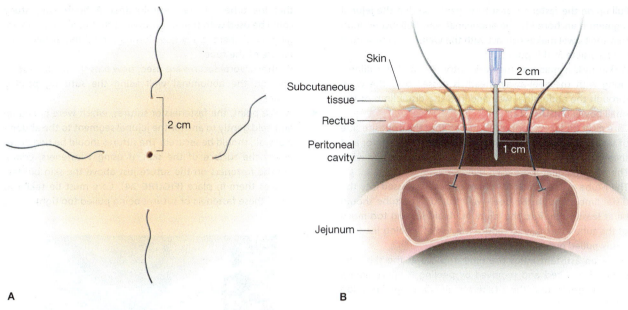

FIGURE 18 • **A,** Diamond configuration of T-fasteners around the tube entry site as seen on the abdominal wall. **B,** Cross-sectional view of trajectory of T-fasteners as they pass through the abdominal wall. Note they enter 2 cm from the tube site at the skin and exit 1 cm from the tube site at the peritoneum.

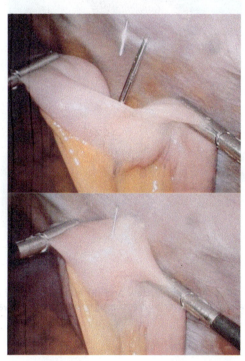

FIGURE 19 • The needle is advanced into the small bowel up to the double marking and the T-fastener is then deployed. Gentle traction after deployment will ensure the T-fastener has engaged the bowel properly.

- in a diamond shape complimentary to the respective sutures on the jejunum. The fourth (medial) suture is placed through the medial portion of the jejunum but not passed through the abdominal wall until the J-tube is inserted (▶ Video 1).
- At this point, the antimesenteric side of the bowel should be almost flush with the abdominal wall in four places (FIGURE 20). A small gap should be left for the next step.

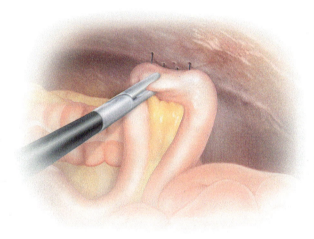

FIGURE 20 • A view of the bowel after all four T-fasteners have been placed. Note the small gap to allow visualization during placement of the J-tube.

- The 18-gauge needle is then advanced into the small bowel in the center of the four T-fasteners or absorbable sutures. Saline, air, or a brief insufflation with carbon dioxide from the laparoscopic insufflator will ensure that the needle is intraluminal. A fluid wave should be seen passing though the bowel. If the needle is submucosal, a local infiltration of saline in the bowel wall will be seen, but it will not pass as a fluid wave within the bowel.
- The wire is then advanced through the needle into the bowel while the assistant uses a blunt grasper to direct the wire into the distal limb of the jejunum. The wire can coil in the bowel easily during this step. This may be avoided if the assistant stretches the distal limb as the wire is passed (FIGURE 21).
- The needle is then removed.

- Pull up on the fasteners or sutures gently so that the jejunal segment is anchored to the abdominal wall. Pull just enough that the bowel makes contact with the wall. The wire should not be visible at this point.
- A skin nick is made at the wire entry site, and the dilator along with the peel-away sheath is passed over the wire, through the abdominal wall and into the distal limb of the small bowel (**FIGURE 22**).
- Care must be taken during this step so that the opposite side of the small bowel is not perforated and that the dilator and sheath should easily follow the path of a gently curved wire.
- The wire and dilator are then removed.
- The J-tube or prepared red rubber catheter is passed into the distal limb through the peel-away sheath. The tube should be at least 10 cm into the jejunum. Avoid leaving too much of the tube externally to reduce the risk of it being inadvertently pulled out.
- While an assistant holds the tube in place at the skin, the sheath is cracked and removed by peeling it apart slowly, making certain that the J-tube remains in proper position (**FIGURE 23**).
- Inject 10 mL of saline or air through the small port to ensure the tube is patent. This also again allows for conformation that the tube is in fact intraluminal. A fluoroscopy study could be used with similar contrast to that used for a cholangiogram if there is any question regarding the intraluminal nature of the tube.
- If intracorporal sutures are used, now pass the medial suture through the abdominal wall using the suturing passing device.
- At this point, the fasteners or sutures, which were pulled up and held gently to anchor the jejunal segment to the abdominal wall, should be secured. The sutures should be tied down below the surface of the skin. If using T-fasteners, crimping the fasteners on the suture just above the skin bolsters secures them in place (**FIGURE 24**). Care must be taken to avoid these fasteners or sutures being pulled too tight as this

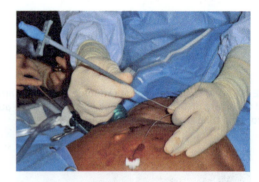

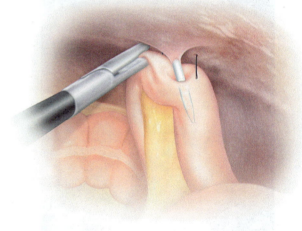

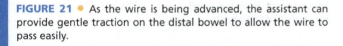

FIGURE 21 • As the wire is being advanced, the assistant can provide gentle traction on the distal bowel to allow the wire to pass easily.

FIGURE 22 • **A,** External view and **(B)** internal view of dilator and sheath passage over a wire, through the abdominal wall, and into the jejunal lumen.

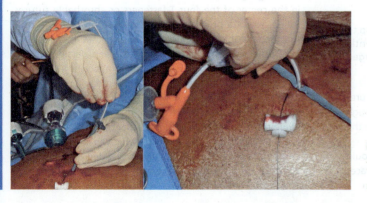

FIGURE 23 • After the dilator and wire are removed, the J-tube is passed through the sheath and into the jejunum. The sheath is then peeled away while the tube is held in place.

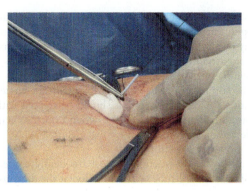

FIGURE 24 • The T-fasteners are crimped into place at the skin level.

could lead to erosion through the bowel. The tube should not be visible at this point from inside the abdominal cavity.
- There should be plenty of room to slide the flange down to the skin and secure it with one or multiple sutures (separate from sutures used to secure the J-tube to abdominal wall if using that method). Be careful not to inadvertently pull the tube out at this step.
- A final evaluation with the laparoscope should reveal no tension or torsion on the bowel as it rests on the anterior abdominal wall.
- The trocar sites are closed in standard fashion, and the procedure is complete.
- An abdominal dressing with tape or abdominal binder is placed over the tube to avoid it snagging during patient transport.

PEARLS AND PITFALLS

Indications	■ Be certain that a J-tube best fits the needs of the patient. Frequently, physicians may request a J-tube when in reality the patient needs a gastrostomy tube (G-tube) or vice versa.
Preprocedure planning	■ Review previous upper abdominal procedures or history of peritonitis that may have scarred another piece of bowel along the proposed track of the J-tube.
Patient position	■ Position the patient supine with the entire abdomen exposed and prepped and draped.
Open G-tube	■ Place the triangle suture and the imbricating sutures carefully to avoid excessively narrowing the lumen of the bowel.
Tube site selection	■ The tube site should be at least 2 cm inferior to the costal margin. ■ Keeping midline retraction on the fascia with clamps while making the incision through the abdominal wall will ensure that the tube does not get kinked as it traverses the abdominal wall once the fascia is closed.
Laparoscopic J-tube	■ Position the patient supine with the right arm tucked to allow a comfortable working space for the surgeon and the laparoscopic assistant on the right side of the patient. ■ Take special care to avoid penetration of the back wall of the jejunum with the needle. ■ Ensure, without question, that the wire and the tube pass intraluminally.
Securing the tube	■ Do not slide the bolster on the tube down tightly against the skin as it may necrose the skin or lead to pulling of the base of the tube through the jejunal wall and into the peritoneum.
Postprocedure care	■ An abdominal binder is helpful for securing the tube and preventing premature or inadvertent removal during patient movement or in a patient with impaired mental status.

POSTOPERATIVE CARE

- Tube feedings can be started the evening of the procedure at a "trophic" or low rate, usually about 10 mL per hour. If the patient tolerates this, they can be advanced by 10 mL per hour every 4 hours until the nutritional goal is reached.
- Care should be taken to avoid the tube catching or pulling while the patient is moving or if the patient's neurologic status is such that they can grab and pull the tube. An abdominal binder or gauze dressing can be used to cover the tube. Hand mittens can be used in the high-risk neurologic patient.
- The patient and their caregiver should receive education regarding proper tube care and simple troubleshooting.

OUTCOMES

- Not applicable

COMPLICATIONS

- Clogged tube
  - A clogged tube can be flushed in essentially every case with a small syringe. Due to the laws of hydraulics, the smaller the diameter of the syringe the more pressure. We recommend the smallest syringe that will tightly fit into the opening in the tube. Carbonated acidic beverages such as Coke may also aid in clearing an obstruction when they are allowed to sit within the tube for an hour or more.

- Dislodged tube
    - It is imperative that patients and caregivers are taught to reinsert the tube immediately if it becomes dislodged so that the tract does not close. If they are unable to reinsert, then they should immediately go to an emergency department where a smaller catheter could be temporarily advanced into place, preserving the tract that could be later dilated, and the proper tube placed.
    - If a tube is reinserted easily without resistance and flushing with water causes no discomfort, the tube may be used per the patient's routine without a conformational radiologic study.
    - However, if the replacement is complicated or if there is discomfort with flushing, the tube position should be checked to ensure proper positioning.
    - For tubes that have been in place for more than 1 month, it is exceptionally unlikely that the tube would not reenter the same bowel and rest in the same functional position where it was dislodged from.
- Fractured tube
    - If a tube is fractured with or without leakage, it may be temporarily patched with a waterproof occlusive tape such as electrical tape or Duct tape. This tube should be electively exchanged for a new tube during a regular clinic appointment. If the tube is new or in complex scenarios, it may need to be exchanged over a glidewire by a gastroenterologist, interventional radiologist, or a surgeon.
- Abdominal wall abscess
    - Tube site infections rarely lead to significant abscess formation, but if this occurs, it should be treated with incision and drainage, leaving the wound open as with any infected open wound.
- Small bowel obstruction
    - Small bowel obstruction is most frequently caused by a balloon on the J-tube or from torsion at the tube insertion site.
    - When an obstruction is evident, any fluid in a balloon should be removed and the bowel obstruction treated with nasogastric decompression as with any bowel obstruction.
    - If this does not resolve the obstruction, a computed tomography scan with oral contrast administered 2 hours prior to the study may be of assistance in assessing torsion of the bowel around the tube insertion site.
    - If torsion is confirmed, an operative exploration either in a laparoscopic or open approach is required to relieve the obstruction.

Chapter 45: Surgical Management of Postgastrectomy Syndrome

Xavier Lyndell Baldwin, Ugwuji N. Maduekwe, and John H. Stewart IV

This chapter will focus on the most commonly used and effective surgical approaches applied when symptoms are persistent, severe, and refractory to dietary or medical interventions.[1-3]

DEFINITION

- Up to 25% of patients who undergo gastric resection and reconstruction will experience a constellation of acute or chronic symptoms referred to as "postgastrectomy syndromes."
- A combination of nausea, emesis, abdominal pain, malnutrition, and vasomotor symptoms such as palpitations, lightheadedness, and tachycardia.
- The majority of post gastrectomy difficulties can take up to a year to resolve and can be managed with dietary modifications and medications (eg, octreotide or acarbose with dumping).
- Dumping syndrome, bile reflux gastritis, afferent/efferent loop syndrome, and Roux stasis syndrome are among the most encountered surgically managed syndromes following gastric surgery.[1]

DIFFERENTIAL DIAGNOSIS

- The differential diagnosis for nausea, vomiting, and abdominal pain following an operation on the stomach includes mechanical or structural causes including small intestinal obstruction, anastomotic stricture, postoperative adhesions, peptic ulcer, gastroparesis, and neoplastic growth with lymphadenopathy.
- The differential diagnosis for malnutrition and vasomotor symptoms also includes inflammatory bowel disease, irritable bowel syndrome, and bacterial overgrowth.

PATIENT HISTORY AND PHYSICAL FINDINGS

- There is no pathognomonic physical finding to diagnose a postgastrectomy syndrome. A careful history focusing on severity and chronicity of abdominal and vasomotor symptoms is important. Physical examination findings regarding abdominal tenderness can help determine urgency of surgical needs and help work through possible syndromes.
- Afferent limb obstruction, marked by immediate nausea, and pain after eating accompanied by bilious emesis leading to relief of the pain. Laboratory findings may include elevated liver function tests and increased amylase from duodenal limb obstruction.
- Dumping syndrome—abdominal pain/discomfort within 15 to 30 minutes (early) or 2 to 3 hours (late) of eating accompanied by vasomotor symptoms (diaphoresis, tachycardia, hypoglycemia in late dumping).
- Bile reflux gastritis—nausea, bilious vomiting, epigastric pain not improved after emesis, testing demonstrating reflux.
- Roux stasis syndrome—vomiting, epigastric pain, weight loss following gastrectomy with Roux-en-Y gastrojejunostomy due to poor motility in the Roux limb.

IMAGING AND OTHER DIAGNOSTIC STUDIES

- The diagnosis cannot be definitively made with physical examination findings or history alone; however, imaging and other ancillary studies can confirm the diagnosis.
- Dumping syndrome—oral glucose challenge, gastric scintigraphy.
- Bile reflux gastritis—esophagogastroduodenoscopy (EGD), gastric pH probe.
- Afferent/efferent loop syndrome—computed tomography (CT), upper gastrointestinal (GI) barium study, EGD, hepatobiliary iminodiacetic acid (HIDA) scan.
- Roux stasis syndrome—upper GI barium study, gastric scintigraphy.

SURGICAL MANAGEMENT

See **TABLE 1**.

Preoperative Planning

- An attempt should be made at pharmacologic management of dumping syndrome and bile reflux gastritis.
- Nutritional assessment:
  - Owing to the significant nutritional abnormalities associated with postgastrectomy syndromes, all patients should have a complete blood count, metabolic panel, and albumin/prealbumin levels collected preoperatively. Micronutrient levels are also essential to assess. Anemias occur in up to one-third of patients, often secondary to iron, folate, and/or B12 deficiencies. Patients who have undergone gastrectomy procedures that divert the food stream away from the duodenum, where calcium is absorbed, may experience calcium deficiencies. Finally, bacterial overgrowth in the afferent limb or inadequate mixing of food with digestive enzymes may lead to poor absorption of fat-soluble vitamins. Supplementation with protein-rich drinks, vitamins, and even parenteral nutrition may be necessary to optimize the patient for surgery.[2]

Table 1: Surgical Management of Postgastrectomy Syndromes

Syndrome	Surgical technique
Dumping	Takedown of a loop gastrojejunostomy, Roux-en-Y gastrojejunostomy
Afferent loop syndrome	Roux-en-Y gastrojejunostomy Excision of redundant loop Braun enteroenterostomy
Bile reflux gastritis	Braun enteroenterostomy, the interposition of 40-cm isoperistaltic jejunal loop between the gastric remnant and duodenum (Henley loop)
Roux stasis syndrome	Excision of original Roux limb

387

- Antibiotics:
  - Routine antibiotic prophylaxis is encouraged, with a first-generation cephalosporin preferred for elective surgeries. In the setting of acute bowel obstruction or perforation, broad-spectrum antibiotic coverage is recommended. All perioperative antibiotics should be administered within 60 minutes of the initial skin incision.
- Venous thrombosis prophylaxis.
- The use of pneumatic compression devices at the start of surgery and continuing through recovery is now the standard of care to prevent deep vein thrombosis. The addition of chemoprophylaxis with the use of heparin or low-molecular-weight heparin may be considered given the length of general anesthesia time depending on the patient's age, body mass index, and other risk factors.

Positioning

- Procedures should be approached minimally invasively or open, depending on the patient's prior abdominal surgical history and surgeon expertise.
- For a minimally invasive approach, the patient is positioned split leg with adequate padding and both arms tucked, footboard to prevent slippage during procedure.
- The patient is positioned supine for the open approach with both arms extending on arm boards.

TECHNIQUES

CONVERSION OF BILLROTH II ANASTOMOSIS TO ROUX-EN-Y RECONSTRUCTION

This technique will describe the revision of a Billroth II gastrojejunostomy to a Roux-en-Y reconstruction (**FIGURE 1**).

Exploration

- Adhesiolysis as necessary.
- Run the small bowel.
- Inspection of the previous gastric anastomosis is essential to isolate the proximal/afferent and distal/efferent limbs.

Takedown of the Gastrojejunostomy

- Divide the bowel proximal to the BII gastrojejunal anastomosis with a blue load linear cutting stapler—this will be the pancreaticobiliary/afferent limb.
- Transect the gastrojejunostomy using sequential loads of the blue load linear cutting stapler.

Creation of New Gastrojejunostomy

- If delayed gastric emptying has been a component of the issues, consider resection of the gastric pouch to <25% remnant.
- Place the patient in steep reverse Trendelenburg position.
- Ensure all tubes are removed from the stomach.
- Use a liver retractor to retract the left lobe of the liver to enhance view of gastric remnant.
- Create gastrotomy and enterotomy on the gastric remnant and the new Roux limb (former efferent limb).
- Focus on preserving orientation of the Roux limb without a twist in the small bowel mesentery.
- Insert the blue load stapler to create a side-to-side gastrojejunostomy.
- Close the common enterotomy using a 2-0 or 3-0 PDS Connell suture and 3-0 silk Lembert sutures overlying.

Creation of Jejunojejunostomy

- Refer to Chapters 37, 41, and 46 as similar techniques and pearls apply here.

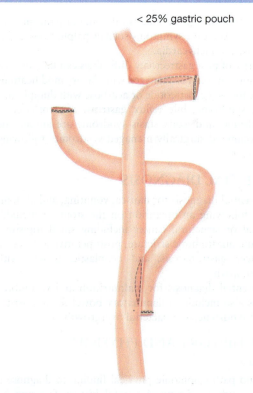

FIGURE 1 Approaches to management of postgastrectomy syndromes by conversion of Billroth II to Roux-en-Y gastrojejunostomy. (Redrawn from Dempsey DT, Milan JE. Postgastrectomy problems: remedial operations and therapy. In: Cameron A, ed. *Current Surgical Therapy*. 13th ed. Elsevier; 2021:85. Figure 6.)

- Swing afferent limb down 40 to 60 cm distal on the Roux limb to create jejunojejunostomy (to prevent bile reflux) using a side-to-side stapled anastomosis using a blue load of the linear cutting stapler.
- Close the common enterotomy with another firing of the linear cutting stapler.
- The mesenteric defect is closed using a running nonabsorbable suture.
- A crotch silk stitch is placed to stabilize the anastomosis.
- Assure hemostasis and no leakage at the jejunostomy site.

BRAUN ENTEROENTEROSTOMY (FIGURE 2)

- Identify the gastrojejunal anastomosis in Billroth II configuration.
- Create side-to-side anastomosis between the afferent and efferent limbs approximately 40 to 60 cm from the gastrojejunal anastomosis. We prefer a hand-sewn anastomosis approximately 3 cm wide using V-Loc sutures.

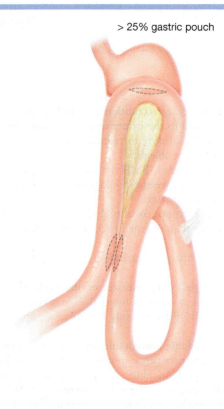

> 25% gastric pouch

FIGURE 2 • Approaches to management of postgastrectomy syndromes by conversion of Billroth II to Braun enteroenterostomy. (Redrawn from Dempsey DT, Milan JE. Postgastrectomy problems: remedial operations and therapy. In: Cameron A, ed. *Current Surgical Therapy*. 13th ed. Elsevier; 2021:85. Figure 6.)

HENLEY JEJUNAL INTERPOSITION

- May be considered for intractable bile reflux after Bilroth I/II gastrectomy reconstruction.
- Isoperistaltic 40-cm segment of proximal jejunum placed between the gastric remnant and the duodenum.

POSTOPERATIVE CARE

- Fluids and electrolytes should be maintained, given the decreased size of the stomach. Therefore, clear liquids are initiated on postoperative day 1 with gradual advancement of oral intake.

OUTCOMES

- About 80% to 90% of patients who undergo Roux-en-Y reconstruction for dumping syndrome will have complete resolution of symptoms. These findings are similar for afferent loop syndrome and bile reflux gastritis as a similar percentage of patients achieve lasting resolution.[3,4]
- Pain is sometimes persistent following reconstruction, and patients should be counseled regarding that possibility.[3]

COMPLICATIONS

Roux-en-Y reconstruction is subject to similar complications of other intra-abdominal operations including infectious complications (abscess, sepsis), structural complications (anastomotic stricture/dehiscence, bowel obstruction), gastric retention, and ulcers.

Also, one must be cognizant of the risk of internal hernia and Roux syndrome.[2,3]

REFERENCES

1. Soriano IS, Dumon KR, Dempsey DT. Benign gastric disorders. In: Zinner MJ, Ashley SW, Hines OJ, eds. *Maingot's Abdominal Operations*. McGraw-Hill Education; 2019:13e.
2. Davis JL, Ripley RT. Postgastrectomy syndromes and nutritional considerations following gastric surgery. *Surg Clin North Am*. 2017;97(2):277-293. doi:10.1016/j.suc.2016.11.005
3. Meilahn JED, Daniel T. Postgastrectomy problems: remedial operations and therapy. In Cameron JL, ed. *Current Surgical Therapy*. 8th ed. Elsevier Mosby; 2004:1343 pages, chap xxxviii; illustrations; 29 cm.
4. Vogel SB, Hocking MP, Woodward ER. Clinical and radionuclide evaluation of Roux-Y diversion for postgastrectomy dumping. *Am J Surg*. 1988;155(1):57-62. doi:10.1016/s0002-9610(88)80258-7

Chapter 46 Laparoscopic Gastric Bypass

Tuesday F. A. Cook, Elizabeth A. Dovec, and Shaneeta M. Johnson

DEFINITION

- Obesity is a medical condition in which excess body fat has accumulated to the extent that it may have an adverse effect on health, leading to reduced life expectancy and/or increased health problems.[1]
- The body mass index (BMI) is a measurement obtained by dividing a person's weight in kilograms by the square of the person's height in meters.[2]
  - BMI greater than or equal to 30 kg/m² is *class I obesity*.
  - BMI greater than or equal to 35 to 39.9 kg/m² is *class II obesity*.
  - BMI greater than or equal to 40 to 49.9 kg/m² is *class III obesity*.
- BMI is one aspect of the measure of obesity; however, metabolic changes can occur at lower BMI in specific ethnicities as well as with different body habitus, e.g., apple vs pear shape.
- Obesity is a leading preventable cause of death worldwide, with increasing prevalence in adults and children. In 2016, more than 1.9 billion adults, 18 years and older, were overweight. Of these, over 650 million were obese. As of 2021, most of the world's population live in countries where overweight and obesity kills more people than underweight.[3]
- A complex, multifactorial disease, with genetic, behavioral, socioeconomic, and environmental origins, and lack of treatment portends an epidemic of overweight and obesity presenting a major challenge to chronic disease prevention and health across the life course around the world.[4]
- Obesity is linked to more than 40 other diseases including type 2 diabetes, heart disease, stroke, and certain types of cancer.[5] Furthermore, in 2013, the American Medical Association recognized obesity as a distinct disease.[6]

PATIENT HISTORY AND PHYSICAL FINDINGS

- Patients should undergo comprehensive preoperative evaluation, with cardiopulmonary workup as needed. Multidisciplinary support with attention to evaluation of behavioral modification, dietary counseling, and exercise medicine is provided for optimum outcome.
- A thorough history should be performed prior to treatment, including a detailed past medical and surgical history, present medications and allergies, family history, social history and previous attempts at weight loss, or an aberrant relationship with food.
- Obesity-related comorbidities include metabolic syndrome, hypertension, dyslipidemia, diabetes mellitus, obstructive sleep apnea, chronic obstructive pulmonary disease, congestive heart failure, coronary artery disease, vascular disease, renal failure, urinary stress incontinence, polycystic ovarian syndrome (PCOS), back pain, joint pain, infertility, pseudotumor cerebri, and anxiety/depression.
- More information continues to develop regarding obesity and its association with metabolic factors including the role of leptin and adiponectin. Adipose tissue in conjunction with the hypothalamic–pituitary–adrenal axis and dysregulation of incretin hormone secretion continues to be studied.[7]

SURGICAL MANAGEMENT

- The goals of the surgical treatment of obesity include
  - Improving health
  - Improving quality of life
  - Increasing the life span
- The American Society of Metabolic and Bariatric Surgery (ASMBS) and the National Institutes of Health (NIH) have reached several conclusions about bariatric surgery and formulated a consensus statement. These organizations agree that metabolic/bariatric surgery is the most effective treatment for morbid obesity.
- For years, gastric bypass had been the gold standard in the treatment of patients with class III obesity (BMI of ≥40 kg/m²) and class II obesity (≥35-39.9 kg/m²) with obesity-associated comorbidities. It has been performed in the United States for more than half a century. It is now the second most commonly performed bariatric operation in the United States.
- A Roux-en-Y gastric bypass is a restrictive and malabsorptive procedure. There are also a myriad of metabolic changes that occur with this operation, including modifications in levels of GLP-1, GLP-2, PYY, insulin, oxyntomodulin, and obestatin, to name a few.[8]

Preoperative Planning

- Preoperative education is a vital part to the success of the patient. Patients must be instructed on what to expect both preoperatively and postoperatively.
- All patients should undergo a surgical evaluation, medical clearances, insurance requirements, psychological evaluation, nutrition education, information seminars, and attend a support group prior to their surgery. In our practice, a preoperative class and bariatric surgery test with discussion is also mandatory.
- A detailed bariatric diet guideline packet is provided to all patients describing each diet phase as well as discussion of vitamins for life. Documented understanding of the dietary expectations is imperative.
- Enhanced Recovery After Bariatric Surgery (ERABS) is paramount to decreased opioid use and early return to activities of daily living as well as decreased length of stay. This includes short preoperative fast, preoperative gabapentin and acetaminophen for preemptive analgesia, preoperative scopolamine patch and intraoperative dexamethasone, and nerve blocks for both pain and nausea control. Encouraging early ambulation in the recovery room, day of surgery

liquid diet and regularly scheduled analgesia and antiemetics instead of PRN, yields excellent outcomes.
- Sequential compression devices are placed and function confirmed prior to the induction of general anesthesia.
- Routine venous thromboembolism (VTE) prophylaxis with subcutaneous anticoagulation administration is administered for all patients in preoperative holding and continues for all patients for at least 14 days postoperation.
- Any patients with obstructive sleep apnea must bring their continuous positive airway pressure machine to the hospital for immediate use upon arrival to the post anesthesia care unit.

Positioning

- The patient is placed on the table in supine position and secured to the bed. The patient confirms comfort prior to general endotracheal anesthesia. After satisfactory anesthesia had been administered, the patient is secured additionally to the bed with care taken to avoid pressure points for neuropathy. A thick, wide strap is placed tightly above the knees and padded well. Support is placed under the patient's knees. A padded footboard is pushed firmly to the patient's feet allowing the feet to turn out slightly, being cognizant not to bow the knees (**FIGURE 1**).
- The left arm is left out at a 75° angle and secured to the arm board with a gauze wrap. The bed is positioned down as low as possible.
- The operating surgeon stands on the patient's right side on an elevated platform, while the assisting surgeon stands on the patient's left side.
- A nasogastric tube is placed in the patient's stomach and allowed to drain. No other devices except the nasogastric tube and endotracheal tube should be in the patient's mouth.

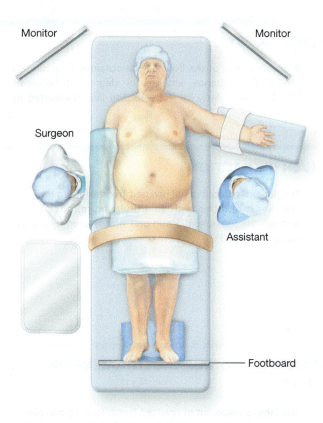

FIGURE 1 • Patient positioning.

- A verbal check for a temperature probe is performed at the initial time out and before any stapling occurs. This is confirmed by the anesthesiologist and circulating nurse.

PLACEMENT OF INCISIONS

- A 5-mm left subcostal trocar is placed 2 cm below the costal margin in the anterior axillary line using an optical entry. Pneumoperitoneum is then established. The abdominal cavity is then inspected for acute pathology, hernias, and adhesions. Additionally, the bowel is inspected to ensure there was no injury from the initial trocar placement. A transversus abdominis plane block is performed bilaterally with bupivacaine and dexamethasone to provide preemptive analgesia. The skin and underlying fascia is injected with local anesthetic for all trocar sites. The remaining five ports are placed under direct visualization. Two 12-mm ports are placed a handsbreadth below the xiphoid on the left and right of the midline. An additional 5-mm port in placed in the right subcostal region followed by a 5-mm liver retractor in the subxiphoid region (**FIGURE 2**).

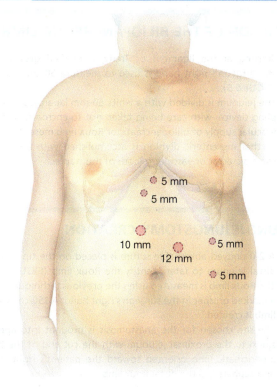

FIGURE 2 • Port placement.

LIVER BIOPSY

- A needle biopsy of the liver may be obtained to accurately predict the presence, absence, or degree of histologic changes due to fatty liver disease. The liver is elevated by two bowel graspers placed through the left lateral ports to ensure the biopsy needle does not go through the liver and cause injury to underlying structures. Two core biopsies are obtained from the left lateral segment of the liver for pathologic examination for the diagnosis and staging of nonalcoholic fatty liver disease.

LIVER RETRACTION

- The patient is placed in full reversed Trendelenburg position. The liver is retracted with an articulating retractor placed through the subxiphoid 5-mm port and secured by a table clamp (FIGURE 3).

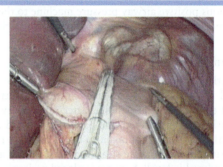

FIGURE 3 • Liver retraction and vertical 60-mm stapler.

IDENTIFICATION OF THE LIGAMENT OF TREITZ

- The table is taken out of reversed Trendelenburg and placed in the supine position. The omentum is retracted cephalad, exposing the transverse mesocolon, which is also elevated and retracted cephalad. The proximal jejunum is retracted to expose the ligament of Treitz and the inferior mesenteric vein (FIGURE 4).

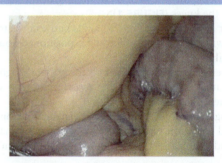

FIGURE 4 • Identification of the ligament of Treitz.

CREATION OF THE BILIOPANCREATIC LIMB

- Starting at the ligament of Treitz, a marked grasper in the surgeon's right hand is used to measure 50 cm distally (FIGURE 5).
- The jejunum is divided with a white 60-mm laparoscopic stapling device, with care being taken not to encroach on the vascular supply of biliopancreatic or Roux limb mesentery.
- Further mesenteric division is accomplished with an ultrasonic dissector or vascular reloads of the stapler.

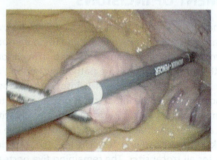

FIGURE 5 • Measurement of the biliopancreatic limb.

JEJUNOJEJUNOSTOMY CREATION

- A 2-0 undyed absorbable suture is placed on the tip of the distal jejunum to later identify the Roux limb (FIGURE 6). The Roux limb is measured using the previous technique with a marked grasper in the surgeon's right hand. A 150-cm Roux limb is created.
- The site chosen for the anastomosis is brought into apposition to the proximal jejunum with the cut end of the biliopancreatic limb oriented toward the patient's right side and cephalad to the distal Roux limb.

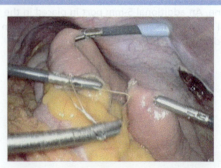

FIGURE 6 • Roux limb identification suture.

- A stay suture of 2-0 absorbable suture is placed through the Roux limb and biliopancreatic limb approximately 3 cm from the biliopancreatic tip.
- An ultrasonic dissector is used to make enterotomies in the biliopancreatic and Roux limbs.
- A white 60-mm laparoscopic stapling device is placed into the enterotomies to construct a side-to-side jejunojejunostomy. Hemostasis of the staple line is assured.
- A suture is placed to appose the common enterotomy in the center. The assistant orients the common enterotomy into a slit rather than a circle oriented at 1 and 7 o'clock.
- A white 60-mm laparoscopic staple reload is used to close the common enterotomy. This enteroenterostomy is also hand-sewn to closure in some instances.
- An antikinking stitch is placed to avoid kinking of the Roux limb at the jejunojejunostomy suturing the biliopancreatic limb to the Roux limb (**FIGURE 7**).

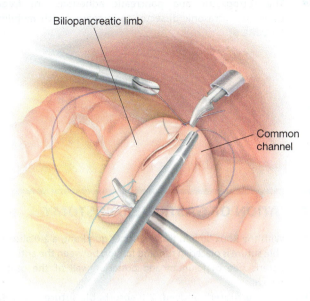

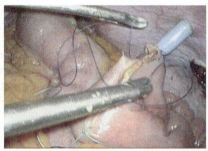

FIGURE 7 • Closure of enterotomy defect before starting to sew.

CLOSURE OF MESENTERIC DEFECT

- The mesenteric defect is closed in a running, locking fashion with 2-0 nonabsorbable suture (**FIGURE 8**).

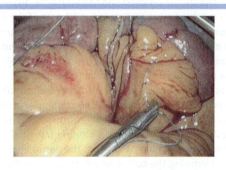

FIGURE 8 • Closure of mesenteric defect.

DIVISION OF GREATER OMENTUM

- The patient is placed in full reversed Trendelenburg position. The omentum is divided vertically, toward the direction of the liver retractor, with the ultrasonic dissector to facilitate bringing the Roux limb up to the gastric pouch. This step can be omitted if the omentum is thin or if the Roux limb is placed in the retrocolic retrogastric position.

GASTRIC POUCH CREATION

- The pars flaccida is opened and the lesser sac is entered. The left gastric artery is identified and preserved. 2 to 4 cm is measured down from the gastroesophageal junction along the lesser curve.
- Successive firings of the laparoscopic stapling device are performed to fashion a gastric pouch.
- With the gastric lavage tube or endoscope retracted into the esophagus by the anesthetist, the angle of His is exposed and dissected with an ultrasonic dissector.
- Identification, dissection, and primary posterior repair of a hiatal hernia is done at this time, if necessary.
- Complete transaction of the stomach and hemostasis are ensured by inspecting the entire staple line. Once divided, the gastric lavage tube is retracted back into the esophagus.

- The retrogastric and pancreatic adhesions are freed using the ultrasonic dissector to increase pouch mobility (**FIGURE 9**).

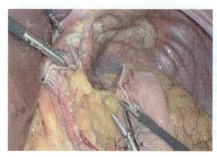

FIGURE 9 • Completed pouch.

CREATION OF GASTROJEJUNOSTOMY

- With the Roux limb in the left upper quadrant, a 2-0 absorbable suture is placed in running fashion between the antimesenteric side of jejunum and posterior wall of the gastric pouch.
- An interrupted, undyed, 2-0 absorbable suture is placed 1.5 cm from the running suture on the antimesenteric side of the Roux limb and posterior wall of the gastric pouch.
- An adequate gastrotomy is created at the transverse staple line of the gastric pouch using an ultrasonic device.
- An adequate enterotomy is created by entering the Roux limb. Care should be taken not to injure the posterior wall of the jejunum.
- A side-to-side gastrojejunostomy is created using the laparoscopic stapler. The assistant orients the tip of Roux limb so that it is in line with the stapler as it is inserted to the 20-mm mark. The stapler is closed and fired (**FIGURE 10**).
- While the assistant continues to hold the tip of the Roux limb in approximation with the gastric pouch, the surgeon places a 2-0 absorbable stitch between the Roux limb and the gastric pouch just beyond the apex of the gastrojejunostomy staple line to suspend the jejunum to the pouch.
- The assistant distracts the absorbable and nonabsorbable sutures to orient the gastrojejunostomy into a slit rather than a circle. The first layer of the gastrojejunostomy is closed using 2-0 absorbable suture in a running fashion. The bougie or endoscope is then passed across the gastrojejunostomy to prevent suturing the back wall and to calibrate the opening. After completion of the first row, an anterior suture layer is placed (**FIGURE 11**).
- Note that the creation of the gastrojejunostomy can be performed using several different techniques.
    - Completely handsewn in two layers (Connell suturing technique)
    - Use of a circular stapler (associated with increased rate of anastomotic stricture, bleeding, wound infection)[9]
    - Linear stapler, with handsewn closure of the resulting opening
    - Linear stapler for both anastomosis and closure of the opening

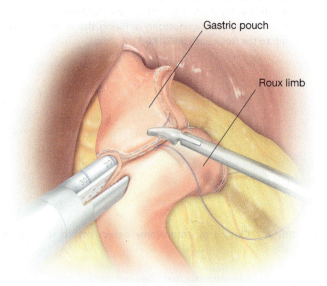

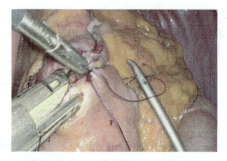

FIGURE 10 • Stapling the gastrojejunostomy.

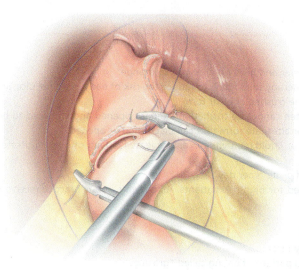
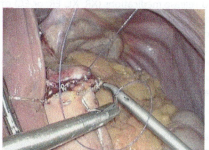

FIGURE 11 • Closure of gastrojejunostomy.

CLOSURE OF PETERSEN DEFECT

- The mesenteries of the biliopancreatic, Roux limb, and transverse mesocolon are all secured with a 2-0 nonabsorbable suture to obliterate a potential hernia site at Petersen defect.

UPPER ENDOSCOPY LEAK TEST

- The Roux limb is occluded with a bowel clamp approximately 2 cm distal to the gastrojejunostomy. The assistant retracts the distal gastric remnant and omentum to keep the gastrojejunostomy in view. With the patient placed in Trendelenburg position, the gastric pouch, gastrojejunostomy, and tip of the Roux limb are submerged under saline (FIGURE 12).
- An endoscope is passed across the gastrojejunostomy to ensure its integrity, hemostasis, and patency. The scope is withdrawn into the pouch, which is inflated with air from the endoscope. The submerged areas are inspected for bubbling indicating an opening, which, if present, is located and repaired with 2-0 absorbable suture. The test is then repeated until there is no further leaking observed. The endoscope is removed, saline is aspirated from the

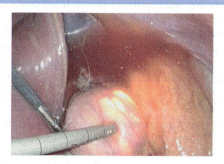

FIGURE 12 • Placement of bowel clamp. Submerged anastomosis with light transilluminating the jejunum.

abdominal cavity, all instruments are removed, and the trocars are removed under direct visualization to ensure hemostasis.

SKIN CLOSURE

- The fascia of the 12-mm trocar sites is closed using 0 absorbable sutures.
- The skin is closed with 4-0 absorbable monofilament suture in a subcuticular fashion. A waterproof sterile adhesive is placed to close the epidermis.

PEARLS AND PITFALLS

Pearls

- The use of sterile adhesive allows the patient to shower and have no dressings to change.
- Patients are maintained on proton pump inhibitor therapy for 30 days to reduce the risk of early marginal ulceration.
- Initially, all medications should be administered in the crushed or elixir form.
- Extended-release medications (XR, XL, ER, or EC) often cannot be crushed, broken, or opened and will need to be changed by their prescribing provider to an immediate release or alternate form that can be crushed or opened.
- Daily supplements with an adult strength chewable or liquid multivitamin and at least 1200 mg of calcium citrate with vitamin D are recommended.
- Long-term dietary goals should include 70 to 90 g of protein per day.
- Home anticoagulation regimen should be considered for high-risk patients. All patients in our practice receive chemical VTE prophylaxis, unless menstruation ensues.

Pitfalls

- Liquid calories and sweets can cause late dumping syndrome.
- Snacking should be avoided to prevent developing a pattern of eating called "grazing."
- Pregnancy is not recommended in the first 18 months after surgery.
- Patient's fertility may increase after surgery and weight loss.
- Birth control pills alone may not be effective for birth control after surgery. Patients are instructed to speak with their gynecologist regarding other methods of birth control.
- Smoking and NSAID use has been associated with higher rates of marginal ulcer.

POSTOPERATIVE CARE

- ERABS protocols are used to accelerate recovery, decrease morbidity, and decrease length of stay. It requires a multidisciplinary approach including the anesthesiologists, nursing, dieticians, and team. It starts preoperatively and extends into the operating room. The postoperative phase includes early feeding, e.g. day of surgery, multimodal analgesic and antiemetic regimen, prophylaxis against atelectasis, and early ambulation.

OUTCOMES

- The long-term average weight loss after a Roux-en-Y gastric bypass is 60% to 70% of excess body weight.
- There is usually rapid resolution of comorbidities such as diabetes mellitus, sleep apnea, hyperlipidemia, and gastroesophageal reflux disease.

COMPLICATIONS

- Early serious complications (<30 days) include gastrointestinal bleeding, bowel obstruction, anastomotic leak, intra-abdominal abscess, deep vein thrombosis, pulmonary embolism, wound infection, and mortality, all of which should be less than 1% in experienced centers.
- Late complications (>30 days) include bowel obstruction, anastomotic stenosis, marginal ulceration, gastrointestinal bleeding, cholelithiasis, internal herniation, gastrogastric fistula, vitamin deficiencies, and mortality.

REFERENCES

1. Haslam DW, James WP. Obesity. *Lancet*. 2005;366(9492):1197-1209.
2. *Healthy Weight, Assessing Your Weight*. CDC." Centers for Disease Control and Prevention. Accessed 15 October 2021. https://www.cdc.gov/healthyweight/assessing/bmi/index.html
3. *Obesity and Overweight Facts*. World Health Organization; 2021. Accessed 15 October 2021. https://www.who.int/news-room/fact-sheets/detail/obesity-and-overweight
4. Hruby A, Hu FB. The epidemiology of obesity: a big picture. *Pharmacoeconomics*. 2015;33(7):673-689. doi:10.1007/s40273-014-0243-x
5. *Adult Obesity Facts, Overweight & Obesity*. CDC." Centers for Disease Control and Prevention; 2018. Accessed 15 October 2021. www.cdc.gov/obesity/data/adult.html
6. *Recognition of Obesity as a Disease H-440.842*. Public Health. AMA Policy Finder; Accessed 24 October 2021. https://policysearch.ama-assn.org/policyfinder/detail/obesity
7. Michałowska J, Miller-Kasprzak E, Bogdański P. Incretin hormones in obesity and related cardiometabolic disorders: the clinical perspective. *Nutrients*. 2021;13(2):351. doi:10.3390/nu13020351
8. Dimitriadis GK, Randeva MS, Miras AD. Potential hormone mechanisms of bariatric surgery. *Curr Obes Rep*. 2017;6(3):253-265. doi:10.1007/s13679-017-0276-5
9. Jiang HP, Lin LL, Jiang X, Qiao HQ. Meta-analysis of hand-sewn versus mechanical gastrojejunal anastomosis during laparoscopic Roux-en-Y gastric bypass for morbid obesity. *Int J Surg*. 2016;32:150-157. ISSN 1743-9191, doi:10.1016/j.ijsu.2016.04.024

Chapter 47 Laparoscopic Sleeve Gastrectomy

Ozanan R. Meireles, Eric G. Sheu, and Matthew M. Hutter

DEFINITION

- Sleeve gastrectomy or partial vertical gastrectomy is defined as the creation of tubular, sleeve-shaped, lesser curve–based stomach by resection of the greater curvature of the gastric body and fundus.
- Laparoscopic sleeve gastrectomy (LSG) has become the most popular bariatric and metabolic procedure due to its relative technical simplicity and excellent safety and efficacy profile. As of 2022, the great majority of insurers have been covering the sleeve gastrectomy, and the number of LSG performed in the United States has grown rapidly in the last several years to become the most performed bariatric and metabolic in the country.
- LSG was initially performed as the first stage of the biliopancreatic diversion–duodenal switch procedure. However, beginning in 2008, LSG has been performed as a stand-alone bariatric operation, and medium-term and long-term follow-up have documented its safety and efficacy.[1]
- In 2010, a Current Procedural Terminology (CPT) code was assigned to the procedure and, in 2017, the American Society for Metabolic and Bariatric Surgery, which has previously recognized LSG as an approved primary bariatric procedure, issued an updated position statement based on long-term outcome data published in the peer-reviewed literature, acknowledging that LSG provides significant and durable weight loss, improvements in medical comorbidities, improved quality of life, and low complication and mortality rates for the treatment of morbid obesity.[2]

PATIENT HISTORY AND PHYSICAL FINDINGS

- A complete history and physical examination should be obtained, with particular attention given to history or identification of metabolic disorders such as diabetes, dyslipidemia, and fatty liver disease; cardiovascular disease; obstructive sleep apnea; venous thromboembolism; and a history of previous abdominal operations.
- Per National Institutes of Health (NIH) consensus guidelines, bariatric surgery is indicated for patients with a body mass index (BMI) greater than 40 or a BMI greater than 35 with obesity-associated comorbidities. Insurers and payers, though, may have other stipulations.
- A detailed nutritional history, including prior attempts at weight loss through dietary, exercise, and medical programs, and psychologic/psychiatric history should be obtained.
- Multidisciplinary evaluation with registered dietitians, psychologists, and medical physicians is critical prior to consideration for any bariatric surgery.

IMAGING AND OTHER DIAGNOSTIC STUDIES

- In the absence of history or physical findings suggestive of upper gastrointestinal (GI) pathology, preprocedural imaging is not mandatory.
- However, symptoms such as dysphagia, early satiety, or odynophagia should prompt further radiologic or endoscopic evaluation.
- In our practice, some find a preoperative barium swallow helpful to rule out gross esophageal motility disorder; assess for hiatal hernias; and exclude mass lesions, stricture, diverticula, and other anatomic abnormalities. Others get a swallow study only if the history and symptoms raise any concerns.
- Subsequent upper endoscopy can then be selectively used to follow up any concerning findings from the swallow study.
- When esophageal dysmotility is suspected based on history or swallow study, preoperative esophageal manometry is obtained.

SURGICAL MANAGEMENT

Preoperative Planning

- Preoperative laboratory, pulmonary, and cardiac evaluation are performed as indicated by patient history, age, and comorbidities as with other major abdominal surgery.
- Patients should be encouraged to lose as much weight as possible leading up to surgery. We place our patients on a low caloric diet 2 to 3 weeks before surgery in order to decrease the volume and rigidity of the left lobe of the liver, facilitate laparoscopic exposure, and allow for a less technically demanding and safer operation.
- Appropriate antibiotic and venous thromboembolism prophylaxis should be administered in a timely fashion.

Positioning

- The patient is positioned supine or in the split-leg position according to the surgeon's preference. Specialized bariatric beds are available to accommodate the super obese and allow for ergonomic positioning of the patient. The arms and legs should be well secured along with a footboard to allow steep reverse Trendelenburg to facilitate visualization of the left upper quadrant intraoperatively. An orogastric tube should be placed to decompress the stomach after endotracheal intubation.

PORT PLACEMENT

- Initial peritoneal access is obtained using the surgeon's preferred method. Pneumoperitoneum is created, and subsequent ports are placed under direct visualization. Many geometric arrangements for port placement will allow adequate exposure for the operation. In general, five ports in the upper abdomen will allow adequate access and visualization for the operation. These will usually include two working ports for the operating surgeon and ports for the camera, liver retractor, and assistant. At least one 12-mm or 15-mm trocar is required to allow introduction of a stapler. Two example diagrams of port placement are shown in **FIGURE 1**.

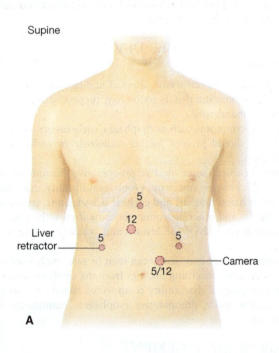
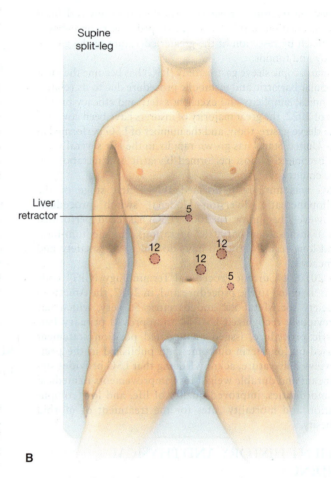

FIGURE 1 • Port placement. Schematic illustration of typical port placements for sleeve gastrectomy in supine positioning **(A)** and split-leg positioning **(B)**.

MOBILIZATION OF THE STOMACH

- After exploration of the peritoneal cavity, the patient is placed into steep reverse Trendelenburg position to drop away the intestines and omentum, and a liver retractor is placed to expose the stomach and hiatus.
- The pylorus is identified and the distal margin of the sleeve is measured within 2 to 6 cm proximal to the pylorus (**FIGURE 2A** and **B**). The greater curvature of the stomach is mobilized by transecting the gastrocolic ligament and short gastric vessels. An ultrasonic or bipolar vessel-sealing device speeds this dissection (**FIGURE 3**). Proximally, the vessels are divided up to the highest short gastric, a reliable landmark which often dives posteriorly toward the pancreas (**FIGURE 4**). We find that complete mobilization of the angle of His from the left crus of the diaphragm and freeing of any lesser sac attachments to the pancreas or posterior gastric space facilitates subsequent formation of the gastric sleeve. These attachments are often avascular and can be taken sharply. Complete mobilization to allow adequate resection of the fundus is believed to be a critical step of sleeve gastrectomy.[3]
- The surgeon should look for a hiatal hernia and fix it should it be readily evident. We do not promote the routine dissection of the hiatus to identify a "hiatal hernia" that is not readily apparent.

Chapter 47 LAPAROSCOPIC SLEEVE GASTRECTOMY 399

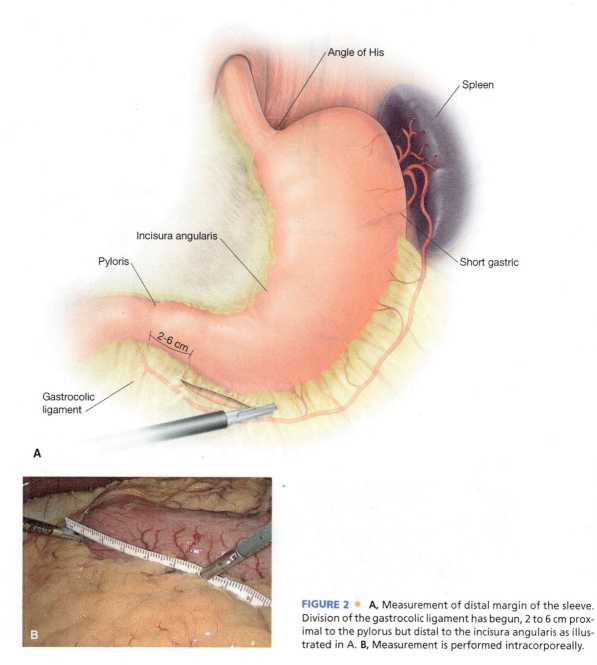

FIGURE 2 • **A,** Measurement of distal margin of the sleeve. Division of the gastrocolic ligament has begun, 2 to 6 cm proximal to the pylorus but distal to the incisura angularis as illustrated in A. **B,** Measurement is performed intracorporeally.

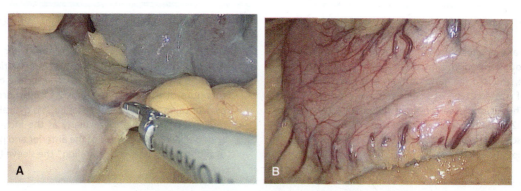

FIGURE 3 • Division of short gastrics and gastrocolic ligament. **A,** The gastrocolic ligament and short gastric vessels are divided using an ultrasonic dissector. **B,** Final view of the distal margin of the dissection as previously measured from the pylorus is shown.

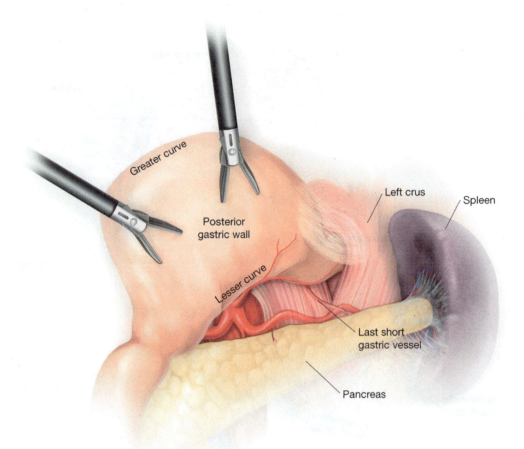

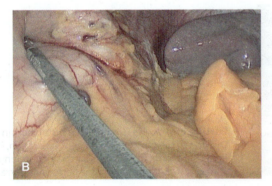

FIGURE 4 • **A,** Complete mobilization of gastric fundus from the diaphragm and lesser sac. The last short gastric vessel often dives posterior and into the pancreas and is a reliable anatomic landmark. **B,** The gastric fundus is fully mobilized up to the left crus of the diaphragm, and lesser sac attachments are dissected to facilitate subsequent stapling.

CREATION OF THE GASTRIC SLEEVE

- Accurate and safe formation of the gastric sleeve is performed using a bougie introduced into the oropharynx, down the lesser curvature, and into the gastric antrum as a guide (**FIGURE 5**). Choice of size and type of bougie remains a surgeon's preference. The recent sleeve consensus statement recommended use of a 32- to 36-Fr bougie.[3] Various Maloney dilators or flexible endoscopes may be used as a bougie. Our practice is to use the therapeutic endoscope (36 Fr in caliber) to size the sleeve, which we find helpful to later perform a provocative leak test and examine our staple line endoluminally.
- With the chosen bougie in place, and after confirmation that no other intragastric tubes (eg, orogastric tubes, temperature probes) remain in place, transection of the greater curvature of the stomach begins 2 to 6 cm proximal to the pylorus using a linear cutting stapler. It is critical to avoid narrowing of the sleeve, particularly at the incisura angularis, and to take equal portions of the anterior and posterior walls of the stomach to avoid "spiraling" the sleeve (**FIGURE 6**).

Chapter 47 LAPAROSCOPIC SLEEVE GASTRECTOMY   401

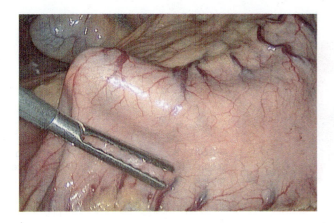

- The gastric sleeve formation is completed with subsequent fires of the linear stapler along the bougie, thus resecting the greater curvature of the stomach. With each staple fire, continued care is made to assure that equal amounts of anterior and posterior gastric wall are resected (**FIGURE 7**). It is often helpful to have the assistant maintain lateral traction on the lateral aspect of the stomach and, at times, toward

FIGURE 5 • Placement of intragastric bougie. A bougie is placed along the lesser curvature into the antrum to guide formation of the sleeve. This illustration shows the use of an endoscope, which is easily manipulated to match the contour of the lesser curvature.

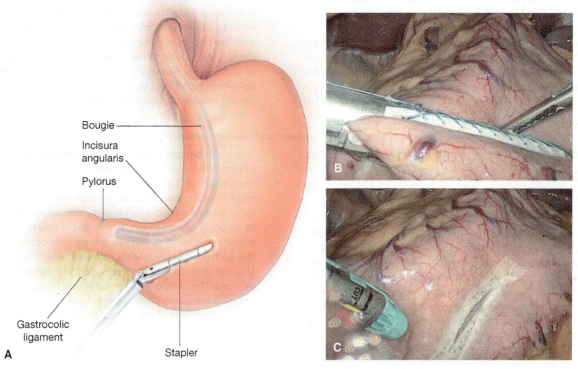

FIGURE 6 • **A,** Initial gastric transection around the incisura angularis. The initial staple fire begins at the previously measured distal division of the gastrocolic ligament and is **(B)** carefully placed to ensure no narrowing or angulation of the stomach at the incisura as well as to resect equal segments of anterior and posterior gastric wall. The initial staple line is shown in **(C)**.

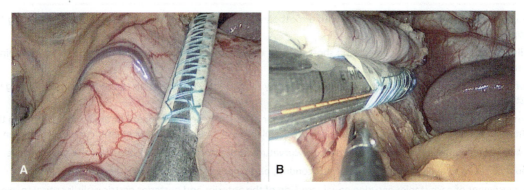

FIGURE 7 • Transection of greater curvature of stomach. Subsequent gastric transection is performed parallel to the lesser curvature, along the bougie, and aimed toward the angle of His. In these photographs, staple line buttressing material is used. The placement of the stapler is examined anteriorly **(A)** and posteriorly **(B)** to ensure equal alignment of the gastric walls.

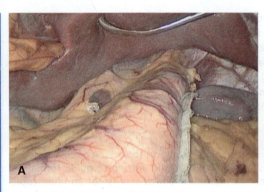
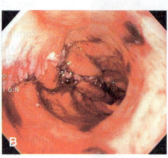

FIGURE 8 • Laparoscopic (A) and endoscopic (B) view of completed sleeve gastrectomy.

the posterior aspect. The final staple line should veer off the gastroesophageal junction as this area is particularly susceptible to leaks.[3] In **FIGURE 8**, a laparoscopic and endoscopic view of the completed sleeve is shown.

- Staple loads should be chosen as appropriate for the thickness of the tissue. The gastric wall is generally thickest on the initial distal staple line at the antrum. The use of staple line reinforcement is controversial. There is some evidence that staple line reinforcement may decrease the incidence of bleeding complications; however, any impact on leak rates is less clear. Several absorbable and permanent staple line buttressing materials are available. Some oversew an unreinforced staple line routinely, which should be performed with the bougie in place to prevent narrowing of the gastric conduit if it is done. Others prefer not to use reinforcements, or to routinely oversew, due to concerns of excessive material where staple lines cross, the added expense, and unclear benefit or potential harms from those practices.

PROVOCATIVE LEAK TEST AND HEMOSTASIS

- A provocative leak test can be performed after the sleeve is created, either with gas or liquid dye. Our practice is to submerge the staple line in saline irrigation while insufflating the sleeve with carbon dioxide (CO_2) via the indwelling endoscope and clamping the distal stomach. A laparoscopic assessment for evidence of leaks or bubbles is done, and simultaneously, an endoluminal examination is performed to exclude intraluminal bleeding and to assess the gastric conduit for any narrowing or kinking. Alternatively, insufflation or instillation with distention via a nasogastric or other device can be done with CO_2, air, or colored liquid; however, oxygen alone should not be used.
- Hemostasis of the staple line and divided gastrocolic ligament from the greater curvature vessels is ensured. Although some surgeons choose to recreate the gastrocolic ligament by suturing the omentum to the staple line in an effort to prevent torsion of the sleeve, we do not routinely do that. The gastrectomy specimen is removed, which can usually be accomplished using a protective bag without enlarging any incisions. The bougie, liver retractor, and trocars are removed under direct vision; pneumoperitoneum is released; and closure is performed of the extraction site with a fascial closure device.

PEARLS AND PITFALLS

- Secure positioning of the patients' extremities with a footboard is imperative to allow steep reverse Trendelenburg to optimize laparoscopic visualization.
- During division of the gastrocolic ligament and short gastrics, care should be taken to avoid injury to the gastroepiploic vessels and spleen.
- It is important to assure that the proximal fundus is completely mobilized by dissecting up to the left crus and taking the highest short gastric vessel.
- Freeing of lesser sac attachments to the pancreas and posterior gastric stomach and release of the angle of His from the left crus give additional mobility of the greater curve to allow precise placement of the stapler for greater curvature resection.
- A 32- to 40-Fr bougie should be placed along the lesser curvature of the stomach to aid in sizing of the gastric sleeve.
- Care should be taken to avoid narrowing the gastric conduit, particularly at the incisura angularis.
- Accurate placement of each stapler ensuring equal resection of the anterior and posterior gastric walls is critical to avoid spiraling of the sleeve, which could result in postoperative obstruction.
- Adequate hemostasis of the staple line and divided gastrocolic ligament from the greater curvature vessels must be ensured.

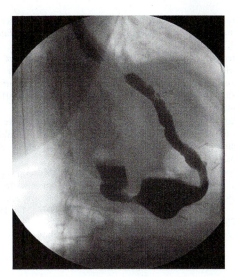

FIGURE 9 • Postoperative barium study of a sleeve gastrectomy.

POSTOPERATIVE CARE

- Postoperative care is similar to other bariatric patients. Early postoperative ambulation, adequate postoperative analgesia, and frequent pulmonary toilet are important to help avoid pulmonary and thrombotic complications. Appropriate perioperative antibiotics and venous thromboembolic prophylaxis are continued. We no longer keep our patients NPO on the first postoperative evening and allow them to start clear liquids oral intake and important oral medications. After 24 hours from the operation, the diet is advanced to full liquids.
- The use of routine postoperative upper GI series is of debatable value. In our practice we used to routinely obtain a Gastrografin and barium swallow examination on postoperative day 1 (**FIGURE 9**); however, after 10 years of experience performing sleeve gastrectomies, we are no longer performing this test after uneventful operations and only ordering it when we find it to be clinically necessary. Furthermore, when a leak is suspected, and the upper GI series is nonconfirmatory, a computed tomography scan of the abdomen with oral contrast is the logical next step. Additionally, use of postoperative upper GI series can be helpful to obtain a baseline study of each patient's anatomy for future reference.
- The patient is started on a clear liquid diet and oral analgesics hours after the operation, or following a negative swallow study, when indicated. We started discharging some patients, who meet the criteria of low postoperative risk and adequate support at home on the same day; however, the majority of our patients are being discharged on postoperative day 1. We maintain our patients on a liquid diet for 9 to 14 days and then introduce soft foods. Multivitamin supplementation is started on discharge, and we keep our patients on acid suppression in the perioperative period.

OUTCOMES AND FOLLOW-UP

- As of 2022, there is sufficient long-term data demonstrating that LSG is a safe and effective bariatric and metabolic operation and provides significant and durable weight loss, improvements in medical comorbidities, improved quality of life, and low complication and mortality rates for the treatment of morbid obesity.[2]
- Additionally, these long-term outcome data show that the LSG has similar outcomes to Roux-en-Y gastric bypass (RYGB), related to weight loss and improvement of comorbidities, including type 2 diabetes.[1,2,4,5]

COMPLICATIONS

- New published data from recent randomized trials show that LSG was associated with significantly fewer major complications within 30 days of surgery, when compared with RYGB. Overall, the incidence of death and more serious complications in the early postoperative period are equivalent for the LSG and the RYGB.[1,2] Most studies have also shown a trend toward decreased rates of late specific complications for the LSG compared to the bypass—for example, obstruction, stricture, and anastomotic ulcer.[6,7]
- The most frequent complications after LSG are bleeding, urinary tract infections, superficial site infections, and deep venous thromboses. They are similar to other bariatric operations in their incidence, diagnosis, and treatment.
- A few LSG-specific complications merit further discussion. Leaks occur overall at a similar incidence as the RYGB. Sleeve leaks can occur both early and late and are most often found at the proximal staple line near the angle of His. Principles and treatment of LSG leaks are similar to other abdominal leaks, including control of sepsis with wide drainage and antibiotics and nutritional optimization. Treatment of leaks after sleeve gastrectomy can be particularly challenging, as the intact pylorus and gastric conduit itself often create a relative distal obstruction and enteral access for nutritional supplementation is more problematic. However, unique to management of LSG leaks is the use of covered stents, which can be placed endoscopically and can be useful to control leaks in combination with intra-abdominal drainage.
- Although extremely infrequent, obstruction after sleeve gastrectomy can occur, and unlike the RYGB, they are not due to internal hernia, as the intestinal spaces are not disturbed, but more commonly due to narrowing or twisting of the gastric conduit. Again, upper endoscopy can be particularly helpful for diagnosing this problem and treatment with endoscopic dilation.
- Chronic gastroesophageal reflux disease could develop after LSG. In a recent position statement from ASMBS, it was recommended that due to the possibility of development of de novo Barrett esophagus after LSG, clinicians should consider a screening EGD for patients 3 or more years after LSG, irrespective of symptoms. Although this recommendation was based on preliminary and significant limited evidence, it is conditionally recommended as a good practice, until better-designed studies could either confirm or refute the current evidence.[8]
- Severe and refractory gastroesophageal reflux has also been described following LSG. Management should include fluoroscopic and endoscopic imaging of the sleeve to assess and treat any defined obstruction. Recalcitrant reflux may even require reoperation with sleeve conversion to RYGB.

REFERENCES

1. Azagury D, Papasavas P, Hamdallah I, Gagner M, Kim J. ASMBS Position Statement on medium- and long-term durability of weight loss and diabetic outcomes after conventional stapled bariatric procedures. *Surg Obes Relat Dis.* 2018;14(10):1425-1441. Epub 2018 Aug 11. PMID: 30242000. doi:10.1016/j.soard.2018.08.001
2. Ali M, El Chaar M, Ghiassi S, Rogers AM; American Society for Metabolic and Bariatric Surgery Clinical Issues Committee. American Society for Metabolic and Bariatric Surgery updated position statement on sleeve gastrectomy as a bariatric procedure. *Surg Obes Relat Dis.* 2017;13(10):1652-1657. Epub 2017 Aug 22. PMID: 29054173. doi:10.1016/j.soard.2017.08.007
3. Rosenthal RJ; International Sleeve Gastrectomy Expert Panel. International sleeve gastrectomy expert panel consensus statement: best practice guidelines based on experience of >12,000 cases. *Surg Obes Relat Dis.* 2012;8(1):8-19.
4. Keidar A, Hershkop KJ, Marko L, et al. Roux-en-Y gastric bypass vs sleeve gastrectomy for obese patients with type 2 diabetes: a randomised trial. *Diabetologia.* 2013;56(9):1914-1918.
5. Schauer PR, Bhatt DL, Kirwan JP, et al. Bariatric surgery versus intensive medical therapy for diabetes—3-year outcomes. *N Engl J Med.* 2014;370(21):2002-2013.
6. Hutter MM, Schirmer BD, Jones DB, et al. First report from the American College of Surgeons Bariatric Surgery Center Network: laparoscopic sleeve gastrectomy has morbidity and effectiveness positioned between the band and the bypass. *Ann Surg.* 2011;254(3):410-420.
7. Carlin AM, Zeni TM, English WJ, et al. The comparative effectiveness of sleeve gastrectomy, gastric bypass, and adjustable gastric banding procedures for the treatment of morbid obesity. *Ann Surg.* 2013;257(5):791-797.
8. Campos GM, Mazzini GS, Altieri MS, et al. ASMBS position statement on the rationale for performance of upper gastrointestinal endoscopy before and after metabolic and bariatric surgery. *Surg Obes Relat Dis.* 2021;17(5):837-847. Epub 2021 Mar 19. PMID: 33875361. doi:10.1016/j.soard.2021.03.007

Chapter 48: Removal and Revision of Laparoscopic Adjustable Gastric Banding

Scott W. Schimpke and Kunoor Jain-Spangler

DEFINITION

- Adjustable gastric banding (AGB) was approved in 2001 for treatment of morbid obesity. It involves placing an adjustable silastic band around the proximal stomach to create a narrowed outflow tract and thus restriction and subsequent weight loss.
- Morbid obesity is a worldwide pandemic and more than one-third of adults in the United States are obese.[1]
- A total of 256,000 bariatric procedures were performed in the United States in 2019, and 16.7% of those were revisional.[2]
- After approval in 2001, there was an exponential increase in volume of AGB in the early 2000s. However, with the introduction of sleeve gastrectomy (SG), and the now known suboptimal long-term outcomes of the AGB, it only comprises 0.9% of bariatric procedures in 2019.[2]
- AGB has a high rate of weight loss recurrence and long-term complications such as band slippage, gastric pouch dilation, band erosion, esophageal dysmotility, gastroesophageal reflux disease (GERD), and port/tubing dysfunction. Up to 60% of patients with a band require removal, with or without conversion to an alternative bariatric procedure.[3]
- Removal of the band and conversion to an alternative bariatric procedure is recommended, when feasible, as weight gain and worsening of a patient's metabolic syndrome is common after removal alone.[4] However, in the setting of a life-threatening complication such as gastric ischemia, perforation, erosion or obstruction, it is prudent to remove the band and address a possible conversion after the patient has recovered.
- Conversion of the AGB to SG, gastric bypass (RYGB), or duodenal switch (DS) are well-established surgical options for the treatment of obesity and associated metabolic syndrome. The most efficacious conversion is debatable but should be tailored based on the reason for conversion and a patient's metabolic profile.
- Conversion of AGB to a secondary procedure can be done in a single-stage (band removal and new bariatric procedure in one setting) or two-stage approach (band removal first followed by interval new bariatric procedure). The approach with the lowest morbidity is debatable.[5]

PATIENT HISTORY AND PHYSICAL FINDINGS

- There are two broad categories for removal and revision of AGB—weight loss recurrence and long-term complications.
- Regardless of the reason, an estimated 10% to 60% of patients with an AGB require reoperation.[6,7]

Weight Loss Recurrence

- The high rate of long-term weight loss failure after AGB is well established and is the most common reason for revision.[4,8-12] Associated with this is the lack of improvement of obesity related comorbidities.[13] Therefore, conversion to a secondary bariatric operation is recommended.
- The gastric bypass has traditionally been considered the revisional procedure of choice, as it adds malabsorptive and hormonal components in patients who failed a purely restrictive procedure. Furthermore, patients with AGB often experience esophageal dysmotility and subsequent GERD. The antireflux properties of the RYGB (along with removing the inciting band) make it a popular choice over the much-debated SG as it relates to GERD.
- SG is the most common bariatric procedure performed in the United States and is increasingly utilized as a conversion following failed AGB. It combines a restrictive component with neurohormonal changes, of which the most widely known is the decrease in plasma ghrelin levels post procedure.[14]
- Conversion to DS is less described with only smaller case series. Because of its superior weight loss and treatment of metabolic syndrome as a primary operation, interest has grown in its utilization. However, the higher rate of complications, as well as the paucity of data as a conversion after failed AGB, limits our recommendations.

Complications of the LAGB

- Port/tubing dysfunction, band slippage, gastric pouch dilation, band erosion, esophageal dysmotility, and GERD are the most common long-term complications and reasons for revision of an AGB. Hardware problems, such as port/tubing dysfunction can be treated with operative revision, although these complications are less common. Therefore, removal and conversion to a new bariatric procedure are most commonly performed.
- Regardless of the reason for removal and/or revision, the first step is to perform a full history and physical examination of the patient. The patient's current BMI and BMI before the AGB, obesity related comorbidities, previous surgeries, short- or long-term complications from the AGB, and if/when the AGB was last adjusted are all important. Social history is of utmost importance to determine the patient's resources and support system, as well as their ability to undergo a procedure that may require intensive pre- and postoperative planning and follow-up. On physical examination the surgeon should identify scars, note where the subcutaneous port is, and look for cellulitis, which can be a sign of band erosion.
- Obtaining the operative note can be extremely helpful to know the type of band inserted, type and number of plicating sutures used, and location of the tubing and port.
- All patients should undergo a psychological evaluation, and if any maladaptive eating disorders or other psychiatric issues are elucidated, those should be treated prior to consideration for surgical revision.

IMAGING AND OTHER DIAGNOSTIC STUDIES

- To determine a patient's candidacy for revision surgery and to formulate an operative plan, a fluoroscopic imaging study of the upper gastrointestinal tract should be performed. This study can show the position of the band, which should be at a 45° angle around the cardia; the foregut anatomy (eg, esophageal size/shape); esophageal motility in the form of peristaltic waves; amount and timing of contrast passing through the band; and the presence or absence of reflux. This can be done concurrently with a band adjustment. For example, decompressing the band is indicated if there is minimal or delayed contrast passage or if the patient is experiencing symptoms of nausea, vomiting, or dysphagia.
- An upper endoscopy is also recommended, in addition to the fluoroscopic study, to evaluate mucosal integrity. Findings of gastritis, esophagitis, Barrett esophagus, and band erosion all would help the surgeon determine the optimal treatment for a patient with failed AGB.

Contraindications

- There are very few contraindications for band removal.
- Absolute contraindications would include any factor that would preclude a patient from undergoing abdominal surgery under general anesthesia.
- A relative contraindication would be if the band was found to be almost completely eroded into the gastric lumen (usually the buckle is not). In this instance an intraluminal stent can be placed to induce complete erosion and then the band can be removed endoscopically sparing the patient a more invasive surgical removal.[15]
- Patients with acute, life-threatening complications such as gastric ischemia, perforation, or obstruction should be treated emergently with band removal and any necessary repairs. Concomitant conversion to a new bariatric procedure should not be considered.
- Lastly, as stated previously, all patients must undergo a thorough nutritional and psychological workup when considering an elective conversion to a new bariatric procedure. Untreated or uncontrolled psychiatric disorders are a contraindication to conversion.

SURGICAL MANAGEMENT

Preoperative Planning

- All patients must complete a surgical evaluation, medical clearances (if necessary), psychological evaluation, dietary evaluation, and any other insurance requirements.
- Every patient is given a bariatric booklet at their first visit that outlines expectations pre- and postoperatively along with a description of each diet phase. At our program, patients start a liquid protein diet 1 week prior to surgery and continue a similar diet 2 weeks postoperatively.
- A venous thromboembolism risk assessment tool is used at each patient's preoperative visit to determine whether

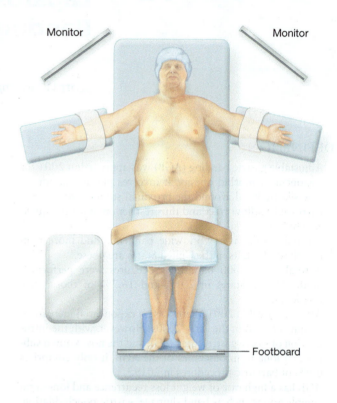

FIGURE 1 • Patient positioning for both a laparoscopic and robotic approach.

extended thromboprophylaxis is required after surgery (either 2 or 4 weeks). On the day of surgery, all patients receive prophylaxis subcutaneous anticoagulation before incision.

Positioning

- See **FIGURE 1**.
- The patient is placed in a supine position. After anesthesia is administered, the patient is secured to the bed with wide Velcro straps around the lower legs and thighs. Both arms are out on arm boards. The heels are padded, and a footboard is secured to allow steep reverse Trendelenburg during the procedure.
- A self-retaining liver retractor is anchored to the bed on the patient's right side either below or above the extended arm depending on the retractor system used.
- The operating surgeon is on the patient's right side and the assisting surgeon on the patient's left if performed laparoscopically. If performed robotically, the robot can be docked from either side of the patient.
- An orogastric tube is placed after induction to decompress the stomach. We perform a separate "time-out" procedure before stapling to ensure all tubes and probes are removed from the patient's mouth except for the endotracheal tube.

PLACEMENT OF INCISIONS

LAPAROSCOPIC

- See **FIGURE 2**.
- A Veress needle is placed in the left upper quadrant to establish pneumoperitoneum, which is then followed by a 5-mm optical port. This can be upsized to a 12-mm port for the conversion procedure, if needed. Inspection of the abdomen is then performed ensuring there was no injury from the initial trocar placement.
- The remaining three ports are then placed under direct visualization after the patient is placed in steep reverse Trendelenburg position. A 5-mm port is placed to the left of the umbilicus for the camera, and a third 5-mm port is placed in the right subcostal region. The 15-mm port is placed in right abdomen between the camera and right subcostal port, through which the AGB is removed.
- A self-retaining liver retractor is placed through a subxyphoid incision.

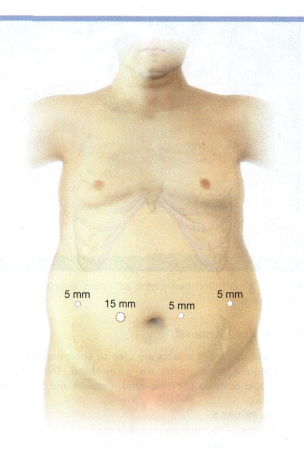

FIGURE 2 • Laparoscopic port placement.

ROBOTIC

- See **FIGURE 3**.
- A Veress needle is placed in the left upper quadrant to establish pneumoperitoneum. The ports are typically placed along a horizontal line about 19 cm caudad to the xyphoid. The abdomen is entered with a 12-mm visual port one handbreadth lateral of the umbilicus in the right abdomen.
- Under visualization, an 8-mm port is placed just left of the umbilicus for the camera. Another 8-mm port is placed in the left lateral abdomen and an 8-mm one between the two aforementioned ports. The latter can be upsized to a 12-mm port depending on the conversion being performed.
- A self-retaining retractor is placed through a subxyphoid incision.

Liver Retraction

- The patient is in steep reverse Trendelenburg position, and self-retaining liver retractor is used.
- This may have to be repositioned as the infrahepatic adhesions are taken down.

Perigastric Lysis of Adhesions

- Often there are infrahepatic and omental adhesions to the band or tubing that must be dissected free.
- See **FIGURE 4**.
- This will expose the fibrous capsule surrounding the band.

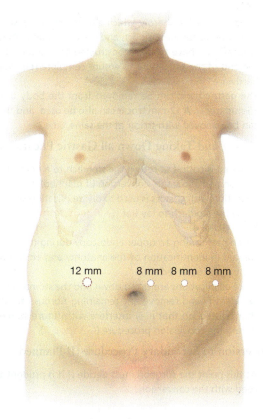

FIGURE 3 • Robotic port placement.

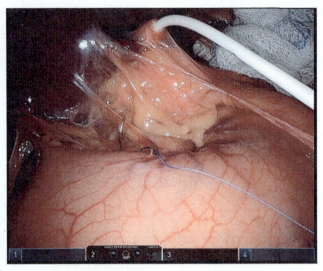

FIGURE 4 • Typical peri-gastric adhesions associated with a gastric band.

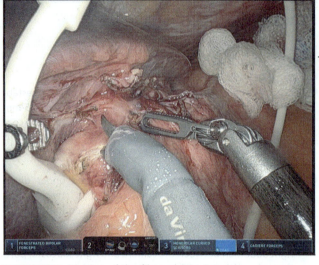

FIGURE 5 • Division of the fibrous capsule.

Gastric Band Removal

- Hook cautery or scissors are used to enter and divide the fibrous capsule around the gastric band. This dissection should continue until the band is mobile and the clasp is freed.
- See **FIGURE 5**.
- It is critical to maintain your dissection directly on the band as inadvertent injury to surrounding structures (eg, stomach, liver, vena cava) can occur due to distorted anatomy (▶ Video 1).
- Divide the tubing sharply, which disconnects the gastric band from the subcutaneous port, and open the band. These two "pieces" will have to be reconstructed on the back table at the end of the procedure to ensure complete removal of all hardware.
- The gastric band can be removed from the body using the 15-mm trocar. A 12-mm trocar can also be used, and the band can be removed with trocar at the same time.

Identifying and Taking Down all Gastric Plications

- This step is critical to return the stomach to a normal configuration and allow safe conversion (if planned). Careful sharp dissection with scissors is used to divide plicating sutures and allow the stomach to lay flat (▶ Videos 1 and 2).
- See **FIGURE 6**.
- Often performing an upper endoscopy during this dissection can aid in identification of the anatomy and ensure no gastric injuries occurred.
- Once all plications are taken down and the stomach lays flat, we identify and remove any remaining fibrous capsule with sharp dissection that may interfere with future staples lines during the conversion procedure (▶ Video 1).

Conversion to Secondary Procedure (If Planned)

- At this point the surgeon must decide if it is prudent to proceed with the conversion.

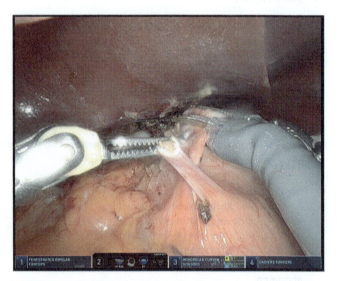

FIGURE 6 • Division of a gastric plication.

- We recommend confirming, often times using endoscopy, that all plications are taken down, there are no gastric injuries, and the tissue is perfused and pliable.

Subcutaneous Port Removal

- The skin and subcutaneous tissue are divided to expose the underlying port. The anchoring sutures must be divided to free the port from the underlying fascia. Beware some ports have sharp hooks instead of sutures.
- The port and tubing is then delivered from the wound and reconstructed on the back table with the previously removed band to ensure complete removal.
- We remove or fulgurate the remaining capsule in the subcutaneous space and ensure all sutures are removed before closing.

PEARLS AND PITFALLS

- Ensure the band, tubing, couplers, and subcutaneous port are removed entirely and reconstructed on the back table to confirm no retained foreign bodies.
- Beware of plicating sutures or metal anchors. All plications and associated sutures/anchors must be taken down or removed before proceeding with conversion (▶ Videos 1 and 2).
- Intraoperative endoscopy is a useful tool to ensure there were no gastric injuries during AGB removal, the stomach is flat with no plications, and the mucosa is well perfused.
- The fibrotic capsule around the now removed AGB should be dissected free from the stomach where your future staple line will be.
- Mobilize the fundus and completely dissect the angle of His to ensure there is no retained fundus, especially when performing SG.
- If complications occur during AGB removal or the gastric tissue quality is poor, then abort the operation and stage the conversion.

POSTOPERATIVE CARE

- AGB removal only
  - This is typically performed as an outpatient surgery, and patients are discharged on a general diet.
  - Early ambulation is imperative, but we limit heavy lifting and strenuous exercise for 2 weeks.
- Conversion to a secondary procedure
  - See Chapters 46 and 47 for technical steps.

CHOICE OF SECONDARY PROCEDURE

Removal Only

- If technically feasible and safe, it is advisable to perform a secondary bariatric procedure rather than AGB removal alone as patients suffer from weight gain and comorbidity recurrence.
- Not only are most patients unable to maintain weight loss after AGB removal but also they regain weight to presurgery levels or higher within 5 years.[4]
- For a subset of patients having band complications, who have lost weight and do not qualify for revisional surgery, band removal alone is advisable.

AGB Revision

- This is typically reserved for patients who are successful with AGB but experience a hardware failure such as a flipped subcutaneous port or complication with the tubing.
- As stated previously, the most common reason for AGB revision is weight loss recurrence followed by slippage, erosion, dysmotility, and GERD, all of which are better addressed by a conversion.

AGB to SG or RYGB

- Weight loss after SG or RYGB as a salvage procedure after failed AGB is similar to each as a primary operation, although not quite as robust. In this meta-analysis, percent excess weight loss was 35% to 65% and 46% to 50%, respectively, for an LAGB conversion to an SG and RYGB at 12 months.[16]
- Both conversion to SG and RYGB can be performed safely with low morbidity. Thirty-day complications, reoperations, and hospitalizations were identified in 3.2%, 1.9%, and 4.5% of patients, respectively.[5] There are still insufficient data to determine which operation carries the lowest risk of complication.[5,12,17]
- There is also limited literature directly addressing choice of revisional surgery for AGB failure. The reason for conversion and a patient's comorbidities must be considered. For example, a patient with esophageal dysmotility, GERD, or diabetes would favor RYGB, while intra-abdominal adhesions and risk factors for marginal ulcer (nonsteroidal anti-inflammatory drugs, steroids, or risk of tobacco use) would favor SG. As for weight loss specifically, some would argue if the initial AGB achieved adequate weight loss, but failure occurred because of a complication (eg, slippage) then another restrictive-like operation such as SG would be appropriate. However, if the reason for reoperation is weight loss recurrence, then RYGB should be considered as it adds malabsorptive and hormonal components and has superior excess weight loss long term.[18,19]

AGB to DS

- As a primary operation, DS offers the most excess weight loss as compared with RYGB and SG. However, despite this, it is estimated that only 0.9% of the total number of bariatric procedures performed in the United States in 2019 were DS due to limited institutions and surgeons who perform the operation, increased morbidity compared with the RYGB and SG, and increased risk of malnutrition and/or vitamin deficiencies.[2] As a secondary operation there are only a few small studies available on conversion from a failed AGB.[20]

Single- or Two-Stage Approach

- Conversion of AGB to RYGB or SG can be performed either as a single-stage (AGB removal and new bariatric procedure in one setting) or two-stage approach (AGB removal first followed by interval new bariatric procedure). The single stage offers the advantage of one general anesthesia episode, limited inconvenience for the patient, and avoids the likely weight gain following AGB removal without conversion.[4] In 2021, Spaniolas et al reported 69.8% of all AGB conversions were performed in a single-stage fashion.[5] However, the historic critique of a single-stage conversion is the potential for increased risk of complication due to fibrosis, which would improve over time and thus favor a two-stage approach. Tan et al found this to not be the case and showed stable histologic changes of the gastric wall in the region of the band capsule over 3 years from band removal.[21]
- In a meta-analysis in 2016, the morbidity rate of conversion to RYGB was 8.3% for single-stage approach and 8.9% for two-stage approach, which is not statistically different.[12]

More recently, a database study with 4330 patients showed a morbidity rate of 9.3% and 18.5% for a one-stage and two-stage conversion, respectively.[5] Both authors concluded AGB to RYGB is a safe operation. Perhaps the increased morbidity rate with the latter study is due to selection bias and/or weight gain of the patient (thus increased difficulty of the operation) before undergoing the second stage.

- The evolution of the optimal approach for AGB to SG parallels that of the RYGB. Earlier studies showed increased complications with the single-stage approach, but more recent studies show no difference or even improved morbidity with the single-stage compared with the two-stage approach.[5,12,17] More controversial is whether conversion to SG is safer than conversion to RYGB. Dang et al reported higher one- and two-stage morbidity rates for the sleeve compared with RYGB (10.9% and 11.2% vs 8.3% and 8.9%, respectively).[12] In contrast, Spaniolas et al reported lower one- and two-stage morbidity rates for the sleeve (5.6% and 12.8% vs 9.3% and 18.5%, respectively).[5]

REFERENCES

1. https://nifa.usda.gov/topic/obesity.
2. https://asmbs.org/resources/estimate-of-bariatric-surgery-numbers.
3. Himpens J, Cadière G-B, Bazi M, et al. Long-term outcomes of laparoscopic adjustable gastric banding. *Arch Surg.* 2011;146(7):802-807.
4. Aarts EO, Dogan K, Koehestanie P, et al. Long-term results after laparoscopic adjustable gastric banding: a mean fourteen year follow-up study. *Surg Obes Relat Dis.* 2014;10(4):633-640.
5. Spaniolas K, Yang J, Zhu C, et al. Conversion of adjustable gastric banding to stapling bariatric procedures: single- or two-stage approach. *Ann Surg.* 2021;273(3):542-547. doi:10.1097/SLA.0000000000003332. PMID: 30998539.
6. Yeung L, Durkan B, Barrett A, et al. Single-stage revision from gastric band to gastric bypass or sleeve gastrectomy: 6- and 12-month outcomes. *Surg Endosc.* 2016;30(6):2244-2250. doi:10.1007/s00464-015-4498-x. http://www.ncbi.nlm.nih.gov/pubmed/26335074
7. Elnahas A, Graybiel K, Farrokhyar F, et al. Revisional surgery after failed laparoscopic adjustable gastric banding: a systematic review. *Surg Endosc.* 2013;27(3):740-745. doi:10.1007/s00464-012-2510-2. http://www.ncbi.nlm.nih.gov/pubmed/22936440
8. Victorzon M, Tolonen P. Mean fourteen-year, 100% follow-up of laparoscopic adjustable gastric banding for morbid obesity. *Surg Obes Relat Dis.* 2013;9(5):753-757.
9. Kindel T, Martin E, Hungness E, Nagle A. High failure rate of the laparoscopic-adjustable gastric band as a primary bariatric procedure. *Surg Obes Relat Dis.* 2014;10(6):1070-1075. doi:10.1016/j.soard.2013.11.014
10. Spivak H, Abdelmelek MF, Beltran OR, Ng AW, Kitahama S. Long-term outcomes of laparoscopic adjustable gastric banding and laparoscopic Roux-en-Y gastric bypass in the United States. *Surg Endosc.* 2012;26(7):1909-1919.
11. DeMaria EJ, Sugerman HJ, Meador JG, et al. High failure rate after laparoscopic adjustable silicone gastric banding for the treatment of morbid obesity. *Ann Surg.* 2001;233(6):809-187.
12. Dang JT, Switzer NJ, Shi X, Karmali S. Response to the letter to the Editor-Re: gastric band removal in revisional bariatric surgery, one-step versus two-step. A systematic review and meta-analysis. *Obes Surg.* 2016;26(6):1321. doi:10.1007/s11695-016-2150-z. PMID: 27021344.
13. Froylich D, Abramovich-Segal T, Pascal G, et al. Long-term (over 10 years) retrospective follow-up of laparoscopic adjustable gastric banding. *Obes Surg.* 2018;28(4):976-980. doi:10.1007/s11695-017-2952-7. https://search.proquest.com/docview/1966294282
14. Anderson B, Switzer N, Almamar A, et al. The impact of laparoscopic sleeve gastrectomy on plasma ghrelin levels: a systematic review. *Obes Surg.* 2013;23(9):1476-1480. doi:10.1007/s11695-013-0999-7. http://www.ncbi.nlm.nih.gov/pubmed/23794092
15. Blero D, Eisendrath P, Vandermeeren A, et al. Endoscopic removal of dysfunctioning bands or rings after restrictive bariatric procedures. *Gastrointest Endosc.* 2010;71(3):468-474. doi:10.1016/j.gie.2009.06.020. PMID: 19748612.
16. Zhou R, Poirier J, Torquati A, Omotosho P. Short-term outcomes of conversion of failed gastric banding to laparoscopic sleeve gastrectomy or Roux-en-Y gastric bypass: a meta-analysis. *Obes Surg.* 2019;29(2):420-425. doi:10.1007/s11695-018-3538-8. PMID: 30293135.
17. Schneck AS, Lazzati A, Audureau E, et al. One or two steps for laparoscopic conversion of failed adjustable gastric banding to sleeve gastrectomy: a nationwide French study on 3357 morbidly obese patients. *Surg Obes Relat Dis.* 2016;12:840-848.
18. Zundel N, Hernandez JD. Revisional surgery after restrictive procedures for morbid obesity. *Surg Laparosc Endosc Percutan.* 2010;20(5):338-343.
19. Ali M, El Chaar M, Ghiassi S, Rogers AM. American Society for metabolic and bariatric surgery Clinical issues Committee. American Society for metabolic and bariatric surgery updated position statement on sleeve gastrectomy as a bariatric procedure. *Surg Obes Relat Dis.* 2017;13(10):1652-1657. doi:10.1016/j.soard.2017.08.007. PMID: 29054173.
20. Elnahas A, Graybiel K, Farrokhyar F, Gmora S, Anvari M, Hong D. Revisional surgery after failed laparoscopic adjustable gastric banding: a systematic review. *Surg Endosc.* 2013;27(3):740-745. doi:10.1007/s00464-012-2510-2. PMID: 22936440.
21. Tan MH, Yee GY, Jorgensen JO, et al. A histologic evaluation of the laparoscopic adjustable gastric band capsule by tissue sampling during sleeve gastrectomy performed at different time points after band removal. *Surg Obes Relat Dis.* 2014;10(4):620-625. doi:10.1016/j.soard.2014.02.037. PMID: 24958647.

Chapter 49

Laparoscopic Biliopancreatic Diversion With Duodenal Switch and Single Anastomosis Duodenal-Ileal Bypass

Dana Portenier

DEFINITIONS

- Biliopancreatic diversion with duodenal switch (BPD/DS), including a gastric resection, was described in 1979 by Dr. Scopinaro and colleagues.[1] This technique combined a distal gastrectomy, a gastrojejunostomy, and a jejunoileostomy, creating a common channel of 50 cm. However, it resulted in a highly malabsorptive bariatric procedure, with complications such as marginal ulcers, dumping syndrome, and postoperative diarrhea. This procedure was later modified: the gastrectomy took the form of a sleeve preserving the pylorus, and the common channel was lengthened to 100 cm. BPD/DS has the highest weight loss but accounts for only 0.8% of the bariatric procedures in the United States, according to the American Society for Metabolic and Bariatric Surgery (ASMBS) estimates from 2018, given its complexity and associated complications.[2]

- In 2007, Sánchez-Pernaute and Torres modified the technique to perform a single anastomosis to reduce complications.[3] This technique is now known as single anastomosis duodenal-ileal bypass, which includes a sleeve gastrectomy (SADI-S), also called stomach intestinal pylorus preserving surgery (SIPS).[4] In this variant of the BPD/DS, the transected duodenum is anastomosed to a loop of the ileum. SADI-S has been endorsed by the ASMBS as a suitable bariatric procedure, although long-term data on safety and efficacy are awaited (see **FIGURE 1**).

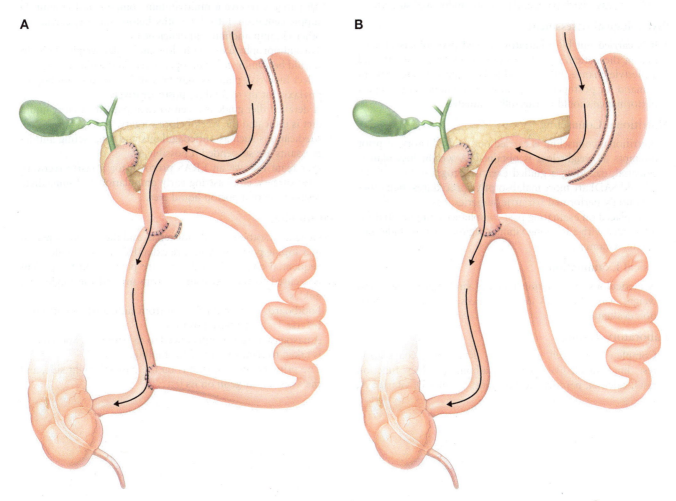

FIGURE 1 • BPDDS (left) vs SADI (right) anatomy.

PATIENT HISTORY AND PHYSICAL FINDINGS

Indications for Bariatric Surgery
- Body mass index (BMI) > 40 kg/m^2
- BMI 35 to 39.9 kg/m^2 with associated comorbidity (diabetes, sleep apnea, hypertension)
- BMI 30 to 34.9 kg/m^2 with diabetes uncontrolled with medical therapy, or metabolic syndrome

General Information
- A preoperative informative meeting is scheduled. In these seminars, several potential candidates for bariatric surgery share an appointment in which nutrition experts, nurses, endocrinologists, and bariatric surgeons explain the surgical alternatives, preoperative planning, and postoperative care potential complications. Focus is on the patient's expectations to align objectives on weight loss.

Patient Evaluation
- Individual patient evaluation should be holistic. A thorough medical history, including medication usage, is obtained to assess preoperative risk factors such as cardiovascular disease, dyslipidemia, diabetes, thrombotic events, obstructive sleep apnea, asthma and COPD, renal failure, gastroesophageal reflux disease, back pain, and previous abdominal surgeries.

Psychological Assessment
- It is carried out by a bariatric trained psychologist, focusing on the patient's predisposition to undergo surgery and a lifestyle change. BPS/DS and SADI require greater patient demand for postoperative follow-up and adherence, so past performance should be carefully evaluated.

Nutritional Counseling
- Nutritional counseling is carried out, and a history of prior attempts at weight loss is obtained. A weight loss plan is essential, including a guided exercise program. Since BPD/DS and SADI are more malabsorptive procedures than other commonly performed bariatric surgeries, particular emphasis is placed on evaluating past compliance and potential for adherence with a life-long vitamin regimen that includes fat-soluble vitamins.

Physical Examination
- A meticulous examination includes vital signs; height and weight; waist, hip, neck circumferences; and body composition evaluation.

Laboratory Testing
- Complete blood cell count with differential, coagulation test, lipid panel, liver enzymes, albumin, kidney function tests, calcium, parathyroid hormone, vitamin D, vitamin A, vitamin B12, and folic acid. Patients are also screened for diabetes.

IMAGING AND OTHER DIAGNOSTIC STUDIES
- Chest x-ray.
- Abdominal ultrasonography (optionally performed based upon symptoms of biliary pathology). The gallbladder is routinely removed at our institution. The rationale is the high prevalence of cholelithiasis after the procedure and the limited options for endoscopic intervention in the case of choledocholithiasis.
- Upper gastrointestinal (GI) endoscopy with biopsy and *Helicobacter pylori* test. If *H. pylori* test is positive, adequate antibiotic and proton pump inhibitor treatment should be administered and resolution should be confirmed before surgery. If moderate to sizable hiatal hernia is noted or duodenal ulcer found patient may be counseled toward alternative procedure or concomitant repair of hiatal hernia.

SURGICAL MANAGEMENT

Preoperative Planning
- Smoking cessation is required before the procedure.
- All patients receive a multivitamin complex and vitamin D supplementation 1 to 3 months before surgery, correcting other vitamin and mineral deficiencies.
- Thromboprophylaxis with low-molecular-weight heparin should be administered preoperatively and while in hospital. Select high-risk patients may be sent home on thromboprophylaxis for up to 30 days postoperatively.
- A detailed diet guide is given to each patient. A clear liquid diet is indicated the week before surgery.
- Medications such as anticoagulants and long-acting antidepressants are suspended if possible.
- Our team follows an ERAS protocol for a faster recovery after surgery, emphasizing early ambulation and immediate resumption of a postop liquid diet.

Positioning
- General anesthesia is administered, and the patient is placed in a supine position. Arms are extended at a 90° angle.
- Sequential compression devices are placed, and the patient is secured to the bed using a strap around the thighs and ankles.
- Footboards prevent the patient from sliding when taken to a reverse Trendelenburg position.
- A nasogastric tube is introduced to the stomach. Special care is taken to remove it prior to stapling.
- The primary surgeon stands on the patient's right side, and the assisting surgeon on its left.

PORT PLACEMENT

- See **FIGURE 2**.
- Pneumoperitoneum is established at 15 mm Hg by introducing the Veress needle into Palmer point.
- The sites of incisions are first marked with a sterile marker. Next, a 5-mm Optiview trocar is inserted left and superior to the umbilicus with the camera in it for direct visualization of the layers of the abdominal wall and abdominal cavity when entering. Next, a 15-mm trocar is superior to the umbilical level on the right midclavicular line. Next, one 12-mm port is placed near Palmer point, and another 5-mm trocar is placed lateral to the 15-mm trocar on the right-sided anterior axillary line. Finally, an additional 5-mm incision is made on the epigastrium for liver retraction.
- Laparoscopic exploration is conducted to rule out any abdominal abnormalities.
- Transverse abdominis plane block is performed with injection of 50 mL solution of 25% bupivacaine + liposomal bupivacaine using a large-bore spinal needle under laparoscopic visualization.

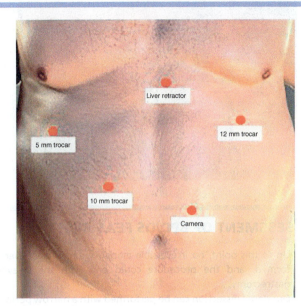

FIGURE 2 • Port placement for BPDDS or SADI.

IDENTIFICATION OF THE ILEOCECAL VALVE

- Omentum is retracted superiorly to reveal the cecum. If the omentum is notably bulky, it is divided to reduce tension on the planned duodenal ileal anastomosis. For this maneuver, the surgeon may optionally stand on the patient's left with the table tilted right side upward. The ileocecal valve is identified. Bowel measurement of the ileum from ileocecal valve to 250 cm (for BPD/DS) or 300 cm (for SADI-S) proximal is carried out by counting 10-cm intervals atraumatic graspers. Care is taken to ensure proper orientation of proximal and distal aspects. A loose approximation suture is placed securing to epiploica of the transverse colon to facilitate easy retrieval later when the operative table is positioned in reverse Trendelenburg position. The ileum proximal to our fixation stitch is painted with a sterile marker introduced laparoscopically to facilitate easy understanding of orientation with stitch being distal and pen marking proximal.

STOMACH MOBILIZATION

- Nathanson liver retractor Mediflex is introduced through the epigastric incision allowing the exposure of the lesser curvature of the stomach and esophageal hiatus. Placement to the right of the falciform ligament elevated the ligament, enhancing the exposure of the pylorus. If the falciform is notably bulky it can be taken down to improve exposure. The patient is put into a steep reverse Trendelenburg position.
- The greater curvature of the stomach is mobilized from the pylorus to the angle of His. A vessel sealer conducts the transection of gastrocolic ligament and short gastric vessels. Gentle traction should be applied to the greater curvature by the surgeon's assistant to avoid avulsion of the short gastric vessels. Care should be taken to fully mobilize short gastric vessels off the base of the right crus muscle to prevent retained fundus on gastric transection.

SLEEVE GASTRECTOMY

- Before beginning the gastrectomy, the surgeon should ask for G-tubes and any other devices to be removed from the patient's mouth to avoid the accidental section of these items with the stapling device.
- Next, a 38- to 40-Fr boogie is inserted into the stomach and slid along the lesser curvature for calibration.
- Longitudinal gastrectomy is performed using a stapler of choice. Care should be taken to provide even consistent retraction that avoids spiraling of the staple line. Each fire stapler should be applied and inspected anteriorly and posteriorly to ensure adequate, consistent tissue retraction. The gastric incisura is a known point of potential narrowing, and narrowing should be avoided. Gastric tissue is known to be thicker in the antrum when compared with the fundus. Staple height should take this thickness difference into account and be individualized for each patient. Our institution typically uses two black staple cartridges followed by purple staple cartridges, all reinforced by the staple line reinforcement methodology of choice (**FIGURE 3**).
- The stomach specimen is retained for later retrieval.

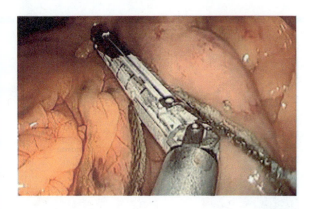

FIGURE 3 • Creation of the sleeve gastrectomy.

ASSESSMENT OF BPD/DS FEASIBILITY

- Up to this point, no irreversible maneuvers have been performed, and the procedure could end with the sleeve gastrectomy.
- Duodenal dissection can be performed with a narrow periduodenal tunnel or a total pyloric mobilization as preferred at our institution. Pyloric mobilization is accomplished by continuing the previous gastrocolic ligament transection down to the pylorus. The pylorus is lifted superiorly, dividing posterior and mesenteric border attachments along pylorus/duodenum up to the level of gastroduodenal artery (GDA). The artery marks the distal extent of dissection to stay well clear of the common bile duct that courses posterior to duodenal dissection through the pancreas. The tunnel behind the duodenum can be performed superior to GDA and facilitated by localized mobilization on antimesenteric border similar to limited kocherization (**FIGURE 4**).
- If deemed technically feasible conventional laparoscopic cholecystectomy is performed. Gallbladder specimen is retrieved later with the resected stomach. The postoperative gluteal rhabdomyolysis rate increases in patients with higher BMI if the surgical duration exceeds 4 hours. Forgoing cholecystectomy can be used to reduce operative time if necessary.

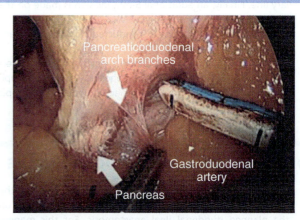

FIGURE 4 • Location of the GDA relative to the duodenum.

DUODENOILEAL ANASTOMOSIS

- The duodenum is divided using a purple 60-mm linear cutting stapler load. The ileum at the previously placed localization stitch site is brought up to assess tension. If necessary, proximal duodenum and pyloric gastrohepatic attachments can be divided to just beyond the right gastric vessel to increase significantly pyloric mobility, decreasing tension on the planned duodenoileal anastomosis.
- The ileum with the 300 cm (SADI-S) or 250 cm (BPD/DS) mark is anastomosed to the proximal duodenal stump in a two-layer end-to-side hand-sewn fashion. Joining of the posterior layer with the staple line of the duodenal stump and the antimesenteric border of the ileum is done using 2.0 absorbable V-loc (Covidien, New Haven, Connecticut) suture. Enterotomy and duodenostomy are performed with a monopolar energy device, and duodenoileal anastomosis is achieved in two full-thickness layers, an internal layer followed by an external layer, using 3-0 Polysorb suture (**FIGURE 5**).
- Up to now, we have accomplished a SADI-S procedure.

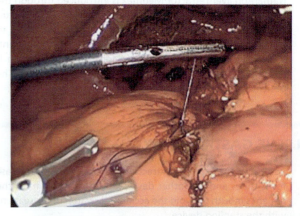

FIGURE 5 • Creation of the duodenoileostomy.

LEAK TEST

- Upper endoscopy is done to check the patency of the duodenoileal anastomosis and perform a leak test by administering air endoscopically while submerging the anastomosis with saline solution laparoscopically (**FIGURE 6**).
- If a SADI is being performed, upper endoscopy is done at this point; if a BPD/DS is being performed, endoscopy may be done after creating the common channel.

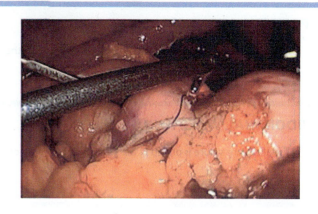

FIGURE 6 • Leak test to evaluate duodenoileostomy.

COMMON CHANNEL CREATION

- The proximal side of the duodenoileal anastomosis is transected near the anastomosis using a 60-mm tan linear stapler load creating our biliopancreatic limb.
- Count back distal from the duodenoileal anastomosis on what will be Roux limb for 150 cm to select the site for jejunojejunostomy, thus creating a 100-cm common channel and 150-cm Roux limb.
- The biliopancreatic limb is anastomosed bidirectionally by creating antimesenteric enterotomy in the biliopancreatic limb and selected jejunojejunostomy site in the previous step. A 45-mm tan load is fired from the right side of the table, and then a second 45-mm tan load is brought in through the Palmer point trocar and fired in opposite direction, creating a large anastomosis (**FIGURE 7**). Common enterotomy can then be safely stapled shut with a 60-mm tan load (**FIGURE 8**).

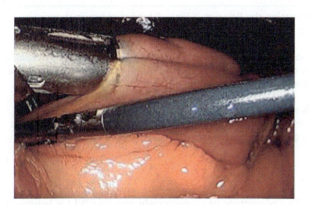

FIGURE 7 • Creation of the jejunojejunostomy.

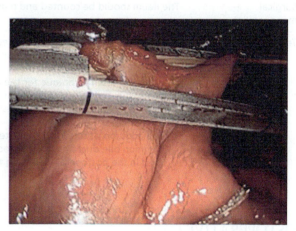

FIGURE 8 • Stapled closure of the common enterotomy.

CLOSURE OF MESENTERIC DEFECT

Mesenteric defects are closed with a 2.0 permanent suture. For BPD/DS, both the jejunojejunostomy and Petersen space are closed. SADI only has Peterson space to close (**FIGURE 9**).

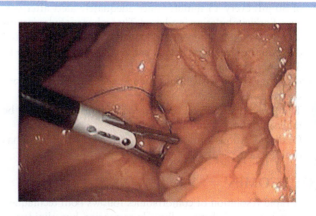

FIGURE 9 • Suture closure of mesenteric defects.

SPECIMEN AND INSTRUMENT RETRIEVAL

- Resected stomach and gallbladder are retrieved through the 15-mm port.
- In addition, the liver retractor is retrieved.
- An optional Jackson Pratt drain can be placed adjacent to the duodenoileal anastomosis, and sleeve staple line, exteriorized through the 5-mm left flank port.

ABDOMINAL WALL AND SKIN CLOSURE

- Fascial closure suture is placed in the 12-mm and 15-mm port sites.
- The skin is closed in a subcuticular fashion with 4-0 absorbable sutures.

PEARLS AND PITFALLS

Patient history and intraoperative findings	▪ The feasibility of performing a BPD/DS is determined before duodenal and ileal transections. If the patient has significant intestinal adhesions, pancreatic or gallbladder inflammation, or other pathological findings, the procedure should be ended. Instead, a sleeve gastrectomy might be accomplished as a sole or two-step surgery.
Duodenoileal anastomosis	▪ BPD/DS is a challenging procedure requiring high dexterity. The duodenoileal anastomosis upgrades the complexity of the procedure, and meticulous dissection of the duodenum is advised to avoid injury to the gastroduodenal artery, common bile duct, and pancreas.
Surgical management	The ileum should be counted and marked methodically to avoid miscount and short common channel.
Technique	▪ In SADI, the procedure is simplified by eliminating the Roux-en-Y limb. A longer common channel is created, seeking to reduce the incidence of postoperative diarrhea, protein caloric malnutrition, and internal hernia. ▪ The hand-sewn technique for the anastomosis of the duodenoileal anastomosis is not the only available technique, but it is strongly encouraged to develop comfort in this technique initially before moving to stapled techniques. If technical issues arise with stapled technique, surgeons need to correct it with a hand-sewn skillset. ▪ The addition of routine cholecystectomy is suggested given the complicated endoscopic access to the common bile duct after these procedures. In cases where cholecystectomy is not performed, ursodiol is used in the postoperative setting to lessen gallbladder pathology.

POSTOPERATIVE CARE

- Postoperative care is similar to that of other bariatric procedures. The patient is started on a full liquid diet at a rate of 30 mL every 15 minutes once adequately alert after surgery. Early ambulation is advised. Thromboprophylaxis with subcutaneous low-molecular-weight heparin is indicated daily during the hospital stay and selectively extended up to 30 days in high-risk patients.
- Upper GI barium swallow is done selectively to rule out strictures and leaks.
- The patients are given oral proton pump inhibitors to be taken daily for 3 months.
- Oral medications may be resumed as soon as the patient has oral tolerance.

OUTCOMES[5]

- A rapid resolution of comorbidities follows both techniques, namely, type 2 diabetes mellitus, hypertension, hyperlipidemia, sleep apnea, and gastroesophageal reflux disease (GERD).
- The percentage of excess weight loss (%EWL) is believed to be similar for BPD/DS and SADI and more significant than the values achieved after other bariatric procedures, with estimates around 70% EWL at 1 year.

COMPLICATIONS

- Short-term serious complications include small bowel obstruction, small bowel perforation, hemoperitoneum, duodenal stump leak, intra-abdominal abscess, and sepsis.
- Long-term serious complications include intractable diarrhea, common channel lengthening, malnutrition, vitamin deficiencies, GERD, anastomotic ulcer, anastomotic stenosis, sleeve stricture, internal herniation, and bowel obstruction.
- BPD/DS-specific complications include vitamin deficiencies and hard-to-treat chronic diarrhea. The reported incidence of internal herniation after this procedure varies from 0 to almost 20% in the literature.
- Concern exists about possible biliary reflux from the afferent limb in SADI, in which the reconstruction follows a Billroth

2 disposition and could ultimately lead to esophageal adenocarcinoma. Published data fail to elucidate the actual incidence of this pathology.[1-5]

REFERENCES

1. Scopinaro N, Gianetta E, Civalleri D, et al. Bilio-pancreatic bypass for obesity: II. Initial experience in man. *Br J Surg*. 1979;66:618-620.
2. Kallies K, Rogers AM, American Society for Metabolic and Bariatric Surgery Clinical Issues Committee. American Society for Metabolic and Bariatric Surgery updated statement on single-anastomosis duodenal switch. *Surg Obes Relat Dis*. 2020;16:825-830.
3. Surve A, Cottam D, Sanchez-Pernaute A, et al. The incidence of complications associated with loop duodeno-ileostomy after single-anastomosis duodenal switch procedures among 1328 patients: a multicenter experience. *Surg Obes Relat Dis*. 2018;14:594-601.
4. Cottam A, Cottam D, Portenier D, et al. A matched cohort analysis of stomach intestinal pylorus saving (SIPS) surgery vs biliopancreatic diversion with duodenal switch with two-year follow-up. *Obes Surg*. 2017;27:454-461.
5. Park CH, Nam S-J, Choi HS, et al. Comparative efficacy of bariatric surgery in the treatment of morbid obesity and diabetes mellitus: a systematic review and network meta-analysis. *Obes Surg*. 2019;29:2180-2190.

Chapter 50
Surgical Management of Bariatric Complications: Internal Hernia and Leak

Elizabeth G. McCarthy, Susan Laura Jao, and Aurora D. Pryor

DEFINITION

- Bariatric surgery has been proven the most effective and sustainable means for the treatment of obesity and its complications.[1,2] Bariatric surgical interventions include sleeve gastrectomy (SG), Roux-en-Y gastric bypass (RYGB), duodenal switch (DS), and single-anastomosis duodenal switch (SADI). With over 250,000 cases being performed each year in the United States, it is important to understand the complications that may arise.[3] Complications include but are not limited to leak, bleeding, venous thromboembolism, internal hernia, intussusception, marginal ulcer, and perforation. Here we will focus on internal hernia and leak along with their associated diagnostic measures and treatments.
- An internal hernia is defined as a protrusion of abdominal viscera through a defect within the abdominal cavity. In bariatric surgery, these defects are surgically created due to rearrangement of the intestine required in the procedure. Closure of this defect at the time of initial operation has shown to reduce incidence.[4-6]
- Internal hernia can occur after RYGB, DS, and SADI. Incidence of internal hernia has been reported from <1% to 9%.[7-12] It has been suggested that the laparoscopic approach leads to a greater incidence of internal hernia due to decreased adhesion formation.[13]
- Areas where a defect can occur depend on the operation performed. An antecolic anastomosis leaves spaces at the jejunojejunostomy and Petersen defect, the area between the transverse mesocolon and the Roux limb mesentery. In a retrocolic anastomosis, there is an additional area for herniation through the transverse mesocolon where the alimentary limb is brought through (**FIGURE 1**).

- Leak has been reported in anywhere from 0.7% to 7% of cases with risks including increased body mass index and revisional surgery.[14-17] It is one of the most feared complications as mortality rate can reach up to 4.3%.[18] Leak is the second most common complication after venous thromboembolism in patients undergoing RYGB.[19]
- Leak generally occurs within 72 hours but can be seen up to 5 to 7 days postoperatively. Early leak is felt to be related to technical error, whereas a leak later is associated with staple line ischemia or anastomotic tension.
- Leak can occur due to improper staple firing as well as retained staples at the apex leading to inadequate approximation of the next staple firing.[19]
- In SG, the most common site of leak is near the esophagogastric junction.[17] In RYGB, leak rates are highest at the gastrojejunostomy followed by the gastric pouch, excluded stomach, and jejunojejunostomy, respectively.[19]

DIFFERENTIAL DIAGNOSIS

- When patients present to the emergency department with abdominal pain after RYGB, the differential diagnosis includes internal hernia, marginal ulcer, maladaptive eating, bacterial overgrowth, constipation, biliary disease, intussusception, anastomotic leak, or stenosis.[7] One should also consider other etiologies for pain that are unrelated to the bariatric surgery.
- If a patient presents with tachycardia and signs of sepsis, you must rule out a leak or perforation if the patient has had bariatric surgery.
- Early complications include leak, bleeding, stenosis, or venous thromboembolism.[11]

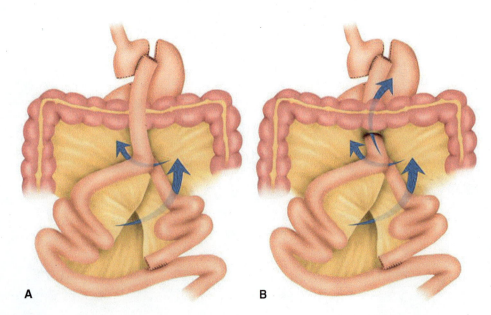

FIGURE 1 • Depiction of possible hernia sites in **(A)** antecolic and **(B)** retrocolic Roux-en-Y gastric bypass. (Drawings courtesy of Susan Laura Jao, BA.)

- Late complications include internal hernia, gallstones, marginal ulcer, perforation, and small bowel obstruction.[11]

PATIENT HISTORY AND PHYSICAL FINDINGS

- Tachycardia is a telltale sign in a patient with leak, and as such, this complication should be investigated early. In postoperative patients with persistent tachycardia, leak should be high on the differential.[11,19]
- Patients can present along a spectrum from stable to septic. Abdominal pain, tachypnea, fever, and oliguria can all be present and should prompt further workup.
- Presentation for an internal hernia can include both acute and chronic pain. Patients will sometimes describe colicky abdominal pain as well as issues with bowel function signifying an obstructive process.
- Patients should be asked about any nausea, vomiting, or obstipation if there is concern for internal hernia and obstruction.
- All patients should be asked about fever or chills at home.
- Physical examination will likely reveal tenderness to palpation, which may or may not include peritoneal signs.

IMAGING AND OTHER DIAGNOSTIC STUDIES

- In a patient with sustained tachycardia postoperatively, early operative intervention prior to imaging should be strongly considered. If the diagnosis is unclear, the study of choice is an upper gastrointestinal series with water-soluble contrast to evaluate for presence of leak.
- A computed tomography (CT) scan can be ordered as this may reveal abscesses or fluid collections adjacent to the site of a leak. This study is also more likely to identify pathology at the jejunojejunostomy.
- Upper endoscopy is an additional modality to look for mucosal disruption. This is typically performed intraoperatively for early leak or as part of a therapeutic procedure for a late leak.
- For patients with suspected internal hernia, a CT scan with PO and IV contrast may elucidate an issue.
- CT scans have been shown to be sensitive but not specific for evaluation of internal hernia.[20]
- Mesenteric swirl is the most common finding on imaging for identification of internal hernia[8,20,21] (**FIGURE 2**).
- Ultimately, if internal hernia is suspected, even with negative imaging, a diagnostic laparoscopy is the next step.

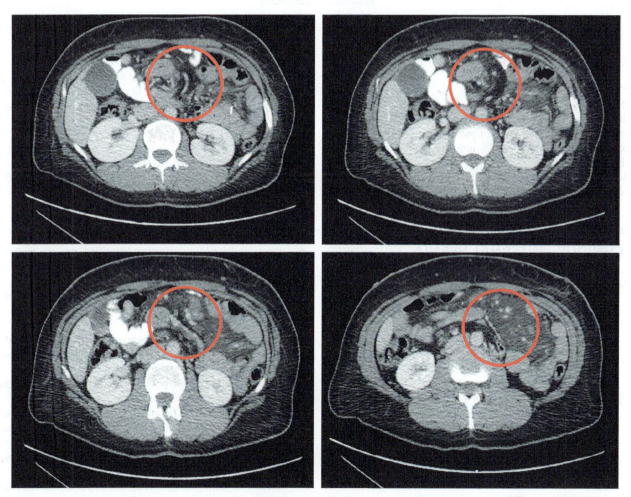

FIGURE 2 • CT imaging demonstrating swirl sign in axial view and vasculature running through defect with mesenteric enhancement in the coronal view.

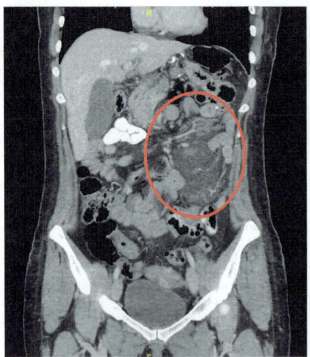 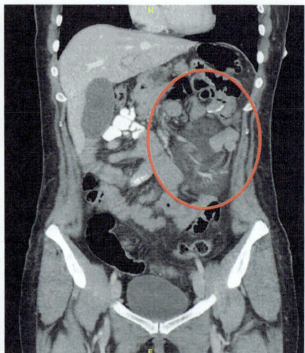

FIGURE 2 • Continued

SURGICAL MANAGEMENT

Preoperative Planning

- If sepsis is suspected in either complication, recommendation should follow surviving sepsis guidelines including IV antibiotics, early fluid resuscitation, pressors to maintain a MAP of 65 mm Hg, and goal-directed therapy.[22]
- Mainstay of treatment for each is resuscitation and source control with early operative intervention.
- Surgical goal for a leak is removal of enteric contents from the abdomen and closure vs drainage at the site of the leak.
- Surgical goal for an internal hernia is reduction of hernia and resection of any compromised bowel along with closure of the defect.

Positioning

- Supine positioning with arms outstretched.
- Reverse Trendelenburg positioning is helpful for evaluation of the hiatus, which is facilitated by a footboard.

TECHNIQUE—INTERNAL HERNIA

LAPAROSCOPIC (▶ VIDEO 1)

- It is safe to start with a Veress needle in Palmer point to achieve pneumoperitoneum. We use an optical trocar into the abdomen once pneumoperitoneum is achieved.
- The abdomen can be briefly inspected at this point prior to placement of additional trocars.
- Trocar placement will be dependent on area of interest, but it may be feasible to place ports at previous incision sites.
- To evaluate for internal hernia, it is necessary to run the small bowel. One can begin at the gastrojejunal anastomosis and run the limb to the jejunojejunostomy (▶ VIDEO 1).
- Inspecting the jejunojejunostomy can reveal a mesenteric defect.
- Lifting the transverse colon will reveal the mesocolon and a potential defect in Petersen space or in the mesocolon itself if the patient underwent a retrocolic anastomosis.
- Once the jejunojejunostomy is identified, one can trace the biliopancreatic limb to the ligament of Treitz. The common channel can also be run to the cecum.
- While running the small bowel, it should move freely. Resistance in an area can signal an internal hernia or adhesion.
- If one has difficulty running the bowel antegrade, it is easiest to identify the cecum and run the bowel from the terminal ileum in a retrograde fashion, working from known to unknown.
- Chylous ascites is commonly encountered with obstructed bowel.
- Often, the bowel can be inflamed and friable making it easily injured. It is advisable to take large bites with an atraumatic grasper when running the bowel. Alternatively, the mesentery can be grasped. This is particularly helpful with dilated bowel.
- Closure of identified defects should be performed with nonabsorbable suture being careful to take shallow bites so as not to disrupt the blood supply.

- Petersen defect can be closed by approximating the Roux limb mesentery to the mesocolon.
- A mesenteric defect can be closed by approximating the mesentery up to the jejunojejunostomy.
- Closure of a mesocolic defect occurs by placing sutures circumferentially around the Roux limb in a running locking fashion to prevent Roux limb obstruction.

OPEN

- Recommend an upper midline incision.
- Overall, steps of the operation should be similar to the laparoscopic procedure.

TECHNIQUE—LEAK

- Intervention will highly depend on the clinical status of the patient.
- In patients with peritonitis, septic shock, or hemodynamic instability, operative intervention is the next step in treatment.
- In stable patients with a contained leak, endoscopic intervention is possible with radiologic drainage of any fluid collection. Please see Chapter 51 for further discussion. Patients may also require laparoscopic or open drainage of fluid collections in conjunction with stent placement.

LAPAROSCOPIC

- As with internal hernia, the safest entry point for abdominal insufflation is at Palmer point or other site away from the symptomatic site.
- The abdomen is evaluated for area of concern. In a gastric sleeve, this is most likely at the angle of His. In a bypass, the gastrojejunostomy is most likely to be the area of concern. The area of focus can also be directed by preoperative imaging. Generally, it is best to inspect each anastomosis, even if imaging provides an area of suspicion.
- Irrigation and suction can be used to drain any purulent fluid.
- Anastomotic disruption can be primarily suture repaired if feasible or stapled off. Patch closure with omentum or bowel can also be helpful.
- Drains should be left in place.

PEARLS AND PITFALLS

- Persistent tachycardia is the most common sign of early leak and should prompt workup for evaluation.
- Clinical stability will guide management for leaks after bariatric surgery.
- Work from known to unknown when running the bowel to identify an internal hernia.
- Surgeons should have a low threshold for diagnostic laparoscopy in patients with concerning symptoms of internal hernia or leak even with negative imaging.

POSTOPERATIVE CARE

- Much of the postoperative care depends on the clinical stability of the patient.
- If the patient has signs of acidosis, was found to have significant necrosis requiring bowel resection, or is hemodynamically unstable, they likely will require a higher level of care and admission to a surgical ICU is appropriate.
- If the patient is clinically stable, no necrotic bowel was found or resected, and reduction of internal hernia was successful, the patient may be started on a full liquid diet postoperatively.
- For patients who required bowel resection, diet can be started with clears and advanced as tolerated.

COMPLICATIONS

- Bleeding
- Anastomotic breakdown
- Postoperative sepsis

REFERENCES

1. Chang SH, Stoll CRT, Song J, Varela JE, Eagon CJ, Colditz GA. The effectiveness and risks of bariatric surgery an updated systematic review and meta-analysis, 2003-2012. *JAMA Surg*. 2014;149(3):275-287. doi:10.1001/jamasurg.2013.3654
2. Schauer PR, Bhatt DL, Kirwan JP, et al. Bariatric surgery versus intensive medical therapy for diabetes—5-year outcomes. *N Engl J Med*. 2017;376(7):641-651. doi:10.1056/nejmoa1600869

3. *Estimate of Bariatric Surgery Numbers, 2011-2019*. Accessed August 20, 2021. https://asmbs.org/resources/estimate-of-bariatric-surgery-numbers
4. Thomas R, Olbers T, Barry JD, Beamish AJ. Closure of mesenteric defects during Roux-en-Y gastric bypass for obesity: a systematic review and meta-analysis protocol. *Int J Surg Protoc*. 2019;15:1-4. doi:10.1016/j.isjp.2019.02.003
5. Aghajani E, Nergaard BJ, Leifson BG, Hedenbro J, Gislason H. The mesenteric defects in laparoscopic Roux-en-Y gastric bypass: 5 years follow-up of non-closure versus closure using the stapler technique. *Surg Endosc*. 2017;31(9):3743-3748. doi:10.1007/s00464-017-5415-2
6. Stenberg E, Szabo E, Ågren G, et al. Closure of mesenteric defects in laparoscopic gastric bypass: a multicentre, randomised, parallel, open-label trial. *Lancet*. 2016;387(10026):1397-1404. doi:10.1016/S0140-6736(15)01126-5
7. Greenstein AJ, O'Rourke RW. Abdominal pain after gastric bypass: suspects and solutions. *Am J Surg*. 2011;201(6):819-827. doi:10.1016/j.amjsurg.2010.05.007
8. Al-Mansour MR, Mundy R, Canoy JM, Dulaimy K, Kuhn JN, Romanelli J. Internal hernia after laparoscopic antecolic roux-en-Y gastric bypass. *Obes Surg*. 2015;25(11):2106-2111. doi:10.1007/s11695-015-1672-0
9. O'Rourke RW. Management strategies for internal hernia after gastric bypass. *J Gastrointest Surg*. 2011;15(6):1049-1054. doi:10.1007/s11605-010-1401-x
10. Nimeri AA, Maasher A, al Shaban T, Salim E, Gamaleldin MM. Internal hernia following laparoscopic roux-en-Y gastric bypass: prevention and tips for intra-operative management. *Obes Surg*. 2016;26(9):2255-2256. doi:10.1007/s11695-016-2267-0
11. Lim R, Beekley A, Johnson DC, Davis KA. Early and late complications of bariatric operation. *Trauma Surg Acute Care Open*. 2018;3(1):e000219. doi:10.1136/tsaco-2018-000219
12. Tartamella F, Ziccarelli A, Cecchini S, et al. Abdominal pain and internal hernias after Roux-en-Y gastric bypass: are we dealing with the tip of an iceberg? *Acta Biomed*. 2019;90(2):251-258. doi:10.23750/abm.v90i2.7145
13. Higa KD, Boone B, Ho T. Complications of the laparoscopic Roux-en-Y gastric bypass: 1,040 patients—what have we learned? *Obes Surg*. 2000;10(6):509-513.
14. Alizadeh RF, Li S, Inaba C, et al. Risk factors for gastrointestinal leak after bariatric surgery: MBASQIP analysis. *J Am Coll Surg*. 2018;227(1):135-141. doi:10.1016/j.jamcollsurg.2018.03.030
15. Chang SH, Freeman NLB, Lee JA, et al. Early major complications after bariatric surgery in the USA, 2003-2014: a systematic review and meta-analysis. *Obes Rev*. 2018;19(4):529-537. doi:10.1111/obr.12647
16. Marshall JS, Srivastava A, Gupta SK, Rossi TR, Debord JR. Roux-En-Y gastric bypass leak complications. *Arch Surg*. 2003;138(5):520-524.
17. Aurora AR, Khaitan L, Saber AA. Sleeve gastrectomy and the risk of leak: a systematic analysis of 4,888 patients. *Surg Endosc*. 2012;26(6):1509-1515. doi:10.1007/s00464-011-2085-3.
18. Daigle CR, Brethauer SA, Tu C, et al. Which postoperative complications matter most after bariatric surgery? Prioritizing quality improvement efforts to improve national outcomes. *Surg Obes Relat Dis*. 2018;14(5):652-657. doi:10.1016/j.soard.2018.01.008
19. Acquafresca PA, Palermo M, Rogula T, Duza GE, Serra E. Early surgical complications after gastric by-pass: a literature review. *Arq Bras Cir Dig*. 2015;28(1):74-80. doi:10.1590/S0102-67202015000100019
20. Altieri MS, Pryor AD, Telem DA, Hall K, Brathwaite C, Zawin M. Algorithmic approach to utilization of CT scans for detection of internal hernia in the gastric bypass patient. *Surg Obes Relat Dis*. 2015;11(6):1207-1211. doi:10.1016/j.soard.2015.02.010
21. Dilauro M, Mcinnes MDF, Schieda N, et al. Internal hernia after laparoscopic roux-en-Y gastric bypass: optimal CT signs for diagnosis and clinical decision making. *Radiology*. 2017;282(3):752-760. doi:10.1148/radiol.2016160956
22. Rhodes A, Evans LE, Alhazzani W, et al. Surviving sepsis campaign: international guidelines for management of sepsis and septic shock—2016. *Intensive Care Med*. 2017;43(3):304-377. doi:10.1007/s00134-017-4683-6

Chapter 51
Endoscopic Management of Bariatric Complications: Leak and Stricture

Megan P. Lundgren and Matthew Kroh

DEFINITION

Leak After Bariatric Surgery

- A *leak* after bariatric surgery is a disruption of the gastrointestinal wall, typically at a staple line or suture.
- The chronic manifestation of a leak is a fistula, once an epithelized tract has formed.
- See **FIGURE 1**.

Stricture After Bariatric Surgery

- A *stricture* after bariatric surgery is otherwise known as a stenosis—stomal stenosis after an anastomotic procedure or sleeve stenosis after a sleeve gastrectomy, to name the most common.

DIFFERENTIAL DIAGNOSIS

Differential of a Leak After Bariatric Surgery

- Systemic inflammatory response syndrome (SIRS)/sepsis due to a gastrointestinal leak
- Postoperative bleeding
- Cardiac events/arrhythmia
- Pulmonary embolism (PE)
- Volume depletion

Differential of a Fistula After Bariatric Surgery

Fistulas and their most commonly associated symptoms are:

- Gastro-gastric (reflux, weight regain, bloating)
- Gastroenteric/colonic (weight loss, diarrhea, feculent breath)
- Gastropulmonary (pneumonia, shortness of breath, chest pain, fever of unknown origin)
- Gastroperitoneal (fever, abdominal pain)
- Enterocutaneous (cutaneous abscess, drainage)

Differential of a Stricture After Bariatric Surgery

- Technical error (especially if the stricture/stenosis is presenting early)
  - If a linear gastrojejunal or duodeno-ileal anastomosis was performed, this can be the result of creation of a false tract.
  - If a small circular stapler was utilized for the gastrojejunal anastomosis.
  - If a sleeve was created over a small bougie.
- Marginal ulcer
  - Nicotine use with cigarettes, cigars, or vaping
  - NSAID use
- Gastro-gastric fistula
- Foreign body reaction to staple or permanent suture
- Malignancy as a remote possibility can be considered

PATIENT HISTORY AND PHYSICAL FINDINGS

Presentation of a Leak

- The presentation of an acute leak includes symptoms such as pain, nausea, emesis, and systemic sepsis.
- Specific physical findings include tachycardia, hemodynamic instability, and fever.
- The patient may show epigastric tenderness, peritonitis, or a normal abdominal examination.

Presentation of a Stricture

- A patient with a stricture will typically present with dysphagia, oral intolerance, epigastric pain worse with oral intake, reflux, increased rate of weight loss and nausea, and emesis.
- Symptoms tend to be progressive and often do not present acutely.

IMAGING AND DIAGNOSTIC STUDIES

- The initial workup for a postoperative patient presenting with pain and tachycardia includes an EKG and chest radiograph and comprehensive laboratory values.
- Typically, a stat computed tomography (CT) scan is ordered inclusive of the chest, abdomen, and pelvis scan with intravascular contrast to rule out PE and with oral contrast to investigate for a leak.
- If these studies are negative and there is still concern for a leak, an upper gastrointestinal study with barium can be performed.
  - Laboratory studies
  - EKG, chest radiograph
  - CT scan of the chest, abdomen, and pelvis with per oral and intravenous contrast (**FIGURE 2A**)
  - Upper gastrointestinal study (**FIGURE 2B**)
  - Upper endoscopy ± fluoroscopy (**FIGURE 2C**)
- The initial workup for a patient presenting with symptoms of a stricture includes:
  - Diagnostic upper endoscopy
  - Upper gastrointestinal contrast study (**FIGURE 2D**)

SURGICAL (AND ENDOSCOPIC) MANAGEMENT

- A patient's presenting symptoms and presence or absence of sepsis will dictate the appropriate need for surgical, endoscopic, and nonoperative management.
- There is no standard or endorsed algorithm for management of leaks and fistulas due to the spectrum of presenting scenarios and heterogeneity of individual patient and previous operations. Refer to **FIGURE 3** for the author's institutions' general algorithm for management of leaks, fistulas, and strictures.
- There may also be a need for recurrent endoscopic or surgical interventions. If repeated endoscopic intervention is performed, consideration must be made of progress and likelihood of achieving definitive management or optimizing a patient for eventual surgery.

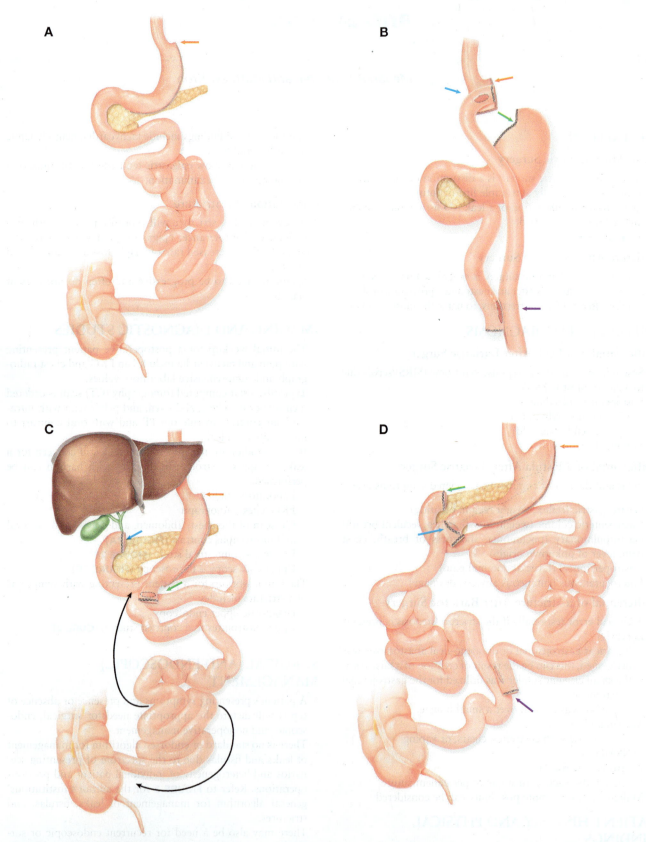

FIGURE 1 Anatomy of leaks. **A,** Sleeve anatomy with most likely leak sites marked. *Orange arrow*: just distal to gastroesophageal junction. **B,** Roux-en-Y anatomy with most likely leak sites marked. (*Orange arrow*: Vertical staple line of pouch. *Blue arrow*: Gastrojejunal anastomosis. *Green arrow*: Remnant stomach staple line. *Purple arrow*: Jejunojejunal anastomosis.) **C,** Single anastomosis duodeno-ileal bypass with sleeve gastrectomy (SADI-S) with most likely leak sites marked. (*Orange arrow*: Just distal to the gastroesophageal junction. *Blue arrow*: Duodeno-ileal anastomosis. *Green arrow*: Duodenal stump staple line). **D,** Biliopancreatic diversion with duodenal switch (BPD-DS) with most likely leak sites marked. (*Orange arrow*: Proximal sleeve staple line. *Blue arrow*: Duodeno-ileal anastomosis. *Green arrow*: Duodenal stump staple line. *Purple arrow*: Distal small bowel staple line.)

Chapter 51 ENDOSCOPIC MANAGEMENT OF BARIATRIC COMPLICATIONS: LEAK AND STRICTURE   425

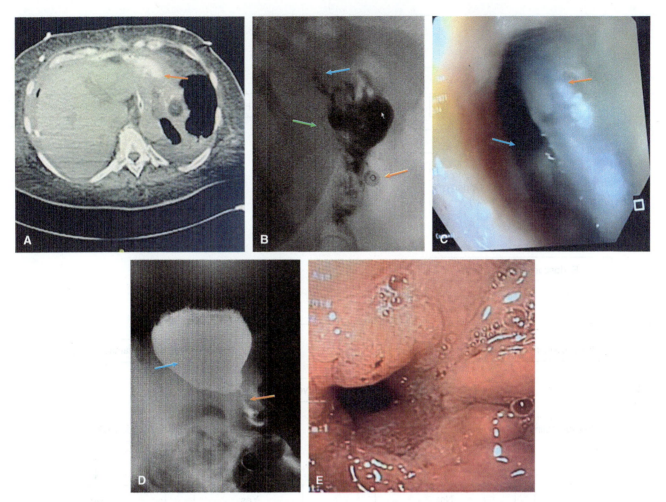

FIGURE 2 Imaging workup. **A,** CT scan with acute leak of enteral contrast and air from the gastrojejunal anastomosis demonstrated (*orange arrow*). **B,** Upper gastrointestinal image (UGI) demonstrating chronic leak/fistula (*blue arrow*), gastrojejunal anastomosis (*green arrow*), PEJ tube (*orange arrow*). **C,** Endoscopic image with defect in gastrojejunal anastomosis (*blue arrow*) and percutaneously placed drain visible (*orange arrow*). **D,** Gastrojejunal stricture (*orange arrow*) with dilated pouch (*blue arrow*) on UGI. **E,** Gastrojejunal stricture on upper endoscopy.

- The following focuses on the endoscopic management of leaks/fistulas. Endoscopic stricture management includes behavioral (stop smoking, stop NSAIDs) and medical intervention (antisecretory medications and mucosal protectants if there is an associated ulcer) and dilation (balloon, rigid) and stent placement (over a wire or through the scope). Balloon dilation and stent placement methods are described in detail within the following technical sections.

Preoperative Planning

- The surgeon should determine the overall status of the patient, including attention to systemic sepsis and malnutrition.
- Source control of sepsis must be obtained first. Ensure antibiotic coverage, including fungal as appropriate, can plan for external drainage if internal drainage is not planned endoscopically.
- Next, nutritional status and frailty should be assessed. If possible, prior to intervention the surgeon should obtain operative reports or speak directly to the index operating surgeon.

Classification of a Leak or Fistula

- The surgeon must ask several questions to plan the endoscopic intervention, including:
  - What is the timing of leak/fistula, site of leak/fistula, and size of the defect? What is the patient's anatomy and why is there a leak?
  - Is there a sleeve stenosis/stricture associated with the leak? (This may require a combination procedure such as balloon dilation or stenting across a sleeve or anastomotic stenosis.)
  - Has a cavity already been drained externally, ie, by interventional radiology? If there is external contamination and the surgical endoscopist plans to close the defect endoluminally (ie, stenting over the defect, over-the-scope clips, endoscopic suture closure of the defect), then the external contamination must be drained (ie, interventional radiology drainage). And importantly, a plan for enteral access/nutrition should be considered preoperatively.
  - Where is the best site for enteral access for nutrition in this patient, relative to the leak or stricture site?

426 SECTION VIII SURGERY OF THE STOMACH AND DUODENUM

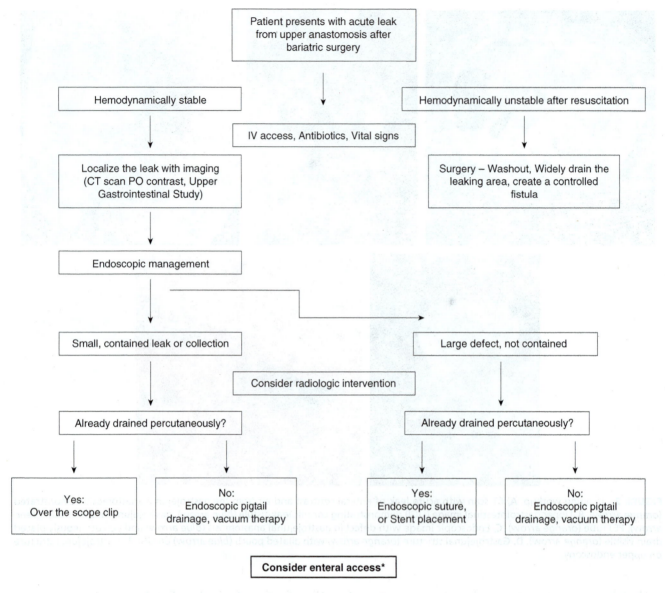

FIGURE 3 • General algorithm for management of leaks.

Positioning and Procedure Setup

- General anesthesia with orotracheal intubation is used in these cases.
- The patients are generally positioned supine.
- It is helpful ergonomically to drop the operating room table to its lowest height and to create a stage to the left of the operating room table out of the several surgical steps.
- Endoscopic screens are positioned to the right of the patient.
- The C-arm is positioned from the start of the case.
- It is important to have available:
  - A standard gastroscope and a therapeutic gastroscope, with the standard scope set up initially
  - Water-soluble contrast
  - Saline
  - Methylene blue
  - Intraoperative fluoroscopy team and C-arm from the start of the case
  - Carbon dioxide insufflation
  - Electrosurgical unit
- An endoscopy cart with:
  - Pigtail drain catheters of various lengths
  - Balloon dilators of various sizes
  - Super stiff and biliary wires
  - Paper clips
  - Partially covered and full covered stents of various lengths
  - Endoscopic clips (over-the-scope clips and hemostatic clips)
  - Methylene blue
  - Feeding tubes

ENDOSCOPIC PIGTAIL DRAINAGE (FIGURE 4A-D)

Indications

- To drain a contained collection internally
- Pigtail drainage can serve as an adjunct to other leak/fistula treatment such as stent placement. Pigtail drainage works best for collection which are not already percutaneously drained.
- Common indications are leaks from postoperative anatomy which upper endoscopy can reach:
    - Gastrojejunal anastomosis
    - Pouch vertical staple line
    - Sleeve staple line leak (frequently located at the proximal staple line)

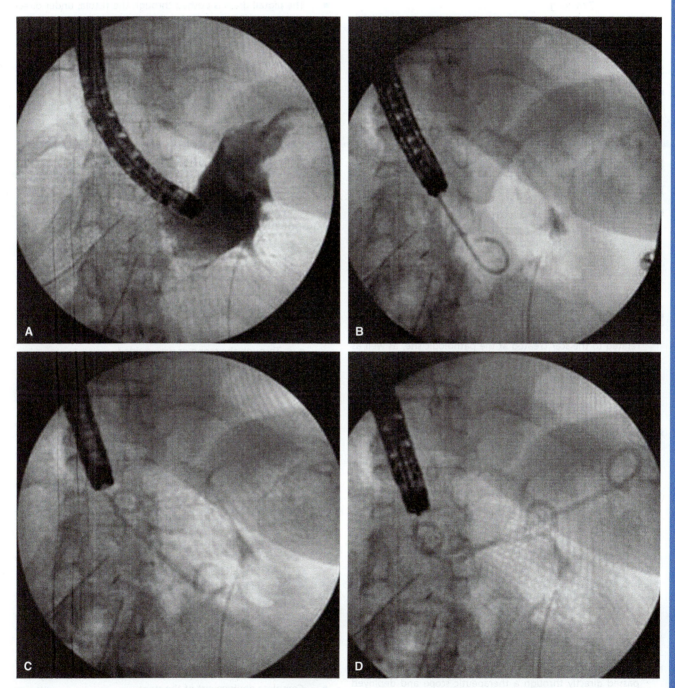

FIGURE 4 • Endoscopic Pigtail Drainage of a leak, with addition of stent placement under fluoroscopy. **A,** Endoscopy with fluoroscopy to confirm the leak site. **B,** Advancement of a distal pigtail drain (7-Fr, 4 mm) into the cavity over a soft biliary type wire with a pusher, allowing it to curl as the scope is pulled back and drain is advanced forward. **C,** The proximal pigtail is pushed off of the wire, allowing it to curl within the lumen. **D,** A second pigtail drain (7-Fr, 7 mm) is placed into the same cavity.

- Duodeno-ileal anastomosis
- Equipment to have in room
  - Standard forward-viewing gastroscope
  - CO_2 insufflation
  - C-arm/fluoroscopy available
  - Water-soluble contrast
  - Double pigtail drains: Pigtail drains come in various sizes (French and length). If the collection can be measured on an imaging study, appropriate length drains can be chosen. Typical sizes include 7- to 10-Fr, 4 to 7 cm long.
  - .035-in biliary wire
  - Pigtail drain "pusher"
  - Paper clips

Steps

- Upper gastrointestinal endoscopy is carried out to identify the fistula/leak site
- Fluoroscopy can be used to identify the site or confirm the site
- The opening is then cannulated with a .035-in guidewire and confirmed to be looped in the cavity using an X-ray
- Mark the pigtail drain with a permanent marker at the site where it will curl.
- Load the double pigtail biliary drain (7-10 Fr, 4-7 cm) onto the wire
- The pigtail drain is then advanced using the "pusher" loaded onto the wire behind the stent
- The pigtail drain is pushed through the fistula, under direct vision, until the marks on the pigtail drain are just outside of the fistula. At this point the distal end will be looped inside of the collection.
- As the scope is pulled back, the proximal pigtail loop is created and lands within the lumen of the gastrointestinal structure
- Fluoroscopy is used to confirm location

ENDOSCOPIC STENTING (FIGURE 5A-D)

Indications

- There are two broad uses for endoscopic stents after foregut surgery:
  1. To divert enteric contents while maintaining gastrointestinal continuity in the management of anastomotic or staple line leaks or in gastrointestinal fistulas.
  2. In the management of postoperative anastomotic or sleeve gastrectomy stenosis/strictures.
- In general, the earlier a stent is placed for a leak, the more likely successful treatment and healing of the leak. This is related to the scar created at the pathologic site, as well as malnutrition associated with chronic anastomotic leaking/fistulas.[1] One large series from Chang et al showed efficacy of stent placement across foregut anastomotic leaks, and one of the great advantages was earlier initiation of enteral feeding as well as avoidance of the morbidity of a major operation.[2]
- Stents are deployed across:
  - Sleeve leaks/fistulas, at any level of the sleeve. Sometimes two stents are required in order to prevent stent migration.
    1. There is a "Mega Stent" designed for sleeve leaks. Mega esophageal stents (Niti-S Mega esophageal stent, Taewoong Medical, Gyeonggido, South Korea) are fully covered metallic stents of 18 to 23 cm in length that are designed for sleeve gastrectomy leaks. These stents can be placed across a stricture in the sleeve, such as across a tight incisura, and simultaneously cover the leak site.[3]
  - Gastrojejunostomy leaks/fistulas
  - Duodeno-ileal leaks after BPD-DS
  - It is more difficult to stent a SADI-S leak due to the afferent and efferent limbs at the loop anastomosis.
- You can choose through the scope stent. These stents are passed directly through a therapeutic scope and deployed under direct vision.
- Alternatively, a fluoroscopic wire-guided stent is possible. In this case a standard gastroscope can be utilized. A super stiff wire is place first, and the gastroscope removed over the wire. The stent is then loaded over the wire and deployed based on the surgeon's radio-opaque marker placement under fluoroscopic guidance.

Equipment

- Standard forward-viewing gastroscope or therapeutic scope
- CO_2 insufflation
- C-arm/fluoroscopy available
- Water-soluble contrast
- Gastrointestinal stents
  - These come in multiple sizes in French and length
  - Fully covered or partially covered
  - Through the scope or wire guided
- Stiff wire
- Paper clips

Steps

- Upper gastrointestinal endoscopy is carried out to identify the fistula/leak site.
- Fluoroscopy can be used to identify the site or confirm the site.
- Mark the leak site with a paper clip on the skin or an endoscopically placed radiopaque clip.
- The scope is advanced beyond the leak site into the target for the distal end of the stent.
  - Beyond the gastroesophageal junction in EGJ leaks.
  - Prepyloric in sleeve gastrectomy leaks depending on the stent and if a sleeve stenosis is present.
  - Roux limb in gastrojejunal leaks.
  - Roux limb.
- Identify the wire and confirm with fluoroscopy that the marker for the distal end of the stent is at the level of your placed marker.
- Slowly deploy the stent under fluoroscopy until near "the point of no return." Adjust the stent as needed at this point.
- Complete deployment of the stent.
- If through the scope:
  - Using a therapeutic scope, pass the stent under direct vision while you are looking at your distal target.

Chapter 51 ENDOSCOPIC MANAGEMENT OF BARIATRIC COMPLICATIONS: LEAK AND STRICTURE

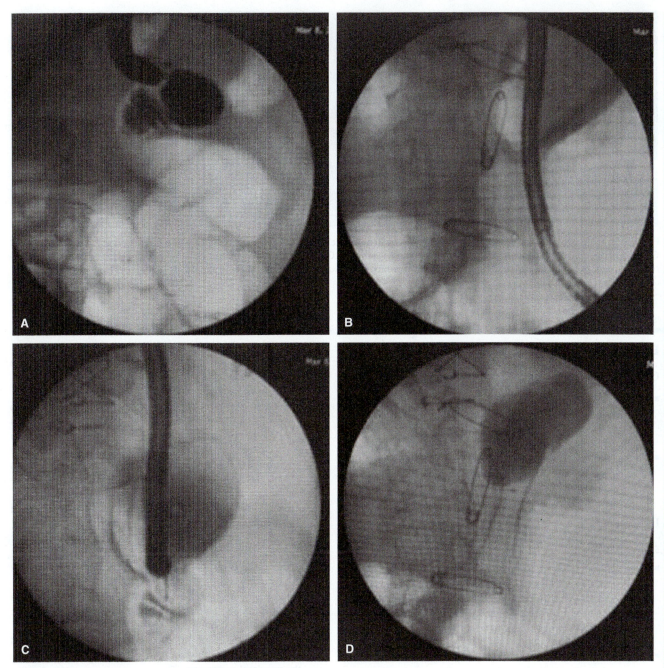

FIGURE 5 • Stenting across a gastrojejunal stricture. **A,** Present endoscopic fluoroscopy to identify a very tight stricture. **B,** After balloon dilation, the scope was able to traverse the stricture. The scope was advanced across the stricture, and paperclips were used to mark the gastroesophageal junction, the stricture, and the distal target in the Roux limb for the stent placement. **C,** A super stiff wire is advanced across the stricture. **D,** Stent is deployed over the wire across the gastrojejunal stricture. At the site of the stricture, the stent can be noted to be slightly stenosed. The stent was clipped into place proximally.

- As you pull the scope back, you can directly visualize the stent deployment.
- You can confirm the stent placement with fluoroscopy.
- You can choose to scope through the stent (preferably with an XP scope) to confirm full coverage of the pathology.
- Fixation of the proximal flange of the stent, with suturing devices, cap-mounted clips, or the nasal bridle technique can be considered.

- Most frequent complications:
  - The most common complication after stent placement was stent intolerance with symptoms of nausea, reflux, epigastric pain, and migration of the stent. Aspiration risk is also increased. Migration of the stent can lead to repetitive trips to the operating room with need for a second stent placement or repositioning or removal.[3]

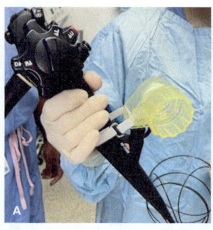 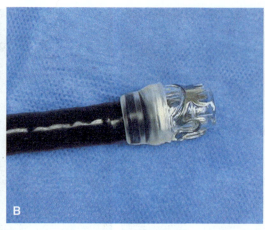 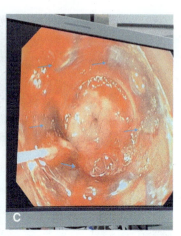

FIGURE 6 • Placement of an over-the-scope clip on a gastro-gastric fistula site. **A,** Over-the-scope clip apparatus attached to standard GIF endoscope. **B,** Over-the-scope clip mounted on end of standard GIF endoscope. **C,** The tines of the over-the-scope clip and seen surrounding and ready to deploy across the small fistula, which had caused a marginal ulcer and a gastrojejunal perforation.

ENDOSCOPIC CLOSURE

Over-the-Scope Clips (FIGURE 6)

- The over-the-scope clipping (OTSC) system (Ovesco Endoscopy AG, Tubingen, Germany) has been used recently for endoscopic closure of defects including fistulae, leaks, and acute perforations.
- The OTSC is a single-use elastic clip mounted on a hood that is placed on the tip of an endoscope and then deployed intraluminal at the site of the defect. This is effective only for defects <2 cm.[4]

Indications

Acute Leaks

- In general, over-the-scope clips work best for small, acute perforations with healthy surround tissue. Success has been shown with over-the-scope clips as a standalone procedure for control of an acute leak—and this was reported in a multicenter study where 73% of acute leaks were controlled with over-the-scope clips alone.[5]
- However, from other authors' perspective, there are not enough studies on the over-the-scope clip as a sole treatment to recommended it as a standalone treatment, especially for nonacute leaks or chronic fistula.

Chronic Fistulas

- One retrospective single institution review did report that over-the-scope clips can have at least short-term success for nonacute defects.[6]

Equipment

- Standard forward-viewing gastroscope
- CO_2 insufflation
- C-arm/fluoroscopy available in the room to do immediate test of efficacy
- Over-the-scope clips—multiple sizes exist
  - Caps of various diameters exist to accommodate endoscopes with tip outer diameters ranging from 8.5 to 14 mm: the choice of diameter of the clip depends on the outer diameter of the gastroscope you are using as well as the defect size. Defects >2 cm cannot be successfully closed with over-the-scope clips.
  - Cap depths can be chosen as well—between 3 and 6 mm.

Steps

- Upper gastrointestinal endoscopy is carried out to identify the fistula/leak site.
- Fluoroscopy can be used to identify the site or confirm the site; this can also be marked with a paper clip on the skin for identification on fluoroscopy later.
- The scope is removed and the over-the-scope clip is mounted on the distal tip of the scope; the hand wheel is mounted to the proximal endoscope.
- The scope with mounted clip is advanced to the defect. The scope must be advanced with care and under direct vision while the clip is mounted. It can be difficult to pass the scope and a jaw thrust is required.
- The tissue of interest is placed in apposition to the clip. An instrument can be used through the working channel to grasp the tissue as needed for better apposition.
- The hand wheel is used to deploy the clip over the defect.
- Fluoroscopy can be used to test the efficacy of the clip placement.

ENDOSCOPIC SUTURING/PLICATION (FIGURE 7A AND B)

- An endoscopic suturing device (OverStitch; Apollo Endosurgery, Austin, Tex, USA) is available in an original form as well as a more recent form. The first requires a double channel endoscope. The new device can be used with a single-channel endoscope. The endoscopic suturing system is mounted onto the endoscope using silicone straps.
- The device use is not entirely intuitive, and demands practice for optimal results. Some defects require complex suturing patterns. Endoscopic suturing for perforations is typically best performed in a right-to-left and distal-to-proximal progression, using a running suture pattern.[7]

Indications

- In the closure of complex or large defects
- Small, acute defects are probably best closed with over-the-scopes clips. Defects associated with stenosis are probably best covered with a stent, with either internal or external drainage of any extraluminal contamination/collection.

Equipment

- Therapeutic forward-viewing gastroscope, with double or single channel depending on the suturing device available
- CO_2 insufflation
- C-arm/fluoroscopy available in the room to do immediate test of efficacy
- Water-soluble contrast
- Endoscopic electrosurgical unit available
  - In case of need to do submucosal dissection prior to suturing
  - In case of need to perform probe coagulation to mark the stitch sites prior to suturing
- Endoscopic suturing device
  - Cap portion
  - Needle driver assembly portion with straps
  - Close the handle of the needle driver to expose the needle and exchange the anchor to perform endoscopic suturing (video link provided).

Steps

- Upper gastrointestinal endoscopy is carried out to identify the fistula/leak site.
- Fluoroscopy can be used to identify the site or confirm the site.
- Remove any nearby foreign bodies like or sutures that will preclude successful closure.
- At this time, depending on the site and indication for suturing:
  - If it is a chronic fistula, an endoscopic submucosal dissection can be performed to remove chronically scarred tissue to allow for re-epithelialization.
  - Argon plasma coagulation or a coagulation probe can be used to mark the target sites for suturing which can be a helpful guide once the distal cap is in place.
- Assemble the needle driver portion to the scope with silicon straps.
- Attach the distal cap portion.
- Suturing
  - Double-channel endoscope or single-channel endoscope.
  - Pass the needle through the right-sided working channel.
  - Squeeze the handle of the needle driver to load the needle and the suture.
  - Once the needle is loaded open the handle to prepare the loaded needle for use.
  - Pass the tissue grasper (helix device) through the left-sided working channel; turn the handle to pull the tissue on one side of the defect toward the end cap.

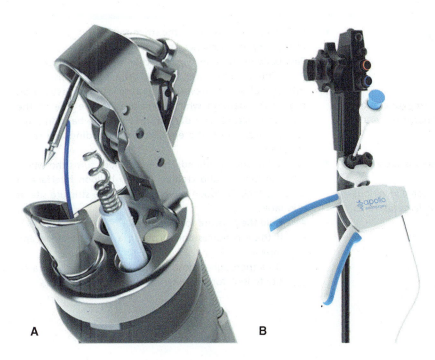

FIGURE 7 Endoscopic suturing with the Overstitch device. The Apollo Endosurgery OverStitch tip with suturing arm and tissue helix on the end of an endoscope **(A)** and Apollo OverStitch handle attached to dual lumen endoscope **(B)** (OverStitch™ Endoscopic Suturing System—Apollo Endosurgery, Inc.)

- Squeeze the needle driver to pass the needle and suture through the tissue.
- Repeat process on the opposite side of the defect.
- Release the needle through the right working port by pushing the blue button which will function as the T fastener.
- Pass the suture end through the eyelet of the cinch device.
- Pass the cinch device through the right-sided working port over the suture.
- Appose this device to the tissue where the closure was started.
- Pull the suture until the tissue edges of the defect are well approximated. Squeeze the handle of the device, which will release the fastener and cut the suture proximal to the fastener.
- Multiple stitches either in interrupted or a running fashion can be placed in a large defect or to take tension of the corners of a small defect closure.[8]

ENDOSCOPIC VACUUM THERAPY

Indications

- In the case of a chronic leak, endoscopic vacuum therapy (EVT), sometimes combined with other modalities such as stenting, can be efficacious.
- EVT is a form of internal drainage.
- EVT is frequently used for gastroesophageal leaks with clinical success higher than 80%. Every 4 to 5 days, the patient undergoes endoscopy to exchange the sponge system.[9]
- The sponge system is anchored either through the nose or alternatively, as has been done at the author's institution, through a percutaneously placed feeding tube.
- Within bariatric surgery, the most successful use of EVT has been for sleeve gastrectomy leaks and fistulas.[10]

Equipment to Have in the Room

- Standard forward-viewing gastroscope
- CO_2 insufflation
- Sponge
- Suture
- 14-Fr nasogastric tube
- Also have available:
- Percutaneous endoscopic gastrostomy tube kit
- Balloon dilation system

Steps

- Upper gastrointestinal endoscopy is carried out to identify the fistula/leak site.
- Evaluate the anatomy for distal obstruction/stenosis.
- Fluoroscopy can be used to identify the site or confirm the site.
- If the defect is small and the collection/abscess cavity is large, the fistula tract can be dilated with a balloon to allow better fit of the sponge.
- Cut the sponge into shape to fit the defect.
- Suture the sponge to the tip of a 14-Fr nasogastric tube, proximally and distally.
- Grasp the sponge with forceps through the working channel of the endoscope and place it in/at the defect under direct vision.
- Apply continuous 100 to 125 mm Hg using an electronic vacuum pump connected transnasally, or percutaneous feeding tube, to the nasogastric tube.
- Replace the sponge every 3 to 5 days.
- If there is a postoperative stricture/stenosis beyond the defect, this must also be treated (ie, balloon dilation).

ENDOSCOPIC BALLOON DILATION (FIGURE 8A-C)

Indications

- This procedure is most frequently used for gastrojejunal anastomosis stricture and sleeve stenosis after bariatric surgery.

Equipment

- Standard forward-viewing gastroscope or therapeutic scope
- CO_2 insufflation
- Continuous radial expansion balloons. These come in various sizes as small as 6 to 8 mm and typically as large as 18 to 20 mm.
- Balloon dilation gun

Steps

- Perform upper endoscopy
- Determine site and size of the stricture
- Choose appropriately sized balloon
- Pass balloon through working channel of the endoscope. Pass it into a "free space" to avoid distal perforation.
- Inflate balloon to level designated on the instruction tag of the balloon which correlates to the size of the balloon/stricture. The person inflating the balloon must communicate with the endoscopist regarding any resistance felt.
- As the balloon is inflated, the endoscopist turns the wheel into the balloon and creates a water-balloon interface in order to look "through the balloon" at the stricture site as it inflates.
- Hold the pressure for 2 minutes.
- If there is no resistance, go up a size of balloon and repeat.
- Do a thorough endoscopic interrogation of the dilated site to look for any potential defects/perforations.

Chapter 51 ENDOSCOPIC MANAGEMENT OF BARIATRIC COMPLICATIONS: LEAK AND STRICTURE 433

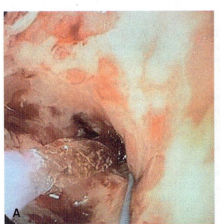 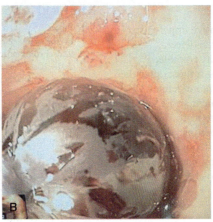 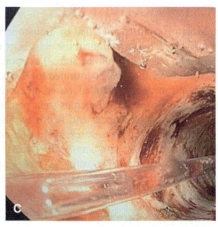

FIGURE 8 • Balloon dilation of a gastrojejunal stricture. **A,** Placement of balloon across stricture. **B,** Partial inflation of the balloon. **C,** Full inflation of the balloon to 20 mm, utilizing size/pressure legend to gauge the pressure. The endoscopist utilizing the balloon-water interface to watch the dilation through the balloon and is watching for signs of perforation (dark spots, muscle tearing).

ENDOSCOPIC SEPTOTOMY

Indications

- This procedure has currently been described with success, within the bariatric literature, for stenosis with leak/fistula after sleeve gastrectomy.
- Endoscopic septotomy is typically a "rescue" method used when a leak is so chronic that a septum has formed between the cavity and the gastric lumen. This septum forms naturally and can be quite fibrotic. Campos et al described their septotomy procedure as a "reshaping." This reshaping occurs between the well-contained abscess cavity and the mucosa of the gastric lumen.[11]

Equipment

- Standard forward-viewing gastroscope
- CO_2 insufflation
- Endoscopic electrical surgical unit
- Electrosurgical knife
- 20 mm balloon or an Achalasia balloon—if there is a sleeve stricture present

Steps

- Upper gastrointestinal endoscopy is carried out to identify the fistula/leak site.
- Evaluate the sleeve for stenosis.
- Locate the septum.
- Place the septum at the 6-o'clock position on the scope.
- Using the electrosurgical knife, cut the septum. Be cautious as the base of the septum is approached. Make cuts toward the staple line.
- Perform balloon dilation of a sleeve stenosis with a 20-mm balloon or an achalasia balloon.

PEARLS AND PITFALLS

- Patience: Endoscopic interventions frequently require multiple trips to the operating room or endosuite. Both the surgeon and the patient should be aware of this. Tolerance of multiple procedures and patience for trial and error is required.
- Use the correct procedure on the correct problem and correct patient: There is no endorsed or standard algorithm for the endoscopic management of leaks and fistulas. There are, however, recommendations for various types of leaks and fistulas depending on the site, the timing from surgery, and the severity of illness of the patient. Refer to the algorithms recommended here and several other published algorithms.
- It is important to have a plan, when to stop/continue endoscopic attempts at management of leaks and fistulas.
- In every case, there must be an immediate consideration of feeding access/nutrition.
- In every case, ensure that the septic source has been controlled and that antibiotics are ordered appropriately.
- Phone a friend—these patients require a multidisciplinary team for optimal management.

POSTOPERATIVE CARE

- Most procedures are aided by a postoperative upper gastrointestinal study to confirm the closure of the defect.
- Enteral feeding should be started as soon as possible.
- Antibiotics should be continued for 4 days at most, after the septic source is controlled, based on current guidelines.
- For some procedures, such as stent placement and EVT and pigtail drainage, repeat endoscopy is inherent to the procedure. For other procedures, such as endoscopic septotomy, especially those associated with sleeve stenosis, a repeat upper gastrointestinal study or endoscopy should be performed within weeks after the procedure to check on healing and progress.

COMPLICATIONS

Stent

- Tolerance: Some patients reporting nausea, vomiting, drooling, and retrosternal discomfort if placed above the gastroesophageal junction.
- Migration: The type of stent used may lead to higher rates of migration. Fully covered stents will have the greatest degree of migration while less covered stents will have a greater degree of tissue ingrowth and must be exchanged more frequently. The high migration rate may been explained by the "unconventional" placement of the stent along the last portion of the esophagus and the gastric pouch. For sleeve, leaks, overlapping stents can be placed to decrease the risk of migration.

Endoscopic Intervention

- Perforation can occur during any endoscopic intervention.
- If a perforation occurs during a procedure, many of the previously described techniques can be utilized to repair the perforation, including over-the-scope clips, endoscopic stent placement, or endoscopic suturing. Of the endoscopic interventions reviewed here, endoscopic dilation of a stricture or stenosis, either rigid or balloon, is most likely to cause a perforation. A thorough endoscopic interrogation of the dilated stricture should occur post dilation. If there is further concern in the post procedural area, a contrast upper gastrointestinal study should be obtained.

REFERENCES

1. Puig CA, Waked TM, Baron TH, et al. The role of endoscopic stents in the management of chronic anastomotic and staple line leaks and chronic strictures after bariatric surgery. *Surg Obes Relat Dis.* 2014;10:613-619.
2. Chang J, Sharma G, Boules M, et al. Endoscopic stents in the management of anastomotic complications after foregut surgery: new applications and techniques. *Surg Obes Relat Dis.* 2016;12(7):1373-1381. doi:10.1016/j.soard.2016.02.041 Epub 2016 Mar 2. PMID: 27317605.
3. Hany M, Ibrahim M, Zidan A, et al. Role of primary use of mega stents alone and combined with other endoscopic procedures for early leak and stenosis after bariatric surgery, single-institution experience. *Obes Surg.* 2021;31(5):2050-2061. doi:10.1007/s11695-020-05211-x Epub 2021 Jan 6. PMID: 33409972.
4. Haito-Chavez Y, Law JK, Kratt T, et al. International multicenter experience with an over-the-scope clipping device for endoscopic management of GI defects (with video). *Gastrointest Endosc.* 2014;80(4):610-622. doi:10.1016/j.gie.2014.03.049
5. Shoar S, Poliakin L, Khorgami Z, et al. Efficacy and safety of the over-the-scope clip (OTSC) system in the management of leak and fistula after laparoscopic sleeve gastrectomy: a systematic review. *Obes Surg.* 2017;27(9):2410-2418. doi:10.1007/s11695-017-2651-4 PMID: 28353180.
6. Winder JS, Kulaylat AN, Schubart JR, et al. Management of non-acute gastrointestinal defects using the over-the-scope clips (OTSCs): a retrospective single-institution experience. *Surg Endosc.* 2016;30(6):2251-2258. doi: 10.1007/s00464-015-4500-7 Epub 2015 Sep 28. PMID: 26416380.
7. Schulman A, Aihara H, Chiang AL, et al. Endoscopic suturing for large colonic perforations. *Gastrointest Endosc.* 2016;83:AB503.
8. Ge PS, Thompson CC. The use of the overstitch to close perforations and fistulas. *Gastrointest Endosc Clin N Am.* 2020;30(1):147-161. doi:10.1016/j.giec.2019.08.010 Epub 2019 Oct 29. PMID: 31739961; PMCID: PMC6885379.
9. Laukoetter MG, Mennigen R, Neumann PA, et al. Successful closure of defects in the upper gastrointestinal tract by endoscopic vacuum therapy (EVT): a prospective cohort study. *Surg Endosc.* 2017;31(6):2687-2696. doi:10.1007/s00464-016-5265-3 Epub 2016 Oct 5. PMID: 27709328.
10. Archid R, Wichmann D, Klingert W, et al. Endoscopic vacuum therapy for staple line leaks after sleeve gastrectomy. *Obes Surg.* 2020;30(4):1310-1315. doi:10.1007/s11695-019-04269-6 PMID: 31792702.
11. Campos JM, Ferreira FC, Teixeira AF, et al. Septotomy and balloon dilation to treat chronic leak after sleeve gastrectomy: technical principles. *Obes Surg.* 2016;26(8):1992-1993. doi:10.1007/s11695-016-2256-3 PMID: 27299918.

Index

Note: Page numbers followed by "*f*" indicate figures and "*t*" indicate tables.

A

Abdominal perforation/repair technique, 143
Abdominal stab wounds, 290
Abdominal wall
 biliopancreatic diversion with duodenal switch, 416
 single anastomosis duodenal-ileal bypass, 416
Achalasia, 21
 complications, 24–25
 diagnostic studies, 21
 differential diagnosis, 21
 imaging, 21
 outcomes, 24
 patient history, 21
 pearls and pitfalls, 24
 physical findings, 21
 postoperative care, 24
 steps, 22–23, 22*f*–23*f*
 surgical management, 21–22
Acute leaks, 430
Adhesiolysis, 212
Adjustable gastric banding (AGB), 405
 contraindications, 406
 duodenal switch (DS) conversion, 409
 imaging and diagnostic studies, 406
 laparoscopic
  patient positioning, 406
  port placement, 407, 407*f*
 patient history and physical findings, 405
 patient positioning, 406, 406*f*
 pearls and pitfalls, 409
 postoperative care, 409
 preoperative planning, 406
 removal only, 409
 revision, 409
 robotic
  gastric band removal, 408, 408*f*
  gastric plications, 408, 408*f*
  liver retraction, 407
  patient positioning, 406
  peri-gastric adhesions, 407, 408*f*
  port placement, 407, 407*f*
  subcutaneous port removal, 408
 single- or two-stage approach, 409–410
AGB. *See* Adjustable gastric banding (AGB)
Airway/pulmonary symptoms, 60
Anastomosis, 293–296, 294*f*–297*f*, 301, 301*f*, 355–356, 356
Anterior component separation technique, 215–217, 216*f*
Antral dissection, 329, 329*f*
Antrectomy
 complications, 313–314, 314*t*
 differential diagnosis, 305, 305*t*
 imaging and diagnostic studies, 306–308, 306*f*, 306*t*–308*t*, 307*f*
 minimally invasive approach, 312
 neoplasms, 305

 patient history, 305–306
 pearls and pitfalls, 313
 peptic ulcer disease (PUD), 305
 physical findings, 305–306
 postoperative care, 313
 reconstruction, 310–311, 311*f*–312*f*
 surgical management, 308–310, 309*f*–310*f*

B

Balloon dilation, gastrojejunal stricture, 433*f*
Bariatric surgery
 internal hernia and leak. *See* Internal hernia and leak, bariatric surgery
 laparoscopic sleeve gastrectomy. *See* Laparoscopic sleeve gastrectomy
 leak and stricture, endoscopic management. *See* Leak/fistula, after bariatric surgery
Barium swallow examination
 for laparoscopic sleeve gastrectomy (LSG), 403
Bassini repair, 158–160, 159*f*
Bile reflux gastritis, postgastrectomy syndrome, 387
Biliopancreatic diversion with duodenal switch (BPD/DS), 411
 abdominal wall and skin closure, 416
 common channel creation, 415, 415*f*
 complications, 416–417
 duodenoileal anastomosis, 414, 414*f*
 duodenoileostomy
  creation, 414, 414*f*
  leak test, 415, 415*f*
 feasibility assessment, 414, 414*f*
 ileocecal valve identification, 413
 imaging and diagnostic studies, 412
 leak test, 415, 415*f*
 mesenteric defect closure, 415, 415*f*
 outcomes, 416
 patient history and physical findings, 412
 pearls and pitfalls, 416
 port placement, 413, 413*f*
 positioning, 412
 postoperative care, 416
 preoperative planning, 412
 sleeve gastrectomy, 413, 414*f*
 specimen and instrument retrieval, 416
 stomach mobilization, 413
Biliopancreatic limb creation, for laparoscopic gastric bypass, 392, 392*f*
Biopsy, upper endoscopy with, 110*f*, 111
Bleeding, after total gastrectomy, 356
Blunt trauma, 290
Bochdalek congenital diaphragmatic hernia (CDH), 33
 complications, 40
 differential diagnosis, 33
 imaging and diagnostic studies, 33–34, 34*f*
 open left repair, 34–37, 36*f*–37*f*

 outcomes, 40
 patient history, 33
 pearls and pitfalls, 39–40
 physical findings, 33
 postoperative care, 40
 surgical management, 34–35, 34*f*
 thoracoscopic left repair, 37–39, 37*f*–39*f*
Body mass index (BMI), 390
Braun enteroenterostomy, 389, 389*f*
Buried bumper syndrome, with gastrostomy tube, 375

C

Caudal dissection, 188
Cephalad dissection, 188
Cervical and upper mediastinal esophageal mobilization, 116–117, 116*f*–117*f*
Cervical esophagus
 complications with, 363
 damage control for, 362
 differential diagnosis for, 358
 drainage, 362
 exposure and evaluation of, 360–361, 360*f*–361*f*
 grading of, 358, 358*t*
 imaging and diagnostic studies for, 358–359, 358*f*–359*f*
 indications for, 359
 nutrition, enteral access for, 362
 patient history and physical findings for, 358, 358*f*
 positioning for, 359
 postoperative care for, 363, 363*f*
 preoperative planning for, 359
 skin incision, 360, 360*f*
 vascularized muscle flap, 362, 362*f*
Cervical perforation/repair technique, 140–141, 141*f*
Chronic gastroesophageal reflux disease, 403
Clogged tube
 gastrostomy tube (G-tube), 374
 jejunostomy feeding tube (J-tube), 385
Collis gastroplasty, 53
 complications, 58
 fundoplication, completion of, 57, 57*f*
 gastroplasty, 54–55, 55*f*
 horizontal staple trajectory, 56, 56*f*
 imaging and diagnostic studies, 53, 53*f*
 intra-abdominal retraction and bougie placement, 55, 55*f*
 outcomes, 58
 patient history, 53
 pearls and pitfalls, 57
 physical findings, 53
 positioning, 54, 54*f*
 postoperative care, 58
 preoperative planning, 54
 vertical staple trajectory, 56, 56*f*

I-1

INDEX

Colocutaneous fistulas, with gastrostomy tube, 374
Colon conduit, 120–121, 120f–121f
Computed tomographic angiography (CTA) for cervical esophagus, 358–359, 359f
Computed tomography (CT)
  internal hernia and leak, bariatric surgery, 419, 419f–420f
  leak/fistula, bariatric surgery, 425f
Concomitant procedures and foreign material removal, 213
Contralateral transversus abdominus release (TAR), 223–224, 224f
Crura, closure of, 72
Crus dissection, 71

D

Dislodged tube
  gastrostomy tube (G-tube), 374
  jejunostomy feeding tube (J-tube), 386
Distal esophageal spasm (DES), 8
  airway management, 9
  complications, 13
  diagnostic studies, 9
  differential diagnosis, 8
  imaging, 9
  outcomes, 13
  patient history, 8
  pearls and pitfalls, 12
  physical findings, 8
  position, 9
  postoperative care, 13
  preoperative planning, 9
  surgical management, 9
  thoracoscopic approach, 9–12, 10f–12f
D2 lymphadenectomy, 336, 336f
Drainage procedures
  complications, 267
  differential diagnosis, 256
  gastrojejunostomy
    laparoscopic, 266, 266f
    open, 263, 263f–264f
  imaging and other diagnostic studies, 256
  outcomes, 267
  patient history, 256
  pearls and pitfalls, 267
  physical findings, 256
  postoperative care, 267
  pyloromyotomy, open, 262–263, 262f
  pyloroplasty
    laparoscopic, 264–265, 265f
    open, 257–260, 257f–261f
  surgical management, 256–257
Dumping syndrome, postgastrectomy syndrome, 387
Duodenal dissection and transection, 335–336, 336f
Duodenal injury, operative management of
  anastomosis, 301, 301f
  complications, 303
  feeding jejunostomy tube, 303
  imaging and diagnostic studies, 300
  jejunal roux limb repair, 302, 302f
  jejunal serosal patch, 301, 302f
  patient history, 299–300
  pearls and pitfalls, 303
  physical findings, 299–300
  postoperative care, 303
  primary repair, 301
  pyloric exclusion, 303, 303f
  resection, 301, 301f
  surgical management, 300, 301f

Duodenal mobilization and transection, 318–319, 318f–319f
Duodenal stump blowout, 356
Duodenal switch (DS) conversion, 409
Duodenoileal anastomosis, 414, 414f
Dysphagia, 60

E

Endoscopic pigtail drainage, leak/fistula, bariatric surgery, 427–428, 427f
Endoscopic suturing, 154
Endoscopic ultrasound (EUS), 111, 112f–113f
  gastric cancer, 348f
Endoscopic vacuum therapy (EVT), 154–155
  leak/fistula, bariatric surgery, 425f
Endoscopy
  adjustable gastric banding (AGB), 406
  gastric cancer, 348f
Enterotomies
  BPD/DS and SADI, 415
  for laparoscopic gastric bypass, 393
  for open jejunostomy feeding tube placement, 377–378, 379f–381f
Epigastric hernia
  complications, 245
  differential diagnosis, 234
  flat mesh, open mesh repair with, 239–240, 240f
  imaging and diagnostic studies, 236, 236f–237f
  laparoscopic mesh repair, 243–244, 243f–244f
  outcomes, 245
  patient history, 234–235, 235f–236f
  pearls and pitfalls, 245
  physical findings, 234–235, 235f–236f
  postoperative care, 245
  surgical management, 236–237, 237f
  suture repair, 238–239, 238f–239f
  ventral patch, open mesh repair with, 240–243, 241f–242f
Epiphrenic diverticulum, 1
  complications, 7
  differential diagnosis, 1
  imaging, 1
  laparoscopic transhiatal approach, 4–5
  open thoracic approach, 4
  outcomes, 6–7
  patient history, 1
  pearls and pitfalls, 5
  physical findings, 1
  positioning, 2
  postoperative care, 6
  preoperative planning, 2
  surgical management, 1
Esophageal achalasia, 15
  diagnostic studies, 15–16, 15f
  imaging, 15–16
  patient history, 15
  physical findings, 15
  surgical management, 16
Esophageal cancer, 365
Esophageal diversion, 143, 144f
Esophageal mobilization, 65
Esophageal perforation
  abdominal perforation/repair technique, 143
  cervical perforation/repair technique, 140–141, 141f
  complications, 145
  conservative management, 144
  differential diagnosis, 138
  endoscopic management of, 146
    conservative management, 153

differential diagnosis, 146
  endoscopic management, 149–153, 149f–153f
  imaging and diagnostic studies, 146–147, 146f–148f
  outcomes, 154–155
  patient history and physical findings, 146
  pearls and pitfalls, 153
  postoperative care, 154
  surgical management, 147–148, 148f
  esophageal diversion, 143, 144f
  imaging and diagnostic studies, 138–139, 139f
  outcomes, 144–145
  patient history, 138
  pearls and pitfalls, 144
  pedicled flap creation, 142, 143f
  physical findings, 138
  postoperative care, 144
  surgical management, 139–140, 140f
  thoracic perforation/repair technique, 142, 142f
Esophagogastrostomy, 119–120, 119f
Esophagography, 359
Exploratory laparotomy, for gastrectomy, 349

F

Fascial defect closure, 224
Feeding jejunostomy, 303, 349
Fistula, bariatric surgery
  chronic, 430
  classification, 425
  differential diagnosis, 423
  endoscopic management. See Leak/fistula, after bariatric surgery
Flank hernias, 196–198, 197f–198f
Fractured tube
  with gastrostomy tube, 374
  jejunostomy feeding tube (J-tube), 386
Fundoplication anchoring, 67, 68f
Fundoplication creation, 67, 67f

G

Gastric cancer, patient history and physical examination findings, 347
Gastric conduit, 118–119, 118f–119f
  formation of, 128, 128f
  mobilization, 127, 127f
Gastric fundus, laparoscopic sleeve gastrectomy, 400f
Gastric injury, 292
  anastomosis, 293–296, 294f–297f
  complications, 298
  differential diagnosis, 290
  exposure, 291
  imaging and diagnostic findings, 290
  injury grading, 291, 291t
  patient history, 290
  pearls and pitfalls, 297
  physical findings, 290
  postoperative care, 298
  surgical management, 290–291
Gastric outlet obstruction
  complications, 273
  differential diagnosis, 268
  endoscopic dilatation, 269, 270f
  endoscopic pyloromyotomy, 271–273, 272f
  endoscopic stenting, 270–271, 271f
  endoscopic stricturoplasty, 270
  with gastrostomy tube, 374
  imaging and diagnostic studies, 268–269
  patient history, 268

INDEX I-3

pearls and pitfalls, 273
physical findings, 268
postoperative care, 273
stricturoplasty, 269, 270f
surgical management, 269
Gastric transection, 319, 320f
Gastrocolic dissection, 335, 335f
Gastrocolic ligament, laparoscopic sleeve gastrectomy, 398, 399f
Gastroduodenal perforation
 complications, 278
 diagnostic laparoscopy, 277
 differential diagnosis, 275
 final steps, 278
 imaging and diagnostic studies, 275
 laparoscopic modified Graham patch repair, 276, 276f
 leak test, 278
 omental patch placement, 277, 277f
 patient history, 275
 pearls and pitfalls, 278
 perforation management, 277, 277f
 peritoneal lavage, 277
 physical findings, 275
 port placement, 277
 postoperative care, 278
 surgical management, 275–276
Gastroesophageal junction, fundus posterior to, 65, 66f
Gastroesophageal reflux disease (GERD)
 after laparoscopic sleeve gastrectomy (LSG), 403
 endoscopic approach
  differential diagnosis, 75
  imaging and diagnostic studies, 75–76, 76f
  lower esophageal sphincter, radiofrequency energy application to, 81–82, 81f–82f
  outcomes, 82–83
  patient history, 75
  pearls and pitfalls, 82
  physical findings, 75
  positioning, 77, 77f
  postoperative care, 82
  preoperative planning, 76–77
  transoral incisionless fundoplication, 77–80, 78f–80f
 laparoscopic partial fundoplication for, 70
  complications, 74
  crura, closure of, 72
  crus dissection, 71
  differential diagnosis, 70
  esophagus, 72
  imaging and diagnostic studies, 70
  outcomes, 74
  partial fundoplication, 72–73, 73f
  patient history, 70
  pearls and pitfalls, 73
  physical findings, 70
  ports placement, 71, 71f, 71t
  postoperative care, 74
  short gastric vessels, 72
  surgical management, 70–71
 magnetic sphincter augmentation (MSA)
  complications, 91–92
  contraindications, 85t
  device selection and placement, 88–89, 88f–89f
  differential diagnosis, 84
  gastroesophageal junction, dissection of, 87–88, 87f–88f
  hiatal hernia repair, 90–91
  imaging and diagnostic studies, 85–86
  medical therapy, 91

minimal hiatal dissection (MHD), 90
Nissen fundoplication, 91
obligatory dissection, 90–91
outcomes, 90–91
patient history, 84–85
pearls and pitfalls, 89–90
port placement, 87
positioning, 87
postoperative care, 90
preoperative planning, 86
surgical management, 86
Gastrojejunal anastomosis, 337, 337f
Gastrojejunostomy, 365
 laparoscopic, 266, 266f
 in laparoscopic gastric bypass, 394, 394f–395f
 open, 263, 263f–264f
 postgastrectomy syndrome, 388
Gastroparesis
 complications, 273
 differential diagnosis, 268
 endoscopic dilatation, 269, 270f
 endoscopic pyloromyotomy, 271–273, 272f
 endoscopic stenting, 270–271, 271f
 endoscopic stricturoplasty, 270
 imaging and diagnostic studies, 268–269
 patient history, 268
 pearls and pitfalls, 273
 physical findings, 268
 postoperative care, 273
 stricturoplasty, 269, 270f
 surgical management, 269
Gastrostomy tube (G-tube), 365
 complications, 374–375
 contraindications, 365
 imaging and diagnostic studies, 365
 indications, 365
 laparoscopic
  equipment and port placement, 371
  tube placement, 371, 372f–373f, 373
 open
  closure, 371
  equipment, 369
  fixation for, 370–371
  gastrotomy and tube placement for, 369–370, 369f–370f
  incision, 369, 369f
 for open gastrostomy tube placement, 369–370, 369f–370f
 patient history and physical findings, 365
 pearls and pitfalls, 373
 percutaneous endoscopic placement of
  equipment, 366
  optional site selection technique for, 366–367, 366f
  pull technique for, 367, 368f
  push technique, 367–368, 368f
  transillumination, 366, 366f
  tube placement, 367, 367f
  tube securing, 368–369, 369f
 positioning, 365
 postoperative care, 374
 preoperative planning, 365
Greater curvature of stomach
 in gastrectomy
  total, 349–350, 349f–350f
 in laparoscopic sleeve gastrectomy, 398

H

Handsewn esophagojejunostomy, 353–354, 353f
Heartburn, 59
Heineke-Mikulicz pyloroplasty, 128
Hemodynamic instability, 365

Henley jejunal interposition, postgastrectomy syndrome, 389
Hepatoduodenal ligament, dissection of, 330
Highly selective vagotomy (HSV), 253–254, 253f–254f
 complications, 255
 differential diagnosis, 246
 imaging and diagnostic studies, 247
 outcomes, 255
 patient history, 246–247
 pearls and pitfalls, 254
 physical findings, 246–247
 postoperative care, 255
 surgical management, 247
Hollow viscus injuries (HVIs), 290
Hypercontractile esophagus (HE), 21
 differential diagnosis, 21
 imaging and diagnostic studies, 21

I

Iatrogenic injury, 275
Ileocecal valve, biliopancreatic diversion with duodenal switch and single anastomosis duodenal-ileal bypass, 413
Incisional hernia
 abdominal wall reconstruction options
  adhesiolysis, 212
  anterior component separation technique, 215–217, 216f
  complications, 218
  concomitant procedures and foreign material removal, 213
  differential diagnosis, 210
  imaging and diagnostic studies, 211
  incision, 212
  outcomes, 218
  patient history, 210
  pearls and pitfalls, 217
  physical findings, 210
  posterior component separation technique, 213–215, 213f–215f
  postoperative care, 217–218
  surgical management, 211–212, 211f–212f
 laparoscopic approaches
  closure, 206, 206f–207f
  complications, 208
  differential diagnosis, 201–202
  dissection, 204, 204f
  imaging and diagnostic studies, 202
  mesh placement and fixation, 205–206, 205f–206f
  outcomes, 208
  pearls and pitfalls, 207
  port placement, 203, 203f–204f
  postoperative care, 208
  surgical management, 202–203, 202f
 open approaches
  anterior onlay and anterior component separation, 191–195, 192f–196f
  complications, 199
  differential diagnosis, 183
  flank hernias, 196–198, 197f–198f
  imaging and diagnostic studies, 184
  modified Rives-Stoppa repair, 186–189, 186f–187f, 189f–191f
  outcomes, 199
  patient history, 183
  pearls and pitfalls, 198–199
  physical findings, 183
  postoperative care, 199
  retrorectus sublay repair, 186–189, 186f–187f, 189f–191f
  surgical management, 184–185

Infection, with gastrostomy tube, 374
Inguinal hernia
  laparoscopic approaches
    anatomy, 169, 169f–170f
    complications, 177
    differential diagnosis, 170
    hernia, reduction of, 173, 174f
    imaging and diagnostic studies, 170
    mesh placement and fixation, 173–174, 175f
    natural history, 170
    nonoperative management, 170–171
    outcomes, 177
    pathogenesis, 170
    patient history, 170
    pearls and pitfalls, 176–177
    peritoneal flap and incisions, 174, 175f
    peritoneal incision, 171–172, 172f
    physical findings, 170
    pneumoperitoneum, 171
    port placement, 171
    postoperative care, 177
    properitoneal plane, 172, 173f
    surgical management, 171
    totally extraperitoneal inguinal hernia repair, 175–176, 176f
  open approaches
    Bassini repair, 158–160, 159f
    complications, 167–168
    differential diagnosis, 156
    imaging and diagnostic studies, 156
    lichtenstein repair, 164, 164f
    McVay repair/Cooper ligament repair, 161–162, 162f–163f
    outcomes, 167
    patient history, 156
    pearls and pitfalls, 167
    physical findings, 156
    postoperative care, 167
    prolene hernia system, 164–166, 165f–166f
    Shouldice repair, 160–161, 160f–161f
    surgical management, 156–158, 157f–158f
Internal hernia and leak, bariatric surgery
  complications, 421
  differential diagnosis, 418–419
  imaging and other diagnostic studies, 419, 419f–420f
  laparoscopic, 420–421
  open, 421
  patient history and physical findings, 419
  pearls and pitfalls, 421
  positioning, 420
  postoperative care, 421
  preoperative planning, 420
Intra-abdominal esophagus, dissection of, 330
Intragastric bougie, in laparoscopic sleeve gastrectomy, 401
Intraoperative endoscopy, 68
Ivor Lewis esophagectomy
  complications, 132
  esophagogastric anastomosis, 129–130, 130f–131f
  esophagus, thoracic mobilization of, 128–129, 129f
  gastric conduit
    formation of, 128, 128f
    mobilization, 127, 127f
  Heineke-Mikulicz pyloroplasty, 128
  imaging and diagnostic studies, 124–125, 124f–125f
  jejunostomy feeding tube, 128
  outcomes, 132
  patient history, 124
  pearls and pitfalls, 131
  physical findings, 124
  postoperative care, 132
  surgical management, 125, 125f–126f

J
Jejunal roux limb repair, 302, 302f
Jejunal serosal patch, 301, 302f
Jejunojejunostomy
  BPD/DS and SADI, 415
  postgastrectomy syndrome, 388
Jejunojejunostomy creation, for laparoscopic gastric bypass, 392–393, 393f
Jejunostomy feeding tube (J-tube), 128, 376
  complications with, 385–386
  imaging and diagnostic studies for, 376
  laparoscopic placement of
    equipment for, 381
    jejunal mobilization for, 381, 382f
    port placement for, 381
    tube placement for, 382–385, 383f–385f
  open placement of
    enterotomy for, 377–378, 379f–381f
    equipment for, 376, 377f
    incision for, 372f, 377
    jejunum mobilization for, 377f, 378f
    tube placement for, 377–378, 379f–381f
  patient history and physical findings, 376
  pearls and pitfalls, 385
  positioning, 376
  postoperative care for, 385
  preoperative planning, 376
  in proximal gastrectomy, 351

L
Laparoscopic adjustable gastric banding (LAGB), 405
Laparoscopic-assisted total gastrectomy, port placement for, 327–328, 327f
Laparoscopic gastric bypass
  biliopancreatic limb creation for, 392, 392f
  complications with, 396
  gastric pouch creation for, 393–394, 394f
  gastrojejunostomy creation in, 394, 394f–395f
  greater omentum division in, 393
  jejunojejunostomy creation for, 392–393, 393f
  ligament of Treitz in, 392, 392f
  liver biopsy for, 392
  liver retraction in, 32, 392f
  mesenteric defect closure in, 393, 393f
  outcomes with, 396
  patient history and physical findings for, 390
  pearls and pitfalls for, 396
  Petersen defect closure in, 395
  port placement for, 391, 391f
  positioning for, 391, 391f
  postoperative care for, 396
  preoperative planning for, 390–391
  skin closure for, 395
  upper endoscopy leak test for, 395
Laparoscopic Heller myotomy (LHM)
  complications, 20
  differential diagnosis, 15
  dissection, 17
  instrumentation for, 17t
  myotomy in, 18
  outcomes, 20
  partial fundoplication, 17t, 18–19
  patient history, 15
  pearls and pitfalls, 19
  physical findings, 15
  ports placement, 16–17
  positioning, 16
  postoperative care, 20
  preoperative planning, 16
  short gastric vessels division, 17
Laparoscopic modified Graham patch repair, 276, 276f
Laparoscopic Nissen fundoplication, 59
  airway/pulmonary symptoms, 60
  anterior stomach, 66, 66f
  complications, 69
  connect left and right hiatal dissections, 64, 64f
  differential diagnosis, 59
  dysphagia, 60
  esophageal mobilization, 65
  fundoplication anchoring, 67, 68f
  fundoplication creation, 67, 67f
  gastroesophageal junction, fundus posterior to, 65, 66f
  heartburn, 59
  imaging and diagnostic studies, 60, 60f–61f
  intraoperative endoscopy, 68
  left crus, 63, 63f
  left phrenogastric ligament, 61, 62f
  open gastrohepatic ligament, 63, 63f
  outcomes, 68–69
  patient history, 59–60
  pearls and pitfalls, 68
  physical findings, 59–60
  posterior crus reapproximation, 65, 65f
  posterior stomach wall marking stitch, 65, 65f
  postoperative care, 68, 69f
  regurgitation, 59
  right crus, 64, 64f
  short gastric vessels, 62, 62f
  surgical management, 60–61, 61f
Laparoscopic sleeve gastrectomy (LSG), 397
  complications, 404
  gastric sleeve creation in, 400–402, 401f–402f
  hemostasis, 402
  imaging and diagnostic studies, 397
  outcomes and follow-up, 403, 403f
  patient history and physical findings, 397
  pearls and pitfalls, 402
  port placement, 398, 398f
  positioning, 397
  postoperative care, 403, 403f
  preoperative planning, 397
  provocative leak test, 402
  stomach mobilization in, 398, 398f–400f
Laparoscopic transhiatal approach, 4–5
Lateral dissection, 187–188
Leak/fistula, after bariatric surgery, 423
  anatomy, 424f
  classification, 425
  differential diagnosis, 423
  endoscopic management, 423
    algorithm, 426f
    balloon dilation, 432, 433f
    closure, 430
    complications, 434
    endoscopic pigtail drainage, 427–428, 427f
    pearls and pitfalls, 433
    positioning, 426
    postoperative care, 434
    procedure setup, 426
    septotomy, 433
    stenting, 428, 429f–430f

suturing/plication, 431–432, 431f
   vacuum therapy, 432
  imaging and diagnosis, 423
  patient history and physical findings, 423
Left crus, 63, 63f
Left gastric artery, division of, 330
Left phrenogastric ligament, 61, 62f
Lesser curvature of stomach, in gastrectomy, 349–350, 349f–350f
LHM. *See* Laparoscopic Heller myotomy (LHM)
Lichtenstein repair, 164, 164f
Ligament of Treitz (LT), 392, 392f
Liver
  in laparoscopic gastric bypass, 392, 392f
  total gastrectomy, 349
Local resectability, esophageal hiatus to, 113–114, 114f
LSG. *See* Laparoscopic sleeve gastrectomy (LSG)
Lumbar hernia
  complications, 245
  differential diagnosis, 234
  flat mesh, open mesh repair with, 239–240, 240f
  imaging and diagnostic studies, 236, 236f–237f
  laparoscopic mesh repair, 243–244, 243f–244f
  outcomes, 245
  patient history, 234–235, 235f–236f
  pearls and pitfalls, 245
  physical findings, 234–235, 235f–236f
  postoperative care, 245
  surgical management, 236–237, 237f
  suture repair, 238–239, 238f–239f
  ventral patch, open mesh repair with, 240–243, 241f–242f
Lymphadenectomy, 320
  in total gastrectomy, 352

M

Magnetic sphincter augmentation (MSA)
  complications, 91–92
  contraindications, 85t
  device selection and placement, 88–89, 88f–89f
  differential diagnosis, 84
  gastroesophageal junction, dissection of, 87–88, 87f–88f
  hiatal hernia repair, 90–91
  imaging and diagnostic studies, 85–86
  medical therapy, 91
  minimal hiatal dissection (MHD), 90
  Nissen fundoplication, 91
  obligatory dissection, 90–91
  outcomes, 90–91
  patient history, 84–85
  pearls and pitfalls, 89–90
  port placement, 87
  positioning, 87
  postoperative care, 90
  preoperative planning, 86
  surgical management, 86
Malignancy, 275
McVay repair/Cooper ligament repair, 161–162, 162f–163f
Mesenteric defect closure, biliopancreatic diversion with duodenal switch and single anastomosis duodenal-ileal bypass, 415, 415f
Mesh implantation, 224

Metastatic disease, abdominal exploration to, 113
Minimally invasive esophagectomy (MIE)
  abdominal, 134–135
  complications, 137
  differential diagnosis, 133
  imaging and diagnostic studies, 133
  patient history, 133
  pearls and pitfalls, 136
  physical findings, 133
  postoperative care, 137
  surgical management, 134
  thoracic, 135–136, 136f
Minimally invasive total gastrectomy (MITG)
  antral dissection, 329, 329f
  complications, 332
  greater curve, dissection of, 328–329, 328f
  hepatoduodenal ligament, dissection of, 330
  imaging and diagnostic studies, 326
  intra-abdominal esophagus, dissection of, 330
  laparoscopic-assisted total gastrectomy, port placement for, 327–328, 327f
  left gastric artery, division of, 330
  outcomes, 332
  postoperative care, 332
  proximal division, 330, 330f
  robotic-assisted total gastrectomy, port placement for, 328, 328f
  stapled esophagojejunostomy, reconstruction with, 331, 331f
  surgical management, 326–327, 327f
Modified Rives-Stoppa repair, 186–189, 186f–187f, 189f–191f
Morgagni congenital diaphragmatic hernia (CDH)
  complications, 32
  differential diagnosis, 26
  imaging and other diagnostic studies, 26
  minimally invasive Morgagni hernia repair, 29–30, 29f–31f
  open Morgagni hernia repair, 27–28, 28f
  outcomes, 32
  patient history, 26
  pearls and pitfalls, 31
  physical findings, 26
  postoperative care, 32
  surgical management, 26–27, 27f
Mucosal closure, 273
Mucosal incision, 271–273
Myotomy, 273

N

Nasomediastinal drainage, 154
Neoplasms, 305
Nutrition, 397
Nutritional assessment, 387, 412
Nutritional deficiencies, after total gastrectomy, 356

O

Obesity, 390
  comorbidities, 390
  laparoscopic gastric bypass for
    biliopancreatic limb creation for, 392, 392f
    complications with, 396
    gastric pouch creation for, 393–394, 394f
    gastrojejunostomy creation in, 394, 394f–395f
    greater omentum division in, 393

    jejunojejunostomy creation for, 392–393, 393f
    ligament of Treitz in, 392, 392f
    liver biopsy for, 392
    liver retraction in, 392, 392f
    mesenteric defect closure in, 393, 393f
    outcomes with, 396
    patient history and physical findings for, 390
    pearls and pitfalls for, 396
    Petersen defect closure in, 395
    port placement for, 391, 391f
    positioning for, 391, 391f
    postoperative care for, 396
    preoperative planning for, 390–391
    skin closure for, 395
    upper endoscopy leak test for, 395
  laparoscopic sleeve gastrectomy for, 397
Omental patch placement, 277, 277f
Omentum
  in gastrectomy, 349, 349f
  in laparoscopic gastric bypass, 393
Open gastrohepatic ligament, 63, 63f
Open left repair, 34–37, 36f–37f
Open thoracic approach, 4
Over-the-scope clipping (OTSC) system, 430

P

Paraesophageal hernia repair, 41
  abdominal entry/port placement, 42–44, 44f
  anterolateral gastropexy, 50, 50f
  antireflux procedure, 49, 49f
  hernia contents, reduction of, 44
  hernia SAC, excision of, 47
  hiatal dissection, 44–45, 45f
  imaging and diagnostic studies, 41, 42f
  intra-abdominal length assessment, 47
  intraoperative upper endoscopy, 49, 49f
  mediastinal dissection, 46, 46f
  mesh reinforcement, 48, 48f
  outcomes, 51
  pearls and pitfalls, 50
  pertinent history, 41
  posterior cruroplasty, 47, 47f
  posterior dissection, 45, 46f
  postoperative care, 51
  preoperative planning, 41–42
Parastomal hernia
  complications, 233
  differential diagnosis, 228
  imaging and diagnostic studies, 228–229, 229f
  laparoscopic mesh underlay technique, 232, 232f
  open underlay technique, 231, 231f
  outcomes, 233
  patient history, 228
  pearls and pitfalls, 233
  physical findings, 228
  postoperative care, 233
  stoma relocation, 230
  surgical management, 229, 230f
Parastomal hernias, 183
Partial fundoplication, 72–73, 73f
Peptic ulcer disease (PUD), 275, 305
Peritoneal cytology, 349
Per-oral endoscopic myotomy (POEM), 21
  differential diagnosis, 21
  imaging and diagnostic studies, 21
Petersen defect closure, in laparoscopic gastric bypass, 395
Plain X-ray imaging, 275

Pneumoperitoneum, 413
Positron emission tomography-computed tomography (CT), 111
Posterior component separation technique, 213–215, 213f–215f
Posterior crus reapproximation, 65, 65f
Posterior stomach wall marking stitch, 65, 65f
Postgastrectomy syndrome, 387
   differential diagnosis, 387
   imaging and diagnostic studies, 387
   patient history and physical findings, 387
   surgical management
      Braun enteroenterostomy, 389, 389f
      complications, 389
      Henley jejunal interposition, 389
      outcomes, 389
      positioning, 388
      postoperative care, 389
      preoperative planning, 387–388
      Roux-en-Y reconstruction, 388, 388f
Postoperative seroma, 183
Preoperative planning, 2
Prolene hernia system, 164–166, 165f–166f
Proximal division, 330, 330f
Proximal gastrectomy
   complications, 345
   diagnostic laparoscopy, 340
   feeding jejunostomy, 344
   imaging and diagnostic studies, 339
   outcomes, 345
   patient history, 339
   pearls and pitfalls, 345
   physical findings, 339
   postoperative care, 345
   pyloromyectomy, 344, 344f
   resection and reconstruction, 342, 343f–344f
   stomach, mobilization of, 340–342, 340f–342f
   surgical management, 339
Proximal gastric transection, 336, 336f
Pseudohernia, 183
Pyloric exclusion, 303, 303f
Pyloromyotomy, open, 262–263, 262f
Pyloroplasty
   laparoscopic, 264–265, 265f
   open, 257–260, 257f–261f

R

Reconstruct esophageal hiatus, 99, 99f
Recurrent hiatal hernia, Roux-en-Y (roux limb reconstruction) for
   complications, 108
   differential diagnosis, 103
   giant paraesophageal hernia, 103f
   imaging and diagnostic studies, 104
   patient history, 103–104
   pearls and pitfalls, 108
   physical findings, 103–104
   postoperative care, 108
   roux limb reconstruction, 104–107, 105f–107f
   subtypes of, 103f
   surgical management, 104
Redo fundoplication, 93
   complications, 101–102
   consider adjuncts, 100
   differential diagnosis, 93, 93f, 93t
   gaining abdominal access, 96, 96f
   identify and expose hiatal anatomy, 96–98, 97f–98f, 97t

imaging and diagnostic studies, 94–96, 95f, 95t
   options for, 99t
   outcomes, 101, 101t
   patient history and physical findings, 94, 94f, 94t
   pearls and pitfalls, 100
   port placement, 96, 96f
   postoperative care, 101
   potential complications, assess for, 100
   reconstruct esophageal hiatus, 99, 99f
   standard technique for, 101t
   surgical management, 96, 96f
   undo previous fundoplication, 98, 99f, 100f
Retrorectus sublay repair, 186–189, 186f–187f, 189f–191f
Right crus, 64, 64f
Rives-Stoppa-Wantz repair, 183
Robotic-assisted total gastrectomy, port placement for, 328, 328f
Robotic inguinal hernia repair
   complications, 182
   differential diagnosis, 179
   imaging and diagnostic studies, 179
   patient history, 179
   pearls and pitfalls, 181–182
   physical findings, 179
   postoperative care, 182
   surgical management, 179–181, 180f–181f
Robotic/minimally invasive distal gastrectomy
   complications, 338
   D2 lymphadenectomy, 336, 336f
   duodenal dissection and transection, 335–336, 336f
   gastrocolic dissection, 335, 335f
   gastrojejunal anastomosis, 337, 337f
   imaging and diagnostic studies, 333
   outcomes, 338
   port placement, 333, 334f–335f
   postoperative care, 337–338
   proximal gastric transection, 336, 336f
   specimen removal, 336
   surgical management, 333, 334f
Robotic ventral hernia repair
   abdominal access/port placement, 220
   alternative approaches, 225
   complications, 225–226, 226f
   contralateral transversus abdominus release (TAR), 223–224, 224f
   imaging and diagnostic studies, 219–220, 220f
   outcomes, 226
   patient history, 219
   pearls and pitfalls, 225
   physical findings, 219
   postoperative care, 225
   retromuscular dissection, 221, 221f
   surgical management, 220, 220f
   transversus abdominis release (TAR), 219–220, 220f, 222, 222f–223f
Roux-en-Y reconstruction
   gastrectomy, 352–354, 353f–354f
   for postgastrectomy syndrome, 388, 388f
Roux limb reconstruction, 104–107, 105f–107f
Roux stasis syndrome, 387

S

Septotomy, 433
Short gastric vessels, 62, 62f, 72, 398
Shouldice repair, 160–161, 160f–161f

Single anastomosis duodenal-ileal bypass (SADI), 411, 411f
   abdominal wall and skin closure, 416
   common channel creation, 415, 415f
   complications, 416–417
   duodenoileal anastomosis, 414, 414f
   duodenoileostomy
      creation, 414, 414f
      leak test, 415, 415f
   feasibility assessment, 414, 414f
   ileocecal valve identification, 413
   imaging and diagnostic studies, 412
   leak test, 415, 415f
   mesenteric defect closure, 415, 415f
   outcomes, 416
   patient history and physical findings, 412
   pearls and pitfalls, 416
   port placement, 413, 413f
   positioning, 412
   postoperative care, 416
   preoperative planning, 412
   sleeve gastrectomy, 413, 414f
   specimen and instrument retrieval, 416
   stomach mobilization, 413
Sleeve gastrectomy, 413, 414f
Sleeve gastrectomy, laparoscopic. See Laparoscopic sleeve gastrectomy
Sleeve leaks, 403
Small bowel injury, 292–293, 293f
   anastomosis, 293–296, 294f–297f
   complications, 298
   differential diagnosis, 290
   exposure, 291
   imaging and diagnostic findings, 290
   injury grading, 291, 291t
   patient history, 290
   pearls and pitfalls, 297
   physical findings, 290
   postoperative care, 298
   surgical management, 290–291
Small bowel obstruction, jejunostomy feeding tube (J-tube), 386
Specimen removal, 336
Spigelian hernia
   complications, 245
   differential diagnosis, 234
   flat mesh, open mesh repair with, 239–240, 240f
   imaging and diagnostic studies, 236, 236f–237f
   laparoscopic mesh repair, 243–244, 243f–244f
   outcomes, 245
   patient history, 234–235, 235f–236f
   pearls and pitfalls, 245
   physical findings, 234–235, 235f–236f
   postoperative care, 245
   surgical management, 236–237, 237f
   suture repair, 238–239, 238f–239f
   ventral patch, open mesh repair with, 240–243, 241f–242f
Staging laparoscopy, 349
Stapled anastomosis, total gastrectomy, 354, 354f
Stapled esophagojejunostomy, reconstruction with, 331, 331f
Stenting, leak/fistula, bariatric surgery, 428, 429f–430f
Stents, 154
Stomach
   in biliopancreatic diversion with duodenal switch, 413

duodenum, mobilization of, 114–115, 114f–116f
greater curvature mobilization of, 318, 318f
in laparoscopic sleeve gastrectomy (LSG), 398, 398f–400f
in single anastomosis duodenal-ileal bypass, 413

Subtotal gastrectomy
closure, 321
complications, 322–324
differential diagnosis, 315
duodenal mobilization and transection, 318–319, 318f–319f
exploratory laparotomy, 317
gastric transection, 319, 320f
imaging and diagnostic studies, 316–317, 316f
lymphadenectomy, 320
outcomes, 322
patient history, 315
pearls and pitfalls, 322
physical findings, 315
postoperative care, 322
reconstruction, 320–321, 320f–321f
staging laparoscopy, 317
stomach, greater curvature mobilization of, 318, 318f
surgical management, 317

T

Thoracic perforation/repair technique, 142, 142f
Thoracoscopic left repair, 37–39, 37f–39f
Total gastrectomy
closure for, 354
complications with, 355–356
esophageal transection in, 352, 352f
exploratory laparotomy for, 349
greater curvature of stomach mobilization for, 349–350, 349f–350f
intestinal continuity restoration in, 352
lesser curvature of stomach mobilization in, 349–350, 349f–350f
liver mobilization for, 349
lymphadenectomy for, 352
outcomes with, 355
patient history and physical findings for, 347
pearls and pitfalls of, 355
positioning for, 348
postoperative care for, 355
preoperative planning for, 348
reconstruction, 352–354, 353f–354f

specimen processing for, 352
staging laparoscopy for, 349
Transhiatal esophagectomy (THE)
biopsy, upper endoscopy with, 110f, 111
cervical and upper mediastinal esophageal mobilization, 116–117, 116f–117f
colon conduit, 120–121, 120f–121f
complications, 123
computed tomography (CT), 111
differential diagnosis, 110–111, 110f, 111t
endoscopic ultrasound, 111, 112f–113f
esophagogastrostomy, 119–120, 119f
gastric conduit, 118–119, 118f–119f
imaging and diagnostic studies, 111
local resectability, esophageal hiatus to, 113–114, 114f
metastatic disease, abdominal exploration to, 113
outcomes, 122–123
patient history, 111
pearls and pitfalls, 122
physical findings, 111
positron emission tomography-computed tomography (CT), 111
postoperative care, 122
stomach and duodenum, mobilization of, 114–115, 114f–116f
surgical management, 111–113, 113f
Transversus abdominis release (TAR), 219–220, 220f, 222, 222f–223f
contralateral, 223–224, 224f
extended totally extraperitoneal, 225
hybrid, 225
Trauma laparotomy
abdomen
open, 283
systematic examination of, 283–286, 284f–285f
complications, 288
contamination, 287
differential diagnosis, 280, 280f
general operative approach, 282–283, 282f, 282t
imaging and diagnostic studies, 281
patient history, 280–281
pearls and pitfalls, 288
physical findings, 280–281
physiologic assessment and planning, 287–288
postoperative care, 288
stop exsanguinating hemorrhage, 283–284
surgical bleeding, 286–287, 286t
surgical management, 281

Truncal vagotomy
complications, 255
differential diagnosis, 246
imaging and diagnostic studies, 247
laparoscopic truncal vagotomy, 250–251
open
anterior (left) vagus nerve, identification and division of, 248, 249f–250f
esophagus, exposure of, 248, 249f
posterior (right) vagus nerve, identification and division of, 248, 250f
retractor positioning, 247, 247f
skin incision, 247, 247f
outcomes, 255
patient history, 246–247
pearls and pitfalls, 254
physical findings, 246–247
postoperative care, 255
surgical management, 247
transthoracic vagotomy, 251–253, 252f–253f
Tumor seeding, gastrostomy tube, 375

U

Umbilical hernia
complications, 245
differential diagnosis, 234
flat mesh, open mesh repair with, 239–240, 240f
imaging and diagnostic studies, 236, 236f–237f
laparoscopic mesh repair, 243–244, 243f–244f
outcomes, 245
patient history, 234–235, 235f–236f
pearls and pitfalls, 245
physical findings, 234–235, 235f–236f
postoperative care, 245
surgical management, 236–237, 237f
suture repair, 238–239, 238f–239f
ventral patch, open mesh repair with, 240–243, 241f–242f

V

Venous thromboembolism risk assessment tool, 406
Vitamin B_{12} deficiency, 356

W

Witzel tunnel, for open jejunostomy feeding tube placement, 378, 380f